HEADACHE

Diagnosis and Treatment

HEADACHE
Diagnosis and Treatment

Editors

C. DAVID TOLLISON, Ph.D.
Pain Therapy Centers
Greenville Hospital System
Greenville, South Carolina

Associate Clinical Professor
Department of Anesthesiology
Medical College of Georgia
Augusta, Georgia

ROBERT S. KUNKEL, M.D.
Head, Section on Headache
Department of Internal Medicine
Cleveland Clinic Foundation
Cleveland, Ohio

Clinical Assistant Professor of Medicine
Pennsylvania State University College of Medicine
Hershey, Pennsylvania

Williams & Wilkins
BALTIMORE • PHILADELPHIA • HONG KONG
LONDON • MUNICH • SYDNEY • TOKYO
A WAVERLY COMPANY

Editor: Jonathan W. Pine, Jr.
Managing Editor: Linda Napora
Copy Editor: Anne K. Schwartz
Designer: Wilma Rosenberger
Illustration Planner: Ray Lowman
Production Coordinator: Barbara J. Felton
Cover Designer: Wilma Rosenberger

Copyright © 1993
Williams & Wilkins
428 East Preston Street
Baltimore, Maryland 21202, USA

Accurate indications, adverse reactions, and dosage schedules for drugs are provided in this book, but it is possible that they may change. The reader is urged to review the package information data of the manufacturers of the medications mentioned.

Printed in the United States of America

Library of Congress Cataloging-in-Publication Data

Headache : diagnosis and treatment / editors, C. David Tollison, Robert S. Kunkel.
    p.   cm.
   Includes index.
   ISBN 0-683-08331-7
   1. Headache.   I. Tollison, C. David, 1949– . II. Kunkel, Robert S.
   [DNLM: 1. Headache—diagnosis. 2. Headache—therapy. WL 342 H43177]
 RB128.H44 1993
 616.8'491—dc20
 DNLM/DLC
 for Library of Congress   93-21787
                                           CIP

93 94 95 96 97
1 2 3 4 5 6 7 8 9 10

To my friend and mentor,
Henry E. Adams, Ph.D.,
who taught me about headaches—
and so very much more
C.D.T.
To Leonard L. Lovshin, M.D., who
first stirred my interest in the
study of patients with headaches
and who has remained a good
friend and colleague for many years
R.S.K.

Preface

Headache is one of the most common health complaints challenging physicians and other health professionals. The vast majority of headaches are not due to any serious underlying pathology, and yet, headaches are a frequent cause of human suffering and disability. Only in recent years have there been attempts to evaluate the time and money lost by chronic headache sufferers and their employers. According to one investigation,* headache represents the greatest single cause of absenteeism from work, with almost 157 million workdays lost per year.

It is essential to diagnose and treat any disease that may be causing headache. However, judicious and proper use of the large array of diagnostic tests available is an important issue in cost containment and concern over the rapidly rising costs of medical care. Taking a complete and detailed history from the headache patient is the most important aspect of the diagnostic work-up. Tests should rarely diagnose conditions not already suspected after the history and physical examination is completed.

The underlying pathophysiology of the "primary headache syndromes" (migraine, cluster, and tension-type headaches) remains poorly understood. Various chapters in this book review the current theories concerning the etiologies of these headaches; however, the primary emphasis throughout this text is on the clinical diagnosis and treatment of headache.

The treatment of headaches with medication has advanced rapidly in the last few years and remains the primary treatment modality. Most pharmacologic agents useful in managing migraine were originally intended for other medical conditions. None of these medications, as far as we know, actually affects the underlying abnormalities that cause one to experience pain in the head. Most of these agents affect the peripheral muscles and vasculature.

While medications remain a front line defense against headache, there is a growing trend by many clinicians and sufferers toward management of headaches with less medication and greater use of nonpharmacologic methods of treatment. We present several chapters on nonpharmacologic treatment of various headache syndromes. Readers should find these a good resource in managing their chronic headache patients.

We have attempted to bring together in this text an interdisciplinary faculty with recognized expertise in the management of head pain. We have encouraged the authors to express their own ideas without extensive editing on our part. Therefore, readers will occasionally find different opinions and even, at times, conflicting statements. Such is the complex and continuing challenge of headache diagnosis and treatment. Our objective is to offer a practical book that will be useful to health professionals. We hope our readers will find this a comprehensive and beneficial source of clinical information for the treatment of headache—both by pharmacologic and nonpharmacologic methods.

C. DAVID TOLLISON, PH.D.
ROBERT S. KUNKEL, M.D.

Contributors

Henry E. Adams, Ph.D.
Research Professor of Psychology
Psychology Clinic
University of Georgia
Athens, Georgia

Joseph H. Arguelles, M.D.
Division of Neurosurgery
Oregon Health Sciences University
Portland, Oregon

Steven M. Baskin, Ph.D.
Co-Director
New England Institute for Behavioral Medicine
Stamford, Connecticut

Ronald Brisman, M.D.
Department of Neurosurgery
College of Physicians and Surgeons
Columbia University
Neurological Institute
Columbia-Presbyterian Medical Center
New York, New York

Kim J. Burchiel, M.D.
Professor and Head
School of Medicine
Division of Neurosurgery
Oregon Health Sciences University
Portland, Oregon

Jerome D. Buxbaum, D.D.S., F.A.G.D., D.A.A.P.M.
Clinical Professor
Department of Physiology
Dental School
University of Maryland
College Park, Maryland

J. Keith Campbell, M.D.
Professor of Neurology
Mayo Medical School
Consultant, Department of Neurology
Mayo Clinic and Mayo Foundation
Rochester, Minnesota

Roger S. Cicala, M.D.
Associate Professor of Anesthesiology
Director, University Pain Treatment Center
University of Tennessee
Memphis, Tennessee

James R. Couch, Jr., M.D., Ph.D.
Professor and Chairman
Department of Neurology
College of Medicine
University of Oklahoma Health Sciences Center
Oklahoma City, Oklahoma

Seymour Diamond, M.D.
Director, Diamond Headache Clinic, Ltd.
Director Inpatient Headache Unit
Weiss Memorial Hospital
Adjunct Professor of Pharmacology and Molecular Biology
The Chicago Medical School
Clinical Associate in Medicine
University of Chicago
Chicago, Illinois

Peter D. Dunne, M.D.
Professor of Neurology
University of South Florida
Tampa, Florida

Arthur H. Elkind, M.D.
Director, Elkind Headache Center
Clinical Assistant Professor of Medicine
New York Medical College
Mount Vernon, New York

David A. Fishbain, M.D., F.A.P.A.
Associate Professor of Psychiatry and Neurological Surgery
University of Miami School of Medicine
Comprehensive Pain Center at South Shore Hospital
Miami Beach, Florida

Frederick G. Freitag, D.O.
Associate Director
Diamond Headache Clinic, Ltd.
Chicago, Illinois

R. Michael Gallagher, D.O.
Director, University Headache Center
Professor of Family Medicine
Associate Dean for Academic and Clinical Affairs
University of Medicine and Dentistry of New Jersey
School of Osteopathic Medicine
Stratford, New Jersey

J. David Gillies, M.D., F.R.A.C.P.
The Prince Henry Hospital
Senior Lecturer in Medicine
The University of New South Wales
Little Bay, Australia

Malcolm Gottesman, M.D.
Acting Chief of Neurology
Winthrop-University Hospital
Mineola, New York

Philip E. Greenman, D.O., F.A.A.O.
Michigan State University
College of Osteopathic Medicine
Department of Biomechanics
East Lansing, Michigan

Thomas E. Gretter, M.D.
Department of Neurology
Cleveland Clinic Foundation
Cleveland, Ohio

Lawrence M. Halpern, Ph.D.
Department of Pharmacology and The Pain Clinic
University of Washington
Seattle, Washington

Kenneth A. Holroyd, Ph.D.
Professor of Clinical Health Psychology
Director, Stress and Health Clinic
Ohio University
Athens, Ohio

Anthony Iezzi, Ph.D.
Department of Psychology
Victoria Hospital
London, Ontario
Canada

Michael R. Jaff, D.O.
St. Vincent Charity Hospital
Cleveland, Ohio

Gary W. Jay, M.D.
Medical Director
Headache Center and Neurological Rehabilitation Institute
Northglenn, Colorado
Medical Director
Center for Brain Injury Rehabilitation
Louisville, Colorado

Jeffrey R. Jernigan, M.D.
Assistant Professor
Department of Anesthesiology
Staff Physician, University Pain Treatment Center
University of Tennessee
Memphis, Tennessee

Patrick R. Johnson, Ph.D.
Clinical Assistant Professor of Psychiatry and Behavioral
    Sciences
Multidisciplinary Pain Center
University of Washington Medical Center
Seattle, Washington

Lee Kudrow, M.D.
Director, California Medical Clinic for Headache
Encino, California

James W. Lance, M.D., F.R.C.P., F.R.A.C.P.
Director
The Institute of Neurological Sciences
The Prince Henry and Prince of Wales Hospitals
Professor of Neurology, The University of South Wales

Howard L. Levine, M.D.
Chief, Section of Nasal-Sinus Surgery
Division of Otolaryngology
Department of Surgery
The Mt. Sinai Medical Center
Cleveland, Ohio

√ Richard B. Lipton, M.D.
Associate Professor of Neurology and Psychiatry
Albert Einstein College of Medicine
Director of Headache Unit (Manhattan Division)
Montefiore Medical Center
Bronx, New York

Michael G. McKee, Ph.D.
Head, Section of Applied Psychophysiology and Biofeedback
Department of Psychiatry and Psychology
Cleveland Clinic Foundation
Cleveland, Ohio

Ninan T. Mathew, M.D.
Director, Houston Headache Clinic
Houston, Texas

Barbara Clark Mims, R.N., M.S.N., CCRN
Coordinator
Critical Care and Trauma Nurse Internship
Parkland Memorial Hospital
Dallas, Texas
Director, Barbara Clark Mims Associates
Lewisville, Texas

Norbert R. Myslinski, Ph.D.
Associate Professor
Department of Physiology
Dental School
University of Maryland
College Park, Maryland

√ Lawrence C. Newman, M.D.
Assistant Professor of Neurology
Albert Einstein College of Medicine
Co-Director of Headache Unit (Manhattan Division)
Department of Neurology
Montefiore Medical Center
Bronx, New York

Burton M. Onofrio, M.D.
Professor of Neurosurgery
Mayo Medical School
Consultant, Department of Neurosurgery
Mayo Clinic and Mayo Foundation
Rochester, Minnesota

Donald B. Penzien, Ph.D.
Associate Professor of Psychiatry (Psychology)
Director of the U.M.C. Headache Clinic
University of Mississippi Medical Center
Jackson, Mississippi

Jeanetta C. Rains, Ph.D.
Assistant Professor of Psychiatry (Psychology)
Associate Director
U.M.C. Headache Clinic
University of Mississippi Medical Center
Jackson, Mississippi

Alan M. Rapoport, M.D.
Assistant Clinical Professor of Neurology
Yale University School of Medicine
New Haven, Connecticut
Co-Director
New England Center for Headache
Stamford, Connecticut

Barry A. Reich, Ph.D.
Director, Comprehensive Pain Program
Nassau Pain and Stress Center
Westbury, New York

A. David Rothner, M.D.
Head, Section of Child Neurology
Cleveland Clinic Foundation
Cleveland, Ohio

George H. Sands, M.D.
Assistant Professor of Neurology
Mount Sinai Hospital
New York, New York
Assistant Professor of Neurology
Albert Einstein College of Medicine
Bronx, New York
Director of Neurology
Queens Hospital Center
Jamaica, New York

Joseph D. Sargent, M.D.
Director of Internal Medicine and Neurology
The Menninger Foundation
Topeka, Kansas

Claren Sheck, M.S.
Department of Psychology
University of Georgia
Athens, Georgia

Fred D. Sheftell, M.D.
Assistant Clinical Professor of Psychiatry
New York Medical College
Valhalla, New York
Co-Director, The New England Center for Headache
Stamford, Connecticut

Marsha M. Silberstein, M.D.
Director of Clinical Studies
Comprehensive Headache Center
The Germantown Hospital and Medical Center
Philadelphia, Pennsylvania

Stephen D. Silberstein, M.D.
Chief of Neurology
Co-Director, Comprehensive Headache Center
Associate Professor of Neurology
Temple University School of Medicine
Philadelphia, Pennsylvania

Glen D. Solomon, M.D., F.A.C.P.
Section of Headache
Department of Internal Medicine
Cleveland Clinic Foundation
Cleveland, Ohio
Professor of Medicine
Pennsylvania State University College of Medicine
Hershey, Pennsylvania
Associate Professor of Medicine
The Ohio State University College of Medicine
Columbus, Ohio

Seymour Solomon, M.D.
Professor of Neurology
Albert Einstein College of Medicine
Director of Headache Unit
Montefiore Medical Center
Bronx, New York

William G. Speed III, M.D., F.A.C.P.
Associate Professor of Medicine
The Johns Hopkins University School of Medicine
Director, Speed Headache Associates
Baltimore, Maryland

Egilius L. H. Spierings, M.D., Ph.D.
Director, Headache Section
Division of Neurology
Brigham and Women's Hospital
Department of Neurology
Harvard Medical School
Boston, Massachusetts

Robert V. Steinmetzer, M.D., F.A.C.P.
Chairman, Department of Internal Medicine
American Hospital of Paris
Paris, France

George A. Ulett, M.D., Ph.D.
Clinical Professor of Psychiatry
University of Missouri—Columbia
School of Medicine
Associate Director for Policy and Ethics
Missouri Institute of Mental Health
Director, Department of Psychiatry
Deaconess Hospital
St. Louis, Missouri

Randall E. Weeks, Ph.D.
Clinical Program Director
The New England Headache Treatment Program at
    Greenwich Hospital
Greenwich, Connecticut

Contents

SECTION

I

FOUNDATIONS

1

Nature and Magnitude of Headache

C. DAVID TOLLISON

Human beings accept without question their predominance within the natural biological order. The human animal, that complex yet adaptable biped, is a triumphant biological phenomenon. It can survive in practically any climate, provide for its nourishment in the midst of barrenness, reproduce in every season, and protect itself against most of the earth's hazards. Many terms have been suggested to differentiate man from the other animals. He has been called thinker, toolmaker, and laugher, and has been credited with countless qualities, all in an attempt to define the essence of humanity. But one especially human attribute has been largely ignored: suffering.

No other animal is thought to suffer the torments of the human being. From itchy dandruff to terminal diseases, from simple anxiety to violent psychosis, humans are thought to spend more of their lives in physical and emotional anguish than any other earthly creature.

Man is almost comical in what appears to be his singular drive to inflict injury and pain upon himself. No other animal is as accident-prone. Humans are forever bumping into objects, tripping, straining muscles, being struck by falling objects, hitting toes against bed rails, burning or cutting themselves, and generally falling victim to every malady from shaving nicks to suicide. At times it appears that the human body seems more dedicated to self-destruction than to self-preservation.

Headache appears to be one of the more innovative and effective means that the human body has available to bedevil itself. Its origin is nonbacterial and nontraumatic in the great majority of cases, yet it thrives as a chronic, often debilitating disorder. Elements of the human metabolic, muscular, neural, and vascular systems cooperate magnificently to produce the torment of a headache. In many ways, headache is an example of an organism turning on itself.

This introductory chapter explores the nature and magnitude of headache through a brief examination of the history of head pain and the incidence and psychosocial impact of headache as a frequently occurring medical disorder.

HISTORY OF HEADACHE

Are common types of headaches a symptom of our contemporary, fast-paced, and stressful lifestyles? The answer is both yes and no. The incidence of headache does seem to increase with mounting stress factors common in modern society. The same may be said for other disorders thought to be partially stress-related, such as coronary artery disease and certain types of ulcers and emotional disorders. Yet headaches have plagued mankind for thousands of years, afflicting generations of our ancestors with the same intense agony and distress that many of us suffer today.

We know that primitive man believed that head pain was the work of evil spirits who invaded the body of unfortunate individuals. Well-intentioned early medical men set about to resolve the suffering of their patients in a most logical manner. If headache was caused by the invasion of evil spirits, then letting the spirits out of the skull should bring relief; thus was born the surgical procedure known as trepanning. In primitive Melanesian colonies on islands in the South Pacific, the custom of trepanning was a popular treatment for insanity, epilepsy, and persistent headaches. Skulls showing signs of trepanning have been found in Europe and on the North and South American continents, particularly in Mexico and Peru, dating back to the Neolithic and Bronze Ages. Many skulls found in Europe have oval openings with edges that appear to be partially healed, suggesting that the patient had surprisingly survived the surgery for some time. If we accept these trepanned skulls as evidence of headache-relief surgery, then the history of headache extends back ten thousand years or more.

Even if we limit ourselves to written accounts, headache still has a history of respectable antiquity. The earliest medical records of many ancient cultures make reference to the disorder. Headache is mentioned in the Atharvaveda of India, for example, a book on the knowledge of magic formulas that was written between 1500 and 800 BC.

A detailed history of headache is outlined in the book *Headache: Understanding, Alleviation* authored by James W. Lance, M.D.(1). Dr. Lance is also coauthor of the chapter "Pathophysiology of Migraine" (Chapter 10) for this text. Portions of the following section are taken from the 1975 book by Dr. Lance.

The scientific age of medicine began with Hippocrates, who was born on the island of Cos in 460 BC. Hippocrates is primarily recognized for his meticulous observation of disease and his recording of details of his patients, including both failures and successes. His formulation of an ethical code of conduct for physicians persists in principle to this day. Hippocrates described a headache that was probably migrainous:

> Most of the time he seemed to see something shining before him like a light, usually in part of the right eye; at the end of a moment, a violent pain supervened in the right temple, then in all of the head and neck, where the head is attached to the spine . . . vomiting, when it became possible, was able to divert the pain and render it more moderate (1).

A detailed description of migraine was submitted by Aretaeus, a physician born in Cappadocia in Asia Minor (now part of Turkey) who practiced in Alexandria, about 81 AD. He emphasized that migraine pain frequently affects one side of the head and named this headache pain heterocrania. His description of headache pain is as follows (2):

> In certain cases the parts of the right side, or those on the left solely, so far that a separate temple, or ear, or one eyebrow, or one eye, or the nose which divides the face into two equal parts; and the pain does not pass this limit, but remains in the half of the head. This is called heterocrania, an illness by no means mild, even though it intermits, and although it appears to be slight. For if at any time it sets in acutely, it occasions unseemingly and dreadful symptoms, spasm and distortion of the countenance takes place; the eyes either fixed intently like horns, or they are rolled inwardly to the side or to that; vertigo, deep-seated pain of the eyes as far as the meninges; irrestrainable sweat; sudden pain of the tendons, as of one striking with a club; nausea, vomiting of bilious matters; collapse of the patient . . . there is much torpor, heaviness of the head, anxiety and ennui. For they flee the light; the darkness soothes their disease: nor can they bear readily to look upon or hear anything agreeable; their sense of smell is vitiated, neither does anything agreeable to smell delight them, and they have also an aversion to fetid things: the patients, moreover, are weary of life and wish to die.

Galen (131 to 200 AD) was a Greek physician and writer who later termed one-sided headache *hemicrania*, this term being the origin of the Old English word *megrim* and the French word *migraine*.

In 600 AD Paul of Aegina, a Greek physician at the Medical School of Alexandria, wrote (2): "Headache, which is one of the most serious complaints, is sometimes occasioned by an intemperament solely; sometimes by a redundance of humors, and sometimes by both." This idea was in keeping with the early Greek medical concept of four humors that were thought to govern health and disease: blood, phlegm, yellow bile, and black bile. Over the centuries, these four humors came to be known as the types of "temperaments"—sanguine, phlegmatic, melancholic, and choleric.

Thomas Willis (1621–1674), a London physician, wrote one of the first textbooks on the anatomy of the brain, *Cerebri Anatome*, which was illustrated by Christopher Wren, the architect of St. Paul's Cathedral. He divided habitual headaches into those that were continuous and those that were intermittent, a distinction that remains of fundamental importance today. In Willis's casebook written in 1683, he reports the case history of a noble lady with migraine, which has often been quoted (3).

> Some twenty years since, I was sent for to visit a most noble lady, for above twenty years sick with an almost continual headache, at first intermitting: she was of a most beautiful form, and a great wit, so that she was skilled in the liberal arts, and in all forms of literature, beyond the condition of her sex, and as if it were thought too much by nature, for her to enjoy so great endowments without some detriment, she was extremely punished with this disease. Growing well of a fevour before she was twelve years old, she became obnoxious to pains in the head, which were wont to arise, sometimes of their own accord, and more often upon every light occasion. This sickness being limited to no one place of the head, troubled her sometimes on one side, sometimes on the other, and often thorow the whole compass of the head. During the fit (which rarely ended under a day and a night's space, and often held for two, three, or four days) she was impatient of light, speaking, noise or any motion, sitting upright in her bed, the chamber made dark, she would talk to no body, nor take any sleep, or sustenance. At length about the declination of the fit, she was wont to lie down with a heavy and disturbed sleep, from which awaking she found herself better, and so by degrees grew well, and continued indifferently well til the time of the intermission. Formerly, the fits came not but occasionally, and seldom under 20 days of a month, but afterwards they came more often: and lately she was seldom free. Moreover, upon sundry occasions, or evident causes (such as the change of the air, or the year, the great aspects of the sun and moon, violent passions, and errors of diet) she was more cruelly tormented with them. But although this distemper, most grievously afflicting this noble lady, above 20 years (when I saw her) having pitched its tents near the confines of the brain, had so long besieged its regal tower, yet it had not taken it: for the sick lady, being free from a vertigo, swimming in the head, convulsive distempers, and any soporiferous symptom, found that the chief faculties of her soul sound enough.

Dr. Willis concludes on a pessimistic note regarding her response to treatment (3).

> There was no kind of medicines both cephalics, antiscorbuticks, hysterical, all forms specificks, which she took not, both from the learned and the unlearned, from quacks, and old women, and yet notwithstanding she professed, that she had received from no remedy, or method of curing, any type of cure or ease, but that the contumacious and rebellious disease, refused to be tamed, being deaf to the charms of every medicine.

The nineteenth century brought in the golden age of description and classification in medicine, although it must be said that treatment modes remained firmly in the Dark Ages. The first major text devoted exclusively to headache was authored by Edward Liveing in 1873 and titled *On*

Megrim, sick headache and some allied disorders, a contribution to the pathology of nerve storms (4). As basic as it was, the text represents a milestone in distinguishing headache as a primary medical disorder.

Acupuncture has been used in traditional Chinese medicine since the technique was devised by Huang Ti, who is said to have lived from 2698 to 2598 BC. Purists maintain that acupuncture penetrates the 12 hypothetical channels of the body that contain the Yang, the active male element, and the Yin, the passive female element, thereby restoring the balance between them. A contemporary perspective of acupuncture is detailed by George A. Ulett, M.D. in Chapter 46 of this text.

With a ten thousand year history, it has been only recently that the investigation of the pathophysiology of headache has generated widespread interest and its treatment has assumed a scientific basis. The general use of aspirin preceded the knowledge that it blocked the action of substances involved in inflammatory processes, including headache. Sir George Pickering further advanced our contemporary knowledge when, in the 1930s, he reported on headache produced by histamine. No single individual, perhaps, has increased our current knowledge of headache more than Harold G. Wolff, M.D. (5), who published his famous text in 1948, which today remains a classic. Many of the current advances in diagnosis and treatment of headache are detailed in subsequent chapters of this book.

MAGNITUDE OF THE HEADACHE PROBLEM

Headache is generally considered the most prevalent of all human diseases; yet severe and especially chronic headache is caused only infrequently by organic disease. Hence it may be inferred that chronic headache, in large part, represents a failure of the headache victim to effectively cope in some measure with the uncertainties of life, a symptom of some obvious or discrete disorder of thought or behavior rather than structural disease of the nervous system. Nonetheless, headache may also be the presenting complaint of catastrophic illness such as cerebral hemorrhage, brain tumor, or meningitis, and to underestimate the headache symptom in this context is to risk the life of the patient. Interestingly, headache may be equally intense whether its source is benign or malignant.

Headache statistics are difficult to compile. This difficulty arises from the fact that headaches affect so many and in such varying degree. As mentioned above, headache may be either an acute or chronic disorder of benign origin, or it may be a symptom of some underlying, serious medical disease.

Despite the inherent complexities, scattered data give us a partial picture of the magnitude of headache. Consider, for example, that an estimated 45 million Americans suffer chronic, recurring headaches (6). Zeigler et al. (7) interviewed 1809 subjects attending meetings of a number of religious and other societies in Kansas City and determined that 41% of men and 50% of women reported having

suffered a "disabling or severe" headache at some time in their lives. Only 4% of women and 9% of men under the age of 35 denied ever having had a headache.

Zeigler et al. (7) estimate that between 5 and 10% of the American population seek intermittent medical treatment of headaches. It is estimated that headache complaints generate over 80 million doctor's office visits each year and cost business and industry over $50 billion annually in employee absenteeism and medical expense (6). The Nuprin Pain Report (8) designated headache as the most frequent pain-related cause of employee absenteeism in the United States, with more than 157 million days lost to work each year. Jones and Harrop (9), in a factory-based survey, reported that the average worker lost 4.3 days of work per annum because of headache.

Medications remain the physician's first line of treatment in the battle against headache, and the cost of this war is high. In excess of $4 billion are spent annually on over-the-counter remedies for headache (6). Over $100 million are spent each year on aspirin (10). To put the figures for aspirin alone in perspective, consider that Americans swallow 20,000 tons each year, or 225 tablets for every man, woman, and child in the United States.

Headache is predominantly a disease of females; 70% of migraine victims are female (6), and approximately 75% of tension-type patients are female (9). Cluster headache, however, overwhelmingly affects males. Pearce (11) reports on a survey study indicating that 84% of cluster headache victims were male. The well-established effects of menstruation, pregnancy, and exogenous hormones may partially explain the higher prevalence of migraine in women, but they do not explain the higher incidence of tension-type headache in the female population.

While migraine and tension-type headaches affect far more females than males during the adult years, the childhood onset of migraine appears to equally affect both boys and girls. Dalsgaard-Nielsen (12) studied 2027 schoolchildren and 390 adults, all with migraine, and determined that migraine is as common among boys as girls up to the age of 10. Thereafter, there is a large predominance of female victims corresponding to the age of menarche. This research further indicates that one-half of adult migraine patients started having headaches before age 12, and one-half of adult female patients started having headaches by 16 years. The great majority of males with migraine develop the disorder before age 32, while females routinely continue to develop migraines until age 42 years.

The frequency of headache episodes, duration of pain, and presence of associated medical symptoms all contribute to the debilitating effects of recurrent headache. In a large-scale study of migraine victims, 9% of the victims reported 3 or more headaches per week, 28% suffered one or two headaches weekly, and 40% claimed one to three severe headache episodes per month (11). Headache pain duration per episode varies. A survey of vascular headache patients indicates that 20% suffered headaches typically lasting less than 6 hours, 16% suffered an average headache duration of between 6 and 12 hours, 19% reported a typical headache episode of between 12 and 24 hours, and a surprising 42% claimed that an average headache lasted longer than 24 hours (11). Nausea, a frequent symptom of migraine attacks, appears to be the most commonly reported symptom associated with recurrent headache. Vahlquist (13), in a survey of pediatric headache patients, reported that only 6.6% of the victims never experience nausea, while 59% vomited on at least some headache occasions.

PSYCHOSOCIAL IMPACT OF HEADACHE

Headache is a recurring nightmare to millions of victims, often becoming the leitmotif of their existence. Countless patients spend the pain-free moments of their lives in dreaded anticipation of the next headache episode. Headache can destroy personal relationships, wreck confidence and self-esteem, and result in vocational disability, depression, and emotional anguish.

There are few more pitiful spectacles than that of the headache victim prostrate on a bed of pain, in a darkened room, a cold towel or ice pack clutched to the head, a frown of agony, the eyes bloodshot, struggling nevertheless to be amiable, to shrug off the perfunctory expressions of concern, to smile away the suffering. Yet though the observer is moved, it is difficult to completely understand the layer upon layer of physical and psychological suffering witnessed. Chronic headache patients are a burden to family and friends, and this knowledge only aggravates the pain. When in the throes of a severe headache, they are incapable of action. Parties, trips, and meetings must be cancelled. Other people are inconvenienced. Guilt and resentment build.

Some victims of severe headaches may even long for death as an end to suffering. The American poet, Emily Dickinson (1830–1886) wrote frequently of pain, some of it mental, some physical. Her poem "I felt a Funeral, in my Brain" suggests the aura and pain of classic migraine.

I felt a Funeral, in my Brain,
And Mourners to and fro
Kept treading—treading—till it seemed
That Sense was breaking through—

And when they all were seated,
A service, like a Drum—
Kept beating—beating—till I thought
My mind was going numb—

And then I heard them lift a Box
And creak across my Soul
With those same Boots of Lead, again,
Then Space—began to toll,

As all the Heavens were a Bell,
And Being, but an Ear,
And I, and Silence, some strange Race
Wrecked, solitary, here—

And then a Plank in Reason, broke,
And I dropped down, and down—
And hit a World, at every plunge,
And Finished knowing—then—

Perhaps the commonest complaints of patients with chronic headaches—aside from the pain itself—are of sleep disturbance, fatigue, and irritability. Patients frequently complain of restless sleep, with frequent waking partly associated with pain. They may arise feeling tired, exhausted, and drained of energy and motivation, not merely from a lack of sleep but also from the deteriorating effects of prolonged pain.

These victims also frequently complain of irritability and may overreact to the slightest actions and minor remarks of those around them. They complain that they find themselves short-tempered and that they snap at friends, family members, and colleagues repeatedly for insufficient reasons. Frequently, chronic headache patients will seek exile by withdrawing from friends to a haven of rest, quiet, darkness, and calm.

Emotional Response to Headache

Many chronic headache patients readily admit to feeling depressed, and in fact, considerable research suggests that the average headache patient does likely suffer a mild depression (14). The relationships that exist between depression and pain are complex and have been investigated by Turk and his colleagues (15–17). In patients suffering the pain of headache, depression appears to be most frequently exhibited in depressed mood, or it may be masked by a preoccupation with the headache and other physical symptoms (fatigue, constipation, etc.). Some evidence suggests that the degree of depression may be proportional to the "headache density" (i.e., the intensity of head pain multiplied by the duration of the headache per unit time) (14).

In addition to depression, the psychosocial impact of recurrent headache is compounded by the conditioning effects of chronic pain. In short, many victims of recurrent headaches soon come to perceive themselves as chronic invalids. They miss increasing hours and days from work and may actually seek medical disability. Commitments are impossible and social activities uncertain because of the unpredictable frequency of the headaches. Life is gradually restricted, bit by bit, until the victim becomes essentially homebound. Excursions out of the home are chiefly to doctors and pharmacies, and the primary interaction of the patient with others is via the sick role.

Chronic headache patients also frequently become preoccupied with the headache as a symptom. Fearful speculations arise about the etiology of the pain, and quiet, dark hours may be spent in rumination of the headache as a "disease." Victims may operate on the premise that pain is always a warning signal of some underlying pathology and the more intense the pain, the more serious the cause. If headache persists chronically or recurrently, patients often fear that physicians have overlooked a potentially fatal diagnosis, such as an aneurysm or brain malignancy. If an acquaintance or family member previously suffered headache prior to death, no matter how removed or incidental to the cause of death, the victim's fears may be intensified. When headache pain is severe and the episode is characterized by associated symptoms such as nausea, vomiting, visual disturbance, and partial paralysis, it may be difficult for the patient to believe that stroke or even death is not imminent.

Behavioral Response to Headache

In addition to the above-noted subjective responses to headache, objective changes occur as well. Social withdrawal and diminished activity, which are easily measured, have already been described. An overreliance on medication may also become a serious problem.

The chronic or recurrent headache patient has more medical contacts than do other patients, soliciting more medical interventions (15). "Doctor shopping" is also a frequent behavioral response.

As previously mentioned, the chronic and recurrent headache victim frequently harbors fears of fatal intracranial pathology as the cause of headache misery. Consequently, many victims seek repeated assurance and a definitive, readily understood diagnosis. In the experience of the author, headache victims have been known to return unexpectedly to the office during the afternoon following a morning appointment or to telephone repeatedly seeking reassurance. Pain, it appears, is easier to bear when it is understood, and the physician errs who thinks the headache victim only seeks pain relief.

Pain relief, however, is also desperately sought, and this understandable drive for relief can compound the victim's symptomatology. If victims delay seeking pharmacological relief until they are deep into the throes of headache pain, such intervention may have no noticeable effect in combating pain intensity. Consequently, the next headache episode calls for larger doses of more powerful drugs, and so on. Physical dependence may be the ultimate outcome. Drug detoxification protocols are outlined in Chapter 41 of this text.

Psychological conditioning (Pavlovian) can further compound the above scenario. With repeated headache, ingestion of analgesics is paired with each occurrence. As headaches become increasingly frequent, the pairing of analgesics with pain occurs with increasing frequency. Soon analgesics are being taken daily in response to nearly daily headache. Yet, such daily headaches are themselves a conditioned response to the need for the analgesic with which they have been paired. The patient may not experience a "craving" for the drug; rather the need (physical dependence) is signaled by the occurrence of headache in a rebound fashion (Table 1.1).

Marital or family dysfunction is another frequent re-

sponse to chronic or recurrent headaches. When headache begins to dominate and control an individual's life, family roles, modes of interactions, and structural organization are frequently altered. Consequently, while the headache patient suffers constant or recurrent pain, the entire family is victimized by the headache experience. The headache patient increasingly withdraws, becomes disabled, and loses some of the status associated with efficient and productive activity. Children are frequently required to assume greater responsibility for the family, two-working-parent households may become dependent on the income of only one parent, and interactions with the headache patient may be gradually altered to that of the sick role. Frustrated and feeling guilty over the gradual change within the family, the headache patient may indirectly and without conscious intent begin to tyrannize other family members through further social withdrawal or temper outbursts. As family members are required to add more and more of the patient's roles and functions to their own, the patient's frustration, irritability, withdrawal, and guilt increase. Nevertheless, the surrender of obligations, the attention, and the acquisition of power in the family can serve to reinforce the adoption of the sick role. Other family members may resent the added burden, yet feel guilty about such resentment and their inability to help the family member find pain relief. It is not infrequent to encounter a chronic or recurrent headache patient who agonizingly describes the negative global impact on the family and yet acknowledges a near inability to function even on "good days" with little or no headache. Sternbach (14) describes this situation as an example of Skinnerian conditioned illness behavior, in which environmental reinforcers maintain and enhance certain behaviors (Table 1.2).

Depression, invalidism, chronic fatigue, work absenteeism and disability, family dysfunction, and medication

Table 1.1.
Drug-conditioned Headache[a]

Stimulus	Response
Headache	Analgesic
Headache	Analgesic (tolerance, dependence)
Withdrawal	Headache

[a]From Sternbach RA. Psychological management of the headache patient. In: Diamond S, Dalessio DJ, eds. The practicing physician's approach to headache. Baltimore: Williams & Wilkins, 1986:160. Reprinted with permission.

Table 1.2.
Environmentally Conditioned Headache[a]

Behavior	Reinforcer
1. Being bedridden	Avoidance of obligations
2. Irritability	Domination of others
3. Headache	Analgesics

[a]From Sternbach RA. Psychological management of the headache patient. In: Diamond S, Dalessio DJ, eds. The practicing physician's approach to headache. Baltimore: Williams & Wilkins, 1986:160. Reprinted with permission.

abuse are only some of the psychosocial ramifications of both chronic and recurrent headache. Yet this assemblage is a woefully insufficient description of the ravages of this disorder. Perched like a flower atop the slender stalk of the spine, the human head and its cradled control center are capable of our greatest joys and our deepest, most intense suffering. Hippocrates (18), one of the first to diagnose migraine, recognized the relationship of pain and our emotions. "From nothing else but the brain come joys, delights, laughter and sport, sorrow and griefs, despondencies and lamentations. And by the brain in a special manner we acquire wisdom and knowledge . . . and by the same organ we become mad and delirious and fears and terrors assail us, some by day and some by night."

The following anecdote (19) may serve as a fitting conclusion to this brief overview of headache and as an introduction to the remainder of this text:

About once a month, until the age of 70, George Bernard Shaw suffered a devastating headache which lasted for a day. One afternoon, after recovering from an attack, he was introduced to Nansen and asked the famous Arctic explorer whether he had ever discovered a headache cure.

"No," said Nansen with a look of amazement.

"Have you ever tried to find a cure for headaches?"

"No."

"Well, that is a most astonishing thing!" exclaimed Shaw.

"You have spent your life in trying to discover the North Pole, which nobody on earth cares tuppence about, and you have never attempted to discover a cure for the headache, which every living person is crying aloud for."

REFERENCES

1. Lance JW. Headache: understanding, alleviation. New York: Charles Scribner's Sons, 1975.
2. Adams F. The extant works of Aretaeus, the Cappadocian. Cited by Lance JW. Headache: understanding, alleviation. New York: Charles Scribner's Sons, 1975:10.
3. Willis T. Cerebri anatome. Cited by Lance JW. Headache: understanding, alleviation. New York: Charles Scribner's Sons, 1975:8.
4. Liveing E. On megrim, sick headache, and some allied disorders: a contribution to the pathology of nerve storms. Cited by Lance JW. Headache: understanding, alleviation. New York: Charles Scribner's Sons, 1975:10.
5. Wolff HG. Headache and Other Head Pain. New York: Oxford University Press, 1948.
6. National Headache Foundation. National Headache Foundation fact sheet. Chicago, 1990.
7. Ziegler DK, Hassanein RS, Couch JR. Characteristics of life headache histories in a nonclinic population. Neurology 1977;27:265–269.
8. Taylor H, Curran NM. The Nuprin Pain Report. New York, Louis Harris and Associates, 1985.
9. Jones A, Harrop C. Study of migraine and the study of attacks in industry. J Intern Med 1980;8:321–325.
10. Tollison CD, Tollison JW. Headache: a Multimodal program for relief. New York: Sterling Publishing, 1982.
11. Pearce JMS. Chronic migrainous neuralgia: a variant of cluster headache. Brain 1980;103:149–159.
12. Dalsgaard-Nielsen T. Some aspects of the epidemiology of migraine in Denmark. Headache 1970;10:14–23.
13. Valquist B. Migraine in children. Int Arch Allergy Appl Immunol 1955;7:348–355.
14. Sternbach RA. Psychological management of the headache patient. In: Diamond S, Dalessio DJ, eds. The practicing physician's approach to headache. 5th ed. Baltimore: Williams & Wilkins, 1986.
15. Turk DC, Rudy TE, Steig RL. Chronic pain and depression: I. Facts. Pain Manage 1987;1(1):17–25.
16. Rudy TE, Turk DC. Chronic pain and depression: II. Five fashionable fads. Pain Manage 1988;1:7–17.
17. Turk DC, Rudy TE. Chronic pain and depression: III. Future directions. Pain Manage 1988;3:113–127.
18. Gould H. Headaches and health. New York: St. Martin's, 1973:6.
19. Lennox WG, Lennox MA. Epilepsy and related disorders. London: Churchill, Livingstone, 1960:216.

2

Taxonomy and Classification of Headache

ROBERT S. KUNKEL

The overwhelming majority of headaches are known as "primary or essential" headaches and include migraine headaches, cluster headaches, tension-type headaches, or combinations thereof. Headaches caused by a specific underlying disease process account for relatively few headaches among those complaining of head pain. When a specific condition is found, the accompanying headache can often be alleviated by treatment of that condition. It is therefore important to look for underlying causes rare as they may be.

Headaches have been described for many hundreds of years. The term migraine is felt to be derived from the term *hemicrania*, first introduced by Galen in the second century AD (1). The term *sick headache* has been extensively used over the years when physicians have written about migraine. Headaches have also been named for their presumed cause. In a book on headaches published early in this century, terms such as congestive headache, emotional headache, neuralgic headache and headaches of monotony are used (2).

The classification and diagnosis of headaches has been and still is difficult because of our lack of knowledge regarding the underlying pathophysiological etiology of the common primary headache syndromes. Migraine, cluster, and tension-type headaches are each very complex conditions. It is becoming increasingly apparent that vascular, neurological, biochemical, hormonal, hematologic, and muscular components may play a role in these headaches. For many years cluster and migraine have been called vascular headaches. Most headache specialists now feel that the vascular dilation noted during the attacks of pain are secondary to a primary neurological dysfunction (3, 4). Blood vessels may therefore not be part of the primary underlying etiology.

Since the diagnosis of a specific type of headache depends almost solely on the symptoms described by the sufferer, classification and diagnosis may be quite imprecise. Many patients are poor observers and cannot give good reliable answers to the physician's questions. It may at times be very difficult to obtain a straightforward history. The inquiring physician needs to ask the right kinds of questions to obtain a reliable history. There are at this time no specific diagnostic tests for migraine, cluster, or tension headache that are reproducible. Some of the newer investigations now going on will undoubtedly lead to some objective findings that will be useful as diagnostic criteria.

The three major problems with devising a headache classification scheme are the lack of knowledge as to the cause of pain in general and headache in particular, the lack of any specific diagnostic test, and the reliance on the patient's history to arrive at a correct diagnosis.

Cluster headache for years was considered to be a variant of migraine, since both were felt to be caused by vascular dilatation. It is now apparent that they are quite distinct entities, although of course both have some common symptoms and they may share some similar pathophysiological abnormalities. Tension-type headache (muscle-contraction headache) is often associated with palpable, tight, tender scalp and cervical muscles, but it may also be present without any clinical or electrical (electromyographic) evidence of increased muscle contraction.

Prior to 1962, just about every treatise on headache used a different classification and different terms. In 1962, a distinguished panel published a headache classification that became universally accepted and was used throughout the world (5). This classification was the result of deliberations of an ad hoc committee of the National Institutes of Health. Virtually all papers published on headache from then until 1989 referred to the ad hoc committee's report when defining the types of headaches discussed.

AD HOC COMMITTEE CLASSIFICATION 1962

1. Migrainous vascular
   - Classic
   - Common
   - Cluster
   - Hemiplegic and ophthalmoplegic
   - Lower-half
2. Muscle contraction
3. Combined: vascular and muscle contraction
4. Nasal vasomotor reaction
5. Delusional, conversion, or hypochondriacal
6. Nonmigrainous vascular
7. Traction
8. Overt cranial inflammation

9–13. Ocular, aural, nasal, sinus, dental, or other cranial or neck structure disorders
14. Cranial neuritides
15. Cranial neuralgias

This classification had 15 categories of headaches, each followed by a brief clinical description. The vascular and muscle-contraction sections also listed some symptoms that are usually present.

The term *classic migraine* was introduced for that migraine headache preceded by a short visual or neurological aura. The migraine occurring without any well-defined aura or warning was called common migraine. What had been known as psychogenic or tension headache was called muscle-contraction headache, implying that the cause of pain was sustained abnormal contraction of scalp and neck muscles. This was also an attempt to get away from the implication that psychological factors were the major cause of headache.

Psychogenic headache is a term that has had different meanings over the years. Many have used the term for what we know as tension headache or muscle-contraction headache. Others use the term psychogenic headache for those rare headaches due to delusional, conversional, or hypochondriacal states. Combined headache was used for those very frequent headaches in which there is both a chronic tension-type headache, and an episodic vascular component. More recently the term *mixed headache* has been preferred for that particular entity.

Other authors, in an effort to simplify headache classification, have developed their own schemes. Diamond and Dalessio have popularized a simple classification that is quite useful for practitioners (6). They divide headaches into three main categories: (*a*) vascular, (*b*) muscle-contraction, and (*c*) traction and inflammatory types. The latter would cover all of the organic headaches caused by diseases or structural abnormalities.

As already noted, combinations of vascular and muscle-contraction headaches are the most common type of headaches seen in headache clinics. Matthew has called these headaches "evolutive," since in most persons they begin with episodic migraine attacks that evolve over the years into this mixed pattern (7). Why so many people with migraine evolve into a mixed type of headache pattern is unknown, but increasingly frequent use of analgesics may be an important factor (8).

In 1988 a committee of the International Headache Society published a new classification of headache after 3 years of deliberations (9). This proposed classification will be used mainly by headache researchers, and it is expected that it will be revised in a few years, after it has been in use. The major reason for an updated headache classification was to develop some diagnostic criteria for the various types of headache so that researchers throughout the world would apply the same criteria when doing clinical research. Research should be more reliable and reproducible if workers follow the same classification and apply the same criteria when doing clinical or physiological studies on headache patients.

The new classification is quite long and complex. It will be used mostly for research purposes. It is, however, a hierarchical outline that can be used by practitioners who need only make use of the major categories. There may be no need to get involved with the detailed diagnostic criteria. The diagnostic criteria will be of help in some patients who present with a headache that is difficult to diagnose by the history alone.

There are some new terms in the IHS classification. Classic and common have been dropped as terms describing migraine, and in their place migraine with aura and migraine without aura are used. The latter two terms are certainly more descriptive. Tension headache, muscle-contraction headache, and psychogenic headache are not used. Tension-type headache is the new proposed term for this type of headache. It is expected that as more studies are done on the etiology of tension-type headache a better term (and, hopefully, a better classification) will be developed.

A couple of new categories are presented in this classification. Headaches caused by metabolic diseases, infection, and drugs are new categories. The rebound phenomenon and "withdrawal headache" seen in persons who frequently use ergotamine tartrate, analgesics, and sedatives is now recognized as a major problem in the development of chronic headaches. The criteria in the new classification are simple and incomplete for this complex area and must be better defined as more studies are published.

The table that follows lists all of the headings in the IHS classification, but none of the specific diagnostic criteria. Many authors of chapters in this book refer to the IHS classification and discuss various aspects of the diagnostic criteria for the particular headache described. The classification of headache will continue to change as we learn more about this very common ailment.

IHS CLASSIFICATION (1988)

1. Migraine
   1.1 Migraine without aura
   1.2 Migraine with aura
      1.2.1. Migraine with typical aura
      1.2.2. Migraine with prolonged aura
      1.2.3. Familial hemiplegic migraine
      1.2.4. Basilar migraine
      1.2.5. Migraine aura without headache
      1.2.6. Migraine with acute onset aura
   1.3 Ophthalmoglegic migraine
   1.4 Retinal migraine
   1.5 Childhood periodic syndromes that may be precursors to or associated with migraine
      1.5.1. Benign paroxysmal vertigo of childhood
      1.5.2. Alternating hemiplegia of childhood
   1.6 Complications of migraine

10.1 Hypoxia
    10.1.1. High-altitude headache
    10.1.2. Hypoxic headache (low-pressure environment, pulmonary diseases causing hypoxia)
    10.1.3. Sleep apnea headache
10.2 Hypercapnia
10.3 Mixed hypoxia and hypercapnia
10.4 Hypoglycemia
10.5 Dialysis
10.6 Headache related to other metabolic abnormality

11. Headache or facial pain associated with disorder of cranium, neck, eyes, ears, nose, sinuses, teeth, mouth, or other facial or cranial structures.
    11.1 Cranial bone
    11.2 Neck
        11.2.1. Cervical spine
        11.2.2. Retropharyngeal tendinitis
    11.3 Eyes
        11.3.1. Acute glaucoma
        11.3.2. Refractive errors
        11.3.3. Heterophoria or heterotropia
    11.4 Ears
    11.5 Nose and sinuses
        11.5.1. Acute sinus headache
        11.5.2. Other diseases of nose or sinuses
    11.6 Teeth, jaws, and related sources
    11.7 Temporomandibular joint disease (functional disorders are coded to group 2)

12. Cranial neuralgias, nerve trunk pain, and deafferentation pain
    12.1 Persistent (in contrast to tic-like) pain of cranial nerve origin
        12.1.1. Compression or distortion of cranial nerves and second or third cervical roots
        12.1.2. Demyelination of cranial nerves
            12.1.2.1. Optic neuritis (retrobulbar neuritis)
        12.1.3. Infarction of cranial nerves
            12.1.3.1. Diabetic neuritis
        12.1.4. Inflammation of cranial nerves
            12.1.4.1. Herpes zoster
        12.1.5. Tolosa-Hunt syndrome
        12.1.6. Neck-tongue syndrome
        12.1.7. Other causes of persistent pain of cranial nerve origin
    12.2 Trigeminal neuralgia (tic douloureux)
        12.2.1. Idiopathic trigeminal neuralgia
        12.2.2. Symptomatic trigeminal neuralgia
            12.2.2.1. Compression of trigeminal root or ganglion
            12.2.2.2. Central lesions
    12.3 Glossopharyngeal neuralgia
        12.3.1. Idiopathic
        12.3.2. Symptomatic
    12.4 Nevus intermedius neuralgia
    12.5 Superior laryngeal neuralgia
    12.6 Occipital neuralgia
    12.7 Central causes of facial pain other than tic douloureux
        12.7.1. Anaesthesia dolorosa
        12.7.2. Thalamic pain
    12.8 Facial pain not fulfilling criteria in groups 11 and 12
13. Headache not classifiable

REFERENCES

1. Lance JW. Mechanism and management of headache. 4th ed. London: Butterworth Scientific, 1982:3.
2. Riley WH. Headache and how to prevent them. Battlecreek, MI: Good Health Publishing, 1916.
3. Lance JW. A personal perspective on the pathogenesis of migraine. In: Saper J, ed. Controversies and clinical varients of migraine. New York: Pergamon Press, 1987:111–118.
4. Raskin NH. On the origin of head pain. Headache 1988;28:254–257.
5. Ad Hoc Committee on Classification of Headache, National Institute of Neurological Diseases and Blindness. Classification of headache. JAMA 1962;179:717–718.
6. Diamond S, Dalassio DJ. The practicing physician's approach to headache. 4th ed. Baltimore: Williams & Wilkins, 1986.
7. Matthew N, Rauveni U, Perez F. Transformed or evolutive migraine. Headache 1987;27:102–106.
8. Kudrow L. Paradoxical effects of frequent analgesic use. Adv Neurol 1982;33:335–342.
9. Headache Classification Committee of the International Headache Society. Classification and diagnostic criteria for headache disorders, cranial neuralgias and facial pain. Cephalalgia 1988;8:(7).

3

Anatomy and Physiology of Headache

PETER B. DUNNE

This chapter outlines and discusses the anatomy, physiology, and certain limited aspects of the biochemistry that currently appear necessary and relevant to understanding headache. It necessarily discusses some of the methods and techniques that have led to advances in our understanding of the mechanisms of headache.

There is now a large body of research concerned with the pathophysiology and biochemistry of headache, particularly migraine. The past decade in particular has produced important advances in our understanding of the mechanisms that produce headache. This basic knowledge has led to the development of more effective headache therapies. Conversely, better understanding of the actions of different medications has led to further insight into headache pathophysiology. This chapter provides background and an introduction to the basic structural and physiological systems that relate to headache, essentially the vascular and neurological systems. The explanation of *how* these systems are involved in the pathogenesis of various types of head pain is the task of later chapters. Nor does this chapter enter into the debate over whether the neurological or the vascular system is the primary or major basis for migraine. The chapter should be used as a ready reference to help interpret and understand the later chapters.

It is beyond the scope of this chapter to discuss the anatomy of the entire nervous system. Certain phenomena, such as spreading depression, that may relate to headache occur without relation to the specific division or area of the nervous system. The discussion focuses on the brain's vascular supply and specific anatomical-physiological systems that presently are important in headache.

VASCULAR-ARTERIAL ANATOMY
Gross Anatomy

Four majors arteries supply the brain. The paired carotid arteries supply the anterior portions of the brain. The vertebral arteries supply the posterior and inferior parts of the brain. The common carotid artery bifurcates in the neck, usually at the level of the thyroid cartilage. This forms in the internal carotid artery to the brain and the external carotid artery to the face and scalp. The internal carotid artery (ICA) goes to the base of the skull and enters the petrous bone via the carotid canal. In the canal it goes anteromedial to the tympanic cavity. It enters the middle cranial fossa covered by dura as it courses through the cavernous sinus, giving off small branches locally and the anterior meningeal artery. The sphenoid bone lies medial to it. As it leaves the cavernous sinus, the ICA sends the ophthalmic artery anteriorly to the eye and adnexa. The ICA follows a reverse loop course beginning in the cavernous sinus so that it is ultimately angulated posteriorly in the carotid siphon. It then goes between the optic and oculomotor nerves and branches into the anterior cerebral artery anteriorly; its largest branch, the middle cerebral artery, which goes laterally; the posterior communicating artery posteriorly; and the anterior choroidal artery.

The vertebral arteries on either side begin from the subclavian arteries. They go cephalad in the foramina of the cervical vertebral transverse processes. The vertebral arteries become intracranial through the foramen magnum. They lie on the anterior surface of the medulla oblongata and come together at the medullary-pontine junction to form the basilar artery. It continues to the upper pons, where it splits into the posterior cerebral arteries. Along the intracranial portion of the vertebral arteries, its major branches are the posterior inferior cerebellar arteries and the posterior and anterior spinal arteries. Branches from the basilar artery are the anterior inferior cerebellar, the internal auditory, and the superior cerebellar arteries.

The circle of Willis is made up of arteries on the base of the brain, encircling the pituitary stalk and the optic chiasm. These vessels form a connection between the anterior and posterior circulations. The posterior communicating arteries bridge between the posterior cerebral artery roots and the final segment of the internal carotid arteries. Anteriorly the anterior communicating artery joins the right and left anterior cerebral arteries, which branch off the internal carotid arteries.

Central (paramedian) and circumferential (cortical) branches emanate from the anterior, middle, and posterior cerebral arteries and the circle of Willis. The former go deep into the brain perpendicularly to supply the diencephalon, corpus striatum, and internal capsule. The circumferential branches lie under the pia mater on the surface of the brain. There are anastamoses between the anterior, middle, and posterior cerebral arteries on the brain surface. The surface vessels give off smaller arteries that penetrate both superficially and deep into the brain.

Next we follow the intracranial branches of the internal carotid artery. The anterior cerebral arteries, after their takeoff from the ICA, go anteriorly and medially toward the longitudinal fissure. After the anterior communicating artery connects them, they follow a parallel course for the right and left hemispheres, curving along the entire course of the corpus callosum superiorly. The anterior cerebral arteries supply the medial portions of the frontal and parietal lobes and reach over their superior-medial territory.

The middle cerebral arteries enter the sylvian fissures in their lateral course, supplying the corpus striatum and internal capsule. Going posterosuperiorly, they then branch over the surface of the frontal and parietal lobes and the superior portions of the temporal lobe.

The posterior cerebral arteries curve laterally around the pons and then the cerebral peduncles to the undersurface of the occipital lobes. They divide into branches going posteriorly to the tip of the occiput and anteriorly and medially to the temporal lobes.

PAIN INNERVATION OF THE HEAD

Not all parts of the head are pain sensitive. Pioneering work done by Ray and Wolff (1) in the 1940s, mainly by stimulating different areas of the head and brain in patients undergoing neurological surgery, mapped out the pain-sensitive areas. Extracranially, pain can be produced in the scalp, the cervical and cranial muscles, and their blood vessels. Intracranially, portions of the dura mater and its meningeal arteries, the venous sinuses, and the proximal portions of the intracerebral arteries, the 2nd and 3rd cervical nerves, and cranial nerves V, VI, and VII are also pain responsive. Extracranially, the skull is not pain sensitive. Intracranially, some portions of dura mater are insensitive. The arachnoid, pia mater, the ependyma lining the ventricular system, choroid plexuses, and the substance of the brain itself are insensitive by these methods.

However, stimulation of certain brainstem structures in man has produced headache similar to migraine. Raskin (2) et al. in 1987 described 15 patients with ventrolateral periaqueductal gray electrode placement (for low back pain) producing head pain. The electrodes were placed adjacent to the dorsal raphé nucleus. Stimulation of other areas of the brain not previously tested, particularly the brainstem, may demonstrate other pain-sensitive areas.

TRIGEMINAL SYSTEM

The trigeminal nerve (5th cranial nerve) is the primary afferent system for pain in the human head. Both intracra-

nially and extracranially, pain perception is carried by its three divisions. These familiar divisions are the ophthalmic, the maxillary, and the mandibular. The ophthalmic provides sensation to the eye and its adnexa, nasal mucous membranes, much of the nose, and the skin of the forehead and scalp, going back to a line drawn from the midauricle of the ear. The maxillary branch innervates the skin of the side of the nose, cheek and upper lips, the upper teeth, oral mucosa, and the antrum. The mandibular division supplies the skin of the mandible, much of the ear, and the temple, plus the lower teeth, the mandible itself, and the anterior two-thirds of the tongue. If an intracranial pain-sensitive structure is located in the anterior cranial fossa, the sensation is carried over the first and second divisions of the trigeminal system. The middle fossa is served by the second and third divisions. Pain from these trigeminally innervated intracranial structures is referred to the frontal, parietal, or temporal areas of the head.

All the trigeminal nerve division's cell bodies lie in the gasserian ganglion. The ophthalmic nerves traverse the superior orbital fissure; the maxillary branch goes cephalad from the structures it innervates, via the inferior orbital fissure and the foramen rotundum, and the mandibular goes through the foramen ovale, to the gasserian ganglion. The central ganglionic axons for pain (and temperature) form the spinal tract and nucleus of V. There they synapse. The nucleus projects down from the pons to the higher cervical cord, where the substantia gelatinosa is continuous with it. The second-order neurons then cross over to the contralateral side and ascend to the arcuate nucleus of the thalamus as the dorsal and ventral trigeminal lemnisci. After synapsing there, axons relay to the postcentral gyrus of the cerebral cortex (3).

NONTRIGEMINAL SYSTEMS

The relatively small areas of the head that are not trigeminally served are innervated by the glossopharyngeal nerve (9th cranial nerve) for the posterior tongue, tonsil, and pharynx, by the vagus nerve (10th cranial) for the pharynx and posterior external ear, while the second and third cervical nerves innervate the intra- and extracranial occipital territory. For the posterior fossa, the above nerves subserve pain. Referred pain is felt in the occiput.

The glossopharyngeal nerve (cranial nerve IX) for the above sensory territories has cell bodies in the petrosal ganglions. The vagus nerve (cranial nerve X) sensory cell bodies lie in the jugular ganglion. The sensory input for the two nerves join in the upper neck and enter the medulla. There they join the spinal tract of the trigeminal nerve and descend with the trigeminal mandibular division to synapse in the cervical cord with the spinal nucleus of V. The second-order axons cross to the other side and reach the thalamus as the ventral ascending tract of the 5th nerve. They synapse there and go along with the trigeminal thalamocortical fibers to the sensory cortex (3).

Briefly, the cervical pain nerves have their cell bodies in the dorsal root ganglia. The proximal axons go to the substantia gelatinosa of the spinal cord, where they synapse. The second-order fibers for pain cross to the contralateral side through the center of the cord and ascend to the ventrolateral thalamus via the lateral spinothalamic tract, where they synapse, and these fibers ascend to the parietal cortex via the internal capsule.

TRIGEMINAL PAIN FIBERS AND NEURONS

In man, free nerve endings are the end organs in the skin, mucous membranes, teeth, cornea, and probably the pain-sensitive intracranial structures such as the dura and proximal arteries of the circle of Willis. These nociceptors are classified based on their activation by different stimuli, either mechanical, chemical, or thermal. The activating stimulus produces a slow-moving action potential going centrally either in small myelinated fibers classified as A alpha or in nonmyelinated C fibers (4, 5).

Studies in the afferents of the monkey face demonstrate that some A alpha fibers are stimulated only by mechanical forces that cause injury, while others have a threshold response to noninjurying pressure but a peak response to injury-producing pressure. Each fiber has a spot receptor field measuring 1 to 2 mm^2. The A alpha heat nociceptor has a spot receptor field of 1 to 4 mm^2 and is activated by noxious thermal or mechanical forces. The C fibers are called polymodal nociceptors, as they are stimulated by damaging chemical, thermal, or mechanical stimuli involving their spot fields of reception (6, 7).

Electron microscopic studies (8) in the cat of the small-diameter nonmyelinated nerve fibers that form a plexus around the great vessels at the base of the brain are consistent with their being C fibers.

Moskowitz (9) has particularly developed the concept that the trigeminal sensory fibers around the great vessels at the base of the brain are the major pathway for headache.

The anatomical-physiological-biochemical sequence involving the "trigeminovascular system" is as follows: Noxious stimulus → calcium-dependent process → activates neuropeptide-containing vesicles located on sensory axons → neuropeptides released → neuropeptides bind to nerve receptor sites → activate sensory nerve ion channels → axon membrane potential generated → goes centrally via trigeminal pathways.

PAIN MODULATION BY THE BRAINSTEM

Several brainstem systems act as modulators and modifiers of pain (10). An ascending and a descending system have been identified.

The ascending system has its neurons of origin in the dorsal raphe nucleus (DRN) located in the midbrain. Studies in primates (11) show that the axons go to the thalamus and cerebral cortex, particularly reaching the somatosen-

sory and visual cortex by well-organized pathways. The neurotransmitter of this system is serotonin.

In the conscious rat, stimulating the ascending system produces increased blood flow in the ipsilateral carotid artery (12) and increases glucose utilization in the areas of somatosensory neocortex that represent the face and neck.

The descending system causes inhibition of cells that transmit pain centrally. Neurotransmission is by enkephalins (13). This system has neurons in the central gray of the midbrain (periaqueductal gray), the medial medulla (raphe nuclei) and the reticular formation of the medulla, and the posterior horns of the spinal cord (14–16). The report by Raskin (2) (mentioned in the anatomy section of this chapter) of head pain occurring shortly after electrode implantation in the ventrolateral periaqueductal gray demonstrates that the brain itself is not invariably pain insensitive and appears to relate to the ascending pain system, as the electrodes were just lateral to the DRN. The implantation itself resulted in first stabbing pain and then throbbing pain in two of the patients reported. Raskin postulates that activation of the serotinergic ascending system may be a primary event in migraine.

SPREADING DEPRESSION

Spreading depression was first described by Leao in 1944. He found that stimulating an area of rabbit cortex electrically produced a marked decrease in the spontaneous and stimulated electrical activity as measured electrocorticographically in that area. After a 10-minute lag period, the depression spread radially over the cortex at 2 to 5 mm/min. Subsequent studies have shown that various chemicals that block metabolism when applied to cortex, mechanical trauma, and hypoxia may produce spreading depression. Increased brain metabolism can be measured ahead of the spreading depression, while at the site of the process, interstitial potassium is first increased and then interstitial sodium, calcium, and chloride decrease. This is compatible with total permeability of the cell membrane to all ions (17). At the same time, nerve and glial cells depolarize. After a plateau phase, the intracellular and interstitial space ions normalize. Invariably blood flow decreases for an hour or more after ionic stabilization (18).

In summary, spreading depression is a physiological response of stimulated neurons. It does not occur spontaneously. Blood flow changes occur secondarily in response to the neuronal changes, not as the primary event.

CEREBRAL BLOOD FLOW AND ITS MEASUREMENTS

There are various methods for evaluating cerebral blood flow changes in migraine. Each technique has temporal and spatial resolution limitations (19, 20). A brief review of the techniques presently used and the resulting data is essential to understanding the pathophysiology of migraine (Table 3.1).

Cerebral angiography has not been of value in the study

Table 3.1.
Techniques for Evaluation of Cerebral Blood Flow Changes in Migraine

Method	Measures	Type–vessels	Time
Angiography	Localization & form of vessels	Arteries, veins	1 sec
Transcranial Doppler sonography	Blood velocity (not flow)	Large arteries	1 sec
Intraarterial regional cerebral blood flow (rCBF)	Fast rCBF components, mainly cortical rCBF	Tissue perfusion	40 sec
Stationary detectors	Mixed cortical, white matter, and extracranial	Tissue perfusion	11 min
Single photon emission computerized tomography	Separated cortical and white matter rCBF	Tissue perfusion	2–4 min
Positron emission tomography	rCBF, glucose and oxygen metabolism	Tissue perfusion	1–3 min
		Tissue metabolism	45 min

of migraine. Transcranial Doppler sonography measures the velocity of arterial flow in the large arteries of the brain. Arterial diameter changes and fluctuations may be calculated when the velocity is added to the regional cerebral blood flow (rCBF) results for the cerebral area of the artery (16, 19, 22).

Increasingly sophisticated methods of measuring rCBF in man, basically using radioisotope uptake or clearance values, have produced information relevant to the pathophysiology of headache. This is equivalent to tissue perfusion of the brain in the areas being monitored. The most widely used isotope is xenon-133, and the most accurate method of delivery of the isotope is by intracarotid rapid bolus injection. Inhalation or intravenous injection has been used, but with lessened sensitivity resulting. This has been improved somewhat by increasing the sensitivity of the recording instrument. In the Scandinavian rCBF studies, with each isotope injection, 254 different areas of cerebral cortex could be measured simultaneously (16, 19, 21).

The intracarotid technique may trigger classic migraine. Studies have been made both following carotid angiography and the intracarotid injection of xenon-133 alone. As the aura develops, six to eight rCBFs are measured and hypoperfusion is seen in the occipital lobe (19, 22). This "oligemia" was also seen without an aura or with an aura that was not visual. The hypoperfusion then advanced at a rate of 2 mm/min anteriorly into the parietal and temporal lobes. It does not conform to arterial territories, nor does it cross the lateral (sylvian) or central (rolandic) sulci. Frontal oligemia was sometimes recorded, presumably traveling via the insula. In some studies (22), focal hyperemia occurred before hypoperfusion. In other studies (23) it did not.

Clinically, headache begins during the oligemic phase. In many subjects, the headache pattern and associated neurological symptoms were identical to their typical migraine.

Intravenous and inhalation techniques have replaced the intracarotid route. Stationary detectors may be used, but interpretative problems may result from isotope detection simultaneously from intra- and extracranial vessels and tissues and even from the other cerebral hemisphere (19). The advantages are that arterial puncture is not used and measurements may be made over a period of hours. The

tomographic feature of single photon emission computerized tomography (SPECT) allows canceling out the extracranial compartment and adequate differentiation intracranially between grey and white matter. Studies (24) by these techniques demonstrate that the oligemic phase may last up to 6 hours. Furthermore, toward or at the end of a migraine, hyperemia has been found in the previously oligemic brain (25).

One other technique is positron emission tomography (PET), which can measure rCBF and the metabolism of oxygen and glucose. Thus far it has proven cumbersome and expensive, with the need for a cyclotron and complicated procedures, and studies have produced few new data in migraine.

The interpretation of these studies so vital to understanding the pathophysiology of headache is controversial. Some (16, 26) postulate that because of the pattern and degree of the oligemia it is a primary neuronal rather than a vascular event. In other words, disordered neurons begin the events, with decreased blood flow in the area a secondary event. Others (27) have postulated a primary vascular event based on various technical corrections to the data, in particular correcting for radiation scatter. Radiation scatter from other brain areas will increase the radiation measurements from an area of reduced rCBF, producing an incorrectly elevated rCBF.

These calculations make the oligemia of an order sufficiently severe to produce actual tissue ischemia, with brain function reduced secondarily.

It has also been theorized that the advancing oligemia is compatible with Leao's spreading depression.

NEUROTRANSMITTERS

Although, strictly speaking, neurotransmitters are biochemical entities, they are so intimately involved in the physiology of migraine that a brief discussion is indicated here. Norepinephrine, acetylcholine, and serotonin (5-hydroxytryptamine) are confirmed neurotransmitters in the CNS. There are now a number of other possibly active and significant neurotransmitters in the CNS. In particular, interest has developed in their potential action as vasomotor neurotransmitters. Table 3.2 outlines some of the more likely compounds, many of which are peptides. The various neuropeptides have been grouped into families. The families of present relevance to migraine are the

Table 3.2.
Neurotransmitters in Migraine

Transmitter	Structure	Origin	Location	Action
Serotonin (5-hydroxytrytophan)		Tryptophan	GI enterochromaffin cells, brain (synthesized), platelets (uptake)	CNS: primarily inhibitory; Vascular: CNS primarily vasoconstriction
Substance P	11-amino-acid peptide	Preprototachykinins	CNS: cord, basal ganglia, hypothalamus; PNS: sensory nerves	CNS: trigeminal nerve → vessels, pial vessels dilate; PNS: primary sensory nerves
Norepinephrine		Tyrosine	CNS sympathetic nerve fibers	Vasoconstriction CNS arteries?
Adenosine triphosphate (ATP)	Adenosine–O–P–O–P–O–P–O	Ribonucleoside from the purine adenine	All cells—including adrenergic neurons	Postsynaptic sympathetic receptors? Vasoconstriction or vasodilation?
Neuropeptide Y (NPY)	Neuropeptide	Synthesized messenger RNA + ribosomes in ganglia cells, etc.	Sympathetic perivascular nerves	CNS vasoconstriction?
Vasoactive intestinal polypeptide (VIP)	Neuropeptide	Synthesized messenger RNA + ribosomes in ganglia cells, etc.	Nerves to CNS blood vessels	Probable neuotransmitter to CNS blood vessels → dilation
Acetylcholine (ACh)	$H_3C–C–O–CH_2–CH_2–N–(CH_3)_3$	Choline + acetyl group from acetyl-CoA	Nonsympathetic cholinergic nerves to vessels in CNS	Vasodilation

opioids, which include the enkephalins; the secretins, of which vasoactive intestinal polypeptide is a member; and the tachykinins, which include substance P. In addition, recent work has enlarged the number of potential transmitter neuropeptides found in sensory nerve vessicles around the great vessels at the base of the brain (9). Calcitonin gene-related peptide (CGRP) (28), neurokinin A (NKA) (29), and galanin (30) are three such neuropeptides.

Serotonin (5-hydroxytryptamine) deserves particular mention because of its possible place in the generation of migraine and recent introduction of sumatriptan, designed to trigger specifically one serotonin subtype (31). Serotonin exerts its effects throughout the body, including the CNS, by binding to cell surface receptors. Three types of receptors have been located for serotonin. Each has further subtypes. The brain has the highest concentration of serotonin 1A receptors (31). Serotonin may act physiologically on CNS vessel diameter in addition to its action on central neutral pathways.

EXTRACEREBRAL MECHANISMS

Headache developing by extracerebral mechanisms must be mentioned in this anatomicophysiological discussion. Much has been written about dilatation of the extracranial arteries as a cause of headache (32). Recent clinical research with digital compression of the superficial temporal artery on the side of the migraine, with transducer-measured pulse amplitude (33), and with facial thermography (34) concludes that in *some* subjects with migraine the scalp arteries do dilate and may contribute to the headache, but the negative results in other headache subjects eliminates scalp vessel dilatation as the basic cause of the pain (35).

Other studies, using a variety of techniques to measure ocular, conjunctival, skin, muscle, and subcutaneous tissues, and arterial blood flow, have produced conflicting data that again suggest that some subjects with vascular headaches have increased extracranial blood flow (36).

This again leads to the conclusion that extracranial vascular changes are not primary in causing headache.

MYOFASCIAL MECHANISMS

Much has been written about possible "myofascial" mechanisms in the production of headache (38). Trigger points, or palpable areas of tenderness in the cervical and occipital muscles, have yielded insignificant or debatable pathological and biochemical abnormalities to date (37). The physiology of pain possibly producing headache from these areas would appear to warrant further study.

REFERENCES

1. Ray BS, Wolff HG. Experimental studies on headache. Pain-sensitive structures of the head and their significance in headache. Arch Surg 1940;41:813–856.
2. Raskin NH, Hosobuchi Y, Lamb S. Headache may arise from perturbation of the brain. Headache 1987;27:416–420.
3. Peele TL. The neuroanatomic basis for clinical neurology. 3rd ed. New York: McGraw-Hill, 1977.

4. Ochoa J. Peripheral unmyelinated units in man: structure, function, disorder, and role in sensation. Adv Pain Res Ther 1984;6:53–68.

5. Torebjork E. Nociceptor activation and pain. Philos Trans R Soc Lond 1985;B308:227–234. Quoted in Yokota T. Anatomy and physiology of intra- and extracranial nociceptive afferent and their central projections. In: Oleson J, Edvinsson L, eds. Basic mechanisms of headache. Amsterdam: Elsevier, 1988.

6. Dubner R, Price DD, Beitel RE, Hu JW. Peripheral neural correlates of behavior in monkey and human related to sensory-discriminative aspects of pain. In: Anderson DJ, Matthews B, eds. Annu Rev Neurosci 1977;6:381–418.

7. Yokota T. Anatomy and physiology of intra- and extracranial nociceptive afferents and their central projections. In: Oleson J, Edvinsson L, eds. Basic mechanisms of headache. Amsterdam: Elsevier, 1988.

8. Liu-Chen L-Y, Liszczack T, King J, et al. An immunoelectron microscopic study of substance P–containing axons in cerebral arteries. Brain Res 1986;369:12.

9. Moskowitz MA. Basic mechanisms in vascular headache. In: Mathew NT, ed. Neurologic clinics. 8 (#4) Philadelphia: WB Saunders, 1990:801–815.

10. Raskin NH. The pathogenesis of migraine. In: Curr Opin Neurol Neurosurg 1989;2:209–211.

11. Molliver ME. Serotenergic neuronal systems: what their anatomic organization tells us about function. J Clin Psychopharmacol 7(suppl 6):3S–23S, 1987.

12. Goadsby PJ, Piper RD, Lambert GA, Lance JW. Effect of stimulation of nucleus raphe dorsalis on carotid blood flow. Am J Physiol 1985;248:R257–262.

13. Pert A. Mechanisms of opiate analgesia and role of endorphins in pain perception, in Critchley M, Friedman AP, Gorini S, Sicuteri F (eds): Adv Neurol 1982;33:107–122.

14. Anthony M. The biochemistry of migraine. In Vinken PJ, Bruyn GW, Klawans HJ, eds. Handbook of clinical neurology. Vol 48. Amsterdam: Elsevier, 1986:85–105.

15. Basbaum AI, Fields HL. Endogenous pain control systems: brainstem spinal pathways and endorphin circuitry. Annu Rev Neurosci 1984;7:309–338.

16. Raskin NH. Headache. 2nd ed. New York: Churchill Livingstone, 1988.

17. Hansen AJ, Lauritzen M. Spreading depression of Leao. In Olesen J, Edvinsson L, eds. Basic mechanims of headache. Amsterdam: Elsevier, 1988:99–107.

18. Lauritzen M, Jorgensen MB, Diemer NH, et al. Persistent oligemia of rat cerebral cortex in the wake of spreading depression. Ann Neurol 1982:12:469–474.

19. Friberg L. Cerebral blood flow changes in migraine: methods, observations and hypotheses. J Neurol 1991;238:S12–S17.

20. Lassen NA, Friberg L. Methods for measurement of regional cerebral blood flow. In: Olesen J, Edvinsson L, eds. Basic Mechanisms of Headache. Amsterdam: Elsevier, 1988:61–68.

21. Friberg L, Roland PE. Functional activation and inhibition of regional cerebral blood flow and metabolism. In: Olesen J, Edvinsson L, eds. Basic mechanisms of headache. Amsterdam: Elsevier, 1988:89–98.

22. Oleson J, Larsen B, Lauritzen M. Focal hyperemia followed by spreading oligemia and impaired activation of rCBF in classic migraine. Ann Neurol 1981;9:344–352.

23. Lauritzen M, Skyhoj Olsen T, Lassen NA, Paulson OB. Changes in regional cerebral blood flow during the course of classic migraine attacks. Ann Neurol 1983;13:633–641.

24. Lauritzen M, Olesen J. Regional cerebral blood flow during migraine attacks by xenon-133 inhalation and emission tomography. Brain 1984;107:447–461.

25. Anderson AR, Friberg L, Skyhoj Olsen T, Olesen J. Delayed hyperemia following hypoperfusion in classic migraine: single photon emission computed tomographic demonstration. Arch Neurol 1988;45:154–159.

26. Oleson J. The pathophysiology of migraine. In: Vinken PJ, Bruyn GW, Klawans HL, eds. Handbook of Clinical Neurology. Vol 48. 1986:59–80.

27. Skyhoj Olsen T, Friberg L, Lassen NA. Ischemia may be the primary cause of the neurologic deficits in classic migraine. Arch Neurol 1987;44:156–161.

28. McCulloch J, Uddman R, Beyerl BD, et al. Calcitonin gene related peptide: functional role in cerebrovascular regulation. Proc Natl Acad Sci USA 1986;83:5731.

29. Saito K, Greenberg S, Moskowitz MA. Trigeminal origin of beta-preprototachykinin in feline pial blood vessels. Neurosci Lett 1987;76:69.

30. Suzuki N. Galanin-positive nerves of trigeminal origin innervate rat cerebral vessels. Neurosci Lett 1989;100:123.

31. Raskin NH. Serotonin receptors and headache. N Engl J Med 1991;325:353–354.

32. Graham JR, Wolff HG. Mechanisms of migraine headache and action of ergotamine tartrate. Am Med Assoc Arch Neurol Psychiatry 1938;39:737–763.

33. Drummond PD, Lance JW. Extracranial vascular changes and the source of pain in migraine headache. Ann Neurol 1983;13:32–37.

34. Drummond PD, Lance JW. Facial temperature in migraine, tension-vascular and tension headache. Cephalgia 1984;4:149–158.

35. Drummond PD, Lance JW. Contribution of the extracranial circulation to the pathophysiology of headache. In: Oleson J, Edvinsson L, eds. Basic mechanisms of headache. Amsterdam: Elsevier, 1988:321–330.

36. Jensen K. Headache and extracerebral blood flow. In: Oleson J, Edvinsson L, eds. Basic Mechanisms of Headache. Amsterdam: Elsevier, 1988:311–320.

37. Langemark M, Jensen K. Myofascial mechanisms of pain. In: Olesen J, Edvinsson L, eds. Basic Mechanisms of Headache. Amsterdam: Elsevier, 1988:330–341.

38. Travell JG, Simons DG. Myofascial Pain and Dysfunction. Baltimore: Williams & Wilkins, 1983.

4

Differential Diagnosis and Related Medical Conditions

ROBERT V. STEINMETZER

While headache remains one of the most common symptoms known to mankind, only a small proportion of headache sufferers will actually seek medical help. Most people, by recognizing the benign character of their headaches, are able to cope and treat the symptoms on their own.

In most instances, it is not all too difficult to classify the headache into one of the categories or subcategories of the IHS (see Chapter 2) defined in a previous chapter. This apparent ease in typing each headache should however not distract from the fact that a small percentage represents serious underlying disease.

Only a very careful history and meticulous physical and neurological examination will give the astute clinician a clue that he may be dealing with something more than a common and benign etiology.

Numerous systemic and local conditions, both intracranial and extracranial, can have headaches as part of their presentation. Rather than compiling another exhaustive list of these possibilities, we shall review some of the points that should raise the index of suspicion and concentrate on some of the more important clinical entities accompanied by headache.

"RED FLAGS" OF HEADACHE

A detailed and properly structured patient interview gives the opportunity to make a correct diagnosis in most instances. A headache present and unchanged for several years is unlikely to represent a serious organic problem. On the other hand, a new onset or a significant change in a previous headache may indicate that something is going wrong. It is particularly important to pay close attention to the chronic sufferer, who may be developing a new and serious condition. Too many times we tend to become complacent in dealing with these patients and think that this is just "one more of their migraines." Unfortunately, in this situation, a new diagnosis is often overlooked, and a delay can have catastrophic consequences.

The pattern of a headache is probably the best indicator of its etiology. The intermittent character of migraine and the episodic recurrence of cluster headaches are quite typical. Daily or almost daily headaches require more careful analysis. While most of these represent chronic muscle contraction or mixed tension-vascular headaches, they are certainly not limited to these conditions. One needs to be particularly attentive to the patient describing a progressive increase in intensity and frequency of symptoms. Also, progressive resistance to usual therapy may indicate underlying trouble.

Nocturnal headache, waking the patient from sleep, may be vascular and represent either migraine or cluster. However, the same pattern can emerge in any condition causing increased intracranial pressure or with infectious processes. Hypoglycemia, sleep apnea, and severe hypertension can also cause nocturnal or early morning headaches.

Effort-related headaches, i.e., those directly precipitated by physical activity, are frequently migrainous and totally benign (1); however, in the absence of other typical characteristics, one should consider the possibility of an intracranial vascular malformation, such as an aneurysm. The same holds true in orgasmic headaches, which fortunately are mostly benign.

Any headache associated with neurological signs or symptoms requires a careful evaluation (2). Subtle clues and previous history will often help differentiate between hemiplegic migraine and a cerebrovascular accident. In most instances and at least initially, these patients all require some form of neuroradiologic imaging. Particular attention should be given to any patient with even minimal cranial nerve dysfunction. This also applies to anyone whose headache is accompanied by a change in mental status.

Any headache associated with fever needs careful observation. While many benign viral and other infectious illnesses are frequently accompanied by headache, one needs to evaluate the patient for the possibility of meningitis or a parameningeal process. If the clinical examination leaves any doubts, one should not hesitate to proceed quickly with a lumbar puncture.

The intensity of a headache may be reason for alarm. A patient describing his "worst headache ever" (3) may give the indication of an impending rupture of an aneurysm. Intensity alone, however, is not a good indicator for the

Table 4.1.
Warning Signs for Potential Danger

New-onset headache
Change in previously existing headache (intensity, frequency, pattern)
Nocturnal headache
Effort-related or positional headache
Previous head trauma
Unusual age of onset for particular diagnosis
Febrile headache
Headache associated with neurologic findings
Headache associated with change of personality or mental status
Headache of unusual intensity

presence or absence of organic disease; for example, the headache of temporal arteritis can be very moderate and nonspecific.

Previous head trauma should raise the possibility of a subdural hematoma, especially in the elderly. Even a minor injury, sometimes forgotten by the patient, can lead to this complication. In small children, physical abuse, including violent shaking, may be the cause of brain trauma and microhemorrhages.

The age of onset is quite helpful in differentiating between some headaches. Although migraine may develop at any age, it would not be the first diagnosis coming to mind in an elderly patient without previous attacks. Temporal arteritis on the other hand would be unlikely under the age of 50. Idiopathic trigeminal neuralgia occurs around the same age. In a younger patient, tic douloureux may be secondary to other conditions, such as multiple sclerosis or brain tumor.

HEADACHE AND ASSOCIATED DISORDERS OF THE CRANIUM

Sensory fibers of the trigeminal nerve, the vagus, and the posterior roots of the 3 first cervical nerves account for most pain transmission from the cranium. Because of interconnection between these systems and the existence of referral pain, a process in one particular area may be perceived as a pain in a different area of the cranium; for example, posterior fossa lesions can produce frontal head pain, and inflammation of the sphenoid sinus may cause referred pain to the vertex.

Because of the frequent lack of correlation between the site of pain and the underlying process, one should beware of making premature assumptions about the cause of a headache. Typically, patients refer to frontal and periorbital pain as "sinus headache," although in most cases, these headaches can be classified differently. The confusion becomes even worse because patients frequently get relief from the usual "sinus medications," which contain a variety of analgesics and decongestants.

Headaches can certainly be caused by both acute and chronic sinusitis. Clinical examination and sophisticated imaging techniques, such as endoscopy and thin-cut computed tomography (CT) scanning, will usually set the record straight and allow specific treatment. Most difficult

to evaluate are those patients who have undergone extensive and repetitive sinus surgeries and continue to have chronic facial pain. Frequently, these patients had unrecognized vascular "lower half" headaches, but by now, the pain has become aggravated by the formation of extensive scar tissue around these highly innervated structures.

The frequency of ophthalmologic causes of headache is also greatly overestimated. Because of the extreme sensitivity of the eye and the neuroanatomy of the orbital and retrorbital structures, the eye is frequently the site of referred pain (4). The first reflex of a parent is to take the child with headache for an eye examination and blame the symptoms on eye strain. Refractive eye disorders, except for astigmatism, rarely cause headaches.

Inflammatory processes such as uveitis may be accompanied by referred pain. Photophobia and lacrimation may be present in these conditions, but they are also typically found in cluster patients. Sometimes, the intensity of the pain makes an office examination very difficult, and one should not hesitate to obtain a full ophthalmologic evaluation under sedation and analgesic coverage.

In acute angle-closure glaucoma, the patient may present with a severe and generalized headache. Further symptoms may include abdominal pain, nausea, and vomiting, mimicking the symptoms of a migraine attack. If not immediately recognized, such patients may rapidly develop irreversible blindness.

Painful ophthalmoplegia needs a careful search for an ipsilateral cerebral aneurysm, which may be enlarging. In the Tolosa-Hunt syndrome (5), progressive cranial nerve paralysis develops in conjunction with retrotorbital pain. The diagnosis may be apparent on CT or magnetic resonance imaging (MRI) of the orbits, and corticosteroid treatment will alleviate the symptoms.

Dental and periodontal causes for facial pain are frequently unrecognized. An impacted wisdom tooth, abcess formation, or trauma to the alveolar nerve endings during dental procedures can become the trigger focus to a neuralgia-type pain. Conversely, many unrecognized cluster patients undergo extensive dental surgeries in an attempt to get relief.

Temporomandibular joint (TMJ) dysfunction is a frequently incriminated mechanism for headache and facial pain. While in some instances the problem truly arises within the joint, most cases seen in headache centers represent myofascial pain with secondary imbalance of the bite mechanism. Many clinicians believe that this represents a localized variant of fibromyalgia and advocate a conservative approach with physical therapy, tricyclics, bite correction, and biofeedback. A later chapter discusses this entity in detail.

Mastoid and ear infections can be responsible for acute and febrile headaches. The examination is usually revealing. The ear and periauricular area may be the site of referred pain from cervical myalgia, occipital neuralgia, TMJ dysfunction, or acoustic neurinoma.

HEADACHES AND ASSOCIATED DISORDERS OF THE CERVICAL STRUCTURES

Arthritic changes of the cervical spine are present in most individuals over the age of 50. There is, however, no linear correlation between the degree of arthritis and the presence of cervical or occipital pain. There is a widespread belief in the lay population that posterior headaches relate to cervical arthritis. In most cases, however, these headaches have a chronic tension-type or tension-vascular character. They usually do not respond to physical therapy, antiinflammatory drugs or muscle relaxants but improve with conventional headache therapy.

It is important to recognize those headaches directly related to cervical spine disorders. Cervical spondylosis and degenerative disc disease cause cervical radiculopathies through foraminal impingement or compression. The posterior roots or C2 and C3 innervate the occipital areas of the scalp. Unilateral inflammation or compression will cause severe pain, localized to the dermatome. Neural blocks, if effective, help make the diagnosis.

Other local abnormalities, such as cervical canal stenosis and cervical spine neoplasms, can produce more diffuse pains but are usually accompanied by other neurological findings.

Cluster patients frequently describe severe cervical pains during the initial phases of their attacks. The symptoms are unilateral, and the patient may notice some crepitation with neck movements. However, there appears to be no correlation between cluster headache and cervical disease.

Sjaastad et al. (6) have identified a separate group of patients, mostly young females, who are sometimes able to provoke their unilateral attacks by certain head and neck movements. These headaches are accompanied by migrainous phenomena, and the belief is that these are truly cervicogenic headaches.

HEADACHE AND CEREBROVASCULAR DISEASE

Headache is a very prominent symptom in subarachnoid hemorrhage. A ruptured aneurysm typically combines severe cephalgia, acute change in mental status, and signs of meningeal irritation. With this picture, the diagnosis is usually clear, and the clinician will institute the appropriate measures without delay.

On the other hand, it is not uncommon to discover on routine imaging a small unruptured berry aneurysm in a headache patient. In most instances, this is asymptomatic and not the reason for the patient's headache. Appropriate testing and neurosurgical referral should be obtained at once.

Aneurysms can present with a warning, or "sentinel" bleeding, preceding the actual rupture (7). The accompanying headaches can be quite severe, acute, and frequently brought on by straining or exertion. MRI scanning followed by lumbar puncture will likely support the diagnosis.

Nonhemorrhagic stroke is associated with a prominent headache in about one-third of cases. With completed stroke, the diagnosis is obvious by neurological examination. The challenge lies in the patient with transient symptoms, combining focal neurological complaints and headache.

The differentiation between transient ischemic attacks (TIA) and transient migraine accompaniments (TMA) can be difficult, as both conditions mostly occur in the age group of 50 and above (8). TIAs typically have a very sudden onset. TMAs, on the other hand, may develop over several minutes and take a "march-like" progression of symptoms. Associated visual symptoms, especially positive phenomena, as well as a previous history of migraine would favor the diagnosis of TMA.

Migraine is a well-recognized risk factor for stroke, especially in the younger population. A recent study indicates that 25% of strokes in those under 50 are direct complications of migraine (9).

Dissection of the internal carotid artery combines an acute headache, neck pain, vascular bruit, and possible Horner's syndrome. Carotidynia or cluster headache could mimic part of this syndrome.

Pituitary apoplexy (10) can present with prominent headache accompanied by oculomotor deficits. The cause can be either ischemic or hemorrhagic, and immediate recognition is crucial to avoid the grave and possible fatal endocrine consequences.

HEADACHE SECONDARY TO INFECTIOUS CAUSES

Any headache combined with fever needs a careful evaluation. It is well known that a high fever (from whatever cause) may induce a severe headache. These headaches are felt to be of the "toxic-vascular" category and are due to intense cerebral vasodilation, as demonstrated in animal experiments.

Influenza, infectious mononucleosis, typhoid, malaria, and rickettsial diseases (to name just a few) may all present with significant headache. Headache can be a prominent symptom in both early and late phases of Lyme disease. The association of chronic headache and persistent Epstein-Barr virus antibodies has been documented.

It is mandatory to maintain a high index of suspicion for meningitis or meningoencephalitis in the presence of fever and headache. If clinical signs suggest a CNS infection, a lumbar puncture and appropriate cultures should be obtained without delay.

It is not uncommon for a headache to persist for weeks or even months after an acute viral illness. If chronic meningitis has been excluded, symptomatic treatment is all that is required.

Herpes zoster can induce severe, persistent neuralgic pain, most often in the upper branch of the trigeminal nerve. Geniculate (Ramsey-Hunt) or occipital nerve involvement can also occur. Most often, the diagnosis can be made on clinical grounds alone.

HEADACHE AND VASCULITIDES

Headache is a presenting symptom in most cases of giant cell or temporal arteritis (TA) (11). The pain can be totally nonspecific and need not be localized over the temporoparietal region. In older studies, headache was present in over 90% of confirmed cases of TA; newer reviews put the frequency at 70 to 80%. The disease is quite common (133/100,000) in the over-50 age group. Systemic symptoms, such as polymyalgia, fever, weight loss, and fatigue, may be absent throughout the disease. Any unexplained, persistent headache in this population requires at least the consideration of temporal arteritis. Although an elevated sedimentation rate will be found in over 90% of cases, a temporal artery biopsy should be obtained to confirm the diagnosis. A prompt diagnosis and treatment are essential as irreversible blindness can develop without warning signs.

In the younger population, headache may be a clue to other systemic or cerebral inflammatory vasculitides (12). Headaches can be very prominent in this group of patients, and can mimic a persistant migraine. If there is a suspicion for systemic lupus erythematosus, the appropriate laboratory tests should be obtained to establish the diagnosis. In the presence of rapidly progressing neurological symptoms, cerebral angiography may be necessary. The symptoms will improve with treatment of the underlying condition; however, permanent sequellae may arise in severe cases of cerebritis.

PSEUDOTUMOR CEREBRI

Pseudotumor cerebri or benign intracranial hypertension affects mostly young women. The presence of papilledema usually initiates an extensive search for an underlying mass lesion. This is a diagnosis of exclusion that usually requires CT or MRI scanning, followed by lumbar puncture. Besides papilledema, these patients may have visual field defects, including increased blind spots and concentric restrictions.

Although in most instances, no specific cause(s) for pseudotumor can be found, this entity has been associated with a variety of endocrine dysfunctions, such as obesity and thyroid, ovarian, and adrenal disease (13). It has also been described in conjunction with excessive ingestion of vitamin A, as well as the use of corticosteroids, oral contraceptives, or tetracyclines. Hematologic conditions (including iron deficiency and thrombocytopenia) have also been associated with this condition.

Treatment consists of removal of the offending agent, correction of the underlying condition, diuretics, and oral corticosteroids. Some patients will require repeat lumbar punctures or even a shunt procedure. Although the prognosis is excellent in most cases, the condition can lead to permanent unilateral or bilateral blindness.

REFERENCES

1. Rooke ED. Benign exertional headache. Med Clin North Am 1978;52:801–808.
2. Edmeads J. The headache of ischemic cerebrovascular disease. Headache 1979;19:345–349.
3. Edmeads J. The worst headache ever. Postgrad Med 1989;86:93–110.
4. Carlow TJ. Headache and the eye. In Dalessio DJ, ed. Wolff's headache and other head pain. 5th ed. New York: Oxford University Press, 1987.
5. Spinnler H. Painful ophtalmoplegia: the Tolosa-Hunt syndrome. Med J Aust 1973;2:645–646.
6. Sjaastad O, Fredriksen TA, Pfaffenrath V. Cervicogenic headache: diagnostic criteria. Headache 1990;30:725–726.
7. Verweij RD, Wijdicks EFM, Van Gijn J. Warning headache in aneurysmal subarachnoid hemorrhage, a case control study. Arch Neurol 1988;45:1019–1020.
8. Couch, JR. Stroke and migraine. In: Saper JR, ed. Controversies and clinical variants of migraine. 1st ed. New York: Pergamon, 1987.
9. Broderick JP, Swanson JW. Migraine related strokes: clinical profile and prognosis in 20 patients. Arch Neurol 1987;44:868–871.
10. Rovit RL, Fein JM. Pituitary apoplexy: a review and reappraisal. J Neurosurg 1972;37:280–288.
11. Huston KA, Hunder GG, Lie JT, et al. Temporal arteritis: a 25 year epidemiologic, clinical and pathologic study. Ann Intern Med 1978;88:162–167.
12. Moore PM, Cupps TR. Neurologic complications of vasculitis. Ann Neurol 1983;14:155–156.
13. Ahlskog JE, O'Neill BP. Pseudotumor cerebri. Ann Intern Med 1982;97:249–256.

5

Headache History and Neurological Examination

LAWRENCE C. NEWMAN, RICHARD B. LIPTON, and SEYMOUR SOLOMON

The large majority of headache patients seen in clinical practice have entirely normal medical and neurological examinations. A comprehensive history is therefore required to ensure appropriate diagnosis. Because head pain and its associated features are difficult to describe, both the physician and patient may become frustrated. Poor descriptions of headache features or inaccurate interpretation by the physician may result in misdiagnosis and mismanagement.

The goal of the headache history is to obtain a comprehensive view of the patient's headache and any associated conditions and problems that might influence diagnosis or treatment. By employing a systematic approach, as outlined in this chapter, the clinician should, in most instances, arrive at the correct diagnosis.

The headache history also provides an opportunity to establish a rapport that will serve as a basis for an ongoing relationship. Many headache patients are embarrassed about their problem and feel that no one understands or cares about their suffering. Rapport is best established by exhibiting a caring, attentive demeanor. Keep the questions simple and patiently wait for a response. Pain sufferers not uncommonly fear that they are afflicted with some terrible malady. Frequently they have rehearsed what they are going to say upon meeting the physician, and they may be easily flustered. Rushing or pressuring patients for an answer may unsettle them and actually prolong the interview. We generally give patients about 10 minutes to give an account of their problem and then systematically explore various features of the headache. Be supportive and nonjudgmental. Occasionally summarizing what the patient has said will help ensure an accurate history and help the patient feel understood. Though obtaining a complete headache history is a time-consuming task, the results are invaluable. We allow a full hour to assess a new headache patient, at least 30 minutes of which are spent on the initial history.

History taking is often complicated by the presence of more than one type of headache or the change in headache pattern over time. It is often helpful to begin with the current headache of greatest concern to the patient and subsequently to explore other current headache patterns and the evolution of those patterns.

We have the patients complete a self-administered questionnaire, sent to their homes prior to the consultation. This tool often helps patients to focus on their symptomatology and course, improving the reliability of the history.

HEADACHE ONSET

Knowing the age of onset can facilitate diagnosis. Migraine most commonly begins prior to age 40, with the highest incidence occurring between the ages of 10 and 30 (1), though it may begin in childhood or late in life. Cluster headaches begin between 20 and 50 years of age, though they too may begin at any age (2). Tension headaches most often have their onset prior to age 50, with 40% of sufferers reporting their first occurrence before age 20.

When headaches begin after age 55, serious disorders such as mass lesions or giant cell arteritis are much more likely. Headaches in the elderly are often associated with ischemic or hemorrhagic cerebrovascular disease (3). Trigeminal neuralgia usually starts in the 6th or 7th decades of life (4, 5). The hypnic headache syndrome is a benign form of headache that begins after age 60 (6, 7).

It is useful to inquire about events associated with the onset of the headache syndrome. Headaches following a blow to the cranium suggest a postconcussive headache disorder or subdural hematoma; contusion, laceration, or traumatic hemorrhage are less likely. However, both migraine and cluster may be triggered by head trauma. Migraine may begin with menarche or (rarely) with menopause. Headaches occurring in the peripartum period may be due to cortical vein or sagittal sinus thromboses. Fever in association with headache onset suggests an infectious etiology. Physical stress may precipitate exertional headache or subarachnoid hemorrhage. Emotional turmoil or depression may trigger migraine or tension-type headache and rarely evokes headaches of psychogenic origin.

LOCATION OF PAIN

The physician must inquire about the localization of maximal pain at the onset of an attack and also note the pattern of spread. Headaches may be diffuse or localized; they may be consistently hemicranial and may or may not alternate sides between attacks. Pain may be experienced as a superficial annoyance or as arising deep within the head.

A unilateral, hemicranial headache usually suggests a vascular mechanism. Migraine headaches are usually unilateral and frontotemporal, but they may become diffuse and are sometimes bilateral at onset. In most migraineurs the pain randomly changes sides from attack to attack, but there is often a predilection for one side. The pain may radiate into the eye, face, neck, shoulder, and arm. Cluster headaches are always unilateral, with the pain centered in or around the eye, temple, cheek, or adjacent areas (8). The pain may spread to involve other areas ipsilaterally, such as the lower jaw or neck, but it does not tend to generalize (9, 10). In contrast to migraine, only 10 to 15% of patients note a change in the side of pain from one attack to another (2). The pattern of pain in tension-type headache is typically bilateral and tends to encompass the cranium in a band-like distribution (11), but it may be maximal bifrontally or bioccipitally. Cervicogenic headache and hemicrania continua are unilateral cephalgias with pains radiating from the neck to the forehead. A similar location of pain may be seen with chronic paroxysmal hemicrania.

Localized pain may also occur with organic diseases. The trigeminal nerve is the major source of innervation to the pain-sensitive structures in the supratentorial space (12). Infratentorial pain-sensitive structures receive innervation from the upper cervical, glossopharyngeal, and vagus nerves (4). For these reasons, supratentorial lesions usually cause frontal headaches, and those situated infratentorially produce pain in the occipital region. When headache is strictly limited to the periorbital region, ocular pathology should be excluded. Trigeminal neuralgia may cause pain in any area of the face innervated by the trigeminal nerve. The mandibular and maxillary branches are the most frequently involved, and the right side of the face is affected more often than the left (5). Pain may occur on both sides of the face, although usually not simultaneously (4). In giant cell arteritis the headache is often located in the temple, but it may occur anywhere (13) and is perceived as being superficial, not deep within the cranium (4). Over half of patients with brain tumors complain of headache (14), and in 80% the site of pain is on the same side as the tumor (15). Headaches associated with cerebrovascular disease may be global or lateralized. When lateralized, the headaches are ipsilateral to the lesion only half of the time (3).

DURATION OF PAIN

Estimating the length of a typical headache and determining the duration of the longest and the shortest headache can yield useful information. Migraines typically last from 4 to 72 hours (16). When they persist for more than 72 hours, the term *status migrainous* is applied. Cluster headaches usually last an average of 15 to 180 minutes (16); they may, however, be as short as 10 minutes or as long as several hours. The headaches of chronic paroxysmal hemicrania typically last 5 to 20 minutes (16), with a range from 2 to 120 minutes (17). Episodic tension-type headaches tend to last from 30 minutes to 7 days (16). When they persist for a number of days, they are likely to evolve into chronic tension-type headaches, becoming continuous and lingering for months or years. The pain paroxysms of trigeminal neuralgia last only 20 to 30 seconds, but a dull ache may be present for several hours (18). As a rule, nonprogressive headaches without associated neurological dysfunction usually imply a benign etiology.

Headaches of organic origin do not have a typical duration, but if the disease progresses, the duration and frequency of the headaches tend to increase.

FREQUENCY AND TIMING OF ATTACKS

The frequency and timing of headaches are helpful in determining both diagnosis and treatment. How often do the headaches occur? Do they have a regular pattern? Are they characterized by nocturnal awakenings? Do they occur in clusters? If no temporal pattern exists, then the average frequency of headaches per day, per week, or per month should be estimated. Determining the longest period of freedom from headache may also be useful. What were the circumstances associated with prolonged remission?

Migraine headaches are episodic and often recur without regular patterns. Frequency ranges from once or twice a year to 4 times per week, but it averages 1 to 3 per month. Distinct patterns may be seen. Women with migraine may note an association with their menstrual cycle; other migraine sufferers develop headaches only on weekends, on vacation, or upon relaxation after stress. Episodic cluster headaches typically occur in a regular pattern. During the cluster period, which usually lasts between 2 weeks and 3 months, headaches may occur as rarely as once every other day or as often as 8 times per day (16). The attacks tend to recur at similar times of the day or night, often waking the patient during REM sleep. A pain-free remission phase follows the cluster period and typically lasts from 1 to 24 months (19). Patients with chronic cluster headache either do not experience remissions or have remissions lasting less than 14 days. In patients with chronic paroxysmal hemicrania, attacks recur as often as 30 times per day (16). Occasionally migraines occur with a periodicity similar to cluster headaches (20). Episodic tension-type headaches recur less than 15 times per month or 180 times per year (16). Patients suffering with hypnic headaches report 1 to 3 headaches per night (6, 7). If a headache pattern is uncovered, potentially useful prophylactic measures may be employed. Menstrual migraines frequently respond to perimenstrual nonsteroidal antiinflammatory medications. Nocturnal cluster attacks may be prevented by administering ergotamine at bedtime.

Chronic daily headaches (chronic tension-type headaches) often evolve in a person who has suffered from long-standing migraines. With the passage of time, these people report a decrease in the frequency of the migrainous features of their headaches, but note a daily persistent global headache. Daily headaches also occur in patients who overuse analgesic medications, barbiturates, ergotamine, or caffeine. These "rebound headaches" are characterized by a constant headache that may wax and wane throughout the day in conjunction with fluctuating blood levels of the drug. Withdrawal headaches may occur upon awakening or actually awaken the patient from sleep.

Organic headaches may be episodic or daily and continuous. Headaches of organic origin do not occur with any set pattern, but if the disease progresses, the frequency of headache increases and may become continuous.

PAIN SEVERITY AND COURSE

It is important to assess the severity of pain as well as the rapidity of onset and resolution. The use of a pain-rating scale that allows patients to grade their pain is invaluable. We advise using a 1 to 10 scale, where 1 represents minimal discomfort and 10 the most excruciating pain the patient can imagine. While these numbers cannot be used to make precise comparisons between individuals, they are very useful for charting improvements in particular patients. As most headaches wax and wane in intensity during the course of an attack and vary in average intensity across different attacks, it is also useful to inquire about the range of pain experienced during a headache.

Migraine headaches usually begin gradually, are of moderate to severe intensity, and resolve slowly or with sleep. Cluster headaches and chronic paroxysmal hemicrania have a rapid onset and climax quickly; they are excruciating. Rarely, migraine headaches have a similar onset (21). Tension-type headaches are usually characterized by a dull ache that may wax and wane over the course of the day. The pain is typically slight to moderate, but brief flare-ups of relatively severe pain may occur. Patients suffering from hemicrania continua, as the name implies, complain of a continuous moderate-intensity headache with occasional exacerbations of more severe pain (22, 23). Trigeminal neuralgia presents with excruciating pains that begin and peak nearly instantaneously and occur in paroxysms lasting less than a minute. Headaches associated with sexual activity may begin as a dull ache and rapidly intensify during orgasm or may present as an explosive, excruciating headache. With the latter, an aneurysmal rupture must be considered. Benign exertional headaches are of moderate to severe intensity and are precipitated by strenuous physical exercise such as lifting weights.

Intracerebral neoplasms most often present with a dull headache of mild to moderate severity but grow in severity as intracranial pressure increases. The headache of subarachnoid hemorrhage (SAH) typically has a sudden, explosive onset and is of excruciating intensity. The headache of giant cell arteritis classically is a low-level, dull ache that intensifies gradually but on occasion may have an explosive onset (4, 24).

The course of "benign" headaches (migraine, cluster, tension-type) varies, but they usually persist for years before tapering off in mid or late adult life. The headache of an intracranial mass lesion increases in severity, duration, and frequency with time. This is also true of the other organic diseases, such as giant cell arteritis. The headache evoked by cerebrovascular disease (including SAH), on the other hand, tends to occur for days or weeks at a time (3); they may precede as well as accompany a stroke.

QUALITY OF PAIN

It is essential for the examiner to obtain a description of the pain, preferably in the patient's own words. At times, this may be a frustrating task, as many patients have difficulty describing their pain and may only report that "it hurts." Prompting the patient by providing descriptive terms such as throbbing, pulsating, pressure-like, burning, boring, or piercing can help elicit a useful response.

The pain of migraine is characteristically throbbing or pulsatile but often begins as a dull steady ache that slowly evolves; it may not acquire a throbbing quality until the pain reaches high intensity. The pain of cluster headaches is usually deep, boring, or piercing. It is sometimes likened to having a red-hot poker thrust into an eye. Similar intense, rapidly climaxing pains are experienced with chronic paroxysmal hemicrania; the pain in most cases is described as throbbing (17). A dull band-like or vice-like sensation is often described by patients with tension-type headaches. Trigeminal neuralgia presents as paroxysms of brief electric shock-like pains. Ice pick headaches have brief, intense, sharp jabbing pains occurring as single episodes or in repeated volleys. They may occur as a separate entity but are more often seen with other headache types. Migraineurs are particularly subject to these head pains (25, 26). When they occur with cluster headaches, their appearance often heralds the end of an attack (8, 27). A moderate throbbing sensation is described with hypnic headaches (6, 7).

The characteristic headache of a brain tumor is a dull ache (14). The headache from a rupture of an aneurysm or arteriovenous malformation is most often a continuous, intense aching or throbbing pain. Headache occurs frequently in patients with cerebrovascular disease. Those with a prior history of recurrent throbbing headaches are more likely to experience a throbbing headache with a cerebrovascular event (3). The pain in giant cell arteritis is usually dull and boring, though it may pulsate (13, 24).

AGGRAVATING OR PRECIPITATING FACTORS

Identifying factors that precipitate or aggravate an attack is useful in establishing a diagnosis. Recognition of these factors may also help control the headaches by allowing the patient to avoid precipitants.

The pain of migraine is worsened or triggered by a myriad of internal or external factors. The most frequently reported include menstruation, stress (especially relaxation after stress), fatigue, too much or too little sleep, skipping a meal, weather changes, high humidity, high altitude, exposure to glare or flickering lights, loud noises, perfumes or chemical fumes, postural changes, physical activity, or coughing. Food triggers occur in approximately 10% of migraineurs and most often include chocolates, cheeses, alcoholic beverages (especially red wine), citrus fruits, and foods containing monosodium glutamate, nitrates, and aspartame (1, 28–30). Cocaine use and cocaine withdrawal may also trigger a migraine-like headache (31). Cluster headaches are triggered by ingestion of alcohol during the cluster period, usually within 30 minutes after imbibing. During the remission phase of the cluster headache, alcohol may be consumed without precipitating an attack. The pain of cluster headaches is often aggravated by lying down. Tension-type headaches are said to be aggravated by the stresses of everyday life and so are worse at the end of the day. Patients with trigeminal neuralgia have trigger points on the face and mucous membranes of the mouth. Slight stimulation of these trigger points by stroking, shaving, or washing the face, brushing teeth, exposure to cold air, eating, or speaking may provoke an attack.

Headaches caused by brain tumors are intensified by exertion, postural changes, bending over, or coughing (14). Aneurysmal rupture may be precipitated by exertion, for example, sexual activity.

AMELIORATING FACTORS

Identifying the factors that ameliorate the discomfort may provide useful diagnostic and therapeutic information. This includes both nonpharmacological and pharmacological factors. Migraineurs commonly volunteer that they must retire to a dark quiet room and lie motionless to obtain relief; many patients find that sleep will clear their attacks. Not infrequently, pressing on the superficial temporal artery brings relief, but only during the period of compression. Hot or cold compresses are often applied. Migraine frequency and severity often decreases during the last 2 trimesters of pregnancy or with the onset of menopause. Cluster headache patients note that sitting upright, rocking in a chair, pacing to and fro, or engaging in vigorous movement seems to lessen the pain. Tension-type headache may be alleviated by relaxation, rest, or sleep.

If analgesics have been used, determine their dosage, frequency, efficacy, and side effects. Inquire how long the prescription has been used. The patient may be using the drug erroneously; either taking a subtherapeutic dosage or taking the medication too infrequently. Conversely, they may be overusing or abusing the medications. Often patients will not recognize how much analgesic they are using until you ask "How long does a bottle of 100 pills last?"

ASSOCIATED FEATURES

Sometimes the symptoms associated with the headache rather than the pain prompt patients to seek help. Associated symptoms may occur prior to, concurrent with, or following the headache; their temporal relationship should be established. We generally begin with open-ended questions such as, "Before the pain begins do you know that you are going to get a headache?" We probe for associated features, according to organ system. For example, under ophthalmologic we ask about scotomata, scintillations, fortification spectra, blurring or loss of vision, tearing, photophobia, etc. If cardinal features are not volunteered, they must be specifically sought, exercising caution to avoid eliciting false-positive responses.

The migrainous prodrome (not to be confused with the aura) refers to symptomatology occurring hours to 1 or 2 days prior to the headache onset. Typical prodromata include mood changes, drowsiness or hyperactivity, food cravings, yawning, or changes in bowel or bladder habits. Frequently, the patients are unaware of prodromata, and questioning close relatives may prove helpful. The aura of migraine refers to a transient neurological phenomenon occurring less than 60 minutes prior to the headache onset (although the aura, in contrast to epilepsy, may occur at the same time as the headache). Most often, the aura of migraine consists of a visual abnormality such as fortification spectra, photopsia, micropsia or macropsia, scintillating scotomata, teichopsia, visual field defects, or obscurations. Among other manifestations of the aura are paresthesias (especially of the face or hand), hemiplegia, aphasia, or symptoms implicating the basilar circulation, such as vertigo.

Migraine may be associated with a multitude of symptoms such as photophobia, phonophobia, osmophobia, and nausea with or without vomiting. In asking about these features, distinguish between a sensitivity that is always present ("I'm always sensitive to light") and a sensitivity that is heightened during a headache ("I'm particularly sensitive to light during an attack"). One must also differentiate nausea that is part of the attack and nausea induced by treatments such as ergot alkaloids. Less often, mood alterations, edema, lightheadedness, polyuria, diarrhea, or other autonomic disturbances are noted. Cluster headache is associated with one or more ipsilateral autonomic symptoms such as lacrimation, injection of the eye, nasal congestion, rhinorrhea, ptosis, miosis, eyelid edema, and perspiration of the forehead and face. While nausea is seen in approximately 40% of cluster sufferers, vomiting is rare

(2). Similar autonomic disturbances are seen in patients with chronic paroxysmal hemicrania. Tension-type headaches usually occur without any associated features. Symptoms, if present, may include only 1 of the following: nausea, photophobia, or phonophobia; vomiting is not a feature of tension-type headache (16). Facial grimacing during a painful spasm is commonly seen in trigeminal neuralgia (hence the term tic douloureux).

A variety of neurological deficits accompany the headache of organic disease, depending upon the localization of the lesion. Intracranial mass lesions are associated with nausea and vomiting or vomiting without nausea (projectile) in half the cases (14). Giant cell arteritis may be associated with localized scalp tenderness, malaise, arthralgias or myalgias (polymyalgia rheumatica), low-grade fevers, depression or other constitutional symptoms, and visual disturbances or stroke. Jaw claudication, if present, is virtually pathognomonic for the disorder. The chronic posttraumatic headache is often accompanied by nonspecific dizziness, malaise, impairment of work efficiency, and anhedonia.

SOCIAL HISTORY

Environmental factors play a large role in headache etiology. The examiner must attempt to explore the patient's interpersonal relationships. These points include the patient's marital and family status, education, occupation, outside interests, and friendships. Are any of these areas a source of stress? Has the patient recently had a major life change such as marriage, divorce, separation, new job, retirement, or death in the family? Is work satisfying or merely drudgery? Is there conflict in the workplace? What is the patient's employment? Occupational exposures (rarely) may be the source of the headache. If ventilation is poor or if workers are exposed to carbon monoxide, headaches may result. Workers in munitions factories may develop nitrite-induced headaches. Inquire about other habits, such as the use of alcohol, tobacco, caffeine, or illicit drugs. A history of homosexual or bisexual activities should prompt a search for a potential infectious cause of the cephalalgia. The sleep habits of the patient may be important. Sleep apnea is not uncommon in middle-aged obese men and may cause morning headache. Depression may be manifested by difficulty in falling asleep or staying asleep, or as early morning awakenings. Likewise, trouble falling asleep may occur with anxiety. Careful questioning about the above possible stressors may uncover a source of conflict or a psychological component to the headache.

FAMILY HISTORY

As some headache disorders are familial, it is useful to obtain a family history. Attempt to get a description of the headache and associated features, rather than accepting the patient's diagnosis of the relative's headache. It would be ideal to get a brief description of the headache from the affected relative, as third-party reports of symptoms are often unreliable. Approximately 50 to 60% of migraineurs have a parent with the disorder, and up to 80% have at least one first-degree relative with these headaches (1, 8). Cluster headaches rarely occur within the same family. Forty percent of patients with tension-type headaches have family members with similar headaches (11). As depressive illnesses may be familial, psychogenic factors may also be found in other family members.

Familial headaches do not necessarily imply a genetic basis. Shared environmental exposures may also cause familial headaches. For example, a leaky furnace may cause familial headaches induced by carbon monoxide.

GENERAL MEDICAL HISTORY AND REVIEW OF SYSTEMS

A medical history and review of systems is an essential part of a complete headache history. This review must include past medical illnesses, injuries, and surgical procedures, as well as current medical conditions. Obtain a list of all medications that the patient uses. Ask specifically about the use of oral contraceptives, vitamins, and other over-the-counter pills, as many patients do not consider these medications. Birth control pills may aggravate migraine; high doses of vitamin A have been implicated in pseudotumor cerebri, and daily use of over-the-counter medications may cause rebound headaches. A variety of disorders affecting the teeth, sinuses, eyes, ears, nose, or throat may produce head pain. Recent lumbar puncture or epidural anesthesia may have induced a low cerebral spinal fluid–pressure headache. A history of recent or remote head trauma suggests a posttraumatic headache syndrome, a cerebral contusion, or a subdural hematoma. Trauma may have also been an initiating factor for migraine or cluster headaches. A past history of carcinoma or infectious illness may provide clues to the etiology of the headache. Prior seizures in a patient suffering from recurrent headaches should elicit a search for an intracranial mass lesion, arteriovenous malformation, or aneurysm. A childhood history of motion sickness, cyclic vomiting, abdominal pains, or vertigo may presage the development of migraine. Mitral valve prolapse occurs in association with migraine. A past history of repeated thromboembolic events, spontaneous abortions, and vascular headaches suggests an antiphospholipid antibody syndrome such as the anticardiolipin syndrome. Pheochromocytomas present as recurrent pulsatile headaches in association with hypertension, diaphoresis, tachycardia, and nausea.

Allergic reactions in the past may have important implications in subsequent therapy. β-Blockers must be used very cautiously if the patient suffers from asthma or diabetes; tricyclic antidepressants must be used carefully in patients with cardiac disease, glaucoma, or prostatic enlargement; ulcer disease is a relative contraindication the use of steroids or the nonsteroidal antiinflammatory agents.

Endocrinologic abnormalities may be associated with headaches. Uncovering a history of galactorrhea or amenorrhea in a headache sufferer should prompt a search for a pituitary tumor. The polycystic ovary syndrome may be associated with pseudotumor cerebri. Thyroid disease (e.g., thyroiditis) may cause pain referral to the ear and could precipitate headaches.

Do not overlook any past history of psychiatric illness. As depression may recur cyclically, this may provide a clue to the etiology of the current headache episode. Loss of libido is more likely a manifestation of depression than an endocrine abnormality.

PAST STUDIES/PAST AND CURRENT HEADACHE TREATMENTS

Many patients with long-standing headaches have had a multitude of diagnostic procedures and have taken a variety of medications. Every reasonable effort should be made to verify prior test results. Obtain a copy of the test report or, better still, a copy of the test itself.

A history of the medications previously prescribed and the dosages in which they were given is useful for many reasons. First, treatment response may help support a diagnosis. Establishing, for example, that ergot-containing medications successfully treated the headache in the past suggests a vascular component to the headache. Second, a detailed history may help explain past treatment failures. Unsuccessful treatment is often the result of incorrect dosing strategies or not allowing enough time to obtain a potential benefit (e.g., discontinuing a β-blocker after only a 1-week trial). Third, the history of benefits and side effects will narrow the future treatment plan. For each past and current medication, ascertain its benefits or side effects and the reason for its discontinuation. Inquire about the use and efficacy of prior nondrug therapies such as psychotherapy, biofeedback, acupuncture, or chiropractic.

Then delve into the patient's current approach to headache treatment. Many headache sufferers overuse medications, willingly or unwittingly. Many over-the-counter pain relievers contain caffeine with acetaminophen or aspirin. Excessive use of these agents as well as narcotics, barbiturates, and ergots can produce withdrawal or rebound headaches. Again, determine the dosages and the frequency of drug use. If subtherapeutic regimens are being employed, correction may lead to better headache control. Conversely, abuse or overuse of medications must be addressed and may require hospitalization for detoxification.

PATIENT'S IDEAS

At this point, having taken a detailed history, again give the patient a chance to speak freely. Ask how the headaches affect their lives or how their lives would be different without the headache. In doing this, you may get a fuller understanding of the patient's concerns and the impact of the headache problem. The patient may report useful information prompted by the more structured interview. Many patients seek the help of a physician for little more than reassurance that they do not have a brain tumor or a leaking aneurysm. Severe or chronic headaches not uncommonly are associated with anxiety and depression. These issues must also be identified and addressed.

HARBINGERS OF SERIOUS DISEASE

Most patients suffer from benign headaches. In taking the history, certain key points suggest that you may be dealing with a serious disorder that requires immediate attention. Headaches occurring with a sudden, explosive onset suggest subarachnoid hemorrhage, pituitary apoplexy, or another serious disorder, and require a prompt and immediate workup that includes a CT scan or MRI, often followed by a lumbar puncture. A new headache or different pattern of pain occurring in a patient with a long-standing headache history must be carefully evaluated. Any new onset of headache occurring in the elderly must be considered to have an organic basis until proven otherwise. Workup should include an erythrocyte sedimentation rate and imaging procedure of the brain to search for giant cell arteritis or intracranial disease. Headaches associated with fever and/or nuchal rigidity should elicit a search for an infectious or hemorrhagic source and may warrant a lumbar puncture. Persistent neurological deficits in association with headaches almost always require further investigations of organic cerebral disease.

PHYSICAL AND NEUROLOGICAL EXAMINATIONS

After completing the history, the patient must be thoroughly examined. Vital signs should be taken, followed by an examination of the heart and lungs with auscultation of the eyes and carotid and vertebral arteries for bruits. Palpate the head and neck, looking for trigger points, other tender areas, masses, bruises, or thickened blood vessels. Examine the temporomandibular joint for tenderness, decreased mobility, asymmetry, or "clicking."

Examination of the nervous system should include evaluation of the mental status, testing of the cranial nerves, motor and sensory systems, deep tendon reflexes, coordination, and gait.

A few key signs bear emphasis. Evidence of papilledema suggests increased intracranial pressure and warrants an imaging procedure to rule out a mass lesion. Nuchal rigidity due to meningeal irritation is seen with intracerebral mass lesions, intraparenchymal or subarachnoid hemorrhages, and meningitis, and prompts a rapid workup. Focal neurological deficits may indicate structural brain disease and likewise require neuroimaging. A thickened or nodular temporal artery, diminished or absent temporal artery pulsations, reddened tender scalp nodules, or necrotic lesions of the scalp or tongue indicate giant cell

Table 5.1.
Historical Features

Headache Type	Age of Onset (years)	Location	Duration	Frequency/Timing	Severity	Quality	Associated Features
Migraine	10–30	Hemicranial	Several hours to 3 days	Variable	Moderate–severe	Throbbing > steady ache	Nausea, vomiting, photo/phono/osmophobia, scotomata, neurological deficits
Tension-type	20–50	Bilateral	30 min to 7 days +	Variable	Dull ache may wax/wane	Vice-like, band-like pressure	Nausea or photo or phonophobia, no vomiting
Cluster	20–40	Unilateral peri/retroorbital	30–120 min	1–8 ×/day, nocturnal attacks	Excruciating	Boring, piercing	Ipsilateral conjunctival injection, lacrimation, nasal congestion, rhinorrhea, miosis, facial sweating
Mass lesion	Any	Any	Variable	Intermittent, nocturnal, upon arising	Moderate	Dull steady/throbbing	Vomiting, nuchal rigidity, neurological deficits
Subarachnoid hemorrhage	Adult	Global, often occipitonuchal	Variable	N.A.	Excruciating	Explosive	Nausea, vomiting, nuchal rigidity, loss of consciousness, neurological deficits
Trigeminal neuralgia	50–70	2nd–3rd > 1st division's trigeminal n.	Seconds, occur in volleys	Paroxysmal	Excruciating	Electric-like	Facial trigger points, spasm of facial muscles ipsilaterally (Tic)
Giant cell arteritis	>55	Temporal, any region	Intermittent then continuous	Constant ? worse at night	Variable	Variable	Tender scalp arteries, polymyalgia rheumatica, jaw claudication

arteritis. Horner's syndrome may be seen with cluster headaches, chronic paroxysmal hemicrania, or intracranial lesions.

While most patients with a chief complaint of headache will have an entirely normal examination, it must be stressed that this portion of the consultation must not be overlooked, for it will help guide subsequent diagnostic and treatment strategies.

HISTORY AFTER THE INITIAL VISIT

On occasion, a diagnosis may not be established on the first visit, or the initial assessment may be incorrect. It is useful to ask the patient to keep a headache diary for both diagnostic and treatment purposes. The frequency, severity, and duration of the headaches are logged, as are the medications that were used and the possible triggers of the headache. On subsequent visits, review of the diary may uncover previously unrecognized patterns of the headaches that can provide clues in diagnosis. Headache triggers identified in this fashion may also suggest behavioral interventions.

CONCLUSIONS

Obtaining a complete and accurate history is an art that takes practice. History taking can be agonizing if the patient is intellectually dull, extremely obsessional, or hypochondriacal. The use of the outline described in this chapter, with modifications tailored to your personal preferences, will be the most effective tool in establishing a diagnosis. Table 5.1 summarizes important features of the various headache disorders discussed in this chapter.

REFERENCES

1. Selby G, Lance JW. Observations on 500 cases of migraine and allied vascular headache. J Neurol Neurosurg Psychiatry 1960;23:23–32.
2. Manzoni G, Terzano MG, Bono G, et al. Cluster headache—clinical findings in 180 patients. Cephalalgia 1983;3:21–30.
3. Portenoy RK, Abissi CJ, Lipton RB, et al. Headache in cerebrovascular disease. Stroke 1984;15:1009–1012.
4. Raskin NH. Headache. 2nd ed. New York: Churchill Livingstone, 1988.
5. Fromm GH. Trigeminal neuralgia and related disorders. Neurol Clin 1989; 7:305–319.
6. Raskin NH. The hypnic headache syndrome. Headache 1988;29:534–536.
7. Newman LC, Lipton RB, and Solomon S. The hypnic headache syndrome: a benign headache disorder of the elderly. Neurology 1990;40:1904–1905.
8. Lance JW, Anthony M. Migrainous neuralgia or cluster headache? J Neurol Sci 1971;13:401–414.
9. Ekbom K, and Kugelberg E. Upper and lower cluster headache (Horton's syndrome). In: Vizioli R, ed. Brain and mind problems. Rome: Il Pensiero Scientifico, 1988:482–489.
10. Solomon S, Karfunkel P, and Guglielmo KM. Migraine-cluster headache syndrome. Headache 1985;25:236–239.
11. Friedman AP, Von Storch TJC, and Merritt HH. Migraines and tension headaches. A clinical study of 2000 cases. Neurology 1954;4:773–788.
12. Coffey RJ, and Rhoton AL. Pain sensitive cranial structures. In: Dalessio DJ, ed. Wolff's headache and other head pain. New York: Oxford University Press, 1987:34–50.
13. Solomon S, and Guglielmo-Cappa K. The headache of temporal arteritis. J Am Geriatr Soc 1987;35:163–165.

14. Rushton JG, Rooke ED. Brain tumor headache. Headache 1962;2:147–152.

15. Kunkle EC, Ray BS, and Wolff HG. Studies on headache: the mechanisms and significance of the headache associated with brain tumor. Bull NY Acad Med 1942;18:400–422.

16. Headache Classification Committee of the International Headache Society. Classification and diagnostic criteria for headache disorders, cranial neuralgias and facial pain. Cephalalgia. 1988;7(suppl 8):1–96.

17. Atonaci F, and Sjaastad O. Chronic paroxysmal hemicrania (CPH): a review of the clinical manifestations. Headache 1990;29:648–656.

18. Jannetta PJ. Cranial nerve vascular compression syndromes (other than tic douloureux and hemifacial spasm). Clin Neurosurg 1981;28:445–456.

19. Kudrow L. Cluster headache: mechanism and management. New York: Oxford University Press, 1981.

20. Solomon S. Variants of cluster headache. In: Rose FC, ed. Handbook of clinical neurology. Vol. 48. Amsterdam: Elsevier, 1986:267–271.

21. Fischer CM. Painful states: a neurologic commentary. Clin Neurosurg 1984;31:32–53.

22. Sjaastad O, and Spierings ELH. "Hemicrania continua": another headache absolutely responsive to indomethacin. Cephalalgia 1984;4:65–70.

23. Zukerman E, Hannuch SNM, Carvalho D, et al. "Hemicrania continua": a case report. Cephalalgia 1987;7:171–173.

24. Goodman BW. Temporal arteritis. Am J Med 1979;67:839–850.

25. Raskin NH, Schwartz RK. Ice pick–like pain. Neurology 1980;30:203–205.

26. Lansche RK. Ophthalmodynia periodica. Headache 1964;4:247–249.

27. Ekbom K. Some observations on pain in cluster headache. Headache 1980;14:219–225.

28. Dalton K. Food intake prior to a migraine attack—study of 2,313 spontaneous attacks. Headache 1975;15:188–193.

29. Schaumburg HH, Byck R, Gerstl R, Mashman JH. Monosodium L-glutamate: its pharmacology and role in the Chinese restaurant syndrome. Science 1969;163:286–288.

30. Lipton RB, Newman LC, and Solomon S. Aspartame as a dietary trigger in migraine. Headache 1989;29:90–92.

31. Lipton RB, Kwong MC, and Solomon S. Headaches in hospitalized cocaine users. Headache 1989;29:225–228.

6

Psychological Factors Influencing Headache

There is now ample evidence, both from published research reports and from the direct clinical experience of a large number of health care providers, that psychological factors often play a significant role in the genesis and maintenance of headache problems. Since Wolff's original description of personality factors related to migraine (1), a number of medical authors and researchers have published attempts to systematically relate behavioral factors to headache. The first general aim of this chapter is to describe some of the interrelationships among behavioral patterns, including cognitive processes and emotional factors, and chronic headaches, based on the existing literature and our own clinical experience at the University of Washington Multidisciplinary Pain Center. This chapter is not intended as a review of the literature, but rather as a more general summary that will provide interested clinicians with an overview of some of what is known in this area.

A second, more practical, aim of this chapter is to present a set of guidelines that practitioners will find helpful in assessing the relationships among psychological factors and headache in clinical settings. Severe, debilitating headaches—and especially mixed headaches that occur on a daily or near-daily basis—are often related to lifestyle factors to a significant degree. Such factors might include the amount and kind of exercise the patients get, how they respond to unpleasant life events and daily hassles, how leisure time is used, and the quality of their primary relationships. This chapter describes such lifestyle factors in detail and provides an outline for assessing the contributions of these patterns and events to headache problems.

For convenience, the chapter is divided into sections, some of which separately review behavioral, cognitive, and affective factors related to headache. This division is not meant to imply that overt behaviors are ever performed independent of thoughts or feelings or that the emotional lives of our patients can ever be experienced irrespective of their attendant cognitions or patterns of activity. Although thoughts, feelings, and behaviors may be considered as conceptually distinct to some extent, they in fact are facets of the individual's personality that are clearly interconnected and overlap in complex ways. Two examples of

headache-related behavior patterns that exemplify this interconnectedness, responses to stress and pacing problems, are also discussed in separate sections below.

Beginning with a short discussion of the issue of medical stability, this chapter follows the course that a clinical interview might take that is intended to elucidate psychological factors related to headache. Throughout the chapter, efforts are made to guide the reader in terms of significant clinical issues, especially those that involve patterns of resistance that patients often demonstrate, and strategies for addressing them. The first clinical issue, though not strictly psychological, concerns the patient's actual medical status.

MEDICAL STABILITY

The question of the medical stability of the patient's headache problem needs to be addressed early in the evaluation, whether or not contributing psychological factors are at issue. To a large degree, the further workup and the eventual treatment plan will be determined by the stability of the problem. In this context, the medical stability means that healing has occurred in those situations in which there was an initial injury or lesion (e.g., in cases of chronic posttraumatic headache) and/or that the condition is not the result of intracranial pathology that may be amenable to medical intervention. It implies as well that, left untreated, the condition will not necessarily follow a deteriorating course, such as would be the case with a slow-growing tumor or low-grade meningitis. Typically, taking a careful clinical history and using scanning procedures (e.g., CT scan or MRI) when indicated is sufficient for ruling out pathology as a primary cause of headache. In this way, making a determination of stability will guide the assessment, since the treating physician will order the tests necessary to rule out ongoing pathology as a cause of headache.

From a psychological perspective, the stability question can also contribute to one's understanding and appreciation of the patient's phenomenological experience of the headaches and the possible contribution of fears and anxieties that headaches are due to an ongoing disease or an unhealed injury, which could have dire implications for long-term well-being. Patients who attribute their headaches to an undetected tumor, for example, are likely to worry about the headaches in a different way than those who relate their headaches primarily to muscle tension.

In assessing chronic pain problems, especially those of musculoskeletal origin, there is now a precedent for making assumptions about the interrelationship between medical stability and the likely source of overt behaviors that communicate suffering related to pain (2). It is typically assumed that a medically stable condition is more likely to be associated with pain behaviors that are under environmental (operant or learned) control than pain behaviors that evince underlying nociception due to an unstable condition. The difference between these two sources of control, environmental factors versus nociception, is, in essence, the difference between operant and reflexive behaviors. A limp resulting from a recent, and yet unhealed, injury to the knee is virtually unavoidable. It is the product of a set of fairly complicated reflexes that exist to protect the individual from further damage. However, a limp that persists for months and years following healing may be a learned reaction to outcomes that were positive to the individual and that outweighed negative outcomes such as not having a normal gait or being able to engage in favorite pastimes. Attempting to differentiate behavioral patterns that reflect nociception from those due to operant patterns is considered important since the latter can be modified through training and rearrangement of contingencies, at least in theory.

The position that stable pain problems are more likely to be controlled by environmental factors is arguable, however, and it is erroneous to maintain that pain behavior that reflects underlying nociception cannot be shaped by operant contingencies. Headaches that have been chronic for a number of years and are clearly not related to intracranial pathology may nonetheless have a significant nociceptive component because of the involvement of pathological muscular, vascular, and neurological activity. And yet, because of the chronicity of the headache problem and the number of headache episodes (or learning trials perhaps) the patient has endured, certain patterns of responding to headaches are developed by both the patient and significant others around him or her.

PATTERNS OF OPERANT HEADACHE BEHAVIOR

In assessing psychological factors related to headache, it is useful to begin with a careful analysis of relevant behavioral patterns, that is, the actual overt behaviors of patients which in some way reflect their headache experience. Such behaviors might include squinting and rubbing the temples, taking medications and lying down, and not attending to work or family functions. Assessment of such behaviors is useful for many reasons. It tells how patients perceive their own level of suffering, assuming that more dramatic displays of pain behavior reflect more suffering.

Moreover, assessing behavior patterns can offer insights about the patient's coping patterns and skills (e.g., how and under what circumstances the patient will opt for emergency room treatment), as well as highlighting inconsistencies in the patient's presentation (e.g., patients who perceive of and describe themselves as getting regular exercise, but whose activity diaries show otherwise). Finally and most importantly, understanding the consequences of headache behaviors for the patient and family sheds necessary light on the patterns of environmental events that may be determining the headache experience to a considerable degree.

To understand the implications of this last point, it may be useful to review some basic tenets of operant theory applied to chronic pain problems. Much of this discussion is based on the pioneering work of Fordyce (3). Established behavioral patterns exist because the positive consequences of the behavior for the individual have consistently outweighed any negative consequences. Behaviors persist because they are reinforced. This is the basic credo of behaviorism, and it is held to be true even if the pattern or nature of the reinforcement is not immediately apparent. For example, a statement such as, "This migraine is killing me," will be made during a headache episode, perhaps, because it has consistently elicited a care-taking response from the patient's spouse during past episodes, even though she has also rolled her eyes and appeared annoyed with the patient. To him, being cared for outweighs any social discomfort produced by his comment, and so some version of the statement, "This is killing me," will likely be repeated next time as well. Eventually, his wife's negative reaction may escalate so that the discomfort it produces for the patient exceeds the value to him of her nurturance; then, his verbal behavior may stop (he may suffer in silence), or it may be joined with more extreme pain behaviors (lying down, taking strong pain killers, or canceling family plans), which would tell her the seriousness of his condition and the need for her to continue to be nurturing, despite her own aggravation with the problem. Behaviors persist when the perception of reinforcement exceeds the perception of negative outcome or punishment.

The basic challenge to clinicians attempting to understand the contribution of behavioral factors to chronic headache is the identification of the relationships between behaviors and outcomes. Essentially, environmental contingencies either support pain behaviors directly, such as by offering emotional support or attention not attainable under other circumstances, or indirectly through avoidance conditioning, i.e., sanctioning time out from aversive activities. Thus, patients may miss time at work or no longer participate in family events that are relatively unpleasant.

In an assessment, two questions are particularly useful in identifying these patterns. The first asks the patient, "What do you not do any more—or do less of—because of your headache?" The answer should reveal both the likely cost to the patient of having headaches, in terms of reinforcing activities that are missed, and the possible reinforcement value of being excused from aversive activities. Obviously, such an assessment can only be made in light of other interview information about job history and job satisfaction, quality of family life, marital status, and so forth.

The second question has two parts. The first is, "When your headaches are really bothering you, what kinds of things do you say or do that let others know you are hurting?" This is followed by, "When others see or hear you doing these things, how do they respond? What do they do?" These questions obviously seek to uncover social reinforcement patterns of pain behavior, particularly within the context of primary relationships. Although we typically think of the response of spouses or significant others in this context, close friends, roommates, parents, and co-workers can also be potent modifiers of pain behavior, usually because their care for the patient inadvertently results in reinforcement of sick-role and disability behavior. It should be noted that significant others, friends, and family can also respond in ways that ultimately punish the pain behavior patterns, though this is rare.

Clinicians need to appreciate that patients are often defensive about discussing operant factors related to their headaches. This is largely because of the erroneous implication that behaviors under social or environmental control are actually being performed willingly by the patient for the procurement of some kind of secondary gain. It is imperative that clinicians help patients understand that this way of construing the relationship between behavior and reinforcement is inaccurate. If the outcome for the patient of performing a particular behavior is perceived as relatively positive, the behavior most likely will be repeated, regardless of the patient's level of intelligence, goals in life, or even the patient's best interest in the long run. Operant reinforcement of behavior often has little to do with what is willed, desired, or intended. Avoidance learning in the context of an aversive work situation illustrates this point well. It is not unusual for headache patients to describe themselves as having stressful, but enjoyable jobs, concurrent with a number of other responsibilities that compete for their time and energy. When headaches necessitate missing work, these patients will honestly report that doing so is aversive since it means loss of income, loss of social and (sometimes) intellectual stimulation, and facing the stigma of calling in sick. As the therapy relationship develops, however, it becomes clear that missing work also provides a necessary break from a demanding routine. Moreover, patients may eventually feel comfortable admitting that their work was in fact more stressful and unpleasant than they initially reported. Thus, a sanctioned time-out from work ultimately has very strong reinforcement value for the behavior of taking time off during subsequent headache episodes, even when such reinforcement is offset by some negative outcome as well, and despite the fact the the reinforcement is not experienced on a conscious level of awareness. Operant learning occurs automatically, irrespective of the personal attributes of the learner, and has nothing to do with malingering or the overt manipulation of others for personal gain.

Patients also tend to be defensive about the reality of their pain, since learning-based factors are being invoked to account for some aspects of their headache problem, in particular its apparent severity. As clinicians, we must convey to our patients that we appreciate both the reality and severity of their discomfort. Also, it is useful for them to understand that reinforcement of their headache behaviors by well-meaning significant others put patients at risk for suffering more than they need to. Pain behavior as a form of social communication can result in erroneous messages about what patients really need or how they really want to be perceived. Fordyce (4) has written about the problem of suffering confounded with pain, which in large part is related to faulty labeling processes (discussed below). In the context of operant learning, treating individuals as if they are sick or disabled risks making them worse, especially if their pain problems are medically stable, as is usually true of chronic headache.

EMOTIONAL FACTORS

To a large extent, we are culturally biased toward avoiding unpleasant emotions. Often, such avoidance takes the form of simply denying feelings we do not like, partly in the apparent belief that by denying such feelings we can eliminate them. Such simplistic defenses often do not stand up to emotionally demanding situations, however, so slightly more sophisticated defenses are used. One subtle way of avoiding or significantly lessening unpleasant emotion is by redistributing the affect, so that it is experienced somatically. Culturally, we tend to condone physical symptoms more than emotional.

Like the other patients we see, headache patients have rich emotional lives that include feelings of disappointment, anger, frustration, depression, and fear, as well as contentment, happiness, joy, and affection. Unlike our other patients, however, headache patients experience a relationship between so-called negative emotions and headache. Anger and depression are probably the emotions that headache sufferers struggle with most commonly.

Anger is the emotional component of our response to frustration, the overall pattern of thoughts, feelings, and behaviors we experience whenever access to a particular goal or set of goals has been blocked. Anger contributes to headaches in two ways primarily. First, a general set of goals that most of us share is to live a productive life that is relatively free of pain and disease. Headaches certainly interfere with the attainment of those goals, so that headache patients often describe feeling angry about the headache problem itself and the tremendous personal cost it involves in terms of feeling bad, loss of productivity, loss of income, and so forth. Second, it is also common for headache patients to have a history of managing anger somewhat ineffectually. Denial of anger as an emotion that nice people do not experience and difficulty expressing angry feelings (that are acknowledged) in a healthy, assertive way both tend to be common problems.

It is important, therefore, for clinicians assessing headache problems to be vigilant in looking for evidence of unresolved or unexpressed anger. In some cases, the intensity and chronicity of the patients' anger may significantly interfere with the overall quality of their life or even be generally debilitating. Even in less extreme cases, though, treatment necessarily includes helping patients develop skills for more effectively resolving long-standing anger and helping them appreciate that emotional reactions to daily life events may be learned to a significant degree but are certainly not willfully chosen. Thus, anger may be construed as an overlearned response to some kinds of events or situations, which occurs nearly automatically. In such situations, our choice is not whether or not to be angry, but rather how to manage the emotion. We do well to remind our patients that, as is true of all feelings, anger is not a sign of personal weakness or a source of chagrin and something to be denied or avoided. Just the opposite, it is a signal that our well-being is somehow being threatened. A more healthy response to anger, therefore, is to acknowledge it, learn more effective skills for managing it, and use the anger as an opportunity for better self-care.

These comments apply equally to depression, which is also common among headache sufferers and merits careful assessment. Diagnosing depression is rather straightforward. Patients are considered to have major depression when they are experiencing at least three vegetative symptoms from a list that includes difficulty falling asleep, maintaining sleep, or sleeping in; appetite change with corresponding weight loss or weight gain; loss of pleasure in normally pleasurable activities, including sexual; decreased memory or concentration; or fatigue throughout the day; in addition to dysphoria, i.e., sadness and depression, or agitation and irritability. Associated features include overall motoric agitation or slowing, difficulty making decisions, pervasive guilt or worthlessness, and of course, suicidality.

In some instances, it is difficult to distinguish symptoms of depression from the patient's direct response to headaches. Poor concentration, sleep disruption, and appetite disturbance, for example, all tend to occur during severe headache episodes. The continued presence of such symptoms during days of less-severe or no headache may indicate that depression is the preeminent problem. In some respects, the distinction is not particularly meaningful, however. Depression is often a reasonable response to loss, and chronic headaches typically result in loss of quality of life, as noted above. Moreover, both depression and headaches may be negatively influenced by maladaptive cognitive patterns (as discussed in the next section), and headaches sometimes improve following administration of antidepressant medications, which suggests a common biochemical substrate. It may be most useful then to point out to patients the typical relationship between headache

and depression—even when the pervasive mood change is agitation or irritability, rather than feeling sad, down, and lethargic—and explain that depression, like anger, has to be admitted to and managed if an optimal treatment outcome is to be achieved.

COGNITIVE FACTORS
Mislabeling/Belief Systems

Assessing medical stability as outlined above also has significant implications regarding cognitive processes associated with headache. Not only does the answer to this fundamental question guide initial approaches to treatment, it also serves the crucial purpose of explaining the nature of the headache to the patients so that they will have some sense of the cause of the headaches, their prognosis, and the available treatment options. The necessity for such explanations should not be underestimated.

We all strive to make sense of our daily experiences, and it is very common for patients to describe their primary treatment goal as simply "to find out what's wrong." Being able to explain, and in limited ways predict, the behavior of ourselves and others allows us to live somewhat orderly and emotionally comfortable lives. To the extent that a headache problem remains unexplained, it disrupts order and creates discomfort. It also places people at risk for generating explanatory models that may be relatively uninformed and ultimately harmful in some respects. "Illness conviction" refers to a well-entrenched system of beliefs that headaches are due to a primarily physical cause, such as a disease, a tumor, or a lesion. Corollary beliefs are: that treatment will involve administration of a potent medication and/or some form of medical procedure, perhaps even a surgery or something equally invasive; that the headache itself is a disease, condition, or syndrome that can and should be fixed; and that psychological factors do not play a role in this problem.

It is striking that these beliefs often persist in the face of overwhelming evidence that underlying intracranial pathology is not the source of the headache, and that lifestyle and behavioral factors are far from irrelevant. It is useful to think of the patients' unflagging adherence to their explanatory models as a type of resistance, born of concerns that they will ultimately be held up as "crocks" who are incompetent to manage their own lives or, worse, as malingerers who are amplifying a set of trivial symptoms, perhaps for some secondary gain. Relating the headache to psychological factors is often perceived as an admission of failure. Rather than having a legitimate disease, patients become their own worst enemy. Unfortunately, health care providers sometimes inadvertently reinforce this erroneous message in the ways we talk to and about our patients.

Also, it is understandably difficult for patients to appreciate the subtle message often given to them that the problem is not that serious, relative to a brain tumor, for example, given the extreme level of pain often associated with headache. Patients often make comments like "I know my body and I know something is wrong in there" or "This pain is so severe, there has to be something in there you can fix." It is difficult to place stock in a clinician's assessment that the headache problem reflects lifestyle issues as much or more than underlying disease, when discomfort is intensely felt and particular beliefs are intently adhered to.

To address these issues, it can first of all be useful to remind patients (and thereby reassure them) that they are being evaluated for a medical problem. And, like most other chronic medical problems, their headaches may well have a significant lifestyle component to them. Heart disease, for example, is a serious medical problem that is significantly improved by simply changing habits. It is also useful to review the results of diagnostic tests, in language suitable to the patient, so that the patient can again be reassured that, despite the intensity of the pain, there is no basis for being worried about some underlying disease or physical pathology. Once assured, patients are likely to be more receptive to a more accurate explanation of their problem.

We have found it helpful to explain that, once a pattern of chronic headaches is established, multiple triggers can produce very similar patterns of symptoms. Such triggers can be predominantly physical or predominantly behavioral. A severe headache occurring at the completion of a major task in a high-pressure work setting is often similar to a menstrual migraine that comes on during a relaxed vacation or the pounding headache that develops following a fight with a spouse. Because patients have often had these varied experiences themselves, they are less threatened by a new model of headache that includes both environmental (physical) and psychological (behavioral or emotional) causes, as compared with a strictly psychological model that does not take into account menstrual, dietary, and perhaps even meteorological influences that patients have observed in the past to be reliable triggering factors.

STRESS

Most chronic headache sufferers have been told, at one time or another in their treatment history, that their headaches may be stress-related. Often patients are also resistant to this notion, in part because of their perception that relating their headaches to stress once again implies a certain level of personal incompetence in their ability to manage their daily responsibilities. Also, patients' beliefs about the relationship between headache and stress tend to reflect a simple-minded understanding about stress as a contributing factor to medical problems that is rampant within our culture, even among many health care professionals. This is the belief that there is a clear, one-to-one correspondence between stress and physical symptoms, so that symptoms will be immediately and reliably exacerbated during periods of relatively higher stress, and will abate when stress is reduced. A corollary to this idea is that only persons whose lives are characterized by extraordinary stressors are at risk for having stress-related symptoms. These notions are inaccurate and contribute to a great deal of misunderstanding between patients and practitioners.

Interactive Model of Stress

Beginning with Selye's pioneering work on what he termed the General Adaptation Syndrome (5), a number of attempts have been made to develop a formal model of stress and its effects on all aspects of everyday life. These have been analyzed and synthesized into a single model of stress, the so-called interactive model of Lazarus and Folkman (6). At the heart of this model is the recognition that personal beliefs, attributions, and perceptions are primary determinants of the seriousness and impact of a stressful experience. By their definition, stress is "a relationship between the person and the environment that is appraised by the person as taxing or exceeding his or her resources and endangering his or her well-being" (6). The individual's appraisal is the key aspect of this definition. An event or situation will be experienced as stressful only if a cognitive appraisal is made that the demands of the situation exceed the individual's ability to handle it and put his or her well-being in jeopardy.

Consistent with Ellis' Rational Emotive Therapy (7) and the cognitive therapy approach of Beck (8) and others, this model emphasizes the role of cognitive mediating processes (e.g., beliefs, perceptions, internal dialogue) in determining the quality of experiences. In evaluating and treating headache patients, awareness of the role of cognitions in mediating stress raises two critical points that are useful to share with patients. The first is that no events or situations are uniformly stressful to all or even most people. Given any particular shared experience, the range of responses will be from total calm and relaxation to nearly total devastation. Thus, it is often not useful to compare your level of stress to that of a co-worker, for example, since, even with similar job descriptions, your beliefs about your ability to meet the demands of the job and the cost to you of not doing so may differ considerably from those of your colleague. Differences in such beliefs determine differences in stress response.

Second, it is useful to point out to patients that stress can be reduced by learning to change beliefs and attributions, which in turn can be accessed by learning to pay attention to one's internal dialogue. Irrational and maladaptive self-statements are typically at the root of a stressful experience, and, as has been taught by cognitive therapists, effective stress management often hinges on learning to detect and modify distorted thoughts and unrealistic expectations and appraisals. Examples of these are given in the section below on pacing.

Major Life Events versus Daily Hassles

It is also useful to highlight stress due to everyday experiences. The initial research on the relationship between stress and physical illness focused on the contribution of major life events such as terminal illness or divorce to the development and maintenance of a variety of medical conditions (9). These studies found consistently strong relationships between stress and disease, which are now considered almost axiomatic. In subsequent research, however, attention has shifted to the relationship of more mundane daily stressors, so-called daily hassles, to disease, with the finding that such hassles may even be more strongly related to illness than are major life events (10). This observation is consistent with patients' reports that it seems unlikely that their headaches are stress-related, since their lives are not marred by major stressful events. Rather, demands such as daily child care, working, paying the bills, and dealing with chronic health problems (e.g., headaches) appear to take a larger toll.

Often, patients systematically underestimate the negative stressful effects of chronic daily hassles, because of what might be termed an accommodation problem. Most of us survive in a competitive, and at times hostile, environment because we have internalized beliefs about the value of work over play, the necessity of being tough, and the ostensible virtue of making delay of gratification a way of life. In the everyday context of "getting by," we may inaccurately appraise ourselves as having just enough in the way of personal resources to meet the world's demands, and then we systematically underestimate the costs we bear for not really being able to meet those demands. Overcommitment and unreasonably high personal performance standards are often observed in headache patients. Mindful of such patterns, the task for clinicians is often to help patients learn to more realistically appraise the match between the demands of their lives and their personal resources, acknowledge the costs of being chronically stressed, and learn to make better decisions about managing time and self-care.

Primary Relationships as a Special Case

One aspect of the daily hassles problem often relates to primary relationships. In a paper entitled "Marital Migraine," Featherstone and Beitman (11) described the particular negative impact that primary relationships often have on headache. In our experience, it is not unusual for the onset or exacerbation of headache symptoms to coincide with changes in a primary relationship. Not surprisingly, headaches are often worse during periods of dissatisfaction or disruption in relationships (e.g., preceding or during a divorce). These are obviously periods of incredible stress, and worse symptoms during these periods are not difficult to explain. Patients who appear to have functional, healthy relationships will also report, however, that their headaches have been worse since the start of their marriage or the birth of a child. Although these events may have overwhelmingly positive valence for the patient, they still represent a class of transactions with the environment that may exceed the patient's own perceptions of his or her

ability to cope. In large part this is because changes in the status of important relationships typically require that a great deal of energy be expended in learning to accommodate a new situation. All change is stressful, and the beginning or ending of an important relationship can be extraordinarily taxing, even though patients may underreport the impact of the relationship since it is not experienced as being overtly aversive. As a practical point in assessing headache history, it is useful to look for temporal relationships between worsening headache symptoms and changes in primary relationships.

Let-Down Phenomenon

It is not uncommon for patients to describe increases in headache pain following a period of high or prolonged stress, such as during a vacation or during leisure time rather than work time. The classic example is the patient whose headaches are only troublesome in the evenings or on weekends or during vacations. Oddly, patients understand this pattern to be further proof that their headaches cannot be stress-related, since they occur only during times of relative relaxation. This well-documented pattern is described in the literature as a "let-down headache." It is a clear example of another kind of interplay between life-style factors and headaches.

Generally, patients have little difficulty appreciating the behavioral implication of "let-down" once the pattern is explained, and, again, they can be reassured that it does not connote incompetence on their part. It is useful to explain that let-down is something like a delayed stress or rebound phenomenon and that, typically, patients with chronic daily headaches do not experience a one-to-one correspondence between increased stress and exacerbations of headache symptoms. A practical suggestion that can be offered to patients is to look for a more general relationship between headaches and stress. If, on average, they have a more stressful month, they might expect that, on average, their headaches will be worse, even if the headaches occur primarily during let-down periods.

PACING

Reinforcement of Excessive Activity

Patients with chronic daily headaches often have what is described as a pacing problem. This problem is characterized by patients overcommitting themselves to more activities than can realistically be accomplished in a given time, corresponding subjective complaints of never having enough time, relative sleep deprivation, tremendous difficulty relaxing, and taking relatively little time for leisure activity and genuine self-care. Patients who do not pace well often describe their lives as busy and full but hectic, with little encouragement. They may also complain of feeling tired much of the time, unappreciated by those for whom they work so hard and resentful that they are taken for granted. Rarely do they describe themselves as depressed, though the irritability, fatigue, poor concentration, and anhedonia they admit to are very consistent with a diagnosis of irritable depression.

Pacing problems occur with surprising frequency among patients with chronic daily headaches, and they really represent one of the cardinal and, therefore, most predictable behavioral patterns among this group of patients. Reinforcers of poor pacing are typically not difficult to identify. They include actually being productive and the social reinforcement of being perceived as industrious, organized, and accomplished. Poor pacers often receive rave performance reviews from others who do not live with or are not close to them. Because such reviews often coincide with the individuals' need to perceive themselves in similar ways (i.e., as being organized and productive), a pattern of poor pacing can be difficult to change.

On the downside, poor pacing is also associated with increased stress, chronic performance anxiety, increased muscle tension, and autonomic nervous system arousal, all based on unreal expectations of one's own performance. These expectations tend to be related to strong feelings of guilt over the prospect of not being organized or productive enough, which in turn are related to maladaptive cognitive distortions (discussed below). Consistent with the maladaptive aspect of this problem, it is very common for patients' families to actually perceive them as stressed, overworked, and unable to relax. Hence, they typically welcome any progress patients make in learning to pace their level of activity more effectively.

Role of Maladaptive Cognitions

Poor pacing is closely related to stress, which (as outlined above) is mediated by cognitions that can be accessed by paying attention to internal beliefs and self-talk. Patients who do not pace well typically do a fair amount of catastrophizing about the supposed negative outcome of not meeting some unrealistic performance goal. "If I am not the perfect wife and mother, my family will desert me" is an extreme and oversimplified version of such a thought process, though it captures the strong belief that an awful thing will happen if a certain level of performance is not maintained.

Helping patients learn to pace effectively involves several steps. Once the pattern is accurately described, patients are often open to making changes, in part because they are being given permission—and, in fact, are being encouraged—to take care of themselves. Maladaptive thoughts are effectively challenged by helping patients develop a plan for better pacing and then taking the risk of putting it into practice. Such a plan typically includes scheduling regular, inviolable breaks into the work day, and patients are often surprised to find that such breaks do not lead to dire outcomes. Productivity remains high and may even be enhanced; they are in no way diminished in the eyes of co-workers or friends, and often their overall quality of life improves.

SUMMARY

It is clear that psychological factors are significant in the development and maintenance of headaches that occur on a daily or near-daily basis. These can include patterns of pain behavior, anger and depression. cognitive processes such as labeling and coping, and difficulty pacing level of activity. Even for patients with strong family histories of headache and for whom dietary and hormonal factors are also relevant, issues related to lifestyle and emotion cannot be overlooked. Effective management of chronic headache must combine changes in patterns of living and interacting with others with appropriate prescriptions for medications and physical therapy.

In assessing psychological factors related to headache as a means of developing an appropriate treatment plan, the following points should be considered:

1. Determining the medical stability of the problem and ruling out intracranial pathology as a cause of headache.
2. Assessing the possibility of controlling nociception through appropriate prescriptions for safe medications and programs of stretch and exercise.
3. Assessing the possible contribution of operant factors.
4. Evaluating the patients' belief system in terms of illness conviction issues and beliefs about the seriousness and cause of their headaches.
5. Assessing the contribution of daily hassles and other stressors, mindful of let-down patterns.
6. Assessing anger and depression issues.
7. Helping patients understand and modify patterns of poor pacing.

Chronic daily headache is amenable to treatment if sufficient attention is given to the complex interplay of medical and psychological factors.

REFERENCES

1. Wolff HG. Headache and other head pain. 2nd ed. New York: Oxford University Press, 1963.
2. Fordyce WE. Behavioral conditioning concepts in chronic pain. In: Bonica JJ, Lindblom U, Iggo A, eds. Advances in pain research and therapy, vol 5. New York: Raven Press, 1983.
3. Fordyce WE. Behavioral methods for chronic pain and illness. St. Louis: Mosby, 1976.
4. Fordyce WE. Pain and suffering: a reappraisal. Am Psychol 1988;43:276–283.
5. Selye H. The stress of life, rev ed. New York: McGraw-Hill, 1976.
6. Lazarus RS, Folkman S. Stress, appraisal, and coping. New York: Springer, 1984.
7. Ellis A, Grieger R, eds. Handbook of rational-emotive therapy. New York: Springer, 1977.
8. Beck AT. Cognitive therapy and the emotional disorders. New York: International Universities Press, 1976.
9. Holmes TH, Masuda M. Life changes and illness susceptibility. In: Dohrenwend BS, Dohrenwend BP, eds. Stressful life events: their nature and effects. New York: Wiley, 1974.
10. Kanner AD, Coyne NC, Schaefer C, Lazarus RS. Comparison of two modes of stress measurement: daily hassles and uplifts versus major life events. J Behav Med 1981;4:1–39.
11. Featherstone HJ, Beitman BD. Marital migraine: a refractory daily headache. Psychosomatics 1984;25:30–38.

7

Psychological Assessment
of the Recurrent Headache Sufferer

DONALD B. PENZIEN, JEANETTA C. RAINS, and KENNETH A. HOLROYD

Contemporary conceptualizations of pain emphasize the interdependence of physiological and psychological systems (1). Recurrent migraine and tension-type headaches are probably best conceptualized as resulting from the interplay of environmental, biological, and psychological factors, with no single factor regarded as a "sole cause" (2). Therefore, assessment of only headache-related physical symptoms to the exclusion of psychological and behavioral factors is apt to inadequately represent the patient's problem. Clinicians equipped with a multidimensional characterization of the patient's problem (i.e., physical symptoms in their psychosocial context) are better able to identify treatments that are optimally suited to the range of problems presented by recurrent headache sufferers.

The multidimensional evaluation of headache patients can be facilitated by using a multiaxial classification scheme such as the one presented here. This multiaxial evaluation requires that every patient be assessed on several "axes," each describing a different class of information that potentially bears on the course and treatment of the presenting headache problem. This is not to suggest that every patient merits extensive evaluation of each dimension, but at least a cursory appraisal of each axis should be undertaken. Multiaxial evaluation of headache ensures appropriate attention to relevant symptoms, aspects of the environment, and areas of functioning that might be overlooked if the focus of the assessment was narrower. Information that may be of value in planning treatment and predicting outcome for an individual headache patient is recorded on each of the following axes:

I. Physical symptoms of headache and headache diagnosis;
II. Psychological/behavioral factors;
III. Other physical symptoms and diagnoses;
IV. Environmental, social, and cultural factors;
V. Functional capacity/disability.

In this chapter, we address the assessment of factors pertinent to axes II and V; the discussion of factors pertinent to the remaining axes is left to other contributors to this volume. First, we provide a review of related empirical

studies, which provides the basis for our specific recommendations for assessment of psychological and behavioral factors germane to recurrent headache. Next we identify the psychological/behavioral complications most frequently seen in recurrent headache sufferers and identify indications for a formal psychological assessment. Finally, we more specifically address assessment of a variety of psychological/behavioral factors including psychological symptoms and psychopathology, neuropsychological functioning, stress and coping, headache medication use and misuse, and headache-related functional impairment.

PSYCHOLOGICAL ASSESSMENT OF HEADACHE PATIENTS: EMPIRICAL STUDIES

Although a great deal has been written about the interrelationships between psychological or behavioral factors and recurrent headache, the exact role of psychological factors in headache is often debated. Published overviews of the empirical literature addressing psychological assessment of headache patients have been limited in scope (i.e., limited number of studies reviewed; issues addressed were narrowly defined), and they have offered contradictory conclusions. Surmising that a great deal remained to be learned from the literature, we undertook a systematic and comprehensive literature review to evaluate the empirical evidence addressing the following three questions:

1. Does the typical headache patient exhibit significant psychopathology?
2. Do psychological treatments improve the psychological functioning of recurrent headache sufferers?
3. Can psychological variables predict response to headache treatments?

Any empirical study meeting the following criteria was included in the review: (a) patients were diagnosed as suffering from recurrent tension-type, migraine, or combined headache; (b) a minimum of five patients who received the same assessment or treatment, and (c) psychological assessment and/or psychological (i.e., nonpharmacological) interventions were employed (e.g., electromyographic (EMG) or thermal biofeedback training, progressive or autogenic relaxation training, stress management training, cognitive-behavior therapy). Of the 317 eligible studies, 229 provided data bearing on the outcome of nonpharmacological treatments for headache; the remaining 88 studies examined psychological factors and headache in the absence of treatment outcome data.

A vast assortment of psychological variables have been measured via the full range of assessment strategies (i.e., interview, patient self-monitoring, questionnaires, behavioral observations, standardized tests; see Table 7.1), but most investigators have relied upon formal tests or questionnaires. The commonly employed psychological tests have included: objective personality measures (e.g., Minnesota Multiphasic Personality Inventory, MMPI, (3); Eysenck Personality Inventory (4)), depression measures (e.g., Beck Depression Inventory, BDI, (5)), anxiety measures (e.g., State-Trait Anxiety Inventory (6)), psychosomatic symptoms measures (e.g., Psychosomatic Symptom Checklist (7)), measures assessing the type of variables patients perceive as influencing their headaches (e.g., Health Locus of Control Scales (8)), stress measures (e.g., Social Readjustment Rating Scale (9)), and measures of the strategies used to cope with stress or pain (e.g., Coping Strategies Inventory (10)). Unfortunately, there has been little consistency across studies in the psychological variables addressed or in choice of assessment instruments.

Does the Typical Headache Patient Exhibit Significant Psychopathology?

Of the 190 studies that reported psychological data, only 77 (42%) compared the psychological test data of recurrent headache sufferers with test data from normative or control samples. Seventy-one percent of the studies that provided such information found increased maladaptive behavior or psychopathology among headache patients, and the remaining 29% specifically reported that headache patients did *not* differ from normative or control samples. Issues pertaining to psychopathology often are *not* addressed in treatment outcome studies evaluating nonpharmacological therapies for headache—only 26% assessed psychopathology prior to treatment. We found it surprising that so few reports addressed psychopathology. We presume that many investigators have compared psychological test scores of headache patients with normative data or normal control samples but may have opted not to report their findings when differences did not emerge.

Most studies reporting increased maladaptive behavior or psychopathology among headache patients used the MMPI or other objective measures of psychological symptoms or personality (i.e., Beck Depression Inventory, Inventory Spielberger State/Trait Anxiety/Eysenck Personality Inventory). Although levels of psychological symptoms observed in headache patients frequently have exceeded those of normal control samples, clinical levels of

Table 7.1.
Psychological Assessment Measures Employed in the Headache Literature

Measure	Number of Studies	Measure	Number of Studies
Minnesota Multiphasic Personality Inventory	50	Rathus Assertiveness Inventory	9
Spielberger State/Trait Personality Inventory	16	Assertiveness Measures—misc.	4
Eysenck Personality Inventory	8	Problem Solving Measures—misc.	2
Derogatis Symptom Checklist-90-revised	7	Tobin et al. Coping Strategies Inventory	7
Hopkins Symptom Checklist	5	Rosensteil & Keefe Coping Strategies Questionnaire	3
Taylor Manifest Anxiety Scale	3	Coping Strategies Measures—misc.	7
Jenkins Activity Survey—type A	3	Blanchard et al. Cognitive Questionnaire	4
Projective Measures—misc.	5	Rosenbaum Self-Control Schedule	3
Personality Measures—misc.	46	Pilowski & Spence Illness Behavior Questionnaire	2
		McGill Pain Questionnaire	12
Beck Depression Inventory	34	Pain Behavior Measures—misc.	13
Centers for Epidemiologic Studies—Depression Scale	9	Disability Measures—misc.	14
Wakefield Depression Inventory	5		
Zung Depression Inventory	4	Holmes & Rahe Social Readjustment Rating Scale	10
Depression Measures—misc.	9	Lazarus Hassles Scale	7
Spielberger State/Trait Anxiety Inventory	26	Brantley & Jones Daily Stress Inventory	3
Anxiety Measures—misc.	14	Stress Measures—misc.	17
Schalling & Sifneos Alexithymia Scale	3		
Cox et al. Psychosomatic Symptom Checklist	14	Moos Family Environment Scale	3
Wahler Physical Symptoms Inventory	13	Cohen et al. Interpersonal Support Evaluation List	3
Mandler et al. Autonomic Perception Questionnaire	7	Family or Marital Functioning Measures—misc.	8
Psychosomatic Symptom Measures—misc.	6		
		Intelligence Measures—misc.	7
Penzien et al. Headache Locus of Control Scales	10	Mental Status Measures—misc.	2
Wallston et al. Health Locus of Control Scales	9	Hypnotic Susceptibility Measures—misc.	6
Rotter Internal/External Locus of Control Scales	8	Treatment Expectancy Measures—misc.	7
Locus of Control Measures—misc.	4	Treatment Credibility Measures—misc.	25
Holroyd et al. Headache Self-Efficacy Scale	5	Measures Not Otherwise Specified	30
Self-Efficacy Measures—misc.	3		
Cognitive Measures—misc.	8		

psychopathology seldom have been observed. When clinical levels of psychological symptoms have been reported, it is usually among only a subset of the headache patient sample. This point is exemplified by the three studies that have employed cluster analytic techniques to identify homogeneous subgroups of headache patients based upon their MMPI profiles (11–13). Each of the three studies identified only one subgroup of patients with "psychopathological" MMPI profiles (i.e., patients exhibiting clinically significant elevations on several psychological symptom scales), and only a small proportion of the patients (between 5 and 13%) have exhibited these psychopathological profiles. Most of the patients were deemed to have an essentially normal MMPI profile (62 to 72% of patients).

Even these figures may overestimate the number of recurrent headache sufferers exhibiting significant psychopathology. Psychopathology typically is identified using measures that in part reflect somatic or vegetative symptoms of chronic headache. For example, patients with higher levels of headache activity endorse more somatic items on the Beck Depression Inventory (e.g., "I am very worried about physical problems and it's hard to think about anything else") but *not* more nonsomatic items (e.g., "I am sad all the time and I can't snap out of it") (14). However, the resulting elevations in BDI scores probably reflect headache symptoms, not depression. Because psychological symptom measures typically do not distinguish the somatic symptoms of psychological disorders from the somatic symptoms of headache, they may overestimate psychopathology in recurrent headache sufferers.

In the assessment of the typical headache patient, measures that assess stress, cognitive and behavioral strategies for coping with stress, beliefs about headaches, factors that influence their perceived personal control of headaches, and headache-related disability may be more useful than measures of clinical psychopathology. The few studies conducted to date have consistently shown that (*a*) the level of daily, minor stress is positively correlated with headache activity level (15–17) and (*b*) headache patients are likely to engage in maladaptive coping behaviors in managing stress or headaches (18–21). Collectively, these findings suggest that we might more profitably shift the focus of psychological assessment from psychopathology toward other, "less pathological" behavioral and cognitive variables in seeking to better delineate the role of psychological factors in recurrent headache.

Do Psychological Treatments Improve the Psychological Functioning of Recurrent Headache Sufferers?

One might expect that studies evaluating nonpharmacological (i.e., psychological or behavioral) interventions for headache would routinely report information pertaining to patients' psychological status. However, only 44% of studies evaluating such treatments (102 of 229 studies) reported any psychological assessment (broadly defined). Treatment outcomes have been operationalized almost exclusively in terms of changes in headache activity; psychological factors typically have been examined as outcome variables of secondary importance, as variables that may be useful for predicting response to treatment or in attempting to elucidate the mechanisms whereby nonpharmacological treatments produce improvements in headache activity.

Of the 102 treatment outcome studies that have reported psychological testing data, 49% reported pre- to posttreatment change in at least one psychological variable, and only 4% reported no change (47% of the studies evaluating nonpharmacological treatments did not examine changes in psychological variables). While very few studies specifically reported no pre- to posttreatment change in any psychological variable, we presume that some investigators may have compared pre- and posttreatment psychological test scores but opted to omit nonsignificant findings. Nevertheless, significant change in psychological variables following nonpharmacological treatment is reported in nearly all of the studies that have addressed this issue.

Improvement with nonpharmacological treatment has been reported on a variety of psychological symptom measures (in every case where change has been observed, patients have shown a reduction in psychological symptomatology from pre- to posttreatment). Most commonly, reductions in depression scores (22) or "psychosomatic" symptoms (23) have been reported. Changes also have been reported in symptoms such as anxiety (24), hysteria (25), neuroticism (26), or improvements in symptom profiles as measured by instruments such as the MMPI (27, 28) or the Derogatis SCL-90-R (29–31).

Although statistically significant, the change in psychological symptoms is usually modest. Of course, prior to treatment, clinical levels of psychopathology seldom have been observed in the average headache patient, so large changes in psychological symptoms would not be expected. For example, in virtually all studies reporting Beck Depression Inventory (BDI) scores, average headache patients' pretreatment scores have fallen in the "non-depressed" range. While some studies have reported a significant reduction in BDI scores from baseline to posttreatment (32, 33), the observed change has been small. Beck and Steer (5) suggest that BDI scores from 0 to 9 are within the normal or asymptomatic range. Blanchard and colleagues reported a mean pretreatment BDI score of 7.8, which fell to 4.8 at posttreatment. Similarly, Holroyd and colleagues reported a mean pretreatment BDI score of 8.5, which fell to 5.4. Clearly, in such instances, there is not a great deal of opportunity for symptom reduction, and such changes in psychological symptom scores probably reflect improvements in headache-related distress and somatic symptoms rather than changes in "psychopathology."

Changes in a variety of other cognitive and behavioral variables also have been examined. Some of these variables have been conceptualized as targets for treatment, e.g., minor stress and pain behavior. (The "pain behavior" construct reflects a patient's verbalizations and nonverbal behaviors (i.e., sounds, expressions, body language, actions) that communicate the experience of pain.) Others are involved in therapeutic mechanisms of the interventions, e.g., headache locus of control (reflecting patients' beliefs about whether their headaches are determined *internally* by their own behavior or *externally* by factors such as fate or the interventions of powerful others) and headache self-efficacy (reflecting a patients' beliefs about their capability of influencing their headaches). Commonly reported changes following nonpharmacological treatments include increased perception that factors influencing headache are more within the patient's control (19, 33–35), greater use of adaptive cognitive and behavioral coping strategies (36–38), reductions in pain behavior (39–41), and reductions in minor stress (42, 43).

Can Psychological Variables Predict Response to Headache Treatments?

Of the 229 studies evaluating behavioral treatments for headache, only 14% (32 studies) have reported the results of their attempts to predict treatment outcome using psychological tests. About one third of the studies failed to identify psychological variables that successfully predicted outcome; the remaining studies predicted outcome using a variety of different variables. Although in nearly every case, greater psychological symptoms at pretreatment (e.g., hypochondriasis, hysteria) have been found negatively related to posttreatment headache improvement, no particular predictor variable stands out as strongly or consistently related to headache improvement. This probably has occurred in part because there has been little consistency across studies in the psychological measures used and because many of the prediction studies are not methodologically rigorous. Although large samples are required to predict treatment outcome reliably, many of the prediction studies have used small samples of headache patients (over 60% of the prediction studies had fewer than 40 patients). In addition, a number of studies have used a disproportionately large number of psychological variables (relative to sample size) in order to only modestly improve prediction of treatment outcome.

Psychological Symptomatology. Of the measures examined to date, depression scores are most often correlated with improvement. Notably, even subclinical scores on psychological tests may prove useful for predicting response to nonpharmacological treatment for headache. For example, two groups of investigators have indicated that Beck Depression Inventory (BDI) scores of 8 or more may be associated with reduced responsiveness to treatment (44, 45). Blanchard and Andrasik (44) found that

only one third of the tension headache patients (16 of 49 patients) with BDI scores of 8 or above were much improved following relaxation training, whereas over half of the patients (41 of 75) with lower BDI scores responded well to this treatment. This finding should *not* be interpreted as indicating that patients with elevated BDI scores will fail to respond to treatment; rather, such patients may fare somewhat more poorly following nonpharmacological treatment than patients with lower scores.

Interestingly, studies have reported that both high and low anxiety predict outcome with nonpharmacological treatment. Whereas two studies have been shown that greater anxiety at pretreatment predicted less headache improvement at posttreatment (46, 47), three studies have shown that greater pretreatment anxiety predicted greater headache improvement (29, 48, 49). One possible interpretation of these inconsistent findings is that there may be an optimal level of anxiety that can facilitate nonpharmacological interventions for headache, which, if exceeded, may interfere with treatment.

Headache-related Beliefs or Cognitions. Cognitive and behavioral variables have been examined less often as predictor variables than measures of psychological symptomatology. Individual headache patients are likely to differ with regard to the factors they believe influence the onset and the course of their headache symptoms. Social psychological research suggests that patients' beliefs are important determinants of their responses to headache episodes and to the health care system, influencing in turn, their responsiveness to available treatment options, the disability and psychological symptoms associated with headaches, and the strategies that are used to cope with headaches (34, 50). Cognitive constructs such as locus of control and self-efficacy have shown promise for predicting treatment outcome.

Of the cognitive constructs, locus of control has been examined as a predictor of treatment outcome most often (9 studies using 6 different locus of control measures (51–53). Most studies show no relationship between locus of control at pretreatment and later outcome. However, the two studies that have measured locus of control specific to headache (53, 54) have found that a more internal headache locus of control was associated with greater headache reduction at posttreatment, suggesting that headache-specific measures of locus of control (e.g., the Headache-Specific Locus of Control Scale (55)) may fare better in predicting treatment outcome than nonspecific locus of control measures (e.g., the Internal-External Locus of Control Scale (56)).

Conclusions Drawn from Review of Empirical Studies

Our review of the empirical evidence yielded several insights into the role of psychological factors in recurrent headache. Although headache patients often differ from control samples, significant psychopathology is seldom reported for the typical headache patient. Headache patients frequently differ from "normals" in less pathological ways (such as the amount of daily stress experienced or the predominant stress coping strategies employed), and this may, in fact, provide a more meaningful way of characterizing recurrent headache patients than traditional indices of psychopathology. Scores on measures of psychopathology (e.g., depression, anxiety) may be reduced following nonpharmacological treatments for headache, but the reported change is usually modest and probably reflects reductions in headache-related distress and somatic symptoms rather than changes in "psychopathology." However, improvement is often noted in cognitive and behavioral functioning (e.g., headache self-efficacy, coping skills) following nonpharmacological treatment. The presence of psychological symptoms at pretreatment has been related repeatedly to poorer treatment outcome. To date, no particular predictor variable has emerged as the most strongly or consistently related to headache improvement; this is at least in part a function of the lack of consistency across studies in the psychological variables addressed and in choice of assessment instruments. Finally, there is some evidence that headache-specific measures of psychological constructs related to treatment (such as locus of control) may enable us to improve our prediction of treatment response.

Psychological/Behavioral Assessment of the Headache Patient

As indicated above, no specific personality traits have been identified which consistently characterize "headache sufferers" as a group or which predispose individuals to develop a headache syndrome. Furthermore, most headache patients have a generally normal psychological adjustment. Thus, extensive psychological testing is probably unnecessary for the typical headache patient. A brief psychological screening should be sufficient to identify the relatively small subgroup who require a more comprehensive psychological evaluation.

At initial evaluation, the clinical should address, at least in a cursory fashion, the headache patient's past and current level of psychosocial functioning. Although this information may be gathered readily as a part of a routine diagnostic interview, the interview can be supplemented by questionnaires completed by the patient prior to interview (cf. the *Headache Patient Information Form* (57)). Psychosocial dimensions of interest include headache-related disability, psychiatric history, mental status examination, behavioral observations, drug use, environmental/lifestyle factors, and family, social, and vocational factors (Table 7.2). A more extensive psychological assessment is probably warranted if any of the following complications are identified or suspected:

Significant disability or decline in psychosocial functioning;
Psychological disturbance (e.g., anxiety disorder, dysthymia, major depression, somatization disorder); gross disturbance in personality organization (e.g., dependent personality disorder, histrionic personality disorder);
Memory of other cognitive deficits (especially following head trauma); intellectual impairment;
Exaggerated or inappropriate pain behaviors; unrealistic beliefs pertaining to pain or disability;
Substance abuse or misuse of medication; overreliance upon the health care system;
Significant stress and reliance upon maladaptive coping skills;
Significant disturbance in family, interpersonal relationships, or vocational functioning; inordinate reinforcement of pain behavior.

Identification of psychological/behavioral complications (such as those listed above) should not necessarily deter the clinician from treating the patient's headache. However, such complications may make headache diagnosis difficult (e.g., significant cognitive deficits), they may have implications for choice of headache therapy (e.g., amitriptyline might be effectively prescribed to treat symptoms of both recurrent headache and major depression), or they may deserve to be addressed independently of headache therapy (e.g., marital discord that may or may not have a marked influence on the patient's headaches). In the following sections, we elaborate upon specific psychological/

Table 7.2.
Psychological/Behavioral Evaluation of Headache Patients

Psychological/Behavioral Domain	Relevant Clinical Features
Headache-related disability	Nature and degree of impairment in ongoing vocational and social activities secondary to headache
Psychiatric history	Psychological adjustment, preexisting psychological disorders, family history of medical/psychiatric illness, prior psychological therapy
Mental status examination	Mood and affect, accuracy of historical information, attitude, speech, thought disorder, cognitive processes, changes in vegetative functions, suicidal or homicidal ideation, intellectual level, insight and judgment
Behavioral observations	Pain-related behaviors, eccentricities of physical behavior, appearance, preoccupation with pain
Drug use	Analgesic medication, psychotropic medication, alcoholic beverages, recreational drugs
Environmental/lifestyle factors	Stress, coping skills, insufficient or excessive sleep, missing meals, dietary precipitants, environmental precipitants such as odors, heat, and noise
Family, social & vocational factors	Family adjustment, familial pain models, reinforcement of pain behavior, current employment, litigation related to injury or disability

behavioral complications that merit assessment in the headache sufferer.

Patients who are identified as requiring formal psychological assessment must be evaluated by a clinician with expertise in psychological testing, and it is preferable that the clinician have experience in assessing patients with chronic or recurrent pain. A broad array of assessment instruments is available, and the task of integrating psychological assessment data into clinical decision-making for the headache patient may require not only an understanding of psychological assessment procedures but also an understanding of pain disorders.

ASSESSMENT OF SPECIFIC PSYCHOLOGICAL/ BEHAVIORAL FACTORS

Assessment of Psychological Symptoms and Psychopathology

Patients with recurrent headache sometimes present with coexisting psychological disorders that merit professional intervention. In such instances, one of the goals of psychological evaluation frequently is to determine the nature of the relationship between psychopathology and the patient's headache problem. There are a number of different possible answers to this question. For example, psychological symptoms (e.g., anxiety, depression) can precipitate or exacerbate headache episodes in headache-prone patients. Psychological symptoms (especially depression) also can result as a consequence of living with chronically disabling headaches. In other instances, headaches may be better understood as a manifestation of a primary psychological disturbance (e.g., when headache is only one of a long list of presenting physical complaints, the diagnosis of somatization disorder might prove more appropriate than a headache diagnosis). Significant psychopathology also may be unrelated to the headache disorder and have little or no impact upon headache treatment (e.g., when a patient presents with schizophrenia or bipolar disorder that is well controlled). Finally, personality disorders can seriously complicate headache evaluation and treatment because of these patients' difficult interpersonal style (e.g., histrionic patients may greatly exaggerate symptom complaints; borderline patients may be inappropriately manipulative; passive/dependent patients may rely excessively upon the health card provider). Consultation with a psychologist or psychiatrist may be used not only to determine whether significant psychopathology is present but also to obtain information about the relationship between psychological problems and headache problems.

Significant psychopathology may be associated with a poor response to both pharmacological and nonpharmacologic headache therapies. When patients exhibit significant psychological symptoms, broad-spectrum behavior therapy or brief psychotherapy should be considered. Intensive psychotherapy is not necessarily indicated; brief, focused attention to the specific adjustment problems that precipitate or exacerbate headache episodes, interfere with

treatment compliance, or interfere with the use of self-regulatory skills often is sufficient.

The research reviewed above revealed that even moderate psychological symptoms may reduce the responsiveness of some headache patients to nonpharmacological treatments, and it is quite likely that more extreme levels of psychopathology will inhibit treatment response. To date, depression has been the psychological symptom that investigators have focused upon most frequently when attempting to predict treatment outcome (29, 44, 45). Some evidence also suggests that patients who report multiple psychosomatic symptoms (58) or exhibit elevations of certain Minnesota Multiphasic Personality Inventory (MMPI) subscale scores are less likely to respond to nonpharmacological treatment than their less symptomatic counterparts (45, 47, 59–62).

Unfortunately, few attempts have been made to identify specific psychological test scores that are useful for predicting an individual patient's response to therapy. In one noteworthy exception, Blanchard and colleagues (58) employed psychological tests to predict patients' response to treatment following 10 sessions of relaxation training. The cutoff scores from the psychological measures that best differentiated patients who improved from patients who failed to improve are presented in Table 7.3. In every case, higher scores (reflecting higher levels of symptoms) predicted a poor response to treatment. As pointed out by Blanchard and Andrasik (44), we have yet to identify ideal predictors, because the tests examined to date have yielded high error rates (i.e., both false-positive and false-negative predictions). In summary, although highly elevated scores on measures of psychopathology may in general portend a relatively poor response to therapy, no specific psychological test is consistently useful for predicting headache patients' responses to any given treatment.

Table 7.3.
Symptom Measures and Cutoff Scores Predicting Response to Relaxation Training[a]

Headache Diagnosis and Symptom Measure	Cutoff Score[b]
Tension headache	
Beck Depression Inventory	8
Psychosomatic Symptom Checklist	8
MMPI scale 2, depression	70
MMPI scale 6, paranoia	58
Migraine headache	
Psychosomatic Symptom Checklist	6
MMPI scale 1, hypochondriasis	60
MMPI scale 3, hysteria	65
MMPI scale 6, paranoia	60
Combined headache	
Trait anxiety	40
Psychosomatic Symptom Checklist	6
MMPI scale 1, hypochondriasis	65
MMPI scale 3, hysteria	65
MMPI scale 8, schizophrenia	50

[a]From Blanchard EB, Andrasik F, Arena JG. Personality and chronic headache. In: Maher B, ed. Progress in experimental personality research, vol 13. New York: Academic Press, 1984.
[b]Patients with higher scores are less likely to respond.

Investigators have only recently begun to examine the usefulness of psychological tests for identifying good and poor candidates for pharmacotherapy. Evidence suggests, however, that patients with high levels of psychological symptoms may fail to respond to at least some abortive and prophylactic medications. For example, Friedman and von Storch (63) characterized patients who failed to respond to both abortive (ergotamine) and prophylactic (vasodilator) therapy as exhibiting signs of "unstable" personality and of a limited ability to "utilize aggression" (p. 442). More recently, Micieli and colleagues (64) found that only a greater occurrence of "clinically marked depressive episodes" (p. 220) distinguished nonresponders from responders to flunarizine. Holroyd and colleagues (42) found that nonresponders to abortive medication obtained higher scores on the Beck Depression Inventory and the Spielberger Trait Anger Scale (65) than patients who responded to abortive pharmacotherapy. In this study, no patient with a trait anger score of 25 or higher on the Trait Anger Scale responded to abortive medication, while 85% of patients with anger scores below 25 did respond to abortive medication. Although these preliminary findings are not adequate to guide clinical practice, they suggest that further research might identify psychological tests that would be helpful in identifying good and poor candidates for different pharmacotherapies and perhaps for aiding clinicians in choosing whether to recommend pharmacological or nonpharmacological headache therapies.

Neuropsychological Assessment

Whereas the mental status examination is a worthwhile component of any intake examination, a more thorough evaluation of the headache patient's cognitive functioning is indicated whenever (a) a diminution of cognitive capacities is observed or (b) the patient presents with posttraumatic headache. Under such circumstances, the patient often requires both a careful neurological examination and neuropsychological testing. Neuropsychological testing provides a more sensitive, comprehensive, and standardized assessment of the cognitive, emotional, and motoric dysfunctions that may be related to brain insult or organicity than that provided by the routine mental status examination (66, 67).

When cognitive deficits are suspected, it is prudent to conduct a careful mental status examination that includes a structured neuropsychological screening test (e.g., Cognitive Capacities Screening Examination, CCSE (68); Mini-Mental State, MMS (69)). Screening tests like the CCSE and the MMS allow rapid evaluation (10 minutes or less for an interviewer to administer) of cognitive functioning and can assist the clinician is deciding whether referral for formal neuropsychological testing is warranted. Such tests evaluate a variety of cognitive capacities (e.g., orientation, immediate and short-term memory, concentration, arithmetic ability, and language). Typically, they are especially sensitive to left hemisphere damage (e.g., verbal and quan-

titative deficits), although they are less sensitive to mild, diffuse cerebral dysfunction and focal right hemisphere lesions (70, 71). Whenever neuropsychological screening indicates cognitive or performance deficits, a thorough neuropsychological examination by a qualified neuropsychologist should be considered.

Neuropsychological deficits are *not* commonly observed in the typical patient with recurrent tension-type and migraine headaches, so extensive neuropsychological evaluation rarely is indicated for these patients (72). The utility of routine neuropsychological screening was evaluated in one study by administering the CCSE to a sample of tension-type and migraine headache patients presenting for treatment to a specialty headache clinic (73). Only 2 of the 88 headache patients scored in the range indicative of organicity of the CCSE. This finding suggests that cognitive and performance deficits are uncommon among recurrent headache patients. However, when such deficits are suspected, careful assessment is warranted.

Assessment of Stress and Coping

Stress has long been recognized as a common precipitant of recurrent tension-type and migraine headaches (74–76). "Stress and worry" was the headache precipitant most frequently endorsed by a clinical sample of 191 patients; 96% of tension-type headache patients and 92% of migraineurs reported that stress precipitated their headache episodes at least some of the time (77). In addition, correlational studies have demonstrated that daily stress levels are positively related to headache activity (15–17). However, there is considerable individual variability in the strength and nature of the temporal relationship between stress and headache (17). A study by Mosley and colleagues provided support for the contention that migraines are more apt to be influenced by minor stressors encountered *prior* to headache onset, whereas muscle-contraction headaches are more influenced by stressors encountered *concurrently* with headache onset.

Measures of minor, daily stress generally have proven more useful than measures of major stressful life events in identifying stressors that appear to precipitate or aggravate headache problems (16–18, 48, 78, 79). For example, Holm and colleagues (18) found that muscle-contraction headache sufferers ($n = 117$) and matched headache-free controls ($n = 174$) did not differ with regard to the number or types of major life events they experienced, but headache sufferers reported more minor stressors than controls. Clinicians interested in examining relationships between stress and headaches are thus likely to find measures of daily, minor stressors such as the Hassles Scale (80) or the Daily Stress Inventory (81) of greater use than measures of major stressful life events such as the Social Readjustment Rating Scale (9).

In addition to assessing the stress patients experience, it can be useful clinically to assess the methods patients choose to manage or cope with stress. A number of studies have suggested that headache patients characteristically may rely upon maladaptive strategies for coping with stress or headaches (18–21, 82). Relative to controls, headache patients have been shown to more frequently use coping strategies such as avoidance and self-blame and to less frequently use social supports in managing stress (18, 20, 82). While this pattern of coping may be effective for some types of stressors (e.g., situations that are out of the patients' control and that cannot be altered), the coping strategies often used by headache patients would be expected to leave most chronically stressful circumstances unchanged, and they are generally associated with less adaptive outcomes. Moreover, the extent to which the above coping strategies are used by recurrent headache sufferers is correlated with the severity of headaches and psychological symptomatology (20, 83). Instruments that have proven useful for assessing the coping strategies of headache patients include the Coping Strategies Inventory (10), the Ways of Coping Checklist (84), and the Coping Strategies Questionnaire (85).

Assessment of Headache Medication Use

An accurate measure of patients' use of headache medications and their compliance with prescribed treatment regimens can be difficult to obtain. Obtaining this information can be important, however, because inappropriate medication use (prescription or nonprescription) can limit the efficacy of both pharmacological and nonpharmacological treatment, and it can exacerbate headache symptoms. Noncompliance with headache medication regimens is a common problem. Packard and O'Connell (86) reported that 52% of headache patients who presented to their clinic were noncompliant with prescribed medication (i.e., failed to take medications or failed to use medications correctly); age, sex, educational level, and headache diagnosis were not predictive of compliance. Similarly, Holroyd and colleagues (42) reported that 70% of migraineurs failed to use ergotamine correctly, even after receiving instruction in medication use by both a neurologist and a psychologist. Regular, especially daily, use of analgesic or abortive medications also can produce paradoxical increases in headache activity (87). (Although there is significant potential for patients to overuse prescribed headache medications, the incidence of other types of drug abuse is probably no greater for the average headache patient than for the general population, and the incidence of physical addiction to narcotic medications among headache patients is low (88).) Such overuse of medication also can limit the benefits obtained from both prophylactic pharmacological (89) and nonpharmacological treatments (90). (Chapter 28 provides additional information about headaches associated with substances and substance withdrawal.)

Routinely, clinicians rely upon retrospective patient reports to assess headache medication use. However, such retrospective self-reports may be inaccurate. When

Johnson and colleagues (91) compared the retrospective reports of headache medication use provided by 89 recurrent headache patients with their daily recordings of medication use, they found that over 20% of the patients consumed medications that they failed to report at intake. In a follow-up study, Johnson and colleagues (92) used urinalysis to assess the validity of patients' self-reports of selected headache medications in 121 recurrent headache patients. Once again, medication self-reports frequently were unreliable. (Thirty-seven percent of patients failed to report ingesting medications within the past 48 hours that were detected by urinalysis. The 37% inaccuracy rate is conservative; their patients were aware of the impending urinalysis and of its purpose (i.e., to examine their headache medication use) when they reported the medications they had recently ingested.) Demographic, headache, or psychological characteristics failed to identify patients whose self-report of medication use was unreliable. This suggests that a significant number of patients may underreport their headache medication use. Inaccurate reporting does not appear to be restricted to any particular type of individual and may be difficult to recognize. Although there is no ideal method for assessing patients' medication use, it appears that patients' daily logs of medication consumption may provide more accurate data than the clinician can obtain via interview.

Assessment of Headache-related Functional Impairment

At present, researchers and clinicians rely most heavily upon patients' reports of pain severity when assessing the severity of the patient's headache problem and when judging headache treatment efficacy. The relationship between pain severity and functional impairment is imperfect, however. Measures of functional capacity (i.e., impairment or disability) provide a better index of the headache sufferer's ability to work or perform other activities than measures of headache frequency, severity, or duration. The assessment of functional impairment resulting from recurrent headache can (a) allow evaluation of the illness's disruptive impact on the patient's life (i.e., work, family, recreational, self-care, and social activities), (b) provide an additional important index of treatment efficacy, and (c) aid in assessing the cost-effectiveness of treatments.

Although the assessment of disability is assuming increasing importance (as evidenced by the recent U.S. federal mandate to study pain and related disability (93)), such measurements are only infrequently reported in the research literature. Only about a dozen studies have reported data specifically bearing on headache-related disability. Half of the available studies required patients to record their headache-related disability on a daily basis using a rating scale (94–96). Most of the latter studies used daily self-monitoring of disability as an index of treatment outcome; all but one study reported a significant reduction in headache-related disability at posttreatment (the exception acknowledged inadequate scaling of the disability dimension).

Although several objective self-report instruments have been developed to measure disability resulting from chronic illness (i.e., the Sickness Impact Profile (97), only four studies have used such measures (55, 98–100). The paucity of results from objective disability measures has occurred because the instruments available until recently were designed to measure comparatively severe levels of disability resulting from chronic, stable conditions such as rheumatoid arthritis, coronary heart disease, and chronic low back pain. Unfortunately, such measures assume that the level of disability is relatively stable, and scores on these measures often do not adequately reflect the intermittent impairment that can result from headache syndromes that have an episodic course.

The Recurrent Illness Impairment Profile (RIIP) (100) was recently developed to fill the gap; it was designed to assess the functional impairment in the social, behavioral, cognitive, and recreational domains that can be associated with episodic or recurrent illnesses such as headache. Wittrock and colleagues administered the "headache version" of the RIIP to 119 recurrent headache patients. Composite Functional Impairment Index scores on the RIIP (representing the average level of impairment during a day when either a typical or a worst headache occurred) revealed that migraineurs were more disabled by headaches than patients with combined headaches, who in turn were more disabled than patients with muscle contraction headaches. In contrast, the RIIP's Total Functional Impairment Index (representing overall average level of impairment regardless of headache severity) revealed no differences among the three headache groups. These data suggest that the diagnostic groups may differ in the amount of impairment they experience during headache episodes but they may *not* differ in overall level of impairment they endure. These initial data suggest that the RIIP is promising as an instrument for assessing functional impairment; it appears to be sensitive not only to the episodic nature of the impairment caused by recurrent headache episodes but also to the differing patterns of impairment experienced by patients with different headache diagnoses. This instrument may prove useful for assessing the impact of recurrent headaches on the patient's life and the ability of different treatments to reduce this disability.

SUMMARY

A multidimensional assessment of the recurrent headache patient—one that addresses not only headache symptoms but also the psychosocial context in which they occur—can assist the clinician in identifying the full range of problems that require intervention. A comprehensive psychological assessment battery is not warranted for most recurrent headache patients because such patients typically do not

present for headache treatment demonstrating clinical levels of psychopathology; instead, routine psychological screening is advisable to determine whether more comprehensive psychological assessment is indicated. In-depth psychological assessment is needed when psychological or behavioral factors are present that may complicate headache evaluation and treatment. Potential complicating factors include psychological or personality disorders, neuropsychological deficits, medication misuse, exaggerated pain behaviors, or decline in psychosocial functioning. Psychological assessment also can identify psychological or behavioral factors that may precipitate or maintain headache. For example, assessment of both the stressors confronting the patient and the patient's usual manner of coping with stress may yield the information needed to successfully intervene with some headache patients.

REFERENCES

1. Melzack, R. The puzzle of pain. New York: Basic Books, 1973.
2. Bakal DA. The psychobiology of chronic headache. New York: Springer, 1982.
3. Hathaway SR, McKinley JC. Minnesota Multiphasic Personality Inventory: manual for administration and scoring. Minneapolis: University of Minnesota Press, 1983.
4. Eysenck HJ, Eysenck SBG. Eysenck Personality Inventory. San Diego: Educational & Industrial Testing Service, 1963.
5. Beck AT, Steer RA. Beck Depression Inventory manual. New York: Psychological Corp, 1987.
6. Spielberger CD, Gorsuch RL, Lushene RE. The State-Trait Anxiety Inventory (STAI) test manual for form X. Palo Alto: Consulting Psychologists Press, 1970.
7. Cox DJ, Freundlich A, Meyer RG. Differential effectiveness of electromyographic feedback, verbal relaxation instructions, and medication placebo with tension headaches J Consult Clin Psychol 1975;43:892–898.
8. Wallston KA, Wallston BS, DeVellis R. Development of the Multidimensional Health Locus of Control (MHLC) Scales. Health Educ Monogr 1978;6:160–170.
9. Holmes TH, Rahe RH. The Social Readjustment Rating Scale. J Psychosom Res 1967;11:213–218.
10. Tobin DL, Holroyd KA, Reynolds RC, Wigal JK. The hierarchical factor structure of the Coping Strategies Inventory. Cognit Ther Res 1988;12:325–339.
11. Kinder BN, Curtiss G, Kalichman S. Cluster analyses of headache-patient MMPI scores: a cross-validation. Psychol Assess 1991;3:226–231.
12. Robinson ME, Geisser ME, Dieter JN, Swerdlow B. The relationship between MMPI cluster membership and diagnostic category in headache patients. Headache 1991;31:111–115.
13. Rappoport NB, McAnulty DP, Waggoner CD, Brantley PJ. Cluster analysis of Minnesota Multiphasic Personality Inventory (MMPI) profiles in a chronic headache population. J Behav Med 1987;10:49–60.
14. Holm JE, Brown TA, Penzien DB, Holroyd KA, Tobin DL. Assessment of depression in headache patients: methodological considerations. Boston: Association for Advancement of Behavior Therapy, 1987.
15. Kohler T, Haimeri C. Daily stress as a trigger of migraine attacks: results of thirteen single-subject studies. J Consult Clin Psychol 1990;58:870–872.
16. Levor RM, Cohen MJ, Naliboff BD, McArthur D, Heuser G. Psychosocial precursors and correlates of migraine headache. J Consult Clin Psychol 1986;54:347–353.

17. Mosley TH, Penzien DB, Johnson CA, Brantley PJ, Wittrock DA, et al. Time-series analysis of stress and headache. Cephalalgia 1991;11:306–307.

18. Holm JE, Holroyd KA, Hursey KG, Penzien DB. The role of stress in recurrent tension headache. Headache 1986;26:160–167.

19. Mizener D, Thomas M, Billings R. Cognitive changes of migraineurs receiving biofeedback training. Headache 1988;28:339–343.

20. Mosley TH, Penzien DB, Johnson CA, Wittrock D, Rubman S, et al. Coping with stress in headache sufferers and no-headache controls. Society of Behavioral Medicine 11th Annual Proceedings 1990:186.

21. Sorbi M, Tellegen B. Stress-coping in migraine. Soc Sci Med 1988;26:351–358.

22. Grazzi L, Frediani F, Zappacosta B, Boiardi A, Bussone G. Psychological assessment in tension headache before and after biofeedback treatment. Headache 1988;28:337–338.

23. Nicholson NL, Blanchard EB, Appelbaum KA. Two studies of the occurrence of psychophysiological symptoms in chronic headache patients. Behav Res Ther 1990;28:195–203.

24. Wooley-Hart A. Biofeedback und entspannungstherapie fur patienten mit migrane und spannungskopfschmerzen [Biofeedback and relaxation therapy in patients with migraine and tension headache]. Psychiatr Neurol Med Psychol 1984;36:649–654.

25. Cram JR. EMG biofeedback and the treatment of tension headaches: a systematic analysis of treatment components. Behav Ther 1980;11:699–710.

26. Janssen K, Neutgens J. Autogenic training and progressive relaxation in the treatment of three kinds of headache. Behav Res Ther 1986;24:199–208.

27. Ellertson B, Troland K, Klove H. MMPI profiles in migraine before and after biofeedback treatment. Cephalalgia 1987;7:101–108.

28. Sovak M, Kunzel M, Sternbach RA, Dalessio DJ. Mechanisms of the biofeedback therapy of migraine: volitional manipulation of the psychophysiological background. Headache 1981;21:89–92.

29. Cox DJ, Lefebvre RC, Hobbs WR. Ancillary symptoms in the biofeedback treatment of headaches. Headache 1982;22:213–215.

30. Steger JC, Harper RG. Comprehensive biofeedback versus self-monitored relaxation in the treatment of tension headache. Headache 1980;20:137–142.

31. Derogatis LR. R-Version manual-I: scoring administration and procedures for the SCL-90. Baltimore: Johns Hopkins University Press, 1977.

32. Blanchard EB, Andrasik F, Appelbaum KA, Evans DD, Myers P, Barron KD. Three studies of the psychologic changes in chronic headache patients associated with biofeedback and relaxation therapies. Psychosom Med 1986;48:73–83.

33. Holroyd KA, Nash JM, Pingel JD, Cordingley GE, Jerome A. A comparison of pharmacological (amitriptyline HCl) and nonpharmacological (cognitive-behavioral) therapies for chronic tension headaches. J Consult Clin Psychol 1991;59:387–393.

34. Holroyd KA, Penzien DB, Hursey KG, Tobin DL, Rogers L, et al. Change mechanisms in EMG biofeedback training: cognitive changes underlying improvements in tension headache. J Consult Clin Psychol 1984;52:1039–1053.

35. Penzien DB, Johnson CA, Carpenter DE, Holroyd KA. Drug vs. behavioral treatment of migraine: long-acting propranolol vs. home-based self-management training. Headache 1990;30:300.

36. Blanchard EB, Appelbaum KA, Radnitz CL, Morrill B, Michultka D, et al. A controlled evaluation of thermal biofeedback and thermal biofeedback combined with cognitive therapy in the treatment of vascular headache. J Consult Clin Psychol 1990;58:216–224.

37. Huber HP, Huber D. Autogenic training and rational-emotive therapy for long-term migraine patients: an explorative study of a therapy. Behav Anal Modif 1979;3:169–177.

38. Murphy AI, Lehrer PM, Jurish S. Cognitive-oriented coping skills training and progressive muscle relaxation in the treatment of tension

headaches: a direct comparison. Society of Behavioral Medicine 11th Annual Proceedings 1986:116–117.

39. Radnitz CL, Appelbaum KA, Blanchard EB, Elliott L, Andrasik F. The effect of self-regulatory treatment on pain behavior in chronic headache. Behav Res Ther 1988;26:253–260.

40. Rains JR, Lohr JM. Changes in illness-related behaviors and dysphoria accompanying behavioral treatment of episodic tension headache (Rep. No. CG03151). Ann Arbor, MI: U Michigan School of Education (ERIC Document Reprod. Serv. No. pending), 1991.

41. Philips C, Hunter M. The treatment of tension headache—II: EMG "normality" and relaxation. Behav Res Ther 1981;19:499–507.

42. Holroyd KA, Holm JE, Hursey KG, Penzien DB, Cordingley, et al. Recurrent vascular headache: home-based behavioral treatment vs. abortive pharmacological treatment. J Consult Clin Psychol 1988;56:218–223.

43. Richardson GM, McGrath PJ. Cognitive-behavioral therapy for migraine headaches: a minimal-therapist-contact approach versus a clinic-based approach. Headache 1989;29:352–357.

44. Blanchard EB, Andrasik F. Management of chronic headaches: a psychological approach. New York: Pergamon Press, 1985.

45. Jacob RG, Turner SN, Szekely BC, Edelman BH. Predicting outcome of relaxation therapy in headaches: the role of "depression." Behav Ther 1983;14:457–465.

46. Blanchard EB, Andrasik F, Neff DF, Teders SJ, Pallmeyer TP, et al. Sequential comparisons of relaxation training and biofeedback in the treatment of three kinds of chronic headache or, the machines may be necessary some of the time. Behav Res Ther 1982;20:469–481.

47. Blanchard EB, Andrasik F, Evans DD, Neff DF, Appelbaum KA, Rodichok LD. Behavioral treatment of 250 chronic headache patients: a clinical replication series. Behav Ther 1985;16:308–327.

48. Andrasik F, Holroyd KA. A test of specific and nonspecific effects in biofeedback treatment of tension headache. J Consult Clin Psychol 1980;48:575–586.

49. Lefebvre RC, Cox DJ, Hobbs W. Predictive value of and effects on ancillary symptoms in the treatment of functional headaches with biofeedback. Society of Behavioral Medicine 3rd Annual Proceedings 1982:63.

50. Bandura A. Social foundations of thought and action: a social cognitive theory. Englewood Cliffs, NJ: Prentice-Hall, 1986.

51. Abramowitz SI, Weiselberg Bell N. Biofeedback, self-control and tension headache. J Psychosom Res 1985;29:95–99.

52. Borgeat F, Hade B, Larouche LM, Bedwani CN. Effect of therapist's active presence on EMG biofeedback training of headache patients. Biofeedback Self Regul 1980;5:275–282.

53. Penzien DB, Ray SE, Holm JE, Brown TA, Allen KA, et al. Home-based behavioral and cognitive-behavioral treatment of recurrent headache: preliminary findings. Society of Behavioral Medicine 9th Annual Proceedings 1988:161.

54. Hudzynski LG, Levenson H. Biofeedback behavioral treatment of headache with locus of control pain analysis: a 20-month retrospective study. Headache 1985;25:380–386.

55. Martin N, Holroyd KA, Penzien DB. The Headache-Specific Locus of Control Scale: adaptation to recurrent headaches. Headache 1990;30:729–734.

56. Rotter JB. Generalized expectancies for internal versus external control of reinforcement. Psychol Monogr 1966;80:1–28.

57. Penzien DB, Andrew ME, Knowlton GE, McAnulty RD, Rains JC, et al. Computer-aided system for headache diagnosis with the IHS headache diagnostic criteria: development and validation. Cephalalgia 1991;11:325–326.

58. Blanchard EB, Andrasik F, Arena JG. Personality and chronic headache. In: Maher B, ed. Progress in Experimental Personality Research, vol. 13. New York: Academic Press, 1984.

59. Collett T, Cottreaux J, Juenet C. GSR feedback and Schultz relaxation in tension headaches: a comparative study. Pain 1986;25:205–213.

60. Stephenson NL, Cole MA, Spann R. Response of tension headache sufferers to relaxation and biofeedback training as a function of personality characteristics. Biofeedback Self Regul 1979;4:39–40.

61. Werder DS, Sargent JD, Coyne L. MMPI profiles of headache patients using self-regulation to control headache activity. Headache 1981;21:164–169.

62. Williamson DE, Thompson JK, Haber JD, Raczynski JM. MMPI and headache: a special focus on differential diagnosis, prediction of treatment outcome, and patient-treatment matching. Pain 1986;24:143–158.

63. Friedman AP, von Storch TJC. Failure in migraine therapy. Neurology 1951;1:438–443.

64. Micieli G, Piazza D, Sinforiani E, Cavallini A, Trucco M, et al. Antimigraine drugs in the management of chronic daily headaches: clinical profiles of responsive patients. Cephalalgia 1985;5(suppl 2):221–224.

65. Spielberger CD, Jacobs G, Crane R, Russel S, Westberry L, et al. State-trait personality inventory. Tampa: Human Resources Institute, University of Florida, 1979.

66. Berg R, Franzen M, Wedding D. Screening for brain impairment: a manual for mental health practice. New York: Springer, 1987.

67. Lezak MD. Neuropsychological assessment. 2nd ed. New York: Oxford University Press, 1983.

68. Jacobs JW, Bernhard MR, Delgado A, Strain JJ. Screening for organic mental syndromes in the medically ill. Ann Intern Med 1977;86:40–46.

69. Folstein MF, Folstein SE, McHugh PR. "Mini-Mental State:" a practical method for grading the cognitive state of patients for the clinician. J Psychiatr Res 1975;12:189–198.

70. Nelson A, Fogel BS, Faust D. Bedside cognitive screening instruments: a critical assessment. J Nerv Ment Dis 1986;174:73–83.

71. Webster JS, Scott RR, Nunn B, McNeer MF, Varnell N. A brief neuropsychological screening procedure that assesses left and right hemispheric function. J Clin Psychol 1984;40:237–240.

72. Sinforiani E, Farina S, Mancusco GC, Bono G, Mazzucchi A. Analysis of higher nervous functions in migraine and cluster headaches. Funct Neurol 1987;2:69–77.

73. Lawson Kerr K, Penzien DB, Hursey KG, Ray SE, Arora R, et al. Caveats in using mental status examinations: factors that may influence performance. New York: Association for Advancement of Behavioral Therapy, 1988.

74. Blau JN, Path FRC, Thavapalan M. Preventing migraine: a study of precipitating factors. Headache 1988;28:481–483.

75. Lance JW, Curran DA, Anthony N. Investigations into the mechanism and treatment of chronic headache. Med J Aust 1965;ii:909–914.

76. Sargent JD. Stress and headaches. In: Goldberger L, Breznitz S, eds. Handbook of stress: theoretical and clinical aspects. New York: Macmillan, 1982.

77. Penzien DB, Allen KD, Johnson CA, Ray SE. Factors precipitating headache: a study of dietary, environmental, and behavioral precipitants. New York: Association for Advancement or Behavioral Therapy, 1988.

78. Penzien DB, Holroyd KA, Holm JE, Hursey KG. Psychometric characteristics of the Bakal Headache Assessment Questionnaire. Headache 1985;25:55–58.

79. Andrasik F, Blanchard EB, Arena JG, Teders SJ, Teevan RC, Rodichok LD. Psychological functioning in headache sufferers. Psychosom Med 1982;44:171–182.

80. DeLongis A, Coyne JC, Dakof G, Folkman S, Lazarus RS. Relationship of daily hassles, uplifts, and major life events to health status. Health Psychol 1982;1:119–136.

81. Brantley PJ, Jones GN. The Daily Stress Inventory professional manual. Odessa, FL: PAR (Psychological Assessment Resources), 1990.

82. Nash JR, Theofanous AG, Pingel JD, Holroyd KA, Tobin DL, et al. Are chronic headache disorders associated with high levels of stress or ineffective coping? Society of Behavioral Medicine 9th Annual Proceedings 1988:162.

83. Tobin DL, Holroyd KA, Holm JE, Hursey KG, Baker A, et al. Headache severity, expectancies and coping as mediators of depression in chronic headache sufferers. Society of Behavioral Medicine 7th Annual Proceedings 1986:116.

84. Lazarus RS, Folkman S. Stress appraisal, and coping. New York: Springer, 1984.

85. Rosensteil, AK, Keefe FJ. The use of coping strategies in chronic lower back pain patients: relationship to patient characteristics and current adjustment. Pain 1983;17:33–44.

86. Packard RC, O'Connell P. Medication compliance among headache patients. Headache 1986;26:416–419.

87. Diener H-C, Wilkinson M, eds. Drug induced headache New York: Springer-Verlag, 1988.

88. Medina JL, Diamond S. Drug dependency in patients with chronic headaches. Headache 1977;17:12–14.

89. Kudrow L. Paradoxical effects of frequent analgesic use. In: Critchley M, Friedman AP, Gorini S, Scuteri F, eds. Advances in neurology: headache: physiopathological and clinical concepts, vol 33. New York: Raven Press, 1982.

90. Michultka DM, Blanchard EB, Appelbaum KA, Jaccard J, Dentinger MP. The refractory headache patient—II: High medication consumption (analgesic rebound) headache. Behav Res Ther 1989;27:411–420.

91. Johnson CA, Mosley TH, Penzien DB, Payne TJ, Carpenter DE. Patterns of drug use in headache sufferers. Society of Behavioral Medicine 10th Annual Proceedings 1989:52.

92. Johnson CA, Penzien DB, Carpenter DE, Mosley TH, Payne TJ, et al. Veridicality of self-reported headache medication use. San Francisco: Association for Advancement of Behavior Therapy, 1990.

93. Osterweis M, Kleinman A, Mechanic D. Pain and disability: clinical, behavioral, and public policy perspectives. Washington, DC: National Academy Press, 1987.

94. Barrios FX. Social skills training and psychosomatic disorders. In: Rathjen DP, Foreyt JP, eds. Social competence interventions for children and adults. New York: Pergamon, 1980.

95. Figueroa JL. Group treatment of chronic tension headaches: a comparative treatment study. Behav Modif 1982;6:229–239.

96. Stout MA. Homeostatic reconditioning in stress-related disorders: a preliminary study of migraine headaches. Psychother 1986;22:531–541.

97. Bergner M, Bobbitt RA, Carter WB, Gilson BS. The Sickness Impact Profile: development and final revision of a health status measure. Med Care 1981;19:787–805.

98. Lacroix R, Barbaree HE. Affective responses to headache pain can predict subsequent headache severity and duration. Society of Behavioral Medicine 11th Annual Proceedings 1990:184.

99. Naliboff BD, Cohen MJ, Yellen AN. Does the MMPI differentiate chronic illness from chronic pain? Pain 1982;13:333–341.

100. Wittrock DA, Penzien DB, Mosley TH Johnson CA. The recurrent illness impairment profile: preliminary results using the headache version. Headache Q. 1991;2:138–139.

8

Sociologic and Cultural Aspects of Headache

BARBARA CLARK MIMS

With a history dating back to the Neolithic and Bronze ages, headache remains a frequent and distressing malady. Though the precise pathophysiological basis of headache remains somewhat elusive, it is widely believed that both psychosocial and humoral factors play a role in etiology. The ramifications of headache have considerable social significance, as headache can cause missed work, disrupted social interactions, and marital and family problems.

HISTORICAL ASPECTS

Although it is commonly thought of as a product of the stress and tension of modern day life, archaeological evidence indicates that the history of headache dates back ten thousand years or more (1). Written evidence of headache is found in the earliest recorded history, with references to it found in the ancient medical records of many great cultures. The following poem (1) was written in the Babylonian era, somewhere between 4000 and 3000 BC.

> Headache roameth over the desert, blowing like the wind,
> Flashing like lightning, it is loosed above and below;
> It cutteth off him who feareth not his god like a reed,
> Like a stalk of henna it slitteth this thews.
> It wasteth the flesh of him who hath no protecting goddess,
> Flashing like a heavenly star, it cometh like the dew;
> It standeth hostile against the wayfarer, scorching him like the day,
> This man it hath struck and
> Like one with heart disease he staggereth,
> Like one bereft of reason he is broken,
> Like that which has been cast into the fire he is shrivelled,
> Like a wild ass . . . his eyes are full of cloud,
> On himself he feedeth, bound in death,
> Headache whose course like the dread windstorm none knoweth,
> None knoweth its full time or its bond.

Another early reference to headache is found in the *Atharvaveda* of India, a book containing magic formulas gathered between 1500 and 1800 BC. The term *heterocrania* was coined by Aretaeus, a physician born in 81 AD. He wrote a detailed description of migraine and emphasized the common pattern of pain affecting one-half of the head. The term *heterocrania* was changed to *hemicrania* by Galen, who lived between 131

and 200 AD. Hemicrania is the origin of the Old English word *megrim* and the French word *migraine* (1).

The notion that headache may result from both nervous tension and humoral agents was put forth by the Greek physician Paul of Aegina in 600 AD. In 1873, Edward Liveing published the first book on headache, *On Megrim, Sick-Headache, and Some Allied Disorders: a Contribution to the Pathology of Nerve Storm* (2). The scientific basis for treating headache was begun in London in the 1930s by Sir George Pickering, who examined the role of histamine in producing headache. During the same era, Dr. Harold G. Wolff and colleagues wrote the classic *Headache and Other Head Pain*.

SOCIOLOGIC FACTORS AND INCIDENCE OF HEADACHE

Age

The incidence of headache is age-related, with fewer headaches reported as age increases (2, 3). Waters has estimated that approximately 30% of Western women aged 21 to 34 years experience migraine at least annually, with the figure declining to 10% at age 75 and beyond. The incidence is lower in men, with approximately 17% of those between 21 and 34 years and only 5% of those 75 and older experiencing migraine (4). A recent report by Cook and colleagues surveyed 3811 persons aged 65 years and older. They report that 53% of women and 36% of men in this age group experienced headache in the year prior to the study (3).

Sex

Before the age of 10 years, boys account for 60% of the migraine population. by age 10, the incidence of migraine is 15% for boys and 22% for girls. In adults, 75% of the migraine population is female (2).

Geographic Location

Headache is commonly thought of as "the wages of stress," a by-product of life in a modern industrial society. Indeed, approximately 40% of individuals residing in the United States and Europe experience severe headache at some time in their lives (5–7). Though the incidence is lower in

China (8) and rural Ecuador (9), Lance makes the interesting observation that headache does occur in countries in which the pace has not increased in 1000 years (1). He comments on the "headache bands" worn by the women working in the rice paddies of Java and the practice of tribes in Papua-New Guinea scarifying their foreheads because of recurrent headache. Lance also notes that the custom of trepanning, which involves making a hole in the skull with a sharp instrument to let out evil spirits, persisted until recently on islands of the South Pacific (1). In addition, the practice of craniotomy for posttraumatic headache persists to a limited extent today in the Kisii tribe in the highlands of Kenya (10).

Social Status

Migraine is commonly assumed to be associated with intelligence and therefore more likely to occur in professional people. The research findings in this area are conflicting. Crisp and colleagues reported a higher incidence of migraine in subjects of higher social class (11). Wadsworth reported no significant differences in the occurrence of headache between social groups (12). Waters reported no difference in the frequency of migraine occurrence between social groups; however, subjects in the higher social groups were more likely to seek medical help than those in the lower groups (13). This may partially explain the perception that the prevalence of migraine increases with social status.

Ethnicity

Ethnicity has been shown to be strongly related to behavior, beliefs, and attitudes associated with pain (14–17). The way in which individuals perceive, respond to, and communicate symptoms is influenced by their ethnic group membership (18, 19). In considering ethnic group influences on pain, two major factors are important. Culture influences the meaning given to symptoms and the treatment individuals seek for health problems. Social factors influence how families and local groups affect people's behavior and relate to illness. Social factors also determine how ethnic expectations affect the relationship between the patient and the health care practitioner (20).

Zborowski was a pioneer in investigating the relationship between ethnicity and the pain experience. In the early 1950s, he interviewed 146 males who were inpatients at a Veterans' Administration Hospital in New York City (16). He was interested in identifying whether or not ethnicity was consistently related to a patient's pain response patterns, attitudes, and beliefs, as well as the meanings attached to the pain symptoms. He hypothesized that responses to pain were learned and patterned as part of the sufferer's heritage. The ethnic groups he studied included Irish, Italian, Jewish, and old American (white, native-born, or Anglo-Saxon origin, usually Protestant, whose grandparents were born in the United States). He found

that the Jewish and Italian patients gave a more emotional description of their pain and tended to "play it up." The Irish and old American patients were less emotional and tended to "play it down." The Jewish and Italian patients exhibited pain by crying, complaining, groaning, and being demanding. Irish and old Americans were more reserved and tended to withdraw from others when experiencing pain. Zborowski studied interethnic differences and did not really address intraethnic differences in response to pain. However, he identified type of pathology, generation American, age, and level of education as important factors in the individual's response to pain (16).

Zola performed another well-known study of interethnic differences in the report of responses to and attitudes toward symptoms such as pain (17). He interviewed 196 patients about their responses to presenting symptoms. He also asked about their families' response. He found that lower-class Irish patients tended to deny pain and emphasize the physical effects of illness. The lower-class Italian patients emphasized the importance of their pain. They had diffuse complaints and multiple symptoms, and were vocal and dramatic in describing the effects of pain on their daily lives. The Anglo-Saxon patients fell between the Irish and Italians in their responses, but were more similar to the Irish (17).

Weisenberg studied the relationship between the ethnic group and the level of anxiety and attitudes toward pain in the head and oral cavity (15). The ethnic groups included in his study were black, Caucasian, and Puerto Rican. He found that Puerto Rican patients tended to avoid dealing with pain by denying it or getting rid of it quickly. Black and white patients were similar in their attitudes toward pain, but differed from the Puerto Rican patients (15).

These studies are widely cited and suggest that cultural background may have a profound influence upon the individual's response to headache. However, Fitzpatrick and Hopkins warn about potential problems with the application of these research findings (21). They point out the possibility that the differences between ethnic groups are caused by educational differences between groups rather than cultural factors. Of considerable risk to the clinician is the danger of stereotyping groups and ignoring the variability in responses to pain within ethnic groups. Fitzpatrick and Hopkins suggest that extreme caution be used in interpreting cultural differences in the expression of illness (21).

CULTURALLY DERIVED TREATMENTS

Many culturally derived treatments for headache exist, ranging from innocuous "headache bands" (1) to ingestion of herbs and invasive surgical procedures (10). Ingestion of native plants in combination with charms, incantations, and witchcraft were widely practiced in primitive times and persist to a limited extent today. An excerpt from the Ebers papyrus, written about 1600 BC, refers to the *Ricinus* (castor oil plant) as a treatment for headache. Headache sufferers in the Cherokee nation sought relief by chewing ginseng while the forehead was rubbed gently with the palm of the right hand as the medicine man sang (10):

The men have just passed by, they have caused relief,
The wizards have just passed by, they have caused relief,
Relief has just been rubbed, they have caused relief,
Sharp!

The medicine man would then blow a mixture of water and ginseng onto the painful area. Herbal medicine is still in use today. Feverfew is a medicinal herb that has recently been used to prevent migraine (22).

Trephination of the skull is the oldest therapeutic procedure for which archaeological evidence exists (10). It involves making a hole in the skull with a sharp instrument, presumably to let evil spirits escape. This practice has been used in Europe, Mexico, Peru, and the islands of the South Pacific (1). It is currently practiced by the Kisii tribe of Kenya, and some claim it has been effective in cases where modern western medicine has failed (23, 24).

Acupuncture has been used in Chinese medicine since it was originated sometime between 2698 and 2598 BC. It has recently been reported to be effective in relieving headache and other pain (1).

SOCIOECONOMIC IMPACT OF HEADACHE

The overall costs of headache to the individual and to the community are significant. The British Office of Health Economics divides the costs of a disease into three categories (4): (a) the direct cost of prevention, diagnosis, and treatment, (b) the indirect cost to the community as a whole for lost productivity, and (c) the personal costs of hardship and disability to the sufferer and his family. Documentation of the costs of headache is scarce. In 1970, the British Office of Health Economics estimated that 0.05% of the hospital service costs, 0.4% of general practice costs, and 0.8% of pharmaceutical costs were attributed to migraine (4). An overall 0.2% of National Health Service costs were attributed to migraine.

Headache and migraine are among the most important causes of absenteeism from work (25). A study by Jones and Harrop showed that, in a population of factory workers, subjects lost an average of 4.3 workdays per year from headache (26). The British Department of Health and Social Security reported 15 days per year of certified incapacity from migraine for males per 1000 population at risk. The female rates were two to three times higher (27). This translates to 295,000 man-days and 167,000 woman-days of recorded absence due to migraine in 1968–1969. This is likely a gross underestimate of morbidity, as absences of less than 3 days were not reported in the Department of Health and Social Security statistics. In the Pontypridd survey, 40 (8%) men of 491 missed work the previous year due to headache. This accounted for a total of 141 days, giving an average of 182 days per year absence per 1000 men (4). The proportion missing work due to

headache fell as age increased, from 12% in those aged 21 to 34 years, to 8% in those aged 35 to 54 years, to 4% in those over 55 years. An interesting point made during the data collection of the Pontypridd study was that several men did not tell their employers that they were calling in sick due to headache. According to one man, "You cannot stay at home with just a bad headache because they will think you are pulling a fast one" (4).

Waters reported that 51 (8%) of 623 men with headache missed work because of headache in the year before the study. Another study of 2018 subjects in northern Finland found that 263 (13%) had missed one or more days work in the previous year because of headache (28). It is likely that productivity among workers is adversely affected when headache occurs during work hours. Fifty-five percent of subjects in one large study indicated that headache had adversely affected their careers (25).

Quantification of personal costs from headache is difficult. Some headaches are trivial, while others are incapacitating. A comment from Black in 1788 (29) is most expressive; "From this calamity, in the extreme, the lives of many are rendered wretched." Recurrent headaches can interfere with social activities and cause marital problems. Family conflicts may also occur, as the family's expectations of what the patient can do may clash with the patient's own expectations (30).

STRESS, HEADACHE, AND SOCIAL SUPPORT

Though stress is frequently implicated as a contributing factor in the etiology of headache, stress is difficult to quantify and somewhat nebulous in definition. Rose and Gawel (31) put it succinctly when they said "stress is one of the most misused words in the English language and its precise meaning is often forgotten." They define stress from the shorter Oxford English Dictionary as simply " a demand upon energy" (31). Selye's classic definition of stress is "the non-specific response of the body to any demand upon it" (32). This definition of stress was modified slightly by Schafer (33) to "an arousal of mind and body in response to demands made upon it." Packard (34) has pointed out that a common thread in the various definitions of stress is the word "demand." He comments that all people are subjected to demands being placed upon energy, body, and mind, and that the response to stress involves all organs and tissues in the body. When the level of arousal becomes too high, symptoms such as trembling hands, churning stomach, tight shoulders, edginess, or poor concentration may occur. If these symptoms are ignored, a stress-related illness such as migraine or muscle contraction headache may occur. Individual reactions to stress are influenced by perception, personality, age, status, life stage, unrealized expectations, prior experiences, social support systems, and the capacity to adapt (35). Packard has stated that stress can contribute to headache development in three ways: (a) by imposing long-term wear and tear on the body and mind, reducing resistance, (*b*) by directly precipitating sustained muscular contraction or changing vascular reactivity in migraine, or (*c*) by aggravating an already existing headache (34).

Numerous stressors occur as part of modern life (34). Unpredictability and change, including both social and personal change, are major sources of stress. Social change involves change in the environment where the individual lives or works. Personal change may involve moving, changing jobs, or retiring. Another stressor involves a fast pace of life, where the individual crams too much into each day and does not get sufficient rest. Although the individual may deny stress, headache is a common occurrence in this setting. Another stressor involves life transitions, such as a geographic move, a promotion, marriage, parenthood, or divorce (34). It is well documented that the greater the clustering of life events, the greater the likelihood that symptoms will develop (36).

Work stress has been identified as a major stressor in today's world (37). To understand the importance of work stress, an individual's feelings about job and roles in life must be examined. "Role" can be defined as the cluster of expectations associated with a social or work position (34). When the individual's desires or abilities do not coincide with what others expect on the job, work stress results. Other factors contributing to work stress include noise (38), improper lighting (39), prolonged staring at computer screens, and extremes of temperature (34).

Other sources of stress may include understimulation (33), social isolation and loneliness (40), financial uncertainty or unemployment (34), and such daily "hassles" as concern about weight, health of a family member, rising prices, home maintenance, and too many things to do (41). Fear of failure, fear of success, or a discrepancy between an individual's self-perception and reality can all lead to stress (34).

The relationship between stress and illness may be mediated by such variables as coping skills and social support (42). It has been argued that individuals who have excellent coping skills and/or strong social support networks are "buffered" from the effects of stress (43, 44). Deficits and changes in social support may constitute stressors (45, 46). A study conducted at the University of Western Australia suggests that low social support leading to elevated stress response contributes to headache development (42). The study further suggests that regular headaches may cause various types of pain behavior and lead to reduced social support networks. Martin and Nathan compared headache prevalence in two groups of psychology students, one at a North American university and one at the University of Western Australia. They found a higher prevalence rate at the North American university, which they attributed to a greater incidence of stressors (particularly examinations) and the relatively deficient social support systems (42).

Budd and Kedesdy have identified situational variables such as emotional stressors or physical antecedents, the provision of social consequences by others, and the child's

use of coping strategies as factors that can affect headache activity in children (47). The tool used in this study was a parent rating scale, the children's headache assessment scale. A review of parental rating indicated that a child's worrying and setting high standards were commonly associated with headache.

SUMMARY

Headache is a frequent and worrisome condition in today's society, with potential costs to the individual, the family, and the community. Though the etiology is complex and multifactorial, it is likely that sociologic and cultural factors play a role. Culturally derived treatments for headache have persisted through the ages, with varying degrees of reported success. Culturally mediated coping skills and social support systems may "buffer" the effects of stress and decrease the incidence of headache. For the clinician faced with the complex challenge of a patient with headache, an appreciation of such concepts is essential. Only within the context of the individual's own sociologic and cultural heritage can an accurate assessment and realistic treatment plan exist.

REFERENCES

1. Lance JW. Headache understanding alleviation. New York: Charles Scribner, 1975.
2. Raskin NH. Headache. 2nd ed. New York: Churchill Livingstone, 1988.
3. Cook NR, Evans DA, Funkenstein HH, et al. Correlates of headache in a population-based cohort of elderly. Arch Neurol 1989;46:1338–1344.
4. Waters NE. Headache (series in clinical epidemiology). London: Croom Helm, 1986.
5. Ziegler DK. Epidemiology of migraine. In: Rose FC, ed. Handbook of clinical neurology. Amsterdam: Elsevier Science Publishers, 1986.
6. Ziegler DK, Hassanein RS, Couch JR. Characteristics of life headache histories in a nonclinic population. Neurology 1977;27:265–269.
7. Goldstein M, Chen TC. The epidemiology of disabling headache. Adv Neurol 1982;33:377–390.
8. Cheng X, Ziegler DK, Li S, et al. A prevalence survey of "incapacitating headache" in the People's Republic of China. Neurology 1986;36:831–834.
9. Sachs H, Sevilla F, Barberis P, et al. Headache in the rural village of Quiroga, Ecuador. Headache 1985;25:190–193.
10. Furnas DW, Sheikh MA, Van den Hombergh P. Traditional craniotomies of the Kisii tribe of Kenya. Ann Plast Surg 1985;15:538–556.
11. Crisp AH, Kalucy RS, McGuiness B, et al. Some clinical, social and psychological characteristics of migraine subjects in the general population. Postgrad Med J 1977;53:54–59.
12. Wadsworth M, Butterfield W, Blaney R. Health and sickness: the choice of treatment. London: Tavistock, 1971.
13. Waters WE. The Pontypridd headache survey. Headache 1974;14:81–90.
14. Mims BC. Sociologic and cultural aspects of pain. In: Tollison CD, ed. Handbook of chronic pain management. Baltimore: Williams & Wilkins, 1989.
15. Weisenberg M, Kreindler ML, Schachat R, Werboff J. Pain, anxiety, and attitudes in black, white, and Puerto Rican patients. Psychosom Med 1975;37:123–135.
16. Zborowski M. Cultural components in response to pain. J Soc Issues 8: 1952;16–30.

17. Zola J. Culture and symptoms—an analysis of patients' presenting complaints. Am Sociol Rev 1966;31:615–630.
18. Kleinman A, Eisenberg L, Good B. Culture, illness, and care. Ann Intern Med 1978;88:251–258.
19. Mechanic D. Medical sociology. New York: Free Press, 1978.
20. Chrisman N, Kleinman A. Health beliefs and practices. In: Thornstrom S, ed. Harvard encyclopedia of American ethnic groups. Cambridge, MA: Harvard University Press, 1980.
21. Fitzpatrick RM, Hopkins A. Illness behavior and headache, and the sociology of consultations for headache. In: Hopkins A. Headache problems in diagnosis and management. London: WB Saunders, 1988.
22. Diamond S. Herbal therapy for migraine. An unconventional approach. Postgrad med 1987;82:197–198.
23. Mukasa P. Surgery: traditional style. Daily Nation (Nairobi), November 21, 1984.
24. Mutahi W. A skull surgeon who never went to medical school. Daily Nation (Nairobi), November 26, 1982.
25. Peatfield R. Headache. New York: Springer-Verlag, 1986.
26. Jones A, Harrop C. Study of migraine and the treatment of acute attacks in industry. J Int Med Res 1980;8:321–325.
27. Office of Health Economics. Migraine, Report No. 41. London: Office of Health Economics, 1972.
28. Nikiforow R, Hokkanen E. An epidemiological study of headache in an urban and a rural population in northern Finland. Headache 1978;18:137–145.
29. Black W. A comparative view of the mortality of the human species, at all ages; and of the diseases and casualties by which they are destroyed or annoyed. London: Rilly, 1788.
30. Roy P. Psychosocial assessment of chronic headache. Health Soc Work 1984;9(4):284–293.
31. Rose CL, Gawel M. What brings on a migraine attack? In: Migraine: the facts. London: Oxford University, 1979:42.
32. Selye H. The stress of life. New York: McGraw-Hill, 1976:412.
33. Schafer W. Wellness through stress management. Davis, CA: International Dialogue Press, 1983:24–26.
34. Packard RC. Life stress, personality factors, and reactions to headache. In: Dalessio DJ, ed. Wolff's headache and other head pain. New York: Oxford University Press, 1987:371.
35. Christensen JF. Assessments of stress: environmental, intrapersonal, and outcome issues. In: McReynolds P, ed. Advances in psychological assessment. San Francisco: Jossey-Bass 1981;5:62–123.
36. Garrity TF, Marx MD, Somes G. Personality factors in resistance to illness after recent life changes. J Psychosom Res 1977;21:23–32.
37. Brodsky CM. Long-term work stress. Psychosomatics 1984;25:361–368.
38. Girdano DA, Everly GS. Controlling stress and tension. Englewood Cliffs, NJ: Prentice-Hall, 1979.
39. Ivancevich JM, Matteson MT. Stress and work. Glenview, IL: Scott, Foresman, 1980.
40. Berkman LF, Syne SL. Social class, susceptibility, and sickness. Am J Epidemiol 1976;104:1–8.
41. Lazarus RS. Little hassles can be dangerous to health. Psychology Today (July): 1981;58–62.
42. Martin PR, Nathan PR. Differential prevalence rates for headaches: a function of stress and social support? Headache 1987;27:329–333.
43. Holroyd KA. Stress, coping and the treatment of stress-related illness. In: McNamara JR, ed. Behavioral approaches to medicine: applications and analysis. New York: Plenum Press, 1979.
44. Dean A, Lin N. The stress buffering role of social support, problems, and prospects for systematic investigation. J Nerv Ment Dis 1977;165:403–417.
45. Andrews G, Tennant C, Hewsar DM, Vaillant GE. Life event stress, social support, coping style, and risk of psychological impairment. J Nerv Ment Dis 1978;9:307–315.
46. Thoits PA. Conceptual, methodological and theoretical problems in studying social support as a buffer against life stress. J Health Soc Behav 1982;23:145–159.
47. Budd KS, Kedesdy JH. Investigation of environmental factors in pediatric headache. Headache 1989;29:569–573.

SELECTED PRIMARY HEADACHE DISORDERS

Migraine

9

Clinical Symptomatology and Differential Diagnosis of Migraine

STEPHEN D. SILBERSTEIN and MARSHA M. SILBERSTEIN

HISTORY OF MIGRAINE

Migraine is an episodic headache disorder often accompanied by neurological, gastrointestinal, and psychological changes. Over the last 5000 years, many authors have described migraine triggers, relieving factors, and the signs and symptoms of the migraine complex including headache, aura, prodrome, nausea or vomiting, and familial tendency (1).

The earliest written reference to migraine is found in an epic poem written in Sumeria around 3000 BC and quoted by Bille (2):

The sick-eyed says not
'I am sick-eyed'
The sick-headed not
'I am sick-headed'

From Mesopotamia comes a description of a form of headache and an associated visual disturbance, in which "the head is bent with pain gripping his temples . . . and his eyes are afflicted with dimness and cloudiness." Hippocrates (400 BC), who was clearly familiar with the syndrome of migraine, described the visual aura that can precede the migraine headache and its relief by vomiting (3).

Celsus (215–300 AD) described migrainous triggers: "drinking wine, or crudity (dyspepsia), or cold, or heat of a fire, or the sun." Because of his classic description of the symptoms, Aretaeus of Cappadocia (2nd century AD) is credited by Critchley as the discoverer of migraine. Migraine clearly was well known in the ancient world (3).

"Migraine" is derived from the Greek word *hemicrania*, introduced by Galen in approximately 200 AD. (He mistakenly believed it was caused by the ascent of vapours, either excessive in amount, too hot, or too cold.) Hemicrania became hemimigranea, migranea, mygrame, myegrym, migram, megrim, and finally migraine, which is French. Popular names evolved over the years for this uncomfortable, sometimes disabling, disorder: sick headache, blind headache, and bilious headache (3, 4).

In modern times, Dr. Thomas Willis (1683) brilliantly described a woman with severe, periodic, migrainous headache preceded by a prodrome and associated with vomiting (3).

> . . . beautiful and young woman, imbued with a slender habit of body, and an hot blood, was wont to be afflicted with frequent and wandering fits of headache . . . On the day before the coming of the spontaneous fit of this disease, growing very hungry in the evening, she eat a most plentiful supper, with an hungry, I may say a greedy appetite; presaging by this sign, that the pain of the head would most certainly follow the next morning; and the event never failed this augury . . . she was troubled also with vomiting.

Tisso (1783) distinguished migraine from common headache (4) and ascribed it to a supraorbital neuralgia "provoked by reflexes from the stomach, gallbladder, or uterus." Over the next century, DuBois Reymond, Mollendorf (1867), and later Eulenburg proposed different vascular theories for migraine. Fothergill (1778) introduced the term *fortification spectra* to describe the visual aura of migraine. Airy (1870) gave a vivid description of the same phenomena, which he called *teichopsia*, quoting Tennyson (6):

> as yonder walls rose slowly to a music slowly breathed, a cloud that gathered shape

James Ware (1814) described bouts of teichopsia without accompanying headache, which he termed *muscoe volitantes* and which have been more recently called migraine equivalents (3).

Liveing (1873), who wrote the first monograph on migraine entitled *On Megrim, Sick-headache, and Some Allied Disorders: A Contribution to the Pathology of Nerve-storms* (7) and was the originator of the neural theory of migraine, ascribed the problem to "disturbances of the autonomic nervous system," which he called "nerve storms." In 1900, Dey (2) suggested that migraine, including menstrual migraine, resulted from intermittent swelling of the hypophysis with compression of the trigeminal nerve. Spitzer (2), in 1901, suggested that headache was produced by recurrent interventricular foramen blockage causing lateral ventricle dilation.

In the 20th century, Harold Wolff (1950) developed the experimental approach to the study of headache (8) and elaborated the vascular theory of migraine, which has come under attack from the work of Blau (9), Olesen (10), Lance (5), Raskin (11), and Welsh (12) as the pendulum again swings back to the neurogenic theory.

MIGRAINE: DEFINITION, EPIDEMIOLOGY, PROGNOSIS

Most migraine definitions stress what Waters (13) refers to as the three features of migraine: the unilateral distribution of the headache; the presence of a warning (often visual); and nausea or vomiting. Vahlquist (14) and later Bille (2) used these features as part of their criteria to diagnose migraine: paroxysmal headaches separated by free intervals and two or more of the following: nausea, scotomata or related phenomena, one-sided pain, and positive family history (parent or sibling). Not all authors agree about the relative emphasis to be placed on these features. Selby and Lance (15) found that only 60% of their migraineurs had hemicranial headache. Other authors have inappropriately included family history as part of the migraine definition and then investigated the prevalence of headache in first-degree relatives of migraine sufferers (13).

The Ad Hoc Committee on Classification of Headache (16) (1962) identified vascular headache of migraine type as

> Recurrent attacks of headache, widely varied in intensity, frequency, and duration. The attacks are commonly unilateral in onset; are usually associated with anorexia and sometimes with nausea and vomiting; in some are preceded by, or associated with, conspicuous sensory, motor, and mood disturbances; and are often familial.

The World Federation of Neurology offered a similar definition (17).

These are not definitions of migraine but rather descriptions of migraine. The uncertainty in the diagnosis of migraine is apparent in an epidemiological study of general practitioners who were asked to diagnose their own migraine (18). Only 41.8% with headache and nausea and 32.7% with unilateral headache self-diagnosed migraine. In the presence of unilateral headache, warning, and nausea, still only 85.9% self-diagnosed migraine. This variability in self-diagnosis by physicians illustrates the difficulty of interpreting any study without strict criteria.

Recent epidemiological studies (19) have attempted to apply uniform criteria to populations to examine the prevalence of headache. These studies have clearly shown that fewer than 50% of migraineurs have ever consulted a doctor for this condition, clearly introducing a bias into all clinic- or physician-based reports of headache prevalence and severity!

Waters (13) developed a migraine questionnaire that he tested against an independent clinical diagnosis by a neurologist. Looking at the population of Rhondda Fach, a town in Wales, Waters found a 19% migraine prevalence in women between the ages of 20 and 64. In analyzing his data, he found that there was no cross-correlation between the three features of migraine (unilateral headache, warning, and nausea), suggesting that these symptoms do not exist as an independent syndrome. (For further discussion see (13)). However, when he looked at the intensity of headache, he found that the three symptoms of migraine occur together more frequently as the headache intensity increases.

Waters (13) states, "The distribution of the headache severity extends as a continuous spectrum from mild attacks, which usually have neither unilateral distribution nor warning nor nausea to severe headaches which are frequently accompanied by the three migraine features." Bakal (20) and Raskin (11) have presented similar arguments.

More recently, Celetano et al. (21), in a telephone interview of 10,000 subjects in Washington County, Maryland, analyzed the frequency of occurrence, pain, and duration of recent (within 4 weeks) headache attacks. They found that symptoms of migraine were frequently experienced concomitantly with tension-type symptoms, and the resultant headaches were moderate in intensity. Symptoms usually associated with migraine (nausea, aura, photophobia) in the absence of concomitant tension-type symptoms were infrequent but resulted in headaches causing the greatest disability. Their data provided additional support for the severity model of headache.

Goldstein and Chen (22) looked at a number of reports of migraine prevalence in children and adults. They found that migraine prevalence was equal in boys and girls prior to puberty. As adolescence approaches, migraine prevalence increases more in girls than in boys, with a peak incidence at menarche. The prevalence of migraine in series of adult men ranges from 2.1 to 14.9% (av 9.19%) and in adult women from 6.3% to 25.4% (av 16.1%).

Linet and Stewart (23) report an even wider variation (range 1 to 31%) in migraine prevalence for both sexes. Thus the source of the sample (clinic vs. population), differences in the age and sex of the sample, the nature of the measure (interview, physician's assessment, questionnaire), and the differences in definition of migraine may account for the large range of reported migraine prevalence.

Prognosis

Migraine prevalence slowly decreases with age after the fourth decade (22). Bille followed a cohort of children with severe migraine for up to 37 years. As young adults, 62%

were migraine-free for more than 2 years, but after 30 years, only 40% continued to be migraine-free, suggesting that migraine is a lifelong disorder (24). Hockaday and Congdon have reported similar long-term remissions (25). For 15 years, Fry (26) collected information on migraine patients in his general practice in Kent. His data showed a tendency for the severity and frequency of attacks to decrease as the patients got older. After 15 years, 32% of the men and 42% of the women no longer had migraine attacks. Waters (13) noted a similar decrease in migraine prevalence.

Migraine: Personality, Intelligence, and Psychopathology

Physician- and clinic-based studies had suggested that migraine occurs more frequently among those with higher "intelligence and education" (24). However, Bille (2), in children, and Waters (13) and Merikangas (27), in adults, found no association between intelligence, social class, and migraine. Migraineurs of a higher social class more readily consult a physician, biasing results of physician-based studies (13).

The reported tendency of migrainous children to be more serious, tidy, vulnerable to frustration and anxiety, and less self-confident may be a function of the pain they experience (28).

In 1982, Geschwind and Behan (29) reported an association between migraine and left-handedness. Because of methodological problems with the study, Messenger et al. (30), in consultation with Geschwind, tested the hypothesis with tighter definitions of migraine. No significant associations were found between migraine and left-handedness.

Brandt et al. (31) in a population study of 162 adults between the ages of 12 and 29 living in Washington County, Maryland, found a higher prevalence of psychological symptoms of anxiety and depression in migraine sufferers, independent of headache frequency. Merikangas (27), in a prospective study of 27- to 28-year-olds in Zurich, Switzerland, found an association between migraine and anxiety, which manifested itself 3 to 4 years before the appearance of migraine. In this age group, depression alone (without anxiety) was more common in nonmigraineurs. Brandt and Merikangas' data suggest that migraine may be part of a distinct syndrome, with different manifestations at different times in the life cycle. Anxiety may appear in early childhood, followed by migraine and then depression. The duration of the disease may be more important than the frequency of the attacks in determining the presence of associated psychological conditions.

Most observers (32–35) have found that MMPI patterns are normal in migraineurs, in contrast to the abnormalities found in patients with chronic tension-type (mixed) headache (33). However, the original MMPI-1 may not be the best instrument for the psychological assessment of migraine patients since it was standardized on samples of psychiatric patients and has a distinct psychopathological bias (31).

Hooker and Raskin (36) found neuropsychological impairment between attacks in patients with either common or classic migraine. These patients, recruited from a neurology or headache clinic, were less able to discriminate forms or analyze spatial relations and showed impaired delayed recall. Personality differences were not considered, and no relationship was noted between degree of impairment and medication use.

Leijdekkers et al. (37), in a community-based study, found no cognitive difference between 37 female migraineurs and 34 nonheadache controls. The patients and control groups differed in measures known to interfere with performance. Patients reported higher trait and state anxiety levels, more depression, and less vigor, but this did not affect cognitive performance. Raskin's (36) suggestion that migraine is associated with a disturbance of cerebral function even when the patient is not having an attack may be a function of the clinic population assessed and the failure to analyze interfering personality characteristics (37).

Familial Factors

Early pedigree studies showed a strong familial history of migraine over several generations, consistent with either dominant or multiple allelic recessive disorder. Most studies show a higher migraine prevalence in migraineur families than in nonmigraineur families (22). When extensive personal interviews were performed on all first-degree relatives of women with migraine, a 90% family history of migraine was found (38). Bille (24) found that the children of migraineurs were more likely to have migraine if the affected parent was the mother. Lucas's and Ziegler's twin studies show a higher concordance ratio for migraine in monozygotic twins than in dizygotic twins (22). Waters's (13) epidemiological study in South Wales gives support for familial and perhaps genetic factors for both headache and migraine. However, a clear genetic pattern is not yet apparent. There may be subsets of migraine, such as the MELAS syndrome (39) with mitochondrial genetics, that may yet be distinguished phenotypically. In particular, familial hemiplegic migraine is most likely an autosomal dominant disorder (11).

Public Health Significance

The National Center for Health Statistics (1960–1962) found a prevalence of headache in 65% of men and 80% of women between the ages of 20 and 30 in the United States (40). About 20% of the adult population suffers from some form of frequent or severe headache (41). In 1977 to 1978, a national ambulatory medical care survey found approximately 4% of all visits to physicians' offices were for severe headache, most commonly migraine, resulting in over 10,000,000 outpatient physician visits per year. An American survey of 40,000 households (112,000 persons) found 5.5 days of restricted activity were due to headache per 100 persons per year—11,572 days in all (41). In the years 1986 to 1987, 8% of men and 14% of women in Washington County, Maryland, missed part or more of a day of work or school because of a headache in the 4 weeks before the interview (42). Disability may not only be caused by migraine itself but also by the drugs used to treat it (43).

NEW IHS CLASSIFICATION OF HEADACHE

In an attempt to clarify the confusion surrounding headache classification, the International Headache Society has proposed and published a new classification of headache, which is a major modification of the classification of headaches proposed by the Ad Hoc Committee in 1962 (16) (Table 9.1).

The new classification of headache attempts to give more precision to the definition of migraine. Migraine headaches were formerly divided into two varieties: classic and common, terms that have been widely used and frequently confused. Previously, either term could be associated with a severe unilateral or bilateral throbbing headache (45). Now common migraine is called migraine without aura (1.1), and classic migraine is called migraine with aura (1.2), the aura being the complex of focal neurological symptoms that initiates or accompanies an attack (44). At most, only 30% of migraine headaches are classic (46). At times the same patient may have the headache without the aura, and the aura without the headache (46–48). Barrie et al. (48) looked prospectively at 71 patients with migraine with aura. They found that 22.5% always had an aura with their attacks, whereas 14.1% usually, 45.1% commonly, and 12.7% occasionally had an aura; 5.6% never had an aura over a 3-month period. Ziegler (40) found a similar variability in reported aura in patients with prior aura.

Migraine without Aura (1.1) (Previously Common Migraine) (Table 9.2)

Separating migraine from tension-type headache may be difficult (49), and therefore at least 5 attacks are required for analysis (A). Part B defines the duration of the attack (4 to 72 hours in adults, 2 to 48 hours in children); part C, the quality of the headache (at least 2 of the following characteristics: unilateral location, pulsating quality, moderate to severe intensity, aggravation by walking stairs or simple routine physical activity); part D, the associated findings (nausea and/or vomiting or photophobia or phonophobia); part E includes all the benign headache definitions to rule out organic causes of headache.

Migraine with Aura (1.2) (Previously Classic Migraine) (Table 9.3)

The diagnostic criteria are at least 2 attacks that have 3 of the 4 characteristics (B): 1) one or more reversible aura symptoms indicating cortical or brain stem dysfunction that 2) develops gradually over more than 4 minutes, 3) a limit to each aura of 60 minutes, and 4) a headache that must occur within 60 minutes of the end of the aura if it occurs at all. These criteria are used to distinguish the aura of migraine from a focal seizure or transient ischemic attack (50). The headache may begin before or simultaneously with the aura. There is a variety of migraine without headache in which only an aura occurs.

There is a subclassification of migraine with typical aura (1.2.1) (Table 9.4) with one or more aura symptoms of the following types: 1) homonymous visual disturbance, 2) unilateral paresthesias and/or numbness, 3) unilateral weakness, and 4) aphasia or unclassifiable speech difficulty. One or more of the above can occur and are charac-

Table 9.1.
Classification of Migraine[a]

1. Migraine
   - 1.1 Migraine without aura (see Table 9.2)
   - 1.2 Migraine with aura (see Table 9.3)
     - 1.2.1 Migraine with typical aura (see Table 9.4)
     - 1.2.2 Migraine with prolonged aura (see Table 9.5)
     - 1.2.3 Familial hemiplegic migraine
     - 1.2.4 Basilar migraine (see Table 9.6)
     - 1.2.5 Migraine aura without headache (see Table 9.7)
     - 1.2.6 Migraine with acute onset aura
   - 1.3 Ophthalmoplegic migraine (see Table 9.10)
   - 1.4 Retinal migraine
   - 1.5 Childhood periodic syndromes that may be precursors to or associated with migraine
     - 1.5.1 Benign paroxysmal vertigo of childhood
     - 1.5.2 Alternating hemiplegia of childhood
   - 1.6 Complications of migraine
     - 1.6.1 Status migrainosus
     - 1.6.2 Migrainous infarction
   - 1.7 Migrainous disorder not fulfilling above criteria

[a]From Spierings ELH. The pathogenesis of the migraine aura: an overview. In: Amery WK, Wauquier A, eds. The prelude to the migraine attack. Philadelphia: Bailliere Tindall, 1986.

Table 9.2.
Migraine without Aura[a,b]

Diagnostic criteria
A. At least 5 attacks fulfilling B–D
B. Headache lasting 4 to 72 hours (untreated or unsuccessfully treated)
C. Headache has at least two of the following characteristics:
   1. Unilateral location
   2. Pulsating quality
   3. Moderate or severe intensity (inhibits or prohibits daily activities)
   4. Aggravation by walking stairs or similar routine physical activity
D. During headache at least one of the following:
   1. Nausea and/or vomiting
   2. Photophobia and phonophobia
E. At least one of the following:
   1. History, physical and neurological examinations do not suggest an organic disorder
   2. History and/or physical and/or neurological examinations do suggest such disorder, but it is ruled out by appropriate investigations
   3. Such disorder is present, but migraine attacks do not occur for the first time in close temporal relation to the disorder

[a]From Headache Classification Committee of the International Headache Society. Classification and diagnostic criteria for headache disorders, cranial neuralgia, and facial pain. Cephalalgia 1988; 8 (suppl 7):1–96.
[b]Previously used terms: common migraine, hemicrania simplex.

Table 9.3.
Migraine with Aura[a,b]

Diagnostic criteria
A.   At least 2 attacks fulfilling B
B.   At least 3 of the following 4 characteristics:
   1.   One or more fully reversible aura symptoms indicating focal cerebral cortical and/or brainstem dysfunction
   2.   At least one aura symptom develops gradually over more than 4 minutes or 2 or more symptoms occur in succession
   3.   No aura symptom lasts more than 60 minutes. If more than one aura symptom is present, accepted duration is proportionally increased
   4.   Headache follows aura with a free interval of less than 60 minutes. (It may also begin before or simultaneously with the aura)
C.   At least one of the following:
   1.   History, physical and neurological examinations do not suggest an organic disorder
   2.   History and/or physical and/or neurological examinations do suggest such disorder, but it is ruled out by appropriate investigations
   3.   Such disorder is present, but migraine attacks do not occur for the first time in close temporal relation to the disorder

[a]From Headache Classification Committee of the International Headache Society. Classification and diagnostic criteria for headache disorders, cranial neuralgia, and facial pain. Cephalalgia 1988; 8 (suppl 7):1–96.
[b]Previously used terms: classic migraine, classical migraine, ophthalmic, hemiparesthetic, hemiplegic or aphasic migraine.

Table 9.4.
Migraine with Typical Aura

Diagnostic criteria
A.   Fulfills criteria for 1.2 including all four criteria under B
B.   One or more aura symptoms of the following types:
   1.   Homonymous visual disturbance
   2.   Unilateral paresthesias and/or numbness
   3.   Unilateral weakness
   4.   Aphasia or unclassifiable speech difficulty

[a]From Headache Classification Committee of the International Headache Society. Classification and diagnostic criteria for headache disorders, cranial neuralgia, and facial pain. Cephalalgia 1988; 8 (suppl 7):1–96.

Table 9.5.
Migraine with Prolonged Aura[a,b]

Description: Migraine with one or more aura symptoms lasting more than 60 minutes and less than a week; neuroimaging is normal

Diagnostic criteria:
   Fulfills criteria for 1.2, but at least one symptom lasts more than 60 minutes and ≤7 days. If neuroimaging reveals relevant ischemic lesion, code 1.6.2 migrainous infarction regardless of symptom duration

[a]From Headache Classification Committee of the International Headache Society. Classification and diagnostic criteria for headache disorders, cranial neuralgia, and facial pain. Cephalalgia 1988; 8 (suppl 7):1–96.
[b]Previously used terms: complicated migraine, hemplegic migraine.

Table 9.6.
Basilar Migraine[a,b]

Description: Migraine with aura symptoms clearly originating from the brain stem or from both occipital lobes

Diagnostic criteria:
A.   Fulfills criteria for 1.2
B.   Two or more aura symptoms of the following types:
   Visual symptoms in both the temporal and nasal fields or both eyes
   Dysarthria
   Vertigo
   Tinnitus
   Decreased hearing
   Double vision
   Ataxia
   Bilateral paresthesias
   Bilateral pareses
   Decreased level of consciousness

[a]From Headache Classification Committee of the International Headache Society. Classification and diagnostic criteria for headache disorders, cranial neuralgia, and facial pain. Cephalalgia 1988; 8 (suppl 7):1–96.
[b]Previously used terms: basilar artery migraine, Bickerstaff's migraine, syncopal migraine.

terized by gradual development, duration of less than 1 hour, and complete reversibility. The visual aura, the most common, is popularly associated with a fortification spectrum near the point of fixation, which spreads laterally with scintillating edges, leaving scotoma in its wake. Next most common are the sensory aberrations. These are characterized by pins and needles moving along one side of the face or body followed by a sense of numbness, or the occurrence of numbness alone. Less common are speech problems and unilateral weakness. Migraine with typical aura (1.2.1) includes the terms ophthalmic, hemiparesthetic, hemiparetic, hemiplegic migraine, or migraine accompaniment.

Migraine with prolonged aura (1.2.2) (Table 9.5) was formerly known as complicated or hemiplegic migraine. Familial hemiplegic migraine (1.2.3) is given a specific IHS code. Both are discussed in another chapter.

Basilar migraine (1.2.4) (Table 9.6) used to be called basilar artery migraine (44) or Bickerstaff's migraine (52). In his early description, Bickerstaff stated that this was mainly a disorder of adolescent girls, but increased experi-

ence showed that it affects all age groups and both sexes, with the usual migraine female predominance. The aura defines the syndrome and consists of combined disturbances of the brain stem, cerebellum, and occipital cortex (53). The attacks generally last less than 1 hour and are usually followed by a headache. The visual aura (see below) frequently begins with a hemianoptic field disturbance but rapidly becomes bilateral, leading at times to temporary blindness. The visual aura is usually followed by ataxia, dysarthria, vertigo, tinnitus, bilateral paresthesia, nausea or vomiting, and change in level of consciousness. Rarer symptoms include nystagmus, diplopia, and decreased hearing. Isolated aura symptoms such as drop attacks or vertigo may occur alone with or without headache. Slater (54) described 7 adults (5 women, 2 men) with the acute onset of vertigo, usually lasting 1/2 to 4 hours and followed by positional vertigo lasting days. Audiograms were normal, but electronystagmography showed spontaneous or positional nystagmus. Four patients had a history of recurrent headache not related to vertiginous attacks, 1 developed headaches and vertigo, 1 had headaches and scotoma, and 1 had visual loss with the vertiginous attack. Moretti et al. (55) described similar cases that responded in part to antimigraine medication. Kuritzky et al. (56) looked at the frequency of vestibular symptoms in 104 headache patients during the headache-free phase. Patients with migraine with aura had more dizzy spells, vertigo, and motion sickness than controls. The common migraine patients showed a non–statistically significant tendency to vestibular impairment.

A syndrome of "occipital lobe epilepsy and interlocated migraine" resembles basilar migraine but has continuous occipital or posterior temporal high-voltage slow and sharp activity that is inhibited by eye opening (25).

Migraine Aura without Headache (1.2.5) (Table 9.7)

Periodic neurological dysfunction that may be part of the migraine aura can occur in isolation without the headache. These phenomena (scintillating scotoma, recurrent sensory, motor, and mental phenomena) can only be accepted as migraine after full investigation and prolonged follow-up. Headache occurring in association with the symptoms will help confirm the diagnosis (25). Headache occasionally is absent in migraine with aura (47). Aura occurring alone is more frequent in the older patient. In Ziegler and Hassanein's series (46), 44% of patients with aura had aura without headache at some time.

Levy (57) (1988) looked at the incidence of transient (<24 hours) neurological loss among neurologists at Cornell. Thirty-two percent (25/80) had transient CNS dysfunction, most commonly visual (15/25) (field cuts), obscurations, scotomata). Ten of 35 had nonvisual symptoms (hemiparesis, clumsiness, paresthesias, dysarthria). Migraine was reported in 29% (23/80). Forty-four percent reporting transient CNS dysfunction (11/25) had migraine, whereas 22% (12/50) of nonreporters had migraine. Follow-up for up to 5 years showed that none developed any residual deficit or chronic neurological disorder, suggesting that these are benign migrainous accompaniments.

Fisher (58) has written extensively about late-life migrainous accompaniments and has reported on 188 patients over the age of 40; 60% were men, and 57% had a history of recurrent headache. They developed an attack or attacks of episodic neurological dysfunction with variable recurrence (1 attack, 27%; 2–10 attacks, 45%; >10 attacks, 28%). The attacks lasted from 1 minute to 72 hours. Fisher considered scintillating scotoma to be diagnostic of migraine even when it occurred in isolation, whereas other episodic neurological symptoms (paresthesias, aphasia, and sensory and motor symptoms) needed more careful evaluation (Table 9.8). Fisher's diagnostic criteria (58) are reproduced in Table 9.9.

When the spells are wholly typical of migraine, particularly if a scintillating scotoma is present, diagnosis is not difficult; extension of the concept to cases without all the characteristics is more tentative. Diplopia, when it occurred, was always episodic and transient. Numbness of the tongue occurred in 20 of 50 cases. Fisher feels that migraine is a prime consideration when isolated tongue numbness is the only neurological symptom. Migrainous numbness can be evanescent, lasting 1 to 10 seconds.

Some of Fisher's patients (59) had sudden onset of severe pain in the head or neck prior to the onset of blindness, blurred vision, or numbness. Others had a feeling of faintness or presyncope.

Fisher feels that transient migrainous accompaniments—scintillating scotomas, numbness, aphasia, dysarthria, and motor weakness—may occur for the first time after the age of 45 and complicate the diagnosis of transient ischemic attacks (TIAs) of cerebrovascular ori-

Table 9.7.
Migraine Aura without Headache[a,b]

Description: Migrainous aura unaccompanied by headache

Diagnostic criteria:
A. Fulfills criteria for 1.2
B. No headache

[a]From Headache Classification Committee of the International Headache Society. Classification and diagnostic criteria for headache disorders, cranial neuralgia, and facial pain. Cephalalgia 1988; 8 (suppl 7):1–96.
[b]Previously used terms: migraine equivalents, acephalgic migraine.

Table 9.8.
Migrainous Accompaniments[a]

Accompaniments (Fisher)	Combined Series
Visual (excluding scintillating scotoma)	
Blindness	17
Homonymous hemianopsia	12
Blurred vision	15
Visual and paresthesias	24
Visual and speech disturbance (dysarthria or aphasia)	9
Visual, paresthesias and speech disturbance	10
Visual, paresthesias, speech disturbance and paresis	27
Visual and brain stem symptoms	17
No visual accompaniments—only paresthesias, etc.	57
Total	188

[a]Adapted from Fisher CM. Late-life migraine accompaniments as a cause of unexplained transient ischemic attacks. Can J Neurol Sci 1980;7:9–17 and Fisher CM. Late-life migraine accompaniments—further experience. Stroke 1986;17:1033–1042.

Table 9.9.
Main Criteria for the Diagnosis of Late-Life Migrainous Accompaniments[a]

1. Scintillations or other visual display in the spell. Next in order, paresthesias, aphasia, dysarthria, and paralysis.
2. Buildup of scintillations. This does not occur in cerebrovascular disease.
3. "March" of paresthesias. This does not occur in cerebrovascular disease.
4. Progression from one accompaniment to another often with a delay.
5. The occurrence of 2 or more similar spells. This helps to exclude embolism.
6. Headache in the spell.
7. Episodes last 15–25 minutes.
8. Characteristic midlife "flurry" of migrainous accompaniments.
9. A generally benign course.
10. Normal angiography. This excludes thrombosis.
11. Exclusion of cerebral thrombosis, embolism and dissection, epilepsy, thrombocythemia, polycythemia, and thrombotic thrombocytopenia.

[a]Adapted from Fisher CM. Late-life migraine accompaniments as a cause of unexplained transient ischemic attacks. Can J Neurol Sci 1980;7:9–17 and Fisher CM. Late-life migraine accompaniments—further experience. Stroke 1986;17:1033–1042.

gin. Diagnosis in all but the most classical cases is still by exclusion (59). Transient global amnesia may be a migraine equivalent and is discussed elsewhere.

Ophthalmoplegic Migraine (1.3) (Table 9.10)

Ophthalmoplegic migraine (44, 52, 60) presents with acute attacks of 3rd nerve palsy associated with a dilated pupil. Rarely, the 4th and 6th cranial nerves are involved. The unilateral eye pain is migrainous. The duration of ophthalmoplegia varies from hours to months.

The differential diagnosis includes berry aneurysm and chronic sinusitis with a mucocele. However, most cases of ophthalmoplegic migraine fit the criteria for the Tolosa-Hunt syndrome of painful ophthalmoplegia (61): (a) steady gnawing, boring, eye pain; (b) involvement of nerves of the cavernous sinus; (c) symptoms lasting days or weeks; (d) spontaneous remission, with recurrent attacks occurring after months or years; (e) CT or MRI limiting disorder to the cavernous sinus, and (f) steroid responsiveness.

Retinal migraine (1.4), childhood periodic syndromes (1.5), and complications of migraine (1.6) are discussed in another chapter.

CLINICAL FEATURES OF MIGRAINE

Selby and Lance (15) looked at the age of onset of migraine in 500 of their patients. Most developed migraine in the 1st, 2nd, and 3rd decades. However, patients continued to develop migraine in the 4th and even the 5th decade. Thus migraine, while a disease of the young, can still develop later in life, with perhaps a different clinical picture (58, 59).

Blau (62) has divided the migraine attack into 5 phases (Table 9.11): the prodrome, which occurs hours or days before the headache; the aura, which immediately precedes the headache; the headache; the headache termination; and the postdrome phase. Migraine without aura consists of the headache, its termination, and the postdrome. Migraine with aura consists of the aura, the headache, its termination, and the postdrome. Both may have associated prodromes. The presence of all 5 phases defines complete migraine. Migraine equivalents consist of fragments of the prodrome or aura in the absence of headache.

Prodrome (Table 9.12) (62, 63)

Premonitory phenomena can occur hours to days before the headache and consist of mental, neurological, or general symptoms. Mental symptoms include depression, euphoria, irritability, restlessness, hyperactivity, and drowsiness. The patient may suddenly become depressed or be euphoric, hyperactive, and talkative, only to have this enhanced mental state crushed by the onset of a severe migrainous headache.

Neurological phenomena include photophobia, phonophobia, and hyperosmia. The patient may complain of dysphasia, yawning, or difficulty concentrating. Episodic bouts of aphasia or difficulty thinking can be a migraine prodrome.

General prodromal symptoms include a stiff neck, a cold feeling, sluggishness, increased thirst, increased urination, anorexia, diarrhea, constipation, fluid retention, and food cravings. Patients with migraine may overindulge in chocolate prior to the attack. Contrary to popular thinking, the chocolate may not be the headache trigger but rather a migraine prodrome producing the craving for chocolate!

The symptoms of the prodrome (64) can continue into the aura, headache, and postdrome phases of the migraine attack, suggesting they are a part of, not only a prelude to, migraine. There may be two types of migraine warning, nonevolutive symptoms that precede the attack by up to 48 hours and evolutive symptoms that start during the last 6 hours before the attack, gradually increase in intensity, and culminate in the attack (65).

When carefully looked for, prodromal migraine is com-

Table 9.10.
Ophthalmoplegic Migraine[a]

Description: Repeated attacks of headache associated with paresis of one or more ocular cranial nerves in the absence of demonstrable cranial lesion

Diagnostic criteria:
A.   At least 2 attacks fulfilling B
B.   Headache overlapping with paresis of one or more cranial nerves III, IV, and VI
C.   Parasellar lesion ruled out by appropriate investigations

[a]From Headache Classification Committee of the International Headache Society. Classification and diagnostic criteria for headache disorders, cranial neuralgia, and facial pain. Cephalalgia 1988; 8 (suppl 7):1–96.

Table 9.11.
Five Phases of Migraine Attack (Complete Migraine)[a]

Prodrome
Aura
Headache
Headache termination
Postdrome

[a]Adapted from Blau JN. Adult migraine: the patient observed. In: Blau JN, ed. Migraine: clinical and research aspects. Baltimore: Johns Hopkins University Press, 1987.

Table 9.12.
Migraine: Prodrome (Premonitory Phenomena)

Mental state	
Depressed	Hyperactive
Euphoric	Talkative
Irritable	Drowsy
Restless	
Neurological	
Photophobia	Difficulty concentrating
Phonophobia	Dysphasia
Hyperosmia	Yawning
General	
Stiff neck	Food cravings
Cold feeling	Anorexia
Sluggish	Diarrhea or constipation
Thirst/urination	Fluid retention

mon—Blau (63) found it in 28/50 cases, while focal aura symptoms were only seen in 6 cases. Isler (66) found 65/100 patients with prodromal migraine. Forty-six had common migraine, 3 basilar, 14 classic, and 2 hemiplegic migraine. Prodromal migraine was as common in migraine without aura (3:4) as in migraine with aura (1:2). Amery et al. (65) found an overall improvement in mood on the day prior to, and a worsening in mood on the day of, the headache. The early warning signs may be of therapeutic importance. Waelkens et al. (68), in a single-blind trial, found that domperidone (an antidopaminergic) given 12 hours before the expected attack blocked 80% of the headache attacks.

Aura (Fig. 9.1)

The migraine aura is the complex of focal neurological symptoms which initiates or accompanies an attack. Most aura symptoms develop over 5 to 20 minutes and usually last less than 60 minutes (44). The aura can be visual, sensory, or motor, and it may involve language or the brain stem (basilar migraine).

    The visual aura is the most common of the neurological symptoms (51, 59). It most often has a hemianoptic distribution (70) and can be associated with paresthesia or aphasic disturbances.

    Photopsia (53, 71), the sensation of unformed flashes of light before the eyes, can consist of flashes of color, wavy lines, spots, or stars. It is the most frequent visual aura, accounting for 89% of the visual symptoms in Lance's series and occurring in 26% of his patients.

    Scotoma (70–72), or partial loss of sight, can occur alone, without the positive phenomenon of scintillations. It is usually hemianoptic, but may consist of "grayouts," "whiteouts," or holes in the visual field.

    Fortification spectrum or teichopsia (15, 70) (Greek; *town wall* and *vision*) (Fig. 9.1) is the visual aura almost diagnostic of migraine. Lance (15) reported a 10.2% incidence of teichopsia in his series. A scotoma beginning near the point of fixation spreads outward into the visual field with a scintillating edge of zigzag, flashing, colored lights, leaving in its wake an enlarging scotoma. Scintillations occur at a rate of 5 to 10 per second. The Abbess Hildegard of Bingen (12th century AD) mystically described her teichopsia (3)

> I saw a great star, most splendid and beautiful, and with it an exceeding multitude of falling sparks with which the star followed southward . . . and suddenly they were all annihilated, being turned into black coals . . . and cast into the abyss so that I could see them no more

Fortification spectra can occur without the headache, particularly in older migraineurs (58) (migraine aura without headache).

    Visual distortions and hallucinations, such as described by Lewis Carroll in *Alice in Wonderland*, can consist of meta-

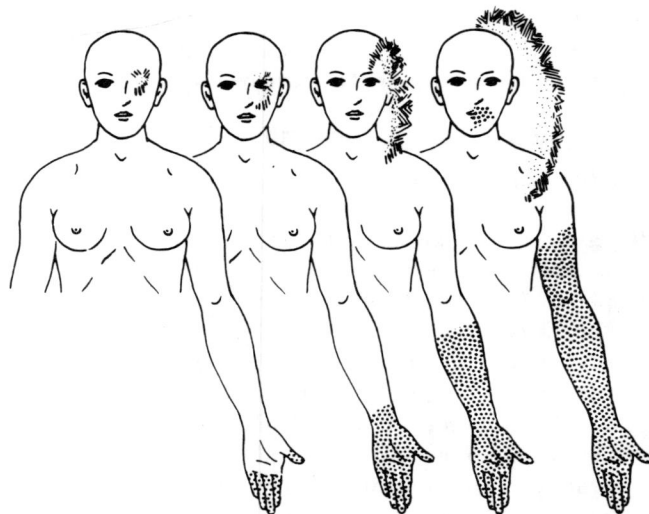

Figure 9.1 Two most characteristic aura symptoms of migraine, the scintillating scotoma and the digitolingual or cheiro-oral syndrome, shown from *left* to *right* in their successive stages of development. (From Spierings ELH. The pathogenesis of the migraine aura: an overview. In: Amery WK, Wauquier A, eds. The prelude to the migraine attack. Philadelphia: Balliere Tindall, 1986. With permission.

morphopsia (or alteration in shape), mosaic vision, microscopia, or macropsia (4). The distortion may be a change in perception—the sufferer may feel very tall or extremely small. Hachinski et al. (72) reported the case of a 6-year-old girl who had episodes beginning with ataxia. Almost immediately, people about her seemed smaller than normal. One time she felt unusually large, and a snowball became huge and turned blue. Hachinski et al. (72) found 16% of the children with auras in his series reported visual distortions and hallucination.

    Sensory phenomena (15, 69) typically begin with a pins-and-needles-like sensation (paresthesias) in the hands, which spreads to the elbow, skips the arm and neck, and then spreads to the tongue (cheiro-oral migraine) (Fig. 9.1). Rarely paresthesias develop simultaneously in the fingers and tongue, but more common is the slow sensory march developing over 10 to 20 minutes. The sensory disturbance may involve the arm and face or the entire side of the body.

Motor Disturbance and Aphasia

A transient mono- or hemiparesis may be part of the aura of migraine (15, 69). When prolonged, it defines hemiplegic migraine. Difficulty in speaking or in understanding language can occasionally occur. Mild anomia or nonfluent dysphasia is the most common symptom. There may be a progression from one aura symptom to another, i.e., from visual aura to paresthesias to dysphasia, with the total migraine aura time proportionally prolonged (44). Most patients with paresthesias also have visual aura. Patients with visual aura commonly have paresthesias (31%). Limb weakness is rarer (46).

HEADACHE

Symptoms typically occurring during the headache of the migraine attack include pain, (which could be unilateral, throbbing, and may be incapacitating), anorexia, nausea and vomiting, phonophobia, photophobia, and mood changes (15, 53, 71, 73).

The headache of migraine can occur at any time of day or night but occurs most frequently on arising (15). The onset of headache is usually gradual; the pain peaks and then subsides. Rarely (crash migraine or thunderclap headache) (74), the headache pain peaks rapidly. This must be differentiated from the headache of a subarachnoid hemorrhage. The headache of a migraine usually lasts between 4 and 72 hours in adults (2 to 48 hours in children). Most patients have 1 to 4 attacks per month. In the remainder, the frequency of headache is very variable, from 1 per year to 10 or more per month (44).

The headache is bilateral in 40%, unilateral in 60%, always on the same side in 20% of patients (15), and it does not become more consistently lateralized with time (75) (Table 9.13). This contradicts the old maxim that patients with persistent unilateral headache should be investigated for an underlying organic cause of their headache. The headache pain is moderate to severe; 50% of the time pulsating, 50% tight or pressure-like! As the pain is typically aggravated by physical activity, patients will frequently lie down in a dark, quiet room (15, 73).

Many patients with migraine will have interictal headaches that do not meet the criteria for migraine (73). Many of these will be shorter and less severe and will meet the criteria of episodic tension-type headache. Some patients note that their headache begins as a tension-type headache and builds into a "migraine" (73, 76). Other patients may have chronic tension-type or chronic daily headache with superimposed bouts of migraine (combination headache).

This is typically seen in patients overusing analgesics or ergotamine (rebound headache) (43).

Patients with migraine may also have short-lived interictal pain lasting for seconds. The pain is described as icepick-, needle-, nail-, or pinprick-like, and it occurs in about 40% of migraineurs (idiopathic stabbing headache (4.1) (Table 9.14)) (77).

Associated Phenomena (Table 9.13)

Gastrointestinal. Sometimes the disability of migraine comes more from the accompanying symptoms than from the headache itself. Gastrointestinal symptoms predominate: anorexia is universal; nausea is extremely common; and vomiting frequent (15, 73). Gastroparesis leads to nausea, vomiting, and poor absorption of oral medication (78, 79). Diarrhea is reported in as many as 16% of patients (15). Abdominal migraine and the periodic syndrome is discussed in Chapter 26.

Cutaneous Manifestations. Skin pallor (8) is common during an attack of migraine and is frequently associated with cold, clammy extremities. Dark rings under the eyes and ecchymoses have been reported (8).

Cardiovascular Manifestations (8, 11). Hypertension secondary to pain is often present during an attack. However, hypotension and bradycardia can also occur.

Neuropsychological Accompaniments. Many patients will have signs of sensory hyperexcitability manifested by photophobia, phonophobia, and osmophobia and will want to escape to a dark, quiet room (15, 82). Lightheadedness and vertigo are not uncommon (56). Some patients have alteration of consciousness in the form of confusion or syncope (15). Mood changes are universal, including lethargy, fatigue, irritability, disorientation, and (in rare cases) exhilaration (15).

Other Findings

In addition to the headache, patients can have scalp tenderness and neck pain, blurred vision, or peripheral edema,

Table 9.13.
Migraine Headache

Symptom	Percentage of Patients	
	Oleson	Selby & Lance
Site		
Holocranial	44	38.2
Hemicranial	56	38.0
Either side		9.4
Always same side		20.6
Both	—	22.6
Quality		
Throbbing/pulsating	47	
Pressure/tightening	56	
Associated features		
Nausea	86	87
Vomiting	47	56
Diarrhea	9	16
Photo/phonophobia	49	82
Dizziness		72
Scalp tenderness	69	65
Lightheadedness		72
Vertigo		33

Table 9.14.
Idiopathic Stabbing Headache[a,b]

Description: Transient stabs of pain in the head that occur spontaneously in the absence of organic disease of underlying structures or of the cranial nerves

Diagnostic criteria:
A.   Pain confined to the head and exclusively or predominantly felt in the distribution of the first division of the trigeminal nerve (orbit, temple, and parietal area)
B.   Pain is stabbing in nature and lasts for a fraction of a second; occurs as single stabs or series of stabs
C.   It recurs at irregular intervals (hours to days)
D.   Diagnosis depends upon the exclusion of structural changes at the site of pain and in the distribution of the affected cranial nerve

[a]From Headache Classification Committee of the International Headache Society. Classification and diagnostic criteria for headache disorders, cranial neuralgia, and facial pain. Cephalalgia 1988; 8 (suppl 7):1–96.
[b]Previously used term: Ice-pick pains

which can begin with the prodrome, hours to days before the migraine attack, or at the onset of the headache (45, 83, 84). This is more common in women with premenstrual syndrome and is followed by a brisk diuresis during the postdrome (83, 84). Nasal congestion and rhinorrhea are less common in migraine than in cluster headache (62).

POSTDROME

Following the headache, there may be a postdrome or hangover phase. The patient may feel tired, washed out, irritable, and listless, or have impaired concentration. Muscle weakness, aching, anorexia, or food cravings can occur (84).

MIGRAINE TRIGGERS (Table 9.15)

Migraine is an episodic disorder frequently triggered by environmental, psychological, and neuroendocrine perturbations. The prodromes of migraine (chocolate craving, anxiety, exhilaration, or depression) can mistakenly be believed to be migraine triggers. Vic denBergh et al. (85) (Table 9.16) collected information on trigger factors in 217 migraineurs (176 women, 41 men). Most patients (85%) were spontaneously aware of one or more trigger factors. The main reported triggers were certain foods (44.7%), menstruation (49%), alcoholic beverages (51.0%), and stress (48.8%).

Diet. Much has been written about the effect of diet on headache. Hunger, fasting, alcohol, certain foods, or additives (in foods or drugs) may trigger migraine. It is controversial whether food allergy can trigger migraine or whether elimination diets can relieve migraine (86). The joint report of the Royal College of Physicians and the British Nutrition Foundation distinguishes between the following (87):

1. *Food aversion*—psychological avoidance of food, or unpleasant bodily reactions caused by emotions associated with food;
2. *Food allergy*—an abnormal immunological interaction with food;
3. *Food intolerance*—broader term—all reactions that are reproduced under blind conditions (chemical, pharmacological, or immunological) (86).

The most common cause of what patients commonly call "food allergy" is food aversion—a psychological response to the food itself. Bix et al. (88) reported on 23 patients who presented to an allergy clinic. Suspected food allergy symptoms included lethargy, head pain, abdominal discomfort, and nausea. Food allergy could not be confirmed in 19 of the 23 patients; this group was almost identical in psychiatric symptomatology and general characteristics with a group of new psychiatric outpatient referrals, except that they were more likely to be professional people and less likely to report and exhibit features of anxiety. There was no evidence of a psychiatric disorder in the 4 of 23 patients with proven food-related atopic symptoms.

Table 9.15.
Migraine: Triggers

1. *Diet:* hunger, alcohol, certain foods or additives, drugs
2. *Sleep:* too much or too little, shift work, jet lag
3. *Hormonal factors:* menstruation, OCs, pregnancy
4. *Environmental factors:* weather or temperature changes, light glare, pungent odors, high altitude
5. *Head or neck pain* of another cause
6. *Physical exertion:* exercise, sexual activity
7. *Stress and anxiety* (poststress or letdown)
8. *Head trauma*
9. *Allergic reactions?*

Table 9.16.
Triggers of Migraine Attacks (217 Patients)

Menstrual cycle (n = 176)	
Menses	85 (48%)
Ovulation	15 (8.5%)
Foods	
Milk/cheese/dairy products/ice cream	54 (24.9%)
Eggs	16 (7.4%)
Chocolate	49 (22.5%)
Other sugar-containing foodstuffs	6 (2.7%)
Fatty food	37 (17%)
Food additives	10 (4.6%)
Beverages	
Alcoholic	112 (51.6%)
With caffeine	14 (6.4%)
Others	
Smoking	9 (4.1%)
Acoustic	6 (2.7%)
Visual	6 (2.7%)
Stress/tension	111 (51.1%)
Fatigue	35 (16.1%)
Acute emotion	15 (6.9%)
Weather	15 (6.9%)

[a]From denBergh VV, Amery WK, Waelkens J. Trigger factors in migraine: a study conducted by the Belgian Migraine Society. Headache 1987;27:191–196.

Some food reactions are chemically mediated, e.g., lactose intolerance or the headache induced by nitrites and monosodium glutamate (89).

Lactose intolerance (90) is a very common genetic disorder occurring in over two-thirds of American blacks, American Indians, and Ashkenazic Jews, and in 10% of whites of Scandinavian ancestry. The most common symptoms of lactose intolerance are abdominal cramps and flatulence, which commonly limits milk and milk product consumption. Children who suffer from abdominal pain and migraine frequently have lactose intolerance. How lactose intolerance triggers migraine in adults and children is uncertain.

Monosodium glutamate (89, 91) (8.1.2) has been shown to produce migraine-like headache and is believed to be responsible for "Chinese restaurant" syndrome. Assorted features include pressure and tightness in the chest and face, facial flushing, dizziness, abdominal discomfort, and a burning sensation in the chest, neck, or shoulders.

Aspartame, a sugar substitute, was found to produce headache in one (92) but not in another controlled study (93). The negative study (93) was tightly controlled (the subjects were inpatients), and no significant effect of aspartame ingestion was found on headache production. The positive study (92) looked at the frequency of migraine in patients consuming aspartame or placebo on a regular basis and found higher migraine frequency on aspartame.

Red Wine (94). Patients with migraine who believed that red wine but not alcohol provoked their headaches were challenged either with red wine or with a vodka mixture of equivalent alcoholic content consumed cold out of dark bottles to disguise color and flavor. The red wine provoked migraine in 9/11 subjects, the vodka in 0/11. Neither provoked headache in other migraine subjects or controls. Alcohol (89) itself may trigger migraine in other migraineurs. It is not known which component of red wine triggers headache, and the study may not have been blinded to oenophiles.

Egger (95) studied 99 children with severe frequent migraine who had been referred to a tertiary care center. Eighty-eight were able to complete an oligoantigenic diet; of these, 48 were atopic, 41 were hyperactive, and 14 had seizures. Only 40 of 74 completed a double-blind trial. Twenty-six of 40 responded to a previously identified food. However, the challenges were not carried out under medical supervision, and not all of the 40 subjects actively developed a headache.

MacDonald (96) used an elimination diet in 60 children with migraine. At most, 15% of the children were found to be food-intolerant. Twenty-three percent showed no benefit from the diet, 28% were noncompliant, 13% had a spontaneous remission as soon as they were given details of the diet, and 17% had a remission while on the diet but did not respond to food challenge.

MacDonald (96) felt that the diet was expensive, difficult to administer, nutritionally inadequate, and not of major benefit in the treatment of migraine.

Moffett et al. (97) looked at the effect of chocolate on a group of volunteer migraineurs who believed that chocolate triggered their migraine. Under double-blind placebo-controlled conditions, subjects did not consistently respond to chocolate. The authors suggested that chocolate on its own rarely is a precipitant of migraine.

Practitioners (98) may diagnose food intolerance by unusual or bizarre techniques of laboratory and clinical investigation such as hair analysis, cytotoxic blood tests, iridology, and sublingual and injection provocation tests. The diagnostic and neutralization procedure used by "clinical ecologists" is performed by injecting extracts of potentially symptom-provoking foods intradermally or subcutaneously. If a symptom is produced (within a few minutes), it can be stopped by injecting a different, neutralizing dose of the same substance.

Jewett et al. (99) attempted to reproduce, in a double-blind manner, allergic symptoms, including headache, by the intradermal injection of extracts of suspected allergens. When the provocation of symptoms to identify food sensitivities is evaluated under double-blind conditions, this type of testing, as well as the treatments based on "neutralizing" such reactions, appears to be the result of

suggestion and chance. Thus, the diagnostic and neutralization procedure, which had been assumed to be fully effective in unblinded use, is in fact based on the placebo response.

In summary, most reactions to food are based on food aversion, chemically, pharmacologically, and (rarely) immunologically mediated. Some "reactions" may be misinterpreted, and the desire for the food may be part of a migraine prodrome.

Sleep (11, 62)

Too much or too little sleep can trigger migraine, as can shift work or jet lag.

Hormonal Factors

Various lines of evidence suggest a link between female sex hormones, estrogens and progestins, and migraine, although the specific mechanisms mediating these effects are uncertain (83).

Menstrual Migraine

Migraine develops most frequently in the second decade, peaking at menarche (15, 100). Women migraineurs outnumber men by at least a 2:1 ratio. This sex difference is not apparent in prepubertal children (13. 22).

Migraine attacks are linked to the period of menses in 60% of women, and exclusively to this period (true menstrual migraine) in 14% (100). It can occur before, during, or after menstruation, or at the time of ovulation. Before menstruation, it may have other features of premenstrual syndrome (PMS), including mood changes, backache, breast tenderness and swelling, and nausea (101). During menstruation, it is often associated with dysmenorrhea (102). Before or during menstruation, migraine is frequently refractory to treatment (103). These are the times of greatest fluctuation in estrogen levels. Unsuccessful attempts have been made to find consistent differences in ovarian hormone levels between women with menstrual migraine and controls. Some authors have reported higher estrogen and progestin levels; others have not (100, 102, 104, 105). However, most find that testosterone, FSH, and LH levels are similar to those of controls.

Somerville (106) reported that the head pain of menstrual migraine occurred during or after the simultaneous fall of estrogens and progesterone. Giving estrogens premenstrually delayed the onset of migraine but not menstruation (106). In contrast, progesterone administration delayed menstruation but did not prevent the migraine attack (107). Somerville concluded that estrogen withdrawal may trigger migraine attacks in susceptible women.

Migraine and Pregnancy

Migraine may worsen in the first trimester of pregnancy; many women become headache-free during later pregnancy, but 25% have no change (53, 108, 109). Menstrual migraine typically improves with pregnancy, perhaps due to sustained high estrogen levels (53, 108, 109).

Migraine and Menopause

The normal menopause results from depletion of follicles that can be stimulated to ovulation. Plasma sex steroid hormone levels are low, whereas gonadotropin levels are elevated. Migraine prevalence decreases with advancing age (22). However, at menopause, migraine can regress, worsen, or remain unchanged (110). Estrogen replacement therapy can exacerbate migraine (110, 111); paradoxically, estrogen alone (113) or with testosterone administration can relieve it (114).

There is no evidence that hysterectomy or oophorectomy is an effective or reasonable treatment of migraine at any age (115, 116).

Migraine and Oral Contraceptives (OCs)

Oral contraceptives (OC) most commonly used in the United States contain combinations of estrogen and progestin taken 21 days each month (117, 118). There is persistent controversy concerning the use of oral contraceptives in migraineurs and the risk of stroke (119). The Collaborative Group for the Study of Stroke in Young Women did not confirm reports that migraine may increase the risk of stroke in women using oral contraceptives but suggested that migraine, itself, may be a risk factor for stroke (120).

OCs can induce, change, or alleviate headache (119). OCs can trigger the first migraine attack, most often in women with a family history of migraine (111, 119, 121). Existing migraine may exacerbate, and headaches may occur on the days off the OC (110, 119, 121, 122). The headache pattern may become more severe and more frequent and may be associated with neurological symptoms (121–123). In most women, however, the headache pattern does not change, and some women may have a distinct improvement in headache (124, 125).

Studies from neurological or migraine clinics (111, 120–122) show an increased incidence and severity of migraine in OC users. Studies from contraceptive clinics and general practitioners are more favorable toward OCs (123–126).

Four double-blind placebo-controlled studies (Nilsson and Solvell (127), Goldzieher (128), Silbergeld (129), and Cullberg (130) showed no difference in headache incidence between OC and placebo. Both groups had a decreasing incidence of headache with continued duration of observation.

OCs may generate new headache or aggravate or ameliorate preexisting headache. These changes in the headache pattern and those that occur during menarche, menstruation, pregnancy, or menopause are related to changes in estrogen levels. These phenomena suggest a relationship between migraine headaches and changes in sex hormone levels in which hormones act as both triggers and modulators.

Other Triggers

Environmental factors including weather or temperature change, light glare, pungent odors, and high altitude can trigger migraine headache in a susceptible individual (85). Head and neck pain of another cause may trigger migraine. Physical exertion from exercise or sexual activity can act as a trigger for headache (62). Stress and anxiety, particularly the poststress letdown phase, and head trauma can precipitate a migraine headache (11, 62, 85).

DIFFERENTIAL DIAGNOSIS OF MIGRAINE

Migraine is a clinical diagnosis, which is made primarily on the history and less on the physical examination and laboratory tests. The temporal pattern of migraine and its associated features are extremely important in the differential diagnosis of headache. Lance (5) differentiates between the acute single headache and the recurrent headache, which are included in the differential diagnosis of migraine, and the subacute headache and the chronic daily headache, which are not.

Acute Single Headache

The first or worst attack of migraine may be very difficult to differentiate from a subarachnoid hemorrhage (SAH), particularly if the pain is of acute onset (thunderclap headache). The typical SAH associated with an acute-onset headache, stiff neck, and obtundation or coma is easily differentiated from migraine. However, Harling et al. (131) could not clinically differentiate between SAH and other benign headaches in patients presenting with the sudden onset of the worst headache of their lives (Table 9.17). Both the SAH and non-SAH groups had neck stiffness and photophobia, but the SAH group had more vomiting (72% vs 28%). An extensive neurological evaluation, including CT or MRI scan and lumbar puncture

Table 9.17.
Acute Onset Headache

Clinical Features: Subarachnoid Hemorrhage (SAH) and Non-SAH Groups[a]			
Feature	SAH ($n = 35$) (%)	Non-SAH ($n = 14$) (%)	
Headache less than 2 hours	1 (2.8)	0 (0)	N.S.
Severe headache after 2 hours	30 (86)	11 (79)	N.S.
Strenuous activity at onset	10 (28)	3 (21)	N.S.
Had to rest after onset	31 (88)	5 (36)	$P < .001$
Vomiting	25 (72)	4 (28)	$P < .02$
Neck stiffness	28 (80)	8 (57)	N.S.
Photophobia	20 (57)	9 (64)	N.S.
Mean blood pressure	114/85	117/83	N.S.
Previous headaches	15 (43)	4 (28)	N.S.

[a]From Harling DW, Peatfield RC, Van Hille PT, Abbott RJ. Thunderclap headache: is it migraine? Cephalalgia 1989;9:87–90.

(LP), is indicated in patients presenting with their first or worst headache, particularly if it is associated with focal neurological signs, stiff neck, or changes in cognition.

Raskin (74) has stated that all patients presenting with intense headache of sudden onset should be evaluated for a suspected aneurysm with angiography, even if the CT, MRI, and LP do not show evidence of a subarachnoid hemorrhage. Day and Raskin (74) reported a case of thunderclap headache in which angiography showed an aneurysm and arterial spasm despite a normal CT scan and bloodless CSF. However, several prospective studies have shown that thunderclap headache is usually benign in the absence of an abnormal neurological examination, CT, MRI, or CSF examination, if performed at the time of the ictus, and angiography is probably not necessary (131, 132).

Other causes of the acute single headache include encephalitis, meningitis, sinusitis, optic neuritis, glaucoma, systemic infection, or the first attack of migraine (5, 133, 134).

The diagnosis of meningitis or meningoencephalitis is not difficult in the presence of severe headache associated with a febrile illness, stiff neck, and changes in cognition. Under these circumstances, neuroimaging and lumbar puncture will confirm the diagnosis (133).

However, nonbacterial meningitis may be more difficult to diagnose. Patients may present with an episodic series of migraine-like headaches associated with sensory, motor, speech, and visual disturbances. Bartleson (135) reported 7 patients with new onset of migraine associated with a lymphocytic CSF pleocytosis, increased CSF protein, increased CSF pressure, and negative CSF cultures who probably had viral meningoencephalitis; similar cases have been described (136). The alternative explanation that an attack of migraine may produce an abnormal CSF is less probable in view of Kovac's (137) series of patients with normal CSF during migraine attacks.

Patients with acute purulent sinusitis are usually acutely ill and febrile, with localized pain and tenderness. This disorder is easy to diagnose except when it involves the sphenoid sinus (138).

Optic neuritis is associated with orbital pain and decreased visual acuity, which should lead to the appropriate diagnosis (139).

Acute glaucoma (140), particularly in the elderly, may be difficult to diagnose when orbital pain is associated with nausea, vomiting, and cognitive changes. The pupil may be nonreactive and the conjuctiva injected. Measurement of intraocular pressure is diagnostic.

Migraine-like headaches can be associated with systemic illness, particularly in patients predisposed to migraine (13). Significant hypertension (systolic BP >120) can produce headache. Since headache pain may raise the blood pressure, it may be difficult to decide what triggered the current headache (141).

Acute recurrent headaches are usually due to migraine or

tension-type headache; subarachnoid hemorrhage, cerebrovascular insufficiency, intermittent hydrocephalus, pheochromocytoma, trigeminal neuralgia, cluster headache, and pseudotumor cerebri are less common causes.

Migraine vs. Acute Tension-type Headache (Table 9.18). Tension-type headache, the most common headache type, occurs at any age, and is covered in more detail in Chapters 16 and 17. The pain is typically bilateral, dull, deep, or bandlike, mild to moderate in severity, not aggravated by exertion, and lasts from 30 minutes to 7 days. Associated symptoms may include anorexia, photophobia or phonophobia, and pericranial muscle tenderness (44). It may be extremely difficult to differentiate between migraine and acute tension-type headache, both clinically (1, 20, 142) and epidemiologically (13): both can recur and be of long duration; both can be bilateral, nonthrobbing, and of moderate severity; both can have associated anorexia, photophobia, and phonophobia. Classic migraine has an associated aura. Migraine with or without an aura may have nausea, vomiting, and diarrhea, symptoms not seen with tension-type headache. Migraine pain is moderate to severe in intensity, may be unilateral, and can be aggravated by movement (44). Both migraine and tension-type headache may be part of the same spectrum of benign headache, differing only in pain severity (11, 13, 141, 142).

Migraine vs. Chronic Tension-type Headache. Chronic tension-type headache is present for at least 15 days a month for at least 6 months. Most patients will have chronic daily headache, which clearly differentiates it from typical episodic migraine (44). The pain is similar to acute tension-type headache, but nausea, photophobia, or phonophobia may be present. Many of these patients have acute exacerbations of headache which fit the criteria for migraine. This used to be called mixed tension-vascular headache. These patients frequently have a history of episodic migraine that became transformed to chronic daily headache by analgesic or ergot overuse (43) (see Chapter 34).

Table 9.18.
Differentiating between Migraine and Acute Tension-type Headache

Characteristic	Common Migraine	Tension-type
Location	Unilateral or bilateral	Bilateral
Frequency	Intermittent	Intermittent
Duration	About 8 hours (2–72 hours)	Variable
Pain	Throbbing (50%)	Often bandlike
Severity	Moderate to severe	Mild to moderate
Associated symptoms	Nausea, vomiting, phonophobia	Uncommon
Sleep pattern	ND[a]	ND
Emotional status	ND	ND
Family history	Often present	Present
Allergy	ND	ND

[a]ND, not different from nonheadache controls.

Cluster vs. Migraine (Table 9.19)

Cluster headache is covered in detail in Chapters 22 and 23. Unlike migraine, cluster is a nonfamilial disorder predominantly affecting men. The attacks are briefer, most frequent, and strictly unilateral; they usually occur in clusters lasting weeks (except for chronic cluster) (44). The pain is excruciatingly severe and is frequently associated with unilateral autonomic signs (nasal stuffiness, lacrimation). There is no prodrome, aura, or postdrome and usually no associated gastrointestinal symptoms. Cluster patients are active during their attacks; migraineurs are passive.

There may be an overlap; attacks of migraine may be clustered or have features of both migraine and cluster.

Recurrent SAH, particularly if due to an arteriovenous malformation (AVM), may mimic migraine. Troost et al. (143) and Kattah and Luessehop (144) have described patients with an unruptured occipital lobe AVM who had bouts of migraine preceded by a visual aura and whose symptoms disappeared upon removal of the AVM. These patients did not have typical fortification spectra, but neither do all patients with classic migraine. Most patients will have signs and symptoms of their AVM or atypical features of migraine (145).

The headache associated with a TIA may simulate either acute tension-type headache or migraine (146). When no headache is present, it may simulate migraine without aura (58). The nature of the neurological symptoms, their rate of buildup, and the presence of typical migrainous features may help differentiate the two. Older patients with atypical features deserve extensive neurodiagnostic evaluation (58, 59).

Migraine-like headaches have been reported in patients with systemic lupus erythematosus (147) and in some cases were the presenting symptoms. Prolonged bouts of migraine have been associated with evidence of arteritis on angiography (148). Whether the vascular changes are due to migraine or whether both the migraine and the vascular changes are a result of a systemic or primary central nervous system arteritis is controversial (149).

Cerebral tumors can (rarely) present with a migraine-like headache unassociated with any focal signs or symptoms of increased cranial pressure for months, particularly in younger children (150). Zammarano et al. (151) found 5 patients who presented with migraine-like headaches among 2416 patients with brain tumors.

Idiopathic intracranial hypertension (152) (pseudotumor cerebri) may present with or without papilledema and may mimic either migraine or tension-type headache. Patients typically are obese women who may have a history of pulsatile tinnitus and may respond to standard antimigraine treatment. The diagnosis is confirmed by lumbar puncture after neuroimaging. In patients with papilledema the major concern is visual loss. In patients without papilledema the diagnosis is more difficult. Headache patients refractory to treatment may have increased intracranial pressure and may warrant neuroimaging and lumbar puncture.

Headache associated with paraoxysms of hypertension (141) can be diagnosed by the associated inordinate increase in blood pressure during the attack. Headaches associated with intermittent hydrocephalus may be associated with an enlarged head or changes in cognition during an attack.

Trigeminal neuralgia (153) is characterized by brief paroxysms of electric shock-like pain and a trigger point and is usually easily distinguishable from migraine. However, it may resemble the "icepick-like" headache that is frequently seen in migraineurs.

Patients with recurrent prodromes of migraine may be thought to have a primary psychological disorder or complex partial seizures. The association of the prodrome with headache should clarify the situation; sometimes prolonged EEG monitoring is needed (154).

Patients who have the aura of migraine but never develop the headache have been discussed under migraine without headache.

Migraine equivalents of childhood, hemiplegic migraine, and migrainous infarction are discussed elsewhere.

Patients with their first headache, particularly if it began during exertion, should be carefully evaluated for symptomatic organic causes. Other warning signs include associated fever, changes in cognition or alertness, stiff neck, focal neurological findings, or a patient who looks ill (131).

Table 9.19.
Differentiating between Migraine and Cluster Headache

Characteristics	Common Migraine	Cluster
Duration	Usually 4 to 24 hours	Brief, ½ to 1 hour
Frequency	Usually 2 to 5 times per month	Multiple daily attacks for several weeks
Sex	Majority female	Majority male
Age	Between 10 and 30	Onset in middle age
Preheadache	Often present	None
Associated disturbances	Present	None
Time of day	Any time	Frequently at night, same time each day
Behavior during attack	Rests in quiet dark room	Paces, bangs head

REFERENCES

1. McHenry LC. Garrison's history of neurology. Springfield: Charles C Thomas, 1969.
2. Bille B. Migraine in school children. Acta Paediatr Scand 1962;51(suppl 136):14–15.
3. Critchley M. Migraine: from Cappadocia to Queen Square. In: Smith R, ed. Background to migraine, vol 1. London: Heinemann, 1967.
4. Sachs O. Migraine: Understanding a common disorder. Berkeley: University of California Press, 1985.
5. Lance JW. Mechanism and management of headache. 4th ed. London: Butterworth Scientific, 1982.
6. Plant GT. The fortification spectra of migraine. Br Med J 1986;293:1613–1617.

7. Liveing E. On megrim, sick headache, and some allied disorders: a contribution to the pathology of nerve-storms. London: Churchill, 1873.
8. Dalessio DJ. Wolff's headache and other facial pain. 5th ed. New York: Oxford University Press, 1987.
9. Blau JN. Migraine pathogenesis: the neural hypothesis reexamined. J Neurol Neurosurg Psychiatry 1984;47:437–442.
10. Olesen J, Edvinsson L, eds. Basic mechanisms of headache. Amsterdam: Elsevier, 1988.
11. Raskin NH. Headache. 2nd ed. New York: Churchill Livingstone, 1988.
12. Welch KMA. Migraine. A behavioral disorder. Arch Neurol 1987;44:323–327.
13. Waters WE. Headache (series in clinical epidemiology). Littleton, MA: PSG Publishing, 1986.
14. Vahlquist B. Migraine in children. Int Arch Allergy 1955;7:348–352.
15. Selby G, Lance JW. Observations on 500 cases of migraine and allied vascular headache. J Neurol Neurosurg Psychiatry 1960;23:23–32.
16. Friedman AP, Finley KH, Graham JR. Classification of headache. Arch Neurol 1962;6:173–176.
17. World Federation of Neurology. In: Cochrane AL, ed. Background to migraine: third migraine symposium. London: Heinemann, 1970.
18. Waters WE. Headache and migraine in general practitioners, the migraine headache and dixarit. Proceedings of a symposium held at Churchill College. Cambridge: Boehringer Ingelheim Brachnell, 1972.
19. Waters WE, O'Connor PJ. Epidemiology of headache and migraine in women. J Neurol Neurosurg Psychiatry 1971;34:148–153.
20. Bakal DA. Psychobiology of chronic headache. New York: Springer, 1982.
21. Celentano DD, Stewart WF, Linet MS. The relationship of headache symptoms with severity and duration of attacks. J Clin Epidemiol 1990;43:983–994.
22. Goldstein M, Chen TC. The epidemiology of disabling headache. In: Critchley M, Friedman AP, Gorini S, Sicuteri F, et al. Advances in neurology, vol 33. New York: Raven Press, 1982.
23. Linet MS, Stewart WF. Migraine headache: epidemiologic perspectives. Epidemiol Rev 1984;6:107–139.
24. Bille B. Migraine in children: prevalence, clinical features, and a 30-year followup. In: Ferrari MD, Lataste X, eds. Migraine and other headaches. Parthenon, NJ, 1989.
25. Silberstein SD. Twenty questions about headaches in children and adolescents. Headache 1990;30:716–724.
26. Fry J. Profiles of disease. Edinburgh: Livingstone, 1966.
27. Merikangas, Angst J, Isler H. Migraine and psychopathology. Results of the Zurich cohort study of young adults. Arch Gen Psychiatry 1990;47:849–853.
28. Hockaday JM. Definitions, clinical features, and diagnosis of childhood migraine. In: Hockaday JM, ed. Migraine in children. London: Butterworth, 1988.
29. Geschwind N, Behan P. Left-handedness: association with immune disease, migraine, and developmental learning disorder. Proc Natl Acad Sci USA 1982;79:5097–5100.
30. Messinger HB, Messinger MI, Graham JR. Migraine and left-handedness: is there a connection? Cephalalgia 1988;8:237–244.
31. Brandt J, Celentano D, Stewart W, Linet M, Folstein MF. Personality and emotional disorder in a community sample of migraine headache sufferers. Am J Psychiatry 1990;147:303–308.
32. Sternbach RA, Dalessio DJ, Kunzel M, Bowman GE. MMPI patterns in common headache disorders. Headache 1980;20:311–315.
33. Invernizzi G, Gala C, Buono M, Cittone L, Tavola T, Conte G. Neurotic traits and disease duration in headache patients. Cephalalgia 1989;9:173–178.
34. Kudrow L, Sutkus GJ. MMPI pattern specificity in primary headache disorders. Headache 1979;19:18–24.
35. Weeks R, Baskin S, Sheftell F, Rapoport A, Arrowsmith F. A comparison of MMPI personality data and frontalis electromyographic readings in migraine and combination headache patients. Headache 1983;23:75–82.
36. Hooker WD, Raskin NH. Neuropsychologic alterations in classic and common migraine. Arch Neurol 1986;43:709–712.
37. Leijdekkers MLA, Passchier J, Goudswaart, Menges LJ, Jacobus FO. Migraine patients cognitively impaired? Headache 1990;30:352–358.
38. Dalsgaard-Nielson T. Migraine and heredity. Acta Neurol Scand 1965;41:287–300.
39. Montagna P, Galassi R, Medori R, et al. MELAS syndrome: characteristic migrainous and epileptic features and maternal transmission. Neurology 1988;38:751–754.
40. Roberts J, Cohrssen J. History of examination findings related to visual acuity among adults: United States, 1960–1962. Vital and Health Statistics, series 11, no. 28, Public Health Service Publication No. 1000. Washington, D.C.: U.S. Government Printing Office, 1968.
41. Ziegler DK. Headache. Public health problem Neurol Clin 1990;8:781–791.
42. Linet MS, Stewart WF, Celentano DD, Ziegler D, Sprecher M. An epidemiologic study of headache among adolescents and young adults. JAMA 1989;261:2211–2216.
43. Mathew NT, Reuveni U, Perez F. Transformed or evolutive migraine. Headache 1987;27:102–106.
44. Headache Classification Committee of the International Headache Society. Classification and diagnostic criteria for headache disorders, cranial neuralgia, and facial pain. Cephalalgia 1988;8(suppl 7):1–96.
45. Silberstein SD. Treatment of headache in primary care practice. Am J Med 1984;77(3A):65–72.
46. Ziegler DK, Hassanein RS. Specific headache phenomena: their frequency and coincidence. Headache 1990;30:152–156.
47. Whitty CWM. Migraine without headache. Lancet 1967;ii:283–285.
48. Barrie MA, Fox WR, Weatherall M, Wilkinson IP. Analysis of symptoms of patients with headaches and their response to treatment with ergot derivatives. Q J Med 1968;146:319–336.
49. Ziegler DK. The headache symptom: how many entities? Arch Neurol 1985;42:273–277.
50. Peatfield RC. Can transient ischemic attacks and classical migraine always be distinguished? Headache 1987;27:240–243.
51. Manzoni GC, Farina S, Lanfranchi M, Solari A. Classic migraine—clinical findings in 164 patients. Eur Neurol 1985;24:163–169.
52. Bickerstaff ER. Migraine variants and complications. In: Blau JN, ed. Migraine: clinical and research aspects. Baltimore: Johns Hopkins University Press, 1987.
53. Lance JW, Anthony M. Some clinical aspects of migraine. Arch Neurol 1966;15:356–361.
54. Slater R. Benign recurrent vertigo. J Neurol Neurosurg Psychiatry 1979;42:363–367.
55. Moretti G, Manzoni GC, Carrara D, Parma M. Benign recurrent vertigo and its connection to migraine. Headache 1980;20:344–346.
56. Kuritzky A, Ziegler KE, Hassanein R. Vertigo, motion sickness and migraine. Headache 1981;21:227–231.
57. Levy DE. Transient CNS deficits: a common, benign syndrome in young adults. Neurology 1988;38:831–836.
58. Fisher CM. Late-life migraine accompaniments as a cause of unexplained transient ischemic attacks. Can J Neurol Sci 1980;7:9–17.
59. Fisher CM. Late-life migraine accompaniments—further experience. Stroke 1986;17:1033–1042.
60. Hosking G. Special forms: variants of migraine in childhood. In: Hockaday JM, ed. Migraine in childhood. London: Butterworths, 1988.
61. Hansen SL, Borelli-Miller L, Strange P, Nielsen BM, Olesen J. Ophthalmoplegic migraine: diagnostic criteria, incidence of hospitalization and possible etiology. Acta Neurol Scand 1990;81:54–60.

62. Blau JN. Adult migraine: the patient observed. In: Blau JN, ed. Migraine: clinical and research aspects. Baltimore: Johns Hopkins University Press, 1987.

63. Blau JN. Migraine prodromes separated from the aura: complete migraine. Br Med J 1980;281:658–660.

64. Blau JN. Clinical characteristics of premonitory symptoms in migraine. In: Amery WK, Wauquier A, eds. The prelude to the migraine attack. London: Bailliere Tindall, 1986.

65. Amery WK, Waelkens J, Vandenbergh V. Migraine warnings. Headache 1986;26:60–66.

66. Isler H. Frequency and time course of premonitory phenomena. In: Amery WK, Wauquier A, eds. The prelude to the migraine attack. London: Bailliere Tindall, 1986.

67. Amery WK, Waelkens J, Caers I. Dopaminergic mechanisms in premonitory phenomena. In: Amery WK, Wauquier A, eds. The prelude to the migraine attack. London: Bailliere Tindall, 1986.

68. Waelkens J, Caers I, Amery WK. Effects of therapeutic measures taken during the premonitory phase. In: Amery WK, Wauquier A, eds. The prelude to the migraine attack. London: Bailliere Tindall, 1986.

69. Jensen K, Tfelt-Hansen P, Lauritzen M, Olesen J. Classic migraine: a prospective recording of symptoms. Acta Neurol Scand 1986;73:359–362.

70. Hupp SL, Kline LB, Corbett JJ. Visual disturbances of migraine. Surv Ophthalmol 1989;33:221–236.

71. Wilkinson M. Clinical features of migraine. In: Rose FC, ed. Handbook of clinical neurology, vol 4. New York: Elsevier, 1986.

72. Hachinski VCC, Porchawka J, Steele JC. Visual symptoms in the migraine syndrome. Neurology 1973;23:570–579.

73. Olesen J. Some clinical features of the acute migraine attack. An analysis of 750 patients. Headache 1978;18:268–271.

74. Day JW, Raskin NH. Thunderclap headache: symptom of unruptured cerebral aneurysm. Lancet 1986;334:1247–1248.

75. Peatfield RC, Bond RA, Rose FC. Do migrainous headaches become more consistently lateralized? Cephalalgia 1987;7:73–75.

76. Drummond PD, Lance JW. Clinical diagnosis and computer analysis of headache symptoms. J Neurol Neurosurg Psychiatry 1984;47:128–133.

77. Raskin NH, Schwartz RK. Icepick-like pain. Neurology 1980;30:203–205.

78. Volans GN. Research review: migraine and drug absorption. Clin Pharmacokinet. 1978;3:313–318.

79. Boyle R, Behan PO, Sutton JA. A correlation between severity of migraine and delayed emptying measured by an epigastric impedance method. Br J Clin Pharmacol 1990;30:405–409.

80. Silberstein SD, Silberstein MM. New concepts in the pathogenesis of migraine headache. Pain Management 1990;3:297–302.

81. Solomon GD. Migrainous periorbital ecchymosis [Abstract]. Headache 1989;29:328.

82. Drummond PD. A quantitative assessment of photophobia in migraine and tension headache. Headache 1986;26:465–469.

83. Silberstein SD, Merriam G. Estrogen, progestogens, and headache. Neurology 1991;41:786–793.

84. Blau JN. Resolution of migraine attacks: sleep and the recovery phase. J Neurol Neurosurg Psychiatry 1982;45:223–226.

85. denBergh VV, Amery WK, Waelkens J. Trigger factors in migraine: a study conducted by the Belgian Migraine Society. Headache 1987;27:191–196.

86. Peatfield RC. Pathophysiology and precipitants of migraine. In: Hockaday JM, ed. Migraine in childhood. London: Butterworths, 1988.

87. Royal College of Physicians and the British Nutrition Foundation. Food intolerance and food aversion. J R Coll Physicians Lond 1984;18:83–123.

88. Bix KJ, Pearson DJ, Bentley SJ. A psychiatric study of patients with supposed food allergy. Br J Psychiatry 1984;145:121–126.

89. Raskin NH. Chemical headaches. Annu Rev Med 1981;32:63–71.

90. Bayless TM, Rothfeld B, Massa C, Wise L, Paige D, Bedine MS. Lactose and milk intolerance: clinical implications. N Engl J Med 1975;292:1156–1159.

91. Schaumberg HH, Byck R, Gerstl R, Mashman JH. Monosodium L-glutamate: its pharmacology and role in the Chinese restaurant syndrome. Science 1969;163:826–828.

92. Koehler SM, Glaros A. The effect of aspartame on migraine headache. Headache 1988;28:10–13.

93. Schiffman SS, Buckley CE, Sampson HA, et al. Aspartame and susceptibility to headache. N Engl J Med 1987;317:1181–1185.

94. Littlewood JT, Glover V, Davies PTG, Gibb C, Sandler M, Rose FC. Red wine as a cause of migraine. Lancet 1988;338:558–559.

95. Egger J, Wilson J, Carter CM, Turner MW, Soothill JF. Is migraine food allergy? Lancet 1983;ii:865–869.

96. MacDonald A, Forsythe I, Wall C. Dietary treatment of migraine. In: Lanzi G, Balottin U, Cernibori A, eds. Headache in children and adolescents. The Netherlands: Elsevier, 1989.

97. Moffett AM, Swash M, Scott DF. Effect of chocolate: a double-blind study. J Neurol Neurosurg. Psychiatry 1974;37:445–448.

98. Ferguson A. Food sensitivity or self-deception? N Engl J Med 1990;323:476.

99. Jewett DL, Fein G, Greenberg MH. A double-blind study of symptom provocation to determine food sensitivity. N Engl J Med 1990;323:429–433.

100. Epstein MT, Hockaday JM, Hockaday TDR. Migraine and reproductive hormones throughout the menstrual cycle. Lancet 1975;i:543–548.

101. Diagnostic and statistical manual of mental disorders. 3rd ed-rev. Washington, DC: American Psychiatric Association, 1987.

102. Davies PTG, Eccles NK, Steiner TJ, Leathard HL, Rose FC. Plasma oestrogen, progesterone and sex-hormone binding globulin levels in the pathogenesis of migraine. Cephalalgia 1989;9(suppl 10):143.

103. Solbach P, Sargent J, Coyne L. Menstrual migraine headache: results of a controlled, experimental, outcome study of non-drug treatments. Headache 1984;24:75–78.

104. Nattero G. Menstrual headache. In: Critchley M, ed. Advances in neurology, vol 33. New York: Raven Press, 1982.

105. Facchinetti F, Sances, G, Volpe A, et al. Hypothalamus pituitary-ovarian axis in menstrual migraine: effects of dihydroergotamine retard prophylactic treatment. Cephalalgia Suppl 1983;1:159–162.

106. Somerville BW. The role of estradiol withdrawal in the etiology of menstrual migraine. Neurology 1972;22:355–365.

107. Somerville BW. The role of progesterone in menstrual migraine. Neurology 1971;21:853–859.

108. Somerville BW. A study of migraine in pregnancy. Neurology 1972;22:824–828.

109. Ratinahirana H, Darbois Y, Bousser MG. Migraine and pregnancy: a prospective study in 703 women after delivery. Neurology 1990;40:437.

110. Whitty CWM, Hockaday JM. Migraine: a follow-up study of 92 patients. Br Med J. 1986;1:735–736.

111. Kudrow L. The relationship of headache frequency to hormone dose in migraine. Headache 1975;15:36–49.

112. Aylward M, Holly F, Parker RJ. An evaluation of clinical response to piperazine oestrone sulphate (Harmogen) in menopausal patients. Curr Med Res Opin 1974;2:417–423.

113. Martin PL, Burnier AM, Segre EJ, Huix FJ. Graded sequential therapy in the menopause: a double-blind study. Am J Obstet Gynecol 1971;111:178–186.

114. Greenblatt RB, Bruneteau DW. Menopausal headache—psychogenic or metabolic? J Am Geriatr Soc 1974;283:186–190.

115. Utian WH. Oestrogen, headache and oral contraceptives. S Afr Med J 1974;48:2105–2108.

116. Alvarez WC. Can one cure migraine in women by inducing menopause? Report on forty-two cases. Mayo Clin Proc 1940;15:380–382.

117. Wentz AC. Contraception and family planning. In: Jones HW, Wentz AC, Burnett LS, eds. Novak's textbook of gynecology. 11th ed. Baltimore: Williams & Wilkins, 1985.

118. Derman R. Oral contraceptives: a reassessment. Obstet Gynecol Surv 1989;44:662–668.

119. Bickerstaff ER. Neurological complications of oral contraceptives. Oxford: Clarendon Press, 1975.

120. Collaborative Group for the Study of Stroke in Young Women. Oral contraceptives and stroke in young women. JAMA 1975;231:718–722.

121. Ryan RE. A controlled study of the effect of oral contraceptives on migraine. Headache 1978;17:250–252.

122. Phillips BM. Oral contraceptive drugs and migraine. Br Med J 1968;2:99.

123. Dalton K. Migraine and oral contraceptives. Headache 1976;15:247–251.

124. Whitty CWM, Hockaday JM, Whitty MM. The effect of oral contraceptives on migraine. Lancet 1966;i:856–859.

125. Larsson-Cohn U, Lundberg PO. Headache and treatment with oral contraceptives. Acta Neurol Scand 1970;46:267–278.

126. Herzberg BN, Draper KC, Johnson AL, Nicol GC. Oral contraceptives, depression, and libido. Br Med J 1971;3:495–300.

127. Nilsson L, Solvell L. Clinical studies on oral contraceptives—a randomized, double-blind, crossover study of 4 different preparations (Anovlar mite, Lyndiol mite, Ovulen, and Volidan). Acta Obstet Gynecol Scand 1967;46(suppl 8):3–31.

128. Goldzieher JW, Moses LE, Averkin E, Scheel C, Taber BZ. A placebo-controlled double-blind crossover investigation of the side effects attributed to oral contraceptives. Fertil Steril 1971;22:609–623.

129. Silbergeld S, Brast N, Noble EP. The menstrual cycle. a double-blind study of symptoms, mood and behavior, and biochemical variables using enovid and placebo. Psychosom Med 1971;33:411–428.

130. Cullberg J. Mood changes and menstrual symptoms with different gestagen/estrogen combinations: a double blind comparison with a placebo. Acta Psychiatr Scand Suppl 1972;236:259–276.

131. Harling DW, Peatfield RC, Van Hille PT, Abbott RJ. Thunderclap headache: is it migraine? Cephalalgia 1989;9:87–90.

132. Wijdicks EFM, Kerkhoff H, Van Gign J. Long-term follow-up of 71 patients with thunderclap headache mimicking subarachnoid hemorrhage. Lancet 1988;ii:68–70.

133. Edmeads J. Emergency management of headache. Headache 1988;28:675–679.

134. Fodden DI, Peatfield RC, Milson PL. Beware the patient with a headache in the accident and emergency department. Arch Emerg Med 1989;6:7–12.

135. Bartleson JD, Swanson JW, Whisnat JP. A migrainous syndrome with cerebrospinal fluid pleocytosis. Neurology 1981;31:1257–1262.

136. Stamboulis E, Spengos M, Rombos A, Heidemenos A. Aseptic inflammatory meningeal reaction manifesting as a migrainous syndrome. Headache 1987;27:439–441.

137. Kovacs K, Bors L, Tothfalugi L, et al. Cerebrospinal fluid (CSF) investigations in migraine. Cephalalgia 1939;9:53–57.

138. Lew D, Southwick FS, Montgomery WW, Weber AL, Baker AS. Sphenoid sinusitis: a review of 30 cases. N Engl J Med 1983;19:1149–1154.

139. Cogan DG. Neurology of the visual system. Springfield IL, Charles C Thomas, 1967.

140. Adler FH. Textbook of ophthalmology. 7th ed. Philadelphia: WB Saunders, 1963.

141. Edmeads J. Headache in cerebrovascular disease. In: Rose CF, ed. Handbook of clinical neurology, vol 4 (48): Headache. Amsterdam: Elsevier, 1986.

142. Featherstone HJ. Migraine and muscle contraction headaches: a continuum. Headache 1985;24:194–198.

143. Troost BT, Mark LE, Maroon JC. Resolution of classic migraine after removal of an occipital lobe AVM. Ann Neurol 1979;5:199–201.

144. Kattah JC, Luessehop AJ. Resolution of classic migraine after removal of an occipital lobe AVM. Ann Neurol 1980;7(1):93.

145. Troost BT, Newton TH. Occipital lobe arteriovenous malformations. Arch Ophthalmol 1975;93:250–256.

146. Portenoy RD, Abissi CJ, Lipton RB, et al. Headache in cerebrovascular disease. Stroke 1984;15:1009–1012.

147. Omdal R, Mellgren I, Husby G. Clinical neuropsychiatric and neuromuscular manifestations in systemic lupus erythematosus. Scand J Rheumatol 1988;17:113–117.

148. Dukes HT, Vieth RG. Cerebral arteriography during migraine prodrome and headache. Neurology 1964;14:636–639.

149. Serdaru M, Chiras J, Cujas M, Lhermitte F. Isolated benign cerebral vasculitis or migrainous vasospasm? J Neurol Neurosurg Psychiatry 1984;47:73–76.

150. Rushton JG, Rooke ED. Brain tumor headache. Headache 1962;2:147–152.

151. Zammarano CB, D'Ancona ML, Miceli MC. Headache and cerebral neoplasm in childood. In: Lanzi G, Balottin U, Cernibori A, eds. Headache in children and adolescents. The Netherlands: Elsevier, 1989.

152. Marcelis J, Silberstein SD. Idiopathic intracranial hypertension without papilledema. Arch Neurol (In press) 1991;48:392–399.

153. Maxwell RE. Clinical diagnosis of trigeminal neuralgia and differential diagnosis of facial pain. In: Rovit RL. Murali R, Jannetta PJ, eds. Trigeminal neuralgia. Baltimore: Williams & Wilkins, 1990.

154. Andermann F, Lugaresi E. Migraine and epilepsy. Boston: Butterworths, 1987.

155. Spierings ELH. The pathogenesis of the migraine aura: an overview. In: Amery WK, Wauquier A, eds. The prelude to the migraine attack. Philadelphia: Bailliere Tindall, 1986.

10

Pathophysiology of Migraine

J. DAVID GILLIES and JAMES W. LANCE

Migraine is a disorder with a diversity of symptoms. Any account of its pathophysiology should explain all the symptoms of migraine with aura (classical migraine), as well as such phenomena as the vague premonitory symptoms, unilateral and alternating headache, nausea, and other associated gastrointestinal symptoms. Further, the action of drugs both in precipitating and controlling headache and other symptoms should be in accord with the proposed mechanisms. In 1963, Wolff (1) summarized clinical and experimental work to that time, concluding that the preheadache phenomena of migraine were associated with cerebral vasoconstriction; the headache phase with increased pulsation and vasodilatation of the cranial arteries, chiefly the external carotid arteries; and that intracranial vasodilatation may occur. This classical view has been partly confirmed and expanded and partly negated.

PAIN-SENSITIVE STRUCTURES IN THE HEAD

Ray and Wolff (2) and Penfield and McNaughton (3) studied the pain sensitivity of the intracranial structures in man. The cerebral arteries at the base of the brain, the dural arteries, the large venous sinuses and their tributary veins from the brain surface, and some parts of the dura at the base of the brain are pain sensitive. The brain tissue itself, most of the pia, arachnoid, and dura, and the cranium, including the emissary and diploic veins, are not sensitive.

Supratentorial structures are innervated by the trigeminal nerve (3–5). The ophthalmic division innervates the tentorium and posterior falx via the intracranial tentorial nerve, and the anterior falx and anterior cranial fossa via meningeal branches entering through the cribriform plate. The mandibular division innervates the anterior middle fossa and sphenoidal ridge via the intracranial middle meningeal branch accompanying the middle meningeal artery. Nervus spinosis, an extracranial branch of the mandibular nerve, enters through the foramen spinosum and innervates the dura of the middle fossa and lateral convexity. Infratentorial structures are innervated by branches of the facial, glossopharyngeal, and vagus nerves, and the upper three cervical segments (6).

Pain from the scalp and galea is sharply localized,

whereas pain from the pial arteries is diffuse and referred to the ipsilateral temporal, frontal, and retroorbital regions. Pain from the anterior fossa is referred to the retroorbital region, the middle fossa to the frontal, retroorbital, and temporal regions, the falx to the temporal-parietal and frontal regions, and the superior surface of the tentorium and adjacent sinuses to the forehead and retroorbital region (2, 3).

INNERVATION OF CRANIAL BLOOD VESSELS

Noradrenaline

There is a plexus of noradrenaline-containing nerve fibers around the arteries, and to a lesser extent the veins, at the base of the brain (7, 8). Most of these fibers originate in the ipsilateral superior cervical ganglion (9) and probably play a part in adjusting the range of arterial pressure in which autoregulation takes place. The vasoconstrictor response of pial blood vessels is dependent on the presence of adequate calcium ions (10, 11) and is blocked by α-adrenoreceptor blockers (8).

Neuropeptide Y

A rich supply of nerve fibers containing neuropeptide Y arises from the superior cervical ganglion and parallels the distribution of noradrenergic fibers (12, 13). The vasoconstrictive effect of this peptide is not antagonized by α-adrenoreceptor blocking agents (12).

Acetylcholine

A network of acetylcholinesterase-containing fibers, originating in the sphenopalatine ganglion (14) surrounds the large vessels at the base of the brain (15). Activation of muscarinic receptors produces relaxation (15).

Serotonin (5-HT)

There are at least 3 types of 5-HT receptor identified by binding studies (16). In the cranial circulation, cerebral arteries have mainly 5-HT1, the superficial temporal arteries mainly 5-HT2, whereas the middle meningeal has all three types (17). Numerous 5-HT-containing fibers surround pial blood vessels, which originate in part from the median and dorsal raphe nuclei in the midbrain, since there is a major reduction in vessel 5-HT after lesions of these nuclei (18–20). 5-HT produces constriction of vessels.

Vasoactive Intestinal Peptide (VIP)

Fibers containing VIP are found in the walls of vessels in the circle of Willis (14, 21–23), and these fibers mostly originate in the sphenopalatine ganglion. Some VIP immunoreactive fibers that innervate pial arterioles on the cortical surface may originate from cortical VIP neurones (24). VIP causes relaxation of pial arterioles (21, 25).

Calcitonin Gene-related Peptide (CGRP)

Fine nerve fibers containing CGRP surround major cerebral arteries, pial arterioles, and veins (26). The trigeminal ganglion contains many cell bodies containing CGRP and section of the trigeminal nerve results in the loss of CGRP immunoreactivity in the pial vessel (26), suggesting that most, if not all, CGRP innervation of the pial vessels is from the trigeminal nerve. CGRP is a potent dilator of cerebral arteries and pial arterioles (27, 28), but, in contrast to substance P; has little effect on pial veins (29).

Substance P (SP)

SP is probably the peptide involved in transmitting nociceptive information to the central nervous system. In man, SP-containing fibers course though the spinal nucleus of the trigeminal nerve (30). Sensory ganglia contain SP (31, 32), and section of the trigeminal ganglion causes loss of SP from the network of fibers surrounding pial arteries (33–36). Dural arterioles (37) and extracerebral cranial vessels (38) also have SP innervation. SP produces relaxation of cat and human cerebral arteries (37).

EXTRACRANIAL BLOOD FLOW STUDIES

Graham and Wolff (39) reported that compression of the carotid artery reduced the pain of migraine and that pain relief by ergotamine was accompanied by reduction in the pulsation of the superficial temporal artery. Recent studies have found that digital compression of the superficial temporal artery or occluding the scalp circulation with a blood pressure cuff relieved the pain of migraine in less than half of the patients studied (40, 41). During scalp compression, shaking or nodding the head augmented the pain, suggesting that the pain of the headache was arising from intracranial structures sensitive to movement (40). Compression of the carotid artery may relieve pain in a few additional subjects who do not respond to digital compression (41), but a significant group of patients had no relief from any form of arterial compression.

Earlier reports (42) suggested that the pulse amplitude of the superficial temporal artery was higher in migrainous subjects and that it increased during headache. Later attempts to replicate these findings gave conflicting results

(43–45). More recently, Drummond and Lance (41) have shown a significant increase in pulsation of the frontal branch of the superficial temporal area during headache, but only in subjects in whom the pain was relieved by digital compression of the artery.

Blood flow in the temporal muscles is normal during migraine (46), and orthostatic regulation is unchanged (47). Ocular blood flow is also unchanged (48). Flow is reduced in dilated conjunctival vessels (42, 49), but this dilatation is seen only in some subjects (50).

Cutaneous blood flow has been studied indirectly by thermography. Earlier studies suggested lower forehead temperatures ipsilateral to the headache (51, 52) or no significant difference (53). More extensive studies (54, 55) have shown a higher temperature in the temporal region during the headache phase on the side of the headache, particularly in subjects whose pain was relieved by superficial temporal artery compression.

From these studies it can be concluded that distension of cerebral blood vessels by normal blood pressure and flow is the factor determining whether a subject experiences pain in no more than half of migrainous patients. This does not negate the possibility that the pain may be arising from blood vessels, but it implies that pain is not induced solely by distension of the extracranial vessels. In a proportion of patients, the site of the pain may be of intracranial or neural origin rather than arising in the scalp vessels.

REGIONAL CEREBRAL BLOOD FLOW IN MIGRAINE
Migrainous Aura

During migraine with aura, there is a unilateral reduction in cerebral blood flow (56). This finding was supported by reports of both focal and global reductions in flow. With the introduction of high-resolution scintillation cameras, all changes have been found to be focal (57–59). Initially, there is a focal reduction in blood flow at the occipital pole. The area of reduced flow spreads gradually forward, progressively involving a greater area of the cerebral cortex. Characteristically, this spreading oligemia advances at a rate of 2 to 3 mm per minute (57), spreading along the cortex. A second focus of low flow commonly appears in the frontal region (58) and spreads at the same rate in all directions. Usually, the cortex in the region of the central sulcus is spared (58). Once initiated, the reduction in blood flow does not follow the distribution of cerebral arteries, and when angiography was performed at the same time as the flow was reduced, occlusion or vasospasm was not observed (60–62). However, these authors observed some retrograde flow of the contrast agent in the basilar artery, suggesting that there was vasoconstriction in the carotid territory although such constriction could not be observed on an angiogram.

Several variations in the nature of the cerebral blood flow changes have been noted. Focal hyperemia preceding the oligemia has been reported in several patients (57, 63), and three patients are reported in whom the focal oligemia originated only in the frontal lobe (63). In none of these patients did the aura involve visual symptoms.

Headache Phase of Migraine with Aura

In most patients studied, the headache has started during the phase of oligemia (57, 59, 64). The period of oligemia may be followed by hyperemia in the areas that previously had low flow. Gulliksen and Enevoldsen (65) observed focal hyperemia 24 hours after migraine with aura. This hyperemia may start as early as 3 to 6 hours after the onset of oligemia (66). These changes appear to be a reactive hyperemia and not related to the headache. Whether the hyperemia accounts for the tiredness and "washed-out" feeling that commonly follows migraine is difficult to prove.

Migraine without Aura

During migraine without aura (common migraine), focal spreading oligemia has not been demonstrated (60, 64, 67, 68). Whether there is any change in cerebral blood flow is a matter of conjecture. Twenty-two patients studied during common migraine have been reported by three groups (64, 67, 68), using 133Xe, SPECT, and PET techniques, without any significant change in cerebral blood flow being demonstrated. Other authors (60, 69) have reported increased blood flow, but in many of these subjects, headache was not present at the time, suggesting that these changes are not related to the pain of the headache. Sakai and Meyer (69) have reported a reduced responsiveness to CO_2 during the headache phase, followed by a period of increased response.

Some of these authors also reported minimal hyperemia during the headache phase. There is one report of reduced flow during common migraine (70). The area was small and did not spread.

Transient Ischemia

Focal spreading oligemia has been reported in patients who have had transient ischemic attacks (71). In these patients the oligemia was induced by angiography or by an intra-carotid injection for the blood flow study, precipitating events similar to the studies of migrainous aura. The symptoms present at the time were similar to those of the previous episode, suggesting that the previously ischemic area was unduly susceptible to precipitating focal spreading oligemia. It is interesting to note that the initial site of the two foci of initial low flow in migraine with aura (58) was in the "watershed" areas between the cortex supplied by the middle cerebral artery and that supplied by the anterior and posterior cerebral arteries, areas commonly involved in cerebral infarction.

In can be concluded that spreading focal oligemia is a feature of migraine with aura, is due to vasoconstriction at the arteriolar level, and is probably responsible for the aura

of migraine but not the ensuing pain. Hyperemic changes are probably reactionary and not related to headache.

SPREADING CORTICAL DEPRESSION

Lashley (72) carefully timed and plotted the position of scintillating scotomas during his migrainous aura. By relating the position of the scotoma to the topographic organization of the visual cortex, he explained the phenomenon as a wave of excitation followed by a longer-lasting inhibition spreading across the cortex at 3 mm per minute. Leão (73) observed that, in the rabbit, cortical neuronal activity may cease suddenly after a minor cortical injury and recover after a few minutes. This cessation of activity spread slowly across the cortex at a rate of 2 to 5 mm per minute, during which time the EEG was markedly depressed. These changes were accompanied by a large negative potential in the affected region (74). A number of biochemical changes have been found during cortical spreading depression in the rat and cat, involving both neurones and neuroglia with calcium, sodium, and chloride entering the cells and potassium and hydrogen ions leaving the cells (75, 76).

In human subjects, negative potential changes have been elicited by injection of KCl into the temporal lobe of patients undergoing surgery for epilepsy (77).

EEG in Migraine

There are many studies of the EEG in migrainous subjects (see review (78)). Nonspecific changes have been reported during the headache-free phase. During the aura, transient slow waves may be seen, usually in the appropriate cortical area. Numerous minor abnormalities are documented in the visual evoked responses. These changes probably reflect no more than minor dysfunction consistent with spreading oligemia. The EEG changes of cortical spreading depression have not been observed in humans undergoing neurosurgical procedures (79), but the spatial resolution of scalp surface EEG may be inadequate to detect the area of change.

The hypothesis, that cortical spreading depression is the mechanism underlying focal spreading oligemia and thus the migrainous aura, is logical but unproven. Several factors support this contention. The duration of oligemia is much longer than that of the migrainous aura, but the duration of the changes in neural activity in the visual cortex of rabbit and cat (73, 80) approximates that of the migrainous aura. Changes in vascular reactivity during focal spreading oligemia, reduced response to CO_2 with normal autoregulation (58, 69, 81, 82), are very similar to those of spreading cortical depression (75, 83).

Possible Role of Serotonin

Over a number of years, evidence has accumulated that changes in serotonin (5-hydroxytryptamine, 5-HT) are associated with migraine. Sicuteri (84) found an excess of the 5-HT metabolite 5-hydroxyindoleacetic acid in the urine during headache. Curran et al. (85) confirmed this rise and showed that there was a drop in platelet serotonin during migraine. A low-molecular-weight releasing factor has been identified in the plasma during headache (86–89), and increased free serotonin has been demonstrated in the plasma during migraine (90). Indirect evidence also suggests that 5-HT is involved in the migrainous process. Reserpine, which releases serotonin, induces a typical headache only in migrainous subjects (86, 91), and the headache is relieved by the intravenous infusion of 5-HT. Methysergide and pizotifen, which are effective prophylactic agents for migraine, are both 5-HT$_2$ antagonists. Sumatriptan, a selective 5-HT$_1$ agonist, is effective in controlling both the pain of the headache and the associated nausea and vomiting (92, 93). The control of pain is dose-related and lasts until the drug level drops. Since Sumatriptan does not cross the blood-brain barrier, its site of action may be on the cranial blood vessels. Whether this represents a direct interference with the migrainous process or simply negates the effect of the migrainous process on terminal pain-sensitive organs is not clear.

NEURAL MECHANISMS

Many symptoms associated with migraine are difficult to explain on the basis of extracranial vascular change or spreading focal oligemia. Premonitory symptoms, occurring 1 to 24 hours (average 10) before the headache, independent of aura, are reported by about half of migrainous subjects, but not necessarily with each headache (54, 94, 95). Irritability or withdrawal, tiredness, yawning, and craving for food are common and suggest a hypothalamic origin (96). Tests of hypothalamic and pituitary function are normal in patients with migraine, but the "triple test" increases prolactin production more in migraineurs than in normals (97), a phenomenon that would be consistent with depressed dopaminergic or increased serotinergic activity. Increased sensitivity of dopaminergic receptors has been suggested because dopamine agonists, such as bromocriptine, cause nausea and postural hypotension more readily in migraineurs. Photophobia, phonophobia, and sensitivity to smell and touch suggest a cerebral phenomenon.

There is an increased propensity for migrainous subjects to experience trigeminal pain. Sudden pain on ingesting ice cream or a cold drink, "ice cream headache" (98), or sudden jabs of pain in the head, "ice-pick pains" (99), are more common in migrainous subjects and tend to be referred to the habitual site of headache (54). The symptoms suggest hyperexcitability in a part of the trigeminal system. The mechanism by which severe headache is limited to one side of the head suggests neural involvement, even if vasodilatation can be demonstrated. For these reasons, hypotheses of the mechanism of migraine have recently focused on the neural control of blood flow and the central pathways of pain.

Trigeminovascular Reflex

Activity in the trigeminal nerve results in a variety of reflex vascular events. Flushing of the face occurs during ablation of the trigeminal ganglion in man, with both thermocoagulation (100, 101) and alcohol injection (102). Increase in skin temperature and capillary dilatation has been observed in the distribution of the division being ablated (41), and substance P and calcitonin gene-related peptide increase in the external jugular artery at this time (103). Extravasation of plasma occurred around vessels in the pia when the trigeminal nerve of the rat was stimulated, and this response was blocked by both ergotamine and Sumatriptan (104, 105). Stimulation of the trigeminal ganglion in the cat increases blood flow in the external carotid artery (106). This reflex response transverses the trigeminal nerve to the brain stem; the efferent limb is the greater superficial (GSP) petrosal nerve, then the pterygopalatine (sphenopalatine) and otic ganglia. The terminal transmitter is VIP (107). Autoradiographic techniques, using iodo[^{14}C]antipyrine, have demonstrated that cerebral blood flow is also increased bilaterally in the frontal and parietal cortex (108). Stimulation of the superior sagittal sinus also induces vasodilatation (108). The efferent limb for reflex dilatation is the GSP branch of the facial nerve, relaying in small ganglia near the carotid artery or turning back from the pterygopalatine ganglion via the deep petrosal nerve to the internal carotid plexus (109).

These vascular changes raise the question of which comes first, the vascular changes? or pain with secondary vascular changes? In either case, there is the possibility of a positive feedback mechanism if vasodilatation evokes nociceptive input to the trigeminal system.

Brainstem Control of Cranial Blood Flow

The locus coeruleus (LC), in the floor of the upper part of the fourth ventricle, contains 97% of the brain noradrenaline (110). Its axons project diffusely to the forebrain, terminating in relation to small intraparenchymal vessels. Electrical stimulation of the LC in the monkey induces a frequency-dependent vasoconstriction in the internal carotid territory (111) with a mean of 20% reduction in blood flow, maximal in the occipital region (112). When the frequency of stimulation is progressively increased above 10 Hz, the intracerebral hyperemia progressively lessens, and there is then a progressive increase in flow in the external carotid circulation. This increase in flow is mediated by the same efferents as the trigeminovascular reflex, that is, the GSP branch of the facial nerve, through the sphenopalatine and otic ganglia (113), with VIP as the transmitter causing vasodilatation (107).

Dorsal Raphe Nucleus

The raphe nuclei in the midbrain are serotonergic. They project to the brainstem, to both dendrites and small blood vessels (114, 115), and to cortical blood vessels (18, 19).

Electrical stimulation of the dorsal raphe nucleus in the monkey produces vasodilatation in both internal and external carotid circulations (116). These effects were not mediated by sympathetic activity, since they are unaffected by cervical sympathectomy or cord section (116). In the cat, the extracranial response is mediated by the facial nerve (GSP) pathway (107). The response was attenuated by depletion of central serotonin (108).

Neuropeptides in Migraine

Goadsby and coworkers (103) reported that calcitonin gene-related peptide (CGRP) and VIP (117) were elevated in external jugular venous blood during the headache of migraine, whether or not there was an aura. This peptide, as well as substance P (SP) and VIP, is found in the extracerebral vessels (103). Electrical stimulation of the trigeminal ganglion, both in man and cat, leads to an increase in extracerebral blood flow and to the release of both CGRP and SP (103). In the cat, VIP is also released (107) by trigeminal stimulation. Stimulation of the superior sagittal sinus has also been shown to release CGRP and SP (118). These findings suggest that migraine is intimately associated with vasodilator peptides, and that these peptides are released in response to trigeminal activation.

GENERAL HYPOTHESIS

Any pathophysiological hypothesis to explain a complex clinical phenomenon is no more than an aggregation and logical ordering of clinical and experimental data. It is essentially ephemeral, since those data on which it must be based are being continually expanded and refined. Nevertheless, a coherent ordering of facts is valuable to the clinician in providing a logical framework for managing the disorder and to the investigator in determining areas for further research. At the center of the current hypothesis of the mechanism of the pain of migraine is the trigeminovascular reflex. This is inherently an unstable reflex, in that trigeminal activation produces vasodilatation in the area supplied by the trigeminal nerve. If the vasodilatation results in any nociceptive input, then the reflex would be augmented by positive feedback, resulting in pain and vasodilatation in the cranial vessels. Transient hyperactivity of the reflex is seen in "ice-pick" headache, where the subject suddenly develops pain in the area of habitual migrainous headache. Excessive afferent input to the reflex, such as a sudden activation of cold receptors in ice cream headache, or pain from occipital neuralgia can also precipitate the sequence of pain, vasodilatation, increased nociceptive input, and thus more pain and reflex vasodilatation. Vasodilatation induced by nitroglycerin may also activate the reflex. Similarly, trauma to the head may distort blood vessels, facilitating a painful reflex.

Drugs that have an effect on the acute attack of migraine reduce the gain of the reflex. Ergotamine and Sumatriptan both cause vasoconstriction, and both block the pial edema induced by stimulating the trigeminal nerve. Aspirin, because of its effect on prostaglandins, reduces edema. Reserpine, which depletes serotonin stores, may induce migraine in susceptible subjects by limiting the transmitter available for vasoconstriction.

There are at least two central nuclei that might precipitate abnormal vasodilatation via the efferent limb of the reflex, the locus coeruleus (LC) and the dorsal raphe nucleus (DRN). The principal sensory input to LC is not well defined, but the DRN receives input from the hypothalamic region. Activity in these nuclei would be expected to produce differing responses in the cerebral vessels, with the LC producing vasoconstriction, and the DRN, vasodilatation.

The aura of migraine is associated with spreading focal oligemia. The mode and rate of progression of the oligemia and the duration of the aura are consistent with the diminished perfusion and neural changes of spreading cortical depression. Possibly, the spreading oligemia and cortical depression is precipitated by vasoconstriction causing focal ischemia in the watershed areas of the cerebral arteries in susceptible subjects, in a manner similar to that observed in patients who have had transient ischemic attacks. The premonitory symptoms of migraine suggest hypothalamic dysfunction preceding the attacks by some hours. It is tempting to suggest that hypothalamic projection to the brainstem may initiate extracranial vasodilatation and intracranial vasoconstriction through the LC and DRN, thus precipitating the headache and aura. Contralateral inhibition at the LC, DRN, or spinal trigeminal nucleus would then make the vasodilatation and trigeminovascular reflex predominate on one side, thus producing unilateral headache. The aura and the headache must rely on separate mechanisms, since there is no constant correlation between the side of the aura and the side of the headache.

CONCLUSION

Migraine may be regarded as a hereditary neurovascular instability in which brain and blood vessels interact to cause neurological syndromes and headache. In some patients, migraine recurs at regular intervals determined by some internal clock, with premonitory symptoms indicating a hypothalamic origin. In others, there is a consistent precipitating factor, an emotional event or excessive afferent input to the nervous system, which triggers the neurovascular changes. On the other hand, some attacks may be initiated from the vascular system by vasodilator drugs or the injection of irritating substances into the carotid or vertebrobasilar arterial systems. Whether the attack is triggered centrally or peripherally, it appears that a vicious cycle is established in the trigeminovascular reflex as described above. Hypothalamic and brainstem activity can induce changes simulating those of migraine. Release of peptides can augment the action of monoamine transmitters, cause a sterile perivascular inflammatory response, and possibly play a part in the sensitization of cranial vessels. The vessels then respond to distension by increasing the discharge of impulses in afferent pain fibers. Whether this afferent barrage is primary or secondary, it enhances the activity of brainstem nuclei and thus completes the vicious circle. It follows that the therapy of migraine must attempt to break the circle, either at the periphery by action on the vascular tree, or centrally by regulating the discharge of monoaminergic, facial, and trigeminal nuclei. 5-HT is known to be implicated in both central and peripheral sites, and the 5-HT1 agonist Sumatriptan has proven to be effective in terminating acute migraine headaches, while 5-HT2 antagonists are useful in their prevention.

REFERENCES

1. Wolff HG. Headache and other head pain. New York: Oxford University Press, 1963.
2. Ray BS, Wolff HG. Experimental studies on headache: pain-sensitive structures of the head and their significance in headache. Arch Surg 1940;41:813–856.
3. Penfield W, McNaughton F. Dural headache and innervation of the dura matter. Arch Neurol Psychiatry 1940;44;43–75.
4. Steiger HJ, Tew JM, Keller JT. The sensory representation of the dura mater in the trigeminal ganglion of the cat. Neurosci Lett 1982;31:231–236.
5. Mayberg MR, Zervas NT, Moskowitz MA. Trigeminal projections to supratentorial pial and dural blood vessels in cats demonstrated by horseradish peroxidase histochemistry. J Comp Neurol 1984;223:46–56.
6. Kimmel DL. Innervation of spinal dura mater and dura mater of the posterior fossa. Neurology 1961;2:800–809.
7. Neilson KC, Owman C. Adrenergic innervation of pial arteries related to the circle of Willis of the cat. Brain Res 1967;6:773–776.
8. Edvinsson L. Sympathetic control of cerebral circulation. Trends Neurosci 1982;5:425–429.
9. Edvinsson L, Owman C. Pharmacological characterization of adrenergic alfa- and beta-receptors mediating the vasomotor responses of cerebral arteries in vitro. Circ Res 1974;35:835–849.
10. McCalden TA, Bevan JA. Sources of activator calcium in rabbit basilar artery. Am J Physiol 1981;241:H129.
11. Skarby T, Hogestatt ED, Andersson K-E. Influence of extracellular calcium and nifedipine on alfa1-and alfa2-adrenoceptor-mediated responses in isolated rat and cat cerebral and mesenteric arteries. Acta Physiol Scand 1984;123:445–456.
12. Edvinsson L, Emson P, McCulloch J, Tatemoto K, Uddman R. Neuropeptide Y: Cerebrovascular innervation and vasomotor effects in the cat. Neurosci Lett 1983;43:79–84.
13. Edvinsson L, Emson P, McCulloch J, Tatemoto K, Uddman R. Neuropeptide Y: Immunocytochemical localization to and effect upon feline pial arteries and veins in vitro and in situ. Acta Physiol Scand 1984;122:155–163.
14. Hara H, Hamill GS, Jacobowitz DM. Origin of cholinergic nerves to the rat major cerebral arteries: Coexistence with vasoactive intestinal polypeptide. Brain Res 1985;14:179–188.
15. Edvinsson L, Falck B, Owman C. Possibilities for a cholinergic action on smooth musculature and on sympathetic axons in brain vessels mediated by muscarinic and nicotinic receptors. J Pharmacol Exp Ther 1977;200:117–126.
16. Humphrey PPA, Feniuk W. Pharmacological characterization of functional neuronal receptors for 5-hydroxytryptamine. In: Nobin A, Owman C, ed. Arneklo-Nobin. Amsterdam, Elsevier, 1987:3–19.
17. Edvinsson L, Jansen I. Characterization of 5-HT receptors mediating contraction of human cerebral, meningeal and temporal arteries: target for GR43175 in acute treatment of migraine. Cephalalgia 1989;9(Suppl.10):39–40.
18. Reinhard JF, Liebmann JE, Schlosbery AJ, Moskowitz MA. Serotonin neurons project to small blood vessels in the brain. Science 1979;206:85–87.
19. Edvinsson L, Degueurce A, MacKenzie ET, Scatton B. Central serotonergic nerves project to the pial vessels of the brain. Nature 1983;306:55–57.
20. Marco EJ, Balfagon G, Salaices M, Sanchez-Ferrer CF, Marin J. Serotonergic innervation of cat cerebral arteries. Brain Res 1985;338:137–139.
21. Larsson L-I, Edvinsson L, Fahrenkrug J, Hakanson R, Owman C, et al. Immunohistochemical localization of a vasodilatory polypeptide (VIP) in cerebrovascular nerves. Brain Res 1976;113:400–404.
22. Kobayashi S, Kyoshima K, Olschowka JA, Jacobowitz DM. Vasoactive intestinal polypeptide immunoreactive and cholinergic nerves in the whole mount preparation of the major cerebral arteries of the rat. Histochemistry 1983;79:377–381.
23. Matsuyama T, Shiosaka S, Matsumoto M, Yoneda S, Kimura K, et al. Overall distribution of vasoactive intestinal polypeptide–containing nerves in the wall of the cerebral arteries: an immunohistochemical study using whole mounts. Neuroscience 1983;10:89–96.
24. Eckenstein F, Baughman RW. Two types of cholinergic innervation in cortex, one co-localized with vasoactive intestinal polypeptide. Nature 1984;309:153–155.
25. Toda N. Relaxant responses to transmural stimulation and nicotine of dog and monkey cerebral arteries. Am J Physiol 1982;243:H145–H153.
26. Uddman R, Edvinsson L, Ekman R, Kingman TA, McCulloch J. Innervation of the feline cerebral vasculature by nerve fibers containing calcitonin gene-related peptide: trigeminal origin and coexistence with substance P. Neurosci Lett 1985;62:131–136.
27. Edvinsson L, Fredholm BB, Hamel E, Jansen I, Verrecchia C. Perivascular peptides relax cerebral arteries concomitant with stimulation of cyclic adenosine monophosphate accumulation of release of an endothelium-derived relaxing factor in the cat. Neurosci Lett 1985;58:213–217.
28. Hanko J, Hardebro JE, Kahrstrom J, Owman C, Sundler F. Calcitonin gene-related peptide is present in mammalian cerebrovascular nerve fibers and dilates pial and peripheral arteries. Neurosci Lett 1985;57:91–95.
29. McCulloch J, Uddman R, Kingman TA, Edvinsson L. Calcitonin gene-related peptide: functional role in cerebrovascular regulation. Proc Natl Acad Sci USA 83:5731–5735.
30. Rikard-Bell GC, Törk I, Sullivan C, Scheibner T. Distribution of substance P–like immunoreactive fibres and terminals in the medulla oblongata of the human infant. Neuroscience 1990;34:133–148.
31. Hökfelt J, Kellerth JO, Nilsson G, Pernow B. Experimental immunohistochemical studies on the localization and distribution of substance P in cat primary sensory neurons. Brain Res 1975;100:235–252.
32. Cuello AC, Del Fiacco M, Paxinos G. The central and peripheral ends of the substance P–containing sensory neurons in the rat trigeminal system. Brain Res 1978;152:400–509.
33. Edvinsson L, McCulloch J, Uddman E: Substance P: immunohistochemical localization and effect upon cat pial arteries in vitro and in situ. J Physiol 1981;318:251–258.
34. Liu-Chen L-Y, Mayberg MA, Moskowitz MA. Immunohistochemical evidence for a substance P–containing trigeminovascular pathway to pial arteries in cats. Brain Res 1983;268:162–166.
35. Uddman R, Edvinsson L, Owman C. Perivascular substance P: occurrence and distribution in mammalian pial vessels. J Cereb Blood Flow Metab 1981;1:227–231.
36. Yamamoto K, Matsuyama T, Shiosaka S, Hayakawa T, Matsumoto M, Tohyama M. Overall distribution of substance P–containing nerves in the wall of the cerebral arteries of the guinea-pig and its origin. J Comp Neurol 1983;215:421–426.

37. Edvinsson L, Uddman R. Immunohistochemical localization and dilatory effect of substance P on human cerebral vessels. Brain Res 1982;232:466–471.

38. Furness JB, Papka RE, Della NG, Costa M, Eskay RL. Substance P–like immunoreactivity in nerves associated with the vascular system of guinea-pigs. Neuroscience 1982;7:447–459.

39. Graham JR, Wolff HG. Mechanisms of migraine headache and action of ergotamine tartrate. Am Med Assoc Arch Neurol Psychiatry 1938;39:737–763.

40. Blau JN, Dexter SL. The site of pain origin during migraine attacks. Cephalalgia 1981;1:143–147.

41. Drummond PD, Lance JW. Extracranial vascular changes and the source of pain in migraine headache. Ann Neurol 1983;13:32–37.

42. Tunis MM, Wolff HG. Analysis of cranial artery pulse waves in patients with vascular headache of the migraine type. Am J Med Sci 1953;224:565–568.

43. Basil P. Craniovascular studies in headache. A report and analysis of pulse volume tracings. Neurology 1956;6:96–102.

44. Heych H. Pathogenesis of migraine. A contribution. Res Clin Stud Headache 1969;2:1–28.

45. Feuerstein M, Bortolussi L, Houle M, Labbe E. Stress, temporal artery activity, and pain in migraine headache: a prospective analysis. Headache 1983;23:296–304.

46. Jensen K, Olesen J. Temporal blood flow in common migraine. Acta Neurol Scand 1985;72:561–570.

47. Jensen K. Subcutaneous blood flow in the temporal region of migraine patients. Acta Neurol Scand 1987;310–318.

48. Horven I, Sjasstad D. Cluster headache syndrome and migraine: ophthalmological support for a two-entity theory. Acta Opthalmol 1977;55:35–51.

49. Tunis M, Clark RG. Studies on headache: further observations on cranial and conjunctival vessels during and between vascular headaches. Trans Am Neurol 1951;76:67–69.

50. Blau JN, Davis E. Small blood vessels in migraine. Lancet 1970;ii:740–742.

51. Lance JW, Anthony M, Sommerville B. Thermographic, hormonal and clinical studies in migraine. Headache 1970;9:93–104.

52. Lance JW, Anthony MA. Thermographic, hormonal and migraine clinical studies in migraine. Headache 1971;9:93–104.

53. Swerlow L, Dieter JN. The value of vascular cold patch in the diagnosis of chronic headache. Headache 1986;26:22–26.

54. Drummond PD, Lance JW. Facial temperature in migraine, tension-vascular and tension headache. Cephalalgia 1984;4:149–158.

55. Giacovazzo M, Martelletti P, Valducci G. Computerized telethermographic assessment in migraine with particular reference to the prodromal phase. Cephalalgia 1986;6:219–222.

56. Skinhøj E, Paulson OB. Regional cerebral blood flow in internal carotid distribution during migraine attack. Br Med J 1969;3:569–570.

57. Olesen J, Larsen B, Lauritzen M. Focal hyperemia followed by spreading olegemia and impaired activation of rCBF in classic migraine. Ann Neurol 1981;9:344–352.

58. Lauritzen M, Skyhøj Olsen T, Lassen NA, Paulson OB. The changes of regional cerebral blood flow during the course of classical migraine attacks. Ann Neurol 1983;13:633–641.

59. Skyhøj Olsen T, Friberg L, Lassen NA. Ischemia may be the primary cause of the neurologic deficits in classic migraine. Arch Neurol 1987;44:156–161.

60. Skinhøj E. Hemodynamic studies within the brain during migraine. Arch Neurol 1973;29:95–98.

61. Norris JW, Hachinski VC, Cooper PW. Changes in cerebral blood flow during a migraine attack. Br Med J 1975;3:676–677.

62. Hachinski VC, Olesen J, Norris JW, Larsen B, Enevoldsen E, Lassen NA. Cerebral hemodynamics in migraine. Can J Neurol Sci 1977;4:245–249.

63. Friberg L, Skyhøj Olsen T, Roland PE, Lassen NA. Cerebrovascular tone instability causing focal ischemia during attacks of hemiplegic migraine. Brain 1987;110:917–934.

64. Lauritzen M, Olesen J. Regional cerebral blood flow during migraine attacks by xenon-133 inhalation and emission tomography. Brain 1984;107:447–461.

65. Gulliksen G, Enevoldsen E. Prolonged changes in rCBF following attacks of migraine accompagnee. Acta Neurol Scand 1984;69:270–271.

66. Andersen AR, Friberg L, Skyhøj Olsen T. Delayed hyperemia following hypoperfusion in classic migraine. Arch Neurol 1988;45:154–159.

67. Olesen J, Tfelt-Hansen P, Henriksen L, Larsen B. The common migraine attack may not be initiated by cerebral ischemia. Lancet 1981;ii:438–440.

68. Herald S, Gibbs JM, Jones EPK, Bookes DJ, Frackowiak RSJ, Legg NJ. Oxygen metabolism in migraine. J Cereb Blood Flow Metab 1985;5(suppl 1):445–446.

69. Sakai F, Meyer JS. Regional cerebral hemodynamics during migraine and cluster headache measured by the 133-Xe inhalation method. Headache 1978;18:122–132.

70. Gelmers HJ. Common migraine attacks preceded by focal hyperemia and partial olegemia in the rCBF pattern. Cephalalgia 1982;2:29–32.

71. Friberg L, Skyhøj Olsen T, Lassen NA. Cerebrovascular tone instability causing focal ischemia in TIA and stroke patients. In: Gagliardi R, Benvenuti L, eds. Controversies in EIAB for cerebral ischemia. Monduzzi Editore. 1987:87–93.

72. Lashley KS. Patterns of cerebral integration indicated by the scutomas of migraine. Arch Neurol Psychiatry 1941;46:331–339.

73. Leão AAP. Spreading depression of activity in cerebral cortex. J Neurophysiol 1944;7:359–390.

74. Leão AAP. Further observations on the spreading depression of activity in the cerebral cortex. J Neurophysiol 1947;19:409–419.

75. Nicholson C, Kraig RP. The behaviour of extracellular ions during spreading depression. In: Zeuthen T, ed. The application of ion-selective microelectrodes. Amsterdam: Elsevier, 1981:217–238.

76. Hansen AJ. The effect of annoxia on iron distribution in the brain. Physiol Rev 1985;65:101–148.

77. Buras J, Buresova O, Krivanek J. The meaning and significance of Leao's spreading depression. Ann Acad Bras Scien 1984;56:385–400.

78. Hockaday JM, Debney L. The EEG in migraine. In: Olesen T, Edvinsson L, eds. Vasic mechanisms of headache. Amsterdam: Elsevier, 1988:365–376.

79. Gloor P. Regional cerebral upflow in migraine. Transneuro Sci 1986;9:21.

80. Leão AAP, Morrison RS. Propagation of cortical spreading depression. J Neurophysiol 1945;8:33–45.

81. Simard D, Paulson OB. Cerebral vasomotor paralysis during migraine attack. Arch Neurol 1973;29:207–209.

82. Skyhøj Olsen T, Friberg L, Ronager J. Cerebral autoregulation and CO$_2$-reactivity are completely abolished during attacks of classic migraine. Further support of the vasopastic theory. Upsala J Med Sci 1986;43(suppl 87)[Abstract].

83. Martins-Ferreira H, De Oliveira Castro G, Struchiner CJ, Rodrigues PS. Circling spreading depression in isolated chick retina. J Neurophysiol 1974;37:773–784.

84. Sicuteri F, Testi A, Anselmi B. Biomedial investigations in headache: increase in hydroxyindoleacetic acid excretion during migraine attacks. Int Arch Allerg 1961;19:55–58.

85. Curran DA, Hinterberger H, Lance JW. Total plasma serotonin, 5-hydroxyindoleacetic acid and p-hydroxy-m-methoxymandelic acid excretion in normal and migrainous subjects. Brain 1965;88:997–1010.

86. Anthony M, Hinterberger H, Lance JW. Plasma serotonin migraine and stress. Arch Neurol 1967;16:544–552.

87. Anthony M, Hinterberger H, Lance JW. The possible relationship of serotonin to the migraine syndrome. Res Clin Stud Headache 1969;2:29–59.

88. Dvilansky A, Rishpon S, Nathan I, Zolotow A, Korczyn AD. Release of platelet 5-hydroxytryptamine by plasma taken from patients during and between migraine attacks. Pain 1976;2:315–318.

89. Mŭck-Seler D, Deanovic Z, Dupelj M. Platelet serotonin (5-HT) and 5-HT releasing factor in plasma of migrainous patients. Headache 1979;19:14–17.

90. Ferrari MD, Odink J, Tapparelli C, Van Kempen GMJ, Pennings EJM, Bruyn GW. Serotonin metabolism in migraine. Neurology 1989;39:1239–1242.

91. Kimball RW, Friedman AP, Vallejo E. Effect of serotonin in migraine patients. Neurology 1960;10:107–111.

92. Ferrari MD, Bayliss EM, Ludlow S, Pilgrim AS. Subcutaneous GR43175 in the treatment of acute migraine. Cephalalgia 1989;9(suppl 10):349–350.

93. Dahlof C, Winter R, Ludlow S. Oral GR43175, a 5-HT1-like agonist, for the treatment of the acute migraine attack: an international study—preliminary results. Cephalalgia 1989;9(suppl 10):351–352.

94. Blau JN. Migraine prodromes separated from the aura: complete migraine. Br Med J 1980;281:658–660.

95. Waelkens J. Warning symptoms in migraine: characteristics and therapeutic implications. Cephalalgia 1985;5:223–228.

96. Herberg LJ. The hypothalamus and aminergic pathways in migraine. In: Pearce J, ed. Modern topics in migraine. London: Heinemann, 1975.

97. Awaki E, Takeshima T, Takahashi KA. Neuroendocrinal study in female migraineurs: prolactin and thyroid stimulating hormone responses. Cephalalgia 1989;9:187–193.

98. Raskin NH, Knittle SC. Ice cream headache and orthostatic symptoms in patients with migraine headache. Headache 1976;16:222–225.

99. Raskin NH, Schwartz RK. Icepick-like pain. Neurology 1980;30:203–205.

100. Sweet WM, Wepsic JG. Controlled thermocoagulation of V ganglion and rootlets for differential destruction of pain fibres Part I. V. Neuralgia. J Neurosurg 1974;40:143–156.

101. Onofrio BM. Radio frequency percutaneous gasserian ganglion lesions. Neurosurgery 1975;42:132–143.

102. Oka M. Experimental study on the vasodilator innervation of the face. Med J Osaka Univ 1950;2:109–116.

103. Goadsby PJ, Edvinsson L, Ekman R. Release of vasoactive peptides in the extracerebral circulation of man and the cat during activation of the trigeminovascular system. Ann Neurol 1988.

104. Saito F, Markowitz S, Moskowitz MA. Ergot alkaloids block neurogenic extravasation in dura mater. Ann Neurol 1988 24:732–737.

105. Buzzi MG, Moskowitz MA. The antimigraine drug Sumatriptan (GR43175) selectively blocks neurogenic plasma extravasation from blood vessels in dura mater. Br J Pharmacol 1990;99:202–206.

106. Lambert GA, Bogduk N, Goadsby PJ, Duckworth JW, Lance JW. Decreased carotid arterial resistance in cats in response to trigeminal stimulation. J Neurosurg 1984;61:307–315.

107. Goadsby PJ, Macdonald GJ. Extracranial vasodilatation mediated by VIP (vasoactive intestinal polypeptide). Brain Res 1985;329:285–288.

108. Goadsby PJ, Lambert GA, Zagami A, Duckworth JW. Comparative effects of activation of the trigeminal ganglion and the superior sagittal sinus on cerebral blood flow and spinal evoked potentials in the cat. Neurosci Abstrs 1987;13:743.

109. Walters DW, Gillespie SA, Moskowitz M. Cerebrovascular projections from the sphenopalatine and otic ganglia to the middle cerebral artery of the cat. Stroke 1986;17:485–494.

110. Amaral DG, Sinnamon HM. The locus coeruleus: neurobiology of a central noradrenergic nucleus. Neurobiol 1977;9:147–196.

111. Goadsby PJ, Lambert GA, Lance JW. Differential effects on the internal and external carotid circulation of the monkey evoked by locus coeruleus stimulation. Brain 1982;249:247–254.

112. Goadsby PJ, Duckworth JW. Low frequency stimulation of locus coerulus reduces regional blood flow in the spinalised cat. Brain Res 1989;476:71–77.

113. Goadsby PJ, Piper RD, Lambert GA, Lance JW. The effect of activation of the nucleus raphe dorsalis (DRN) on carotid blood flow. I. The monkey. Am J Physiol 1985;248:R257–R262.

114. Di Carlo V. Serotoninergic innervation of extrinsic brainstem blood vessels. Neurology 1981;31:104.

115. Di Carlo V. Perivascular serotonergic neurons somatodendritic contacts and axonic innervation of blood vessels. Neurosci Lett 1984;51:295–302.

116. Goadsby PJ, Macdonald GJ. The effect of infusion of various peptide antisera on vasodilatation in the cat common carotid vascular territory. Clin Exp Neurol 1985;21:115–121.

117. Goadsby PJ, Edvisson L, Ekman R. Vasoactive peptide release in the extracerebral circulation of the human during migraine headache. Ann Neurol 1990;28:183–187.

118. Zagami AS, Goadsby PJ, Edvisson L. Stimulation of the superior sagittal sinus in the cat causes release of vasoactive peptides. Neuropeptides 1990;16:69–75.

11

Medical Management of Acute Migraine Episode

ROBERT S. KUNKEL

When treating migraine, one should try to identify any trigger factors, the avoidance of which will diminish the frequency of the attacks. Prophylactic agents may be necessary in those with frequent attacks in an effort to decrease both the severity and frequency of the attacks. Even if the number or severity of the attacks is lessened, acute therapy will be needed for those attacks of migraine that do occur. Many different types of pharmacological agents have been used over the years in an effort to decrease the pain and associated symptoms that accompany an acute attack of migraine. Nonpharmacological measures and the use of biofeedback in migraine are discussed in Chapters 14 and 15, respectively.

It is important to realize that absorption can be greatly reduced during a migraine attack (1). This decreased absorption is probably largely due to decreased gastric functioning. Studies with barium have shown gastric stasis and prolonged gastric emptying (2, 3). This accounts for the ineffectiveness of oral agents such as the analgesics, ergotamine tartrate, and even strong narcotics in easing the pain of migraine. In general, the quicker the abortive medication is taken, the more effective it is. This is not only because the pain is less intense early on but also because of the disturbed absorption from the gastrointestinal tract, which may develop. Vomiting will also account for ineffectiveness of oral medication.

ANTIEMETIC AGENTS

Antiemetic agents such as chlorpromazine, prochlorperazine, promethazine, hydroxyzine, and trimethobenzamide are useful in controlling nausea and vomiting. Metoclopramide, which promotes gastric emptying, can be useful as an acute emetic as well as enhancing the effectiveness of other oral agents. Studies have shown that it will increase blood levels of analgesics (4, 5). Metoclopramide can be given orally in a dosage of 10 to 20 mg prior to the use of analgesics or ergotamine and may enhance the effectiveness of these agents. It can also be used intravenously in the office or emergency room. A recent report demonstrated effectiveness of IV metoclopramide alone in reducing the pain of migraine headache, whereas a previous study did not demonstrate any

effectiveness on the pain of migraine (6, 7). Metoclopramide can cause extrapyramidal reactions, so it must be used with caution.

Most of the other antinauseants are available in oral and suppository form. Parenteral (IV or IM) administration of these agents is often a useful adjunct to narcotics.

ANALGESICS AND NARCOTICS

Undoubtedly most migraine sufferers take simple analgesics for the attacks and try to sleep them off. They do not consult a physician. Aspirin, in my clinical experience, is more efficacious than acetaminophen for migraine attacks. Double-blind studies have not found aspirin to be very effective in migraine. Tfelt-Hansen and Olesen found that effervescent aspirin alleviated migraine in only 37% of patients (8). Ross-Lee and colleagues found that aspirin was "highly effective" in 44% of patients (9). The overwhelming majority of patients presenting to the physician have tried aspirin and acetaminophen many times and come to the physician requesting something "stronger."

Such analgesics as propoxyphene, carisoprodol, and chlorzoxazone are at times helpful in alleviating migraine pain. In persons unable to take vasoconstrictors, they may be worth trying. Combinations of a barbiturate, caffeine, and aspirin or acetaminophen are often quite effective, and when used periodically and sparingly, they are satisfactory and adequate treatment for migraine attacks. Problems frequently arise with these combinations, however, when they are abused and tolerance develops. Codeine combined with aspirin or acetaminophen is an effective oral agent in many cases of migraine. Meperidine, which is used so often by the parenteral route, is not a very effective oral agent. Other oral narcotics such as oxycodone or hydrocodone bitartrate are a little stronger than codeine and meperidine when used orally. These narcotics should not be used in patients with frequent migraine attacks because of the frequent development of dependency.

NONSTEROIDAL ANTIINFLAMMATORY DRUGS

NSAIDs are quite useful in migraine. The faster-acting agents should be used for the acute attack. These drugs decrease platelet aggregation, inhibit prostaglandin synthesis, and have analgesic properties. When used acutely and episodically, they are generally well tolerated. Pradalier and associates reviewed the use of NSAIDs and found that in most drug trials they have been efficacious (10).

In an unpublished trial in which the author participated, meclofenamate sodium was as effective as ergotamine tartrate in the acute attack of migraine but had fewer side effects. The dosage is 200 mg at the onset of the headache, followed by 100 to 200 mg in 1 hour, if needed. Naproxen, naproxen sodium, and ibuprofen are more effective than placebo and have fewer side effects than ergotamine tartrate in double-blind trials (11–14). The NSAIDs may be used in conjunction with other agents such as metoclopramide or even ergotamine tartrate and be very effective. I prefer to use meclofenamate sodium at the dosage mentioned above, since it acts very rapidly. I often combine this drug with ergotamine orally. Ketorolac, (Toradol) a parenteral and oral nonsteroidal agent that has potent analgesic properties, has been very effective in treating acute migraine attacks. It is being used frequently in the emergency room with dihydroergotamine and meperidine for the patient coming in with acute migraine.

VASOCONSTRICTIVE AGENTS
Isometheptene Mucate

Isometheptene mucate is a mild vasoconstrictive agent. It is usually combined with acetaminophen and a nonbarbiturate sedative (dichlorphenazone) (Midrin, Isocom) or with caffeine (Migralam). It is very well tolerated, although it is not as effective as ergotamine tartrate in its constricting effect on blood vessels. Since perhaps 50% of persons using ergotamine tartrate have gastrointestinal side effects, I usually start with isometheptene mucate and then move on to use ergotamine tartrate, if necessary. It is important to take enough to abort the attack. Two capsules should be taken at the very earliest sign of the headache, followed by one or two capsules in an hour. It may be repeated in another hour, but as with ergotamine tartrate, the attack is usually aborted after the first couple of doses or there is very little effect on that particular attack. Since the isometheptene products contain acetaminophen, it can also be used as an analgesic every 4 hours or so.

Ergotamine Tartrate

Ergotamine tartrate is the "gold standard" for the alleviation of an acute migraine attack. All other agents are usually compared to ergotamine tartrate when studies are done. It is usually combined with caffeine and can be used orally, rectally, sublingually. The sublingual form does not contain caffeine. The most effective means of using ergotamine tartrate is by rectal suppository, but this is also the least convenient form.

Ergotamine tartrate is a potent vasoconstrictor with a selective effect on the external carotid system (15). There has been some concern about using this agent in persons

with visual or neurological symptoms prior to or during a headache attack, because of the fear that the vasoconstriction might prolong the symptoms. However, ergotamine tartrate has no significant constrictive effects on the intracranial circulation (16). It therefore should be used at the initial symptoms of the attack, whether that is an aura or the pain itself. Ergotamine tartrate should not be used in persons with known ischemic disease, liver disease, or any chronic illness.

Like all drugs, ergotamine tartrate has multiple effects, and some of these may be important in addition to the vasoconstrictive effects. It reduces neurogenic inflammation in the dura mater and has central effects on serotonin metabolism (17, 18). Sterile inflammation is felt to play a role in the pain of migraine, and serotonin is felt to be a key substance in the initiation of the migraine attack.

The dosage of ergotamine that is needed varies, because some persons are very sensitive to this drug. Standard regimens are recommended and described here. One or two ergotamine tartrate tablets (1 mg) are taken at the very onset of the migraine attack, and one is repeated in one-half hour increments for two or three additional doses, if necessary. The suppository form contains 2 mg of ergotamine, and one should be used at the onset and repeated in 1 hour, if needed. Many persons, however, find that a half or a third of a suppository is sufficient to abort the headache.

The sublingual form of ergotamine does not contain caffeine, as the tablets and suppositories do. The sublingual tablets contain 2 mg of ergotamine tartrate, and one is used under the tongue at the very onset of the attack and repeated in 1 hour, if needed. The bitter taste of the sublingual tablets greatly limits their acceptance by patients.

The most common side effects of ergotamine tartrate are nausea and vomiting, which occurs in perhaps 40 to 50% of persons. Less frequent effects are abdominal pain, diarrhea, muscle cramping, and tingling in the extremities. Some people are very sensitive to the drug and have symptoms due to vasoconstriction, such as tingling in the extremities and chest pain, even with a very small dose. Others may take very large amounts for many years without any vasospastic symptoms (19). The amount of caffeine (100 mg in ergotamine tartrate tablets and suppositories) will cause nervousness and restlessness in many people.

A rebound headache, occurring 12 to 48 hours after the use of ergotamine tartrate, develops in a substantial number of persons using the drug on a regular basis (20, 21). The total amount doesn't have to be excessive, but frequent use will likely lead to dependency, causing a withdrawal or rebound headache. Ergotamine tartrate use should be limited to twice weekly, with 3 to 4 days between usage. Because ergotamine tartrate is usually combined with caffeine and persons are often taking daily analgesics, the cause of the "rebound" headache is complex, since analgesics and caffeine can cause rebound or withdrawal headaches as well. Daily or regular use of ergotamine needs to be discontinued. Naproxen may help reduce the withdrawal effects when ergotamine tartrate is stopped (22).

Dihydroergotamine

Dihydroergotamine mesylate (DHE-45) is a vasoconstrictive agent that has enjoyed wider use recently for the acute treatment of migraine (23). It is available in parenteral form and has also been found to be effective as a nasal spray (24). DHE-45 does not seem to produce the rebound headache that ergotamine tartrate may. It can be used subcutaneously or intravenously. Treatment with IV DHE is usually used following metoclopramide or prochlorperazine. The usual dosage is 0.5 to 1 mg, which can be repeated in 30 to 60 minutes. In many cases, the use of perenteral narcotics in the emergency room can be avoided by the use of DHE-45 along with other agents (25).

Sumatriptan

Sumatriptan succinate is a serotonin receptor agonist which has been found in studies done in the United States and Europe to be a very effective treatment of acute migraine attacks (26, 27). Sumatriptan has a specific effect on the 5 HT1D receptor site. Stimulation of these receptors causes vasoconstriction. Sumatriptan also blocks plasma extravasation from blood vessels in the dura mater (28). Other effects of this agent undoubtedly occur, since sumatriptan seems to alleviate some of the associated symptoms of migraine such as nausea, vomiting, photophobia, and phonophobia even more effectively than it does the actual pain of migraine.

This pharmacological agent has been extensively studied. One hour after treatment with 6 mg of Sumatriptan given subcutaneously, 70% of persons were significantly improved (26). Eighty percent of patients were significantly improved in 2 hours, some of whom were given a second injection 1 hour after the first (26, 27). The differences seen after the second injection were not statistically significant.

Sumatriptan is well tolerated. Transient symptoms of warmth and flushing, pressure sensation, and irritation at the site of injection occur in a few patients. A significant number of patients had a reoccurrence of headache within 24 hours necessitating "rescue medication" (26, 27). The nature and reason of reoccurrence of head pain is not well understood at this time. It is expected that other methods of administering sumatriptan will be developed.

OTHER THERAPIES

Phenothiazines

Intravenous use of the phenothiazines, chlorpromazine and prochlorperazine has been reported to abort acute migraine attacks (29, 30). These agents are often used in the emergency room when a patient comes in with acute migraine. Prochlorperazine is perhaps less likely to cause significant hypotension and probably is safer to use. Parenteral use of the phenothiazines, dihydroergotamine, ketorolac, and sumatriptan has made a great impact on our usual treatment of acute migraine. Narcotics can now be avoided completely in many persons, whereas formerly, they were the usual agents used in an emergency.

Corticosteroids

Corticosteroids are frequently helpful in acute migraine but cannot be used too often on a repetitive basis. Oral prednisone, methylprednisolone, or dexamethasone in short courses often will control a migraine that has been going on for a few days. Dexamethasone 1.5 mg twice daily for 2 to 3 days has proven to be very effective in my practice. If the migraineur is vomiting and a parenteral agent would seem appropriate, 40 to 80 mg of the long-acting form of methylprednisolone acetate or 12 to 16 mg of the long-acting form of dexamethasone can be used with good results. Intravenous hydrocortisone in a dosage of 100 mg may be helpful acutely, but it doesn't usually break the attack. The corticosteroids probably are effective because of their reduction of the perivascular inflammation that occurs in migraine.

Vasodilating Agents

There are times when a quick-acting vasodilating drug may be very useful. When the aura symptoms are prolonged or quite disabling, a vasodilator will often clear the symptoms rapidly and usually will not aggravate the headache (31). Many times the headache does not develop. Vasodilators are often very effective for migraine aura that occurs without subsequent headache. Nitroglycerin and nifedipine have been shown to be effective, as has isoproterenol (31–33). Although these are potent vasodilators, like every other drug they also have other effects in the body, which may contribute to their effectiveness in stopping the visual and neurological symptoms that precede the migraine attack or those symptoms that occur without a subsequent headache. In my experience, they are underused because of the fear of aggravating the headache. If the aura symptoms last more than 15 or 20 minutes, it would be worth trying sublingual nifedipine or nitroglycerin to see if the attack can be aborted.

STATUS MIGRAINOSUS

A migrainous attack that continues longer than 72 hours is termed "status migrainosus." Most patients with this condition require parenteral medication (34). Most have used vasoconstrictors, analgesics, antiemetics, and narcotics without breaking the headache. These patients are usually vomiting and may be dehydrated. Occasionally electrolyte abnormalities occur as well.

Parenteral corticosteroids are very useful in aborting a prolonged migraine attack. The long-acting form of dexamethasone, 12 to 16 mg, or methylprednisolone, 40 to 80 mg, is usually given intramuscularly. Antiemetics and sedatives are usually warranted as well. Gallagher demonstrated that the use of dexamethasone with meperidine and promethazine was better than meperidine and promethazine or meperidine and DHE-45 in a group of patients with status migrainosus (35).

Raskin has shown good results with dihydroergotamine (DHE-45) used repetitively by the intravenous route (36). DHE-45 1 mg after an initial test dose of 0.5 mg is given every 8 hours for a total of 6 to 8 doses. Metoclopramide 10 mg can be used along with the DHE-45 to control nausea and vomiting. One of the phenothiazines could also be used and will provide a sedative effect. In contrast to ergotamine tartrate, DHE-45 seems to be effective even when used late in the headache attack.

SUMMARY

A wide variety of medications are available to treat the acute migraine attack. Specific therapy to affect the vascular component of the pain is used with agents that control inflammation and nausea. The development of new drugs that are well tolerated and effective will allow even better treatment of the patient with migraine.

REFERENCES

1. Volans GN. Migraine and drug absorption. Clin Pharmacokinet 1978;3:313–318.
2. Carstairs LS. Headaches and gastric emptying time. Proc R Soc Med 1958;51:790–791.
3. Kaufman J, Levine I. Acute gastric dilatation of the stomach during attack of migraine. Radiology 1936;27:301–302.
4. Volans GN. The effect of metoclopramide on the absorption of effervescent aspirin in migraine. Br J Clin Pharmacol 1975;2:57–63.
5. Tokola R, Neuvonen P. Effects of migraine attack and metoclopramide on the absorption of tolfenamic acid. Br J Clin Pharmacol 1984;17:67–75.
6. Tek DS, McCellan DS, Olshaker JS, et al. A prospective, double-blind study of metoclopramide hydrochloride for the control of migraine in the emergency department. Ann Emerg Med 1990;19:1083–1087.
7. Tfelt-Hansen P, Olesen J, Krabbe A, et al. A double-blind study of metoclopramide in the treatment of migraine attacks. J Neurol Neurosurg Psychiatry 1980;43:369–371.
8. Tfelt-Hansen P, Olesen J. Effervescent metoclopramide and aspirin (Migravess) vs. effervescent aspirin or placebo for migraine attacks: a double-blind study. Cephalalgia 1984;4:107–111.
9. Ross-Lee L, Eadie MJ, Tyrer JH. Aspirin treatment of migraine attacks: clinical observations. Cephalalgia 1982;2:71–76.
10. Pradalier A, Clapin A, Dry J: Treatment review: non-steroidal anti-inflammatory drugs in the treatment and long-term prevention of migraine attacks. Headache 1988;28:550–557.
11. Johnson E, Ratcliff D, Wilkinson M. Naproxen sodium in the treatment of migraine. Cephalalgia 1985;5:5–10.
12. Sargent J, Baumel B, Peters K, et al. Aborting a migraine attack: naproxen sodium vs. ergotamine plus caffeine. Headache 1988;28:263–266.
13. Pearce T, Frank G, Pearce J. Ibuprofen compared with paracetamol in migraine. Practioner 1983;227:465–467.
14. Havanka-Kannainen H. Treatment of acute migraine attack: ibuprofen and placebo compared. Headache 1989;29:507–509.
15. Lance JW, Spira PJ, Mylecharane EJ, et al. Evaluation of the drugs applicable to treatment of migraine in the cranial circulation of the monkey. Res Clin Stud Headache 1978;6:13–18.
16. Edmeads J. Cerebral blood flow in migraine. Headache 1977;17:148–152.
17. Saito K, Markowitz S, Moskowitz MA. Ergot alkaloids block neurogenic extravasation in dura mater, proposed action in vascular headaches. Ann Neurol 1988;24:732–737.
18. Sofia RD, Vassar HB. The effect of ergotamine and methysergide on serotonin metabolism in the rat brain. Arch Int Pharmacodyn Ther 1975;216:40–50.
19. Friedman AP, Von Storch TJC, Araki S. Ergotamine tartrate: its history, action, and proper use in the treatment of migraine. NY State J Med 1959;59:2359–2366.
20. Saper JR, Jones JM. Ergotamine tartrate dependency: features and possible mechanisms. Clin Neuropharmacol 1986;9:244–256.
21. Wainscott G, Volans G, Wilkinson M. Ergotamine-induced headaches. Br Med J 1974;2:724.
22. Mathew NT. Amelioration of ergotamine withdrawal symptoms with naproxen. Headache 1987;27:130–133.
23. Callahan M, Raskin N. A controlled study of DHE in the treatment of acute migraine headache. Headache 1986;26:168–171.
24. Krause K, Blecher M. DHE nasal spray in the treatment of migraine attacks. Cephalalgia 1985;5(suppl 3):138–139.
25. Belgrade M, Ling L, Schleevogt M, et al. Comparison of single dose meperidine, butorphanol, and DHE in the treatment of vascular headache. Neurology 1989;39:590–592.
26. Cady RK, Wendt JK, Kirchner JR, et al. Treatment of acute migraine with subcutaneous sumatriptan. JAMA 1991;265:2831–2835.
27. Ferrari MD, Melamed E, Gawel M. Treatment of migraine attacks with sumatriptan. N Engl J Med 1991;325:316–321.
28. Buzzi MG, Moskowitz MA. The anti-migraine drug, sumatriptan (GR43175), selectively blocks neurogenic plasma extravasation from blood vessels in dura mater. Br J Pharmacol 1990;99:202–206.
29. Lane P, Ross R. Intravenous chlorpromazine—present research in acute migraine. Headache 1985;25:302–304.
30. Jones J, Sklar D, Dougherty J, White W. Randomized double-blind trial of IV prochlorperazine for the treatment of acute headache. JAMA 1989;261:1174–1176.
31. Kunkel RS. Vasodilator therapy for classic migraine headache. In: Rose FC, ed. Advances in migraine research and therapy. New York: Raven Press, 1982:205–209.
32. Tucker RM. Sublinguinal nifedipine relieves migraine prodromes. Headache 1984;24:285.
33. Coopersmith MJ, Hass WK, Chase NE. Isoproterenol treatment of visual symptoms in migraine. Stroke 1979;10:299–305.
34. Couch JR, Diamond S. Status migrainosus: causative and therapeutic aspects. Headache 1983;23:94–101.
35. Gallagher RM. Emergency treatment of intractable migraine. Headache 1986;26:74–75.
36. Raskin N. Repetitive intravenous DHE as therapy for intractable migraine. Neurology 1986;36:295–297.

12

Medical Management of Recurrent Migraine

SEYMOUR DIAMOND

The main concern of a patient seeking a physician's help for either sporadic headache or unrelenting status migraine, is that no life-threatening event is the cause of the problem. The physician should focus on the origin of the headaches, as well as what is available to relieve the patient's pain.

The headache patient usually seeks a quick and efficient remedy, a wonder drug, which would cure the headaches once and forever. Unfortunately, as is generally the case throughout medicine, no miracle cure for headache exists. At the present time, however, we are more cognizant of the pathophysiological mechanisms of migraine. Any prejudice regarding the fear that migraine is an untreatable disorder must be rejected. The patient should be reassured and the physician educated that migraine is indeed a controllable problem. This possible resolution must be emphasized, especially in patients with numerous psychological problems and/or with neurotic, hypochondriac, or histrionic traits. Also, the clinician must recognize that migraine and especially coexisting migraine and tension-type headaches, are complex disorders with many triggers and provoking factors. In many cases, they require complex and combined treatment. A therapeutic approach to the migraine patient must be comprehensive and may require a variety of treatment modalities.

Approximately 45 to 50 million people in the United States experience chronic headache. This fact should indicate to the reader the quantity of analgesics consumed daily and the frequency of emergency room visits for headache complaints. One can only imagine the amount of money spent annually for analgesics and emergency room visits due to headaches.

Therefore, it is very important to consider prophylactic treatment. Potential habituation problems with narcotics and analgesics must be avoided. The anguish of migraine sufferers and their families or co-workers should be alleviated to return them to normal life without physical, psychological, or social limitations.

Contrary to the concept that all headaches are similar, the first issue to be addressed in treating headache is obvious: what type of headache is it? The next step is determining if this particular patient requires abortive or prophylactic therapy.

Provocative factors must be identified and avoided. The patient should be tried on a diet limiting foods containing vasoactive substances, such as tyramine, as well as restricting alcohol and excessive amounts of caffeine. Certain physical activities and emotional or stress factors should be avoided if they have been identified as the factors triggering the headaches. Maintaining a regular meal and sleep schedule may benefit some patients. External stimuli such as bright light, scintillating screens, and other strong sensory provocateurs should be avoided. Supplemental estrogen therapy or oral contraceptives may be deleterious in migraine patients, as these drugs are known to increase the frequency, severity, and complications of migraine.

When to Initiate Prophylactic Therapy?

The decision to use a daily pharmacological regimen is based on the frequency and duration of attacks and the degree of impairment of the patient's quality of life. Prophylactic treatment is indicated in patients with more than two migraine attacks per month. This type of therapy should also be considered if a single attack of disabling intensity lasts more than one day and causes regular absences from work, school, or social activity. Contraindications or intolerance of abortive therapy also warrant prophylactic treatment (Table 12.1).

Treatment must be individualized. The risk-benefit ratio must be considered, with the benefits of prophylaxis outweighing the inconvenience and side effects of the prescribed medication. In preventing migraine attacks, several drugs have been used with varying degrees of success. The benefit of these drugs, however, may be delayed by several days or weeks. This latency should be explained to the patient, for assurance about the slow initial progress.

Mechanism of Action of Prophylactic Drugs

The pathogenesis of the migraine has been poorly understood for centuries. This resulted in a lack of effective preventive medications. Some agents used for disorders other than headache have proved effective in migraine prophylaxis, giving a better understanding of migraine on the basis of receptor theories.

Agents used in the prophylactic treatment of migraine include extracranial vasoconstrictors, β-blockers, calcium channel blockers, serotonin antagonists, antidepressants, antiprostaglandins, and vasodilators. It has been suggested that the probable mode of action of these drugs is complex. These agents do not act exclusively as vasoactive components and antidepressants but possibly at the site of brain serotonin and noradrenergic receptors (Table 12.2).

Unified Theory of Migraine

To better understand the role of receptors in migraine, the concept of a unified theory of migraine (1) needs to be summarized. Migraine is a complex disorder involving the release of several neurotransmitters, platelet aggregation with release of platelet serotonin, and vasodilation of cerebral and extracerebral arteries. Subsequently, in response to certain specific or nonspecific stimuli, a cascade of dynamic processes takes place. The preheadache vasoconstrictor phenomenon represents a neurogenic vasospasm of the innervated intracranial vascular system. This vasoconstriction produces a relative reduction in local cerebral blood flow (2, 3), with the consequent local metabolic tissue abnormalities (4) with prodromal symptoms. The parenchymal arteries responsive to focal metabolic demands, as well as cranial arteries on the outside of the head, subsequently dilate, producing the familiar throbbing headache of migraine. The change in tone of the extracranial arteries provokes the release of multiple local chemical and vasoactive substances, producing edema, sterile inflammation, a lowering of pain threshold, and clinical headache.

Many neurotransmitters and vasoactive substances are involved in the migrainous process including: catecholamine, histamine, serotonin, tyramine, substance P, the slow-reacting substance of anaphylaxis (SRSA), prostaglandins, peptide kinin, enkephalins, and the beta endorphin, tryptophan. The serotonin levels of plasma fall at the onset of a migraine attack, and platelets containing almost all of the serotonin present in blood, aggregate more readily (5, 6).

Anselmi and co-workers (7) found in migraine sufferers, decreased levels of CSF enkephalins, increased serum beta-endorphin-like immunoreactivity at the end of attack, and increased CSF and free plasma tryptophan. Recent work of Solomon (8) and others (9) also confirmed a fall in free plasma serotonin and an elevation in plasma substance P levels during an acute migraine attack.

Receptors, Synapses, and Neurotransmitters

Generally, neuroactive drugs act through specific receptors within the CNS (10). Receptors are proteins located in the plasma membrane that recognize and selectively bind drugs, thus enabling them to exert their effects. Drugs may also influence the propagation of regulatory signals from the receptor to the target cell, either by a direct intracellular effect or by affecting the release of a second messenger, such as cyclic AMP (cAMP) (11). Transmission in the nervous system occurs over the chains of anatomically distinct neurons linked together by the apposition of the axon terminals, the synapses. (Fig. 12.1)

Neurotransmitters that function as chemical messengers, including serotonin, acetylcholine, and norepinephrine, are stored in and secreted from presynaptic vesicles. The release of the neurotransmitters to the synaptic cleft is induced by calcium influx resulting from depolarization of

Table 12.1.
Guidelines for Prophylactic Treatment of Migraine

More than two headaches per month
Regular single attack of disabling intensity lasting more than 24 hours
Contraindication to symptomatic (abortive) therapy
Substance abuse tendencies
Regular absences from work or school, substantial disruption of household and social responsibilities.
Intolerance or failed abortive therapy

Table 12.2.
Binding Capacities of Antimigraine Drugs[a]

Drug	Serotonin	Adrenergic		
		α₁	α₂	β
Methysergide	5+	2+	2+	0
Cyproheptadine	5+	3+	2+	0
Ergotamine	4+	4+	4+	+
DHE	4+	4+	4+	0
Ergonovine	4+	2+	2+	0
Amitriptyline	4+	4+	+	0
Propranolol	2+	0	0	4+

[a]Adapted from Raskin NH. Headache. 2nd ed. New York: Churchill Livingstone, 1988:135–213.

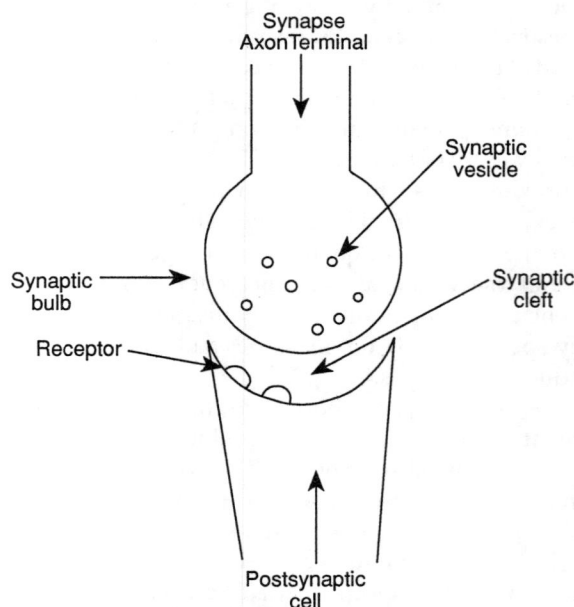

Figure 12.1. Synapse—site of communication between neurons in the central nervous system and site of drug action. Schematic drawing of anatomy of synapse.

the nerve terminal, which action potentiates and binds to its receptors on the postsynaptic cell. The nature of the receptor determines the final character of postsynaptic potentials, thus inhibiting or activating the postsynaptic neuron. Transmitters are resynthesized de novo in axon terminals. Neurotransmitters that are bound to postsynaptic receptors are actively reuptaken, making them available for further release.

Drugs possessing effects on chemical transmitters may act in a variety of ways (Table 12.3) (6, 12–14):

Selective inhibition of the reuptake mechanism, which prolongs the survival and availability of the transmitter close to its receptor;

Table 12.3.
Possible Mechanisms of the Agents Used in Migraine Treatment[a]

Agent	Mechanism
Amitriptyline	Inhibition of synaptic reuptake of serotonin
Papaverine, caffeine	Inhibition of PDE, cyclic AMP activation
Ergot alkaloids, methysergide	Serotonin receptor agonism at presynaptic autoreceptors
β-Blockers	Inhibition of forebrain postsynaptic serotonin receptor
Calcium channel blockers	Decrease serotonin release from brain tissue and inhibit platelet serotonin uptake and release
Prostaglandin	Modulation of serotoninergic neurotransmission
MAOIs	Inhibition of serotonin catabolism
Oxygen	Activation of tryptophan hydroxylase

[a]Modified from Raskin NH. Headache. 2nd ed. New York: Churchill Livingstone, 1988:135–213.

Augmentation of transmitter synthesis;
Inhibition of catabolism of the transmitter, which prolongs its survival;
Imitation of the effect of a transmitter, with direct effect upon receptor;
Alteration of the turnover of a cAMP, which modulates some of the postsynaptic effects of certain transmitters;
Inhibition of phosphodiesterase (PDE), which increases the intracellular levels of a cAMP and thus potentiates the effect of the transmitter on postsynaptic receptors (Fig. 12.2);
Change in intracellular calcium concentration and calcium entry into neurons, with calcium ions then increasing the number of serotonin-binding sites in brain membranes so that eventually the calcium channel blockers inhibit serotonin release;
Inhibition of the release of neurotransmitters from terminals of descending monoaminergic pathways, thus affecting pain transmission.

Appenzeller has recently proposed a very intriguing theory that does not exclude the role of other pathological mechanisms and neurotransmitters in migraine (15). He describes a significant action of the endothelial cells that not only form a barrier between the blood and the vascular smooth muscles but also are highly active metabolic endocrine organs. These cells produce several important substances, including prostacyclin; endothelium-derived relaxing factor, which is identical to nitric oxide (EDRF-NO), and endothelin-1 (ET-1). EDRF-NO, generated by L-arginine, relaxes vascular smooth muscle and inhibits platelet aggregation and adhesion. The release of EDRF-NO has been observed in association with heavy exercise and infections. ET-1 has ten times more vasoconstrictor action than angiotension II and acts as a neurotransmitter resembling serotonin. Endothelial cells also interact with

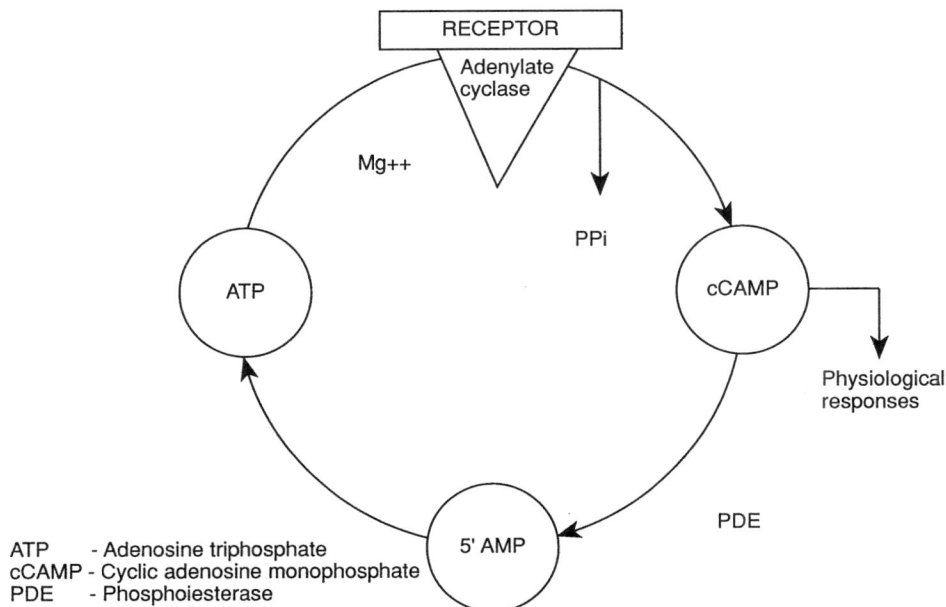

ATP - Adenosine triphosphate
cCAMP - Cyclic adenosine monophosphate
PDE - Phosphoiesterase

Figure 12.2. Metabolism of cAMP. Postsynaptic receptor activates adenylate cyclase, triggering cycle of synthesis and degradation of cAMP.

perivascular nerves that modulate vessel diameter and change the paracrine function of endothelial cells.

Role of Serotonin

The central serotonergic system is contained in clusters of cell bodies located mainly in the raphe nuclei of the brainstem. Some of the nuclei also contain catecholamine, GABA, and neuropeptides (16, 17).

There appear to be both presynaptic and postsynaptic serotonin receptors. Currently, four subtypes of $5\text{-}HT_1$ receptors are recognized, including 1A, 1B, 1C, 1D, as well as $5\text{-}HT_2$ and $5\text{-}HT_3$ receptors. These receptors may be linked to different second messenger's systems and may be found in different states of excitability.

The predominant action of serotonin is inhibitory, the suppression of cerebral neuronal firing postsynaptically. However, since 5-HT receptors are on both sides of the synapses, certain drugs may modulate release of serotonin. Drugs with a structure similar to that of serotonin, including ergot alkaloids and cyproheptadine, initiate the central action of serotonin by suppressing the electrical discharge of serotonergic neurons through a predominately presynaptic action (18).

Chronic administration of certain drugs changes the number of 5-HT receptors—down-regulation—which may explain delayed response to most antidepressant therapy. Trazodone, for example, appears to acutely antagonize $5\text{-}HT_2$ receptors and down-regulate these receptors upon chronic administration (19). Reduction of the number of $5\text{-}HT_2$ receptors may provide more $5\text{-}HT_2$ receptors available for a pool of serotonin.

According to Aghajanian (20), serotonin receptors and the rate of firing of raphe neurons are regulated by a feedback loop. Stimulation of the receptors by the serotonin agonist also results in a depression of the firing rate of raphe neurons. This is consistent with a reciprocal relationship between serotonergic neuronal activity and synaptic serotonin levels. Thus, the monoamine oxidase inhibitors (MAOIs) that block a catabolic pathway of serotonin (Fig. 12.3), elevate the concentration of intrasynaptic serotonin, and in turn depress the firing rate of the raphe neurons. Similarly, amitriptyline, which inhibits synaptic reuptake of serotonin, produces higher intrasynaptic concentration of 5-HT and a reduced firing rate of the raphe neurons (21).

Cyclic AMP has a substantial role in mediation of the effect of serotonin at its receptors (13). Inhibition of phosphodiesterase (PDE), the catalytic enzyme that degrades cAMP (Fig. 12.2), results in an increase in intracellular cAMP, and thus potentiates the effect of the neurotransmitter in activating the postsynaptic receptor. This mechanism of action is attributed to caffeine and papaverine (22, 23).

Costa and Meek (24) observed substantial elevation of serotonin synthesis in rats exposed to 100% oxygen. The oxygen, by its hydroxylative role in metabolism of tryptophan to 5-hydroxytryptophan (Fig. 12.3) and serotonin, augments the metabolic pool of intrasynaptic serotonin.

The dorsal raphe neurons receive stimulatory adrenergic input. Agents that block noradrenergic transmission or suppress norepinephrine cell firing inhibit serotonin cell firing and thus the metabolism of serotonin (25). Conversely, serotonin has a major role in modulation of the function as well as a number of central β-adrenoceptors. In addition, it appears that β-blocking drugs bind to brain serotonin receptors (26). The mode of action of the antimigraine therapy is summarized in Figure 12.4.

VASOACTIVE DRUGS

Most prophylactic antimigraine agents possess vasoactive properties. Although a vast majority of drugs from this heterogenous group are used in treatment of many medical problems, only two (propranolol and timolol) have been approved by the Food and Drug Administration (FDA) for long-term migraine prophylactic therapy. Empirical use has proven their ability to prevent migraine or lessen the intensity or frequency of migraine attacks. The mechanism of these agents in migraine prophylaxis is not very well understood. However, it is not limited to regulation of the lumen of the intracranial and extracranial vasculature (Table 12.4).

METABOLISM OF 5-HT (Serotonin)

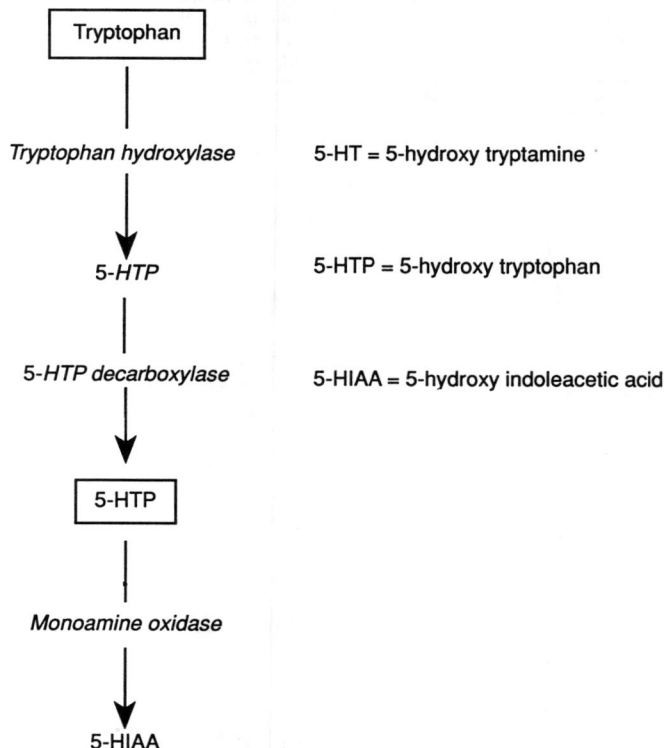

Tryptophan hydroxylase	5-HT = 5-hydroxy tryptamine
5-HTP	5-HTP = 5-hydroxy tryptophan
5-HTP decarboxylase	5-HIAA = 5-hydroxy indoleacetic acid
5-HTP	
Monoamine oxidase	
5-HIAA	

Figure 12.3. Metabolism of 5-HT (serotonin) from tryptophan. Notice the position of monoamine oxidase in this cycle.

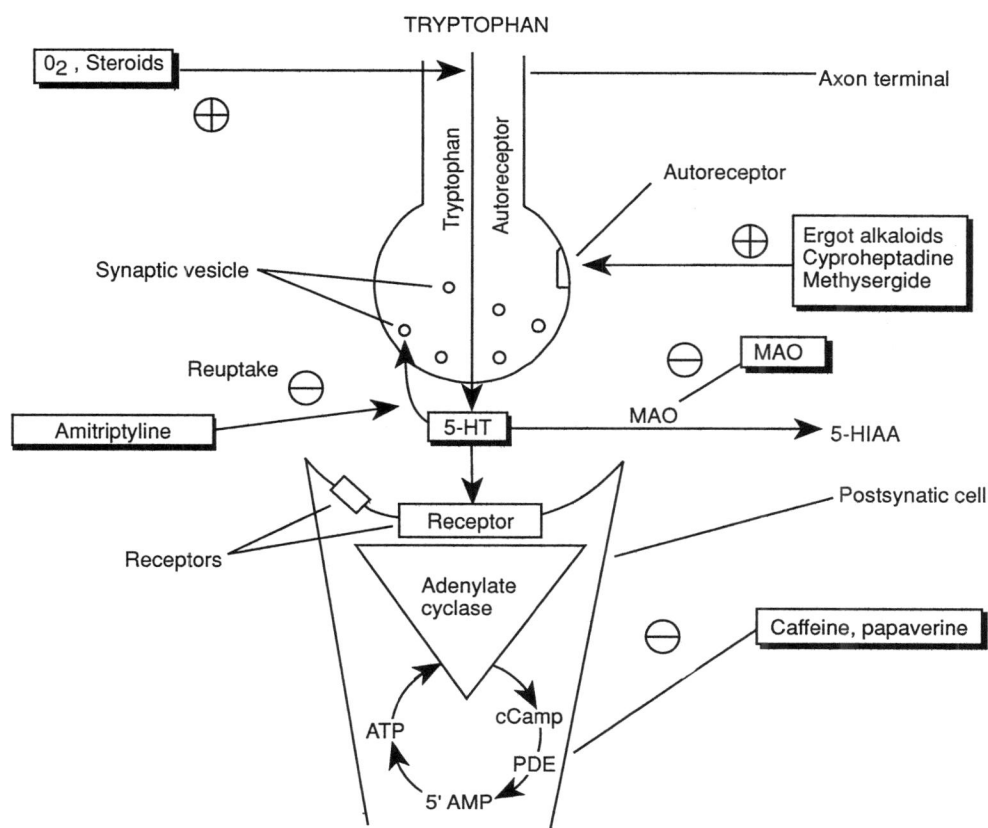

Figure 12.4. Mode of action of antimigraine therapy—site and action of some antimigraine drugs at synaptic level. *Symbols,* $\oplus$ indicates agonist effect, $\ominus$ indicates inhibitory effect.

Table 12.4.
Vasoactive Drugs

β-Adrenergic blockers
Calcium channel blockers
Ergot alkaloids
Clonidine
Papaverine

Table 12.5.
β-Blockers in Migraine Prophylaxis

Generic/Trade Name	Plasma Half-Life (hours)	Lipid Solubility	Dose (mg/day)
Propranolol/Inderal, Inderal LA	1–6	+ + +	40–320
Nadolol/Corgard	16–24	0	40–160
Timolol/Blocadren	4–5	+	10–40
Metroprolol/ Lopressor (cardioselective)	3	+	50–250
Atenolol/Tenormin (cardioselective)	6–9	0	50–200

β-Blockers

The effectiveness of β-blocking drugs in migraine therapy (see Table 12.5) was discovered serendipitously. Rabkin and his colleagues (27) observed the disappearance of concomitant migraine headaches in a cardiac patient treated with propranolol. Several controlled studies have confirmed that certain β-blockers have definitive beneficial effect in the prevention of migraine (Table 12.5) (28–32). β-Blockers have numerous indications. Although originally designed for treatment of angina, hypertension, cardiac arrhythmias, and acute myocardial infarction, these drugs also have a definitive role in the therapy of thyrotoxicosis, anxiety states, glaucoma, and migraine.

All β-blockers act competitively by inhibiting catecholamine at receptor sites. The exact mechanism of action of β-blockers in migraine is unknown. One explanation is the blockade of peripheral vasodilatation. Stimulation of β_2 receptors located in vascular smooth muscle causes vasodilation. Thus, the prevention of peripheral vasodilation by β-blockers is considered one of the pathogenic mechanisms of migraine headache. This theory, however, is questionable, as demonstrated in Olesen's study of propranolol's effects on cerebral blood flow (33).

β-Blockers may exert their effect through several biochemical processes (Table 12.6). The inhibition of lipolysis produces a decrease in arachidonic acid, a precursor of prostaglandin, thus resulting in a decrease in prostaglandins. The decrease in prostaglandins accounts for the inhibition of platelet aggregation. Increases in platelet aggregation parallels an increase in plasma serotonin levels during the prodromal phase of migraine. Similarly, platelet adhesiveness increases during the prodromes (34). The membrane-stabilizing effect is thought to contribute to migraine relief by reducing the pain caused by vasodilation and precapillary edema.

PROPRANOLOL

As stated previously, propranolol has been approved by the FDA with an indication for long-term prophylactic treatment of migraine. There are two optical isomers of propranolol, and only the *l*-form is β-blocking, although both possess membrane-stabilizing activity (35). Both isomers pass the blood-brain barrier almost immediately.

After the accidental discovery by Rabkin and his co-workers (27), several prospective studies were conducted to confirm their observations. In their controlled study, Diamond and Medina (36) demonstrated the efficacy of propranolol in the prophylaxis of migraine headache in 55 to 80% of cases. Long-acting propranolol has also been found effective for migraine prophylaxis, with results comparable to those observed with regular propranolol (37). Obviously, the long-acting form is more convenient for the patients, increases compliance, and is less expensive. In contrast, the long plasma half-life prevents rapid adjustment of the dose in the case of an adverse reaction.

Propranolol is a nonselective β-blocker with high lipid solubility, resulting in high brain penetration. This agent may be associated with some CNS side effects. It has extensive first-pass liver metabolism, very short plasma half-life, and no intrinsic sympathomimetic activity. The biological half-life of propranolol and all other β-blockers considerably exceeds the plasma half-life (35).

Propranolol is completely absorbed from the gastrointestinal tract and is almost completely metabolized in the liver. Levels of the drug are lower in smokers and in blacks. However, plasma levels are not closely correlated with therapeutic responses. Some of the metabolites of propranolol are pharmacologically active and may contribute to the effects of propranolol (35).

Propranolol is considered one of the most effective drugs in migraine prophylaxis and is the most widely used. The usual initial dose is 80 mg/day in three to four divided doses. Maintenance doses may range from 100 to 240 mg/day. The dosage must be individualized, as some migraineurs need a dosage as low as 40 mg a day, whereas others may require up to 320 mg, with tolerance. Duration of propranolol administration varies, but Diamond and Medina (36) have shown that 46% of patients who discontinued the use of propranolol after at least 6 months of efficacy had no significant recurrence of attacks during the subsequent follow-up period. The long-acting form of propranolol has been developed in doses of 60, 80, 120, and 160 mg. This single-daily-dose preparation has been especially effective in promoting patient compliance (37).

If no response occurs within 4 to 6 weeks, another agent should be used. Propranolol is contraindicated in heart failure because of negative inotropic effect, in severe bradycardia, high-degree heart block, and asthma or bronchospasm because of the β₂-blocking effect on the bronchial tree. In patients with insulin-dependent diabetes mellitus, propranolol masks autonomic reactions to hypoglycemia. This drug is also contraindicated in severe peripheral vascular disease.

The three major mechanisms of side effects to propranolol and other β-blockers are through (*a*) central nervous penetration (vivid dreams, insomnia, depression, impotence); (*b*) smooth muscle spasm (bronchospasm, vasoconstriction); and (*c*) exaggeration of the cardiac therapeutic actions (bradycardia, heart block, excess of negative inotropic effects, hypotension). There are isolated reports of peripheral vasoconstriction due to concurrent use of propranolol and ergotamine ((38) and personal observation). β-Blockers cross the placental barrier and are excreted in breast milk. Avoidance of these drugs is advisable during pregnancy and postpartum (Table 12.7).

Propranolol should not be withdrawn suddenly, especially in patients with coronary artery disease, to avoid exacerbation of angina, with potential danger of myocardial infarct. Withdrawal symptoms consist of tachycardia, ventricular arrhythmia, angina, nervousness, tremulousness, and exacerbation of hyperthyroidism. A tapering period of 14 days minimizes the withdrawal symptoms, and the patient should be closely observed.

Interaction between β-blockers and other drugs should also be considered. Combination of β-blockers and MAOIs is generally not recommended because of the potentiating hypotensive effect, and masking the signs and symptoms

Table 12.6.
Mechanism of Action of β-Blockers

Block β-receptors and thus prevent arterial dilation
Inhibit catecholamine-induced platelet aggregation
Decrease platelet adhesiveness
Block catecholamine-induced lipolysis
Prevent elevation of coagulation factors during epinephrine release
Inhibit renin secretion
Shift the hemoglobin-oxygen dissociation curve, promoting release of oxygen to tissue
Inhibit forebrain postsynaptic serotonin receptors

Table 12.7.
Side Effects of β-Blockers

CNS	Vivid dreams, nightmares, insomnia, fatigue, depression, hallucination, acute psychosis, impotency
CVS	Bradycardia, hypotension, lightheadedness, palpitation, heart block, exacerbation of heart failure, claudication, cold extremities, paresthesias, Raynaud's phenomenon
Others	Bronchospasm, dyspnea, abdominal cramps, diarrhea, dry mouth, blurred vision

of orthostatic hypotension. However, the Diamond Headache Clinic has extensive and successful experience with this combination. As a rule, treatment should be initiated in a closely monitored setting, preferrably in a specialized hospital unit with experienced nursing staff.

Cimetidine reduces hepatic blood flow and, therefore, increases blood levels of propranolol. This effect is not observed with β-blockers, such as nadolol and atenolol, that are not metabolized in the liver. Nonsteroidal antiinflammatory drugs (NSAIDs) attenuate the antihypertensive effects of β-blockers and thiazide diuretics (39).

OTHER β-BLOCKERS

The selection of a β-blocker in migraine prophylaxis (Table 12.5) depends on the patient's basic medical condition. Awareness of contraindications, side effects, and the pharmacokinetic properties of these drugs is essential. Agents with low lipid solubility should be used in individuals complaining of vivid dreams, insomnia, depression, and memory disturbances.

Cardioselective drugs, such as metoprolol and atenolol, are less likely to produce bronchospasm or mask hypoglycemic reaction in diabetic patients. β-Blockers with intrinsic sympathomimetic activity, such as acebutol and pindolol, have not been found useful in migraine prophylaxis (28).

Nadolol

Nadolol is noncardioselective β-blocker with long plasma half-life that permits once-daily dosing. It is less lipid soluble than propranolol, so CNS side effects are less frequently reported. The reported contraindications are similar to those of propranolol.

Initial dosage is 40 mg once a day, with an average dose of 120 mg. Dosage should be increased in weekly increments of 40 mg. Peak plasma levels are achieved 3 to 4 hours after administration, and 75% of the drug is excreted unchanged in the urine.

If switching from propranolol to nadolol, the propranolol does not need to be slowly withdrawn. The dosage of nadolol should be 20 to 40 mg less than the daily dose of propranolol. Efficacy of nadolol is comparable to that of propranolol (12, 28–29), but it is reportedly better tolerated.

Timolol

Timolol has also been approved for long-term migraine prophylactic therapy. It is a nonselective β-blocker with a short plasma half-life of 4 to 5 hours, low lipid solubility, and thus, low blood-brain penetration. Peak plasma levels are achieved in 1 to 2 hours. The initial dosage is 10 mg twice a day, with weekly increments of 10 mg daily. The average daily dose of timolol is 60 mg in two divided doses.

Stellar and his associates (30) confirmed the efficacy of timolol in 94 patients in a double-blind crossover study. Although a substantial decrease in frequency of headache attacks was achieved, no significant changes were noted in duration and severity of headaches. The side effects and contraindications are similar to those of propranolol.

Metoprolol

Metoprolol is a cardioselective β-blocker with a short plasma half-life of 3 to 4 hours, requiring twice-daily dosing. It penetrates the CNS well and is readily metabolized in the liver. Only 15% of the drug is plasma bound.

The starting dosage is 50 mg twice a day. If no response is noted, dosage may be increased to 100 mg twice a day. Because of its cardioselective properties, metoprolol may be used with considerable safety in diabetic and asthmatic patients.

Atenolol

Atenolol, like metoprolol, is cardioselective and may also be used in asthmatic and diabetic patients. The plasma half-life is 6 to 9 hours, with peak blood levels 2 to 4 hours after administration. Atenolol has very low lipid solubility and is excreted by the kidneys. Therefore, dosage adjustment is necessary in a patient with renal insufficiency. The initial dosage is 50 mg in a once-daily regimen, with an average daily dose of 100 mg.

CALCIUM CHANNEL BLOCKERS

The calcium channel blockers enjoy great popularity in Europe for the prophylactic treatment of migraine and cluster headache. These agents were originally designated for treatment of hypertension, angina, and arrhythmias. Their introduction to migraine prophylaxis was due to their vasospasm-inhibiting properties. However, several additional mechanisms for calcium blocker activity were discovered as a possible mode of action in migraine prophylaxis. Studies evaluating efficacy of this group of drugs are controversial. Nevertheless, use of calcium entry blockers is gaining popularity.

Role of Calcium in Vascular Smooth Muscle

Intracellular calcium is about 10 times less abundant than extracellular, indicating that some mechanism is responsible for maintaining a concentration gradient. This mechanism involves the calcium channel–proteins located in the cell membrane, which provide a route for the passage of ions. Intracellular calcium regulates muscle contraction, secretion of hormones and neurotransmitters, and the activity of a variety of enzymes.

Ions move through the calcium channel via an electrochemical gradient that requires an open channel. There are two types of channels, voltage-dependent channels that open by changes in membrane potential and ligand-gated channels that open by binding channel-associated receptors by ligands (40). Calcium channel blockers occupy these receptor sites and thus interfere with the influx of calcium into cells via voltage-dependent channels. Calcium channel receptors in the brain are primarily associated with certain synaptic areas, thus regulating serotonin release. Blocking of serotonin release at forebrain terminals may be one of the calcium channel blockers' modes of action in migraine.

Calcium channel blockers also block platelet serotonin release and aggregation (41), probably protecting the brain from ischemia and hypoxia. This action, thereby, decreases the chances of a migraine attack and prevents hypoxia-induced increases in blood viscosity. These agents also have an antihistaminic effect (42).

Several conflicting theories and studies exist regarding the mechanism and activity of calcium channel blockers in migraine prophylaxis (28, 41, 43–46). One of the theories, based on a proposed neuronal hypothesis of migraine, has been documented on animal experimental models. It shows that calcium entry blockers, namely flunarizine, have a potency to inhibit the spreading depression of Leao (44, 47). Spreading depression is an experimental phenomenon consisting of gradually spreading depolarization of neurons and glial cells. It explains the typical feature of the aura, enlarging fortification spectrum, or the gradual march of paresthesia in complicated migraine (48). However, there is no evidence that this spreading depression causes headache.

Some experimental findings indicate that flunarizine may interfere with central dopaminergic systems. The relationship between calcium channels and neurotransmitters is not simple. Flunarizine can reduce the K^+-induced release of dopamine and metenkephalin in corpus striatum, which may be responsible for induction of the extrapyramidal side effects and increase both basal and stimulated prolactin levels (49, 50).

Calcium channel blockers may act on different sites within the vascular smooth muscle cells. Verapamil is thought to inhibit calcium influx through receptor-operated channels, blocking the trigger release of sarcolemnal calcium. Flunarizine presumably inhibits intracellular calcium overload. Diltiazem decreases intracellular calcium concentrations through effects on the sodium-potassium pump and energy-dependent calcium extrusion (43).

Calcium blockers of "first-generation" as well as novel calcium entry blockers, consist of five different, unrelated classes: (a) dihydropyridines—nifedipine, nimodipine, and nicardipine; (b) phenylalkylamines—verapamil; (c) benzothiazepines—diltiazem; (d) piperazines—flunarizine; and (e) diphenylalkylamines—prenylamine (Table 12.8).

Verapamil

Verapamil, a prototype of calcium antagonists, is a papaverine-derived agent that possibly has multiple mechanisms

Table 12.8.
Calcium Channel Blockers

Drug	Average Daily Doses (mg)
Verapamil	240–480
Diltiazem	90–270
Nifedipine	30–90
Nicardipine	90–120
Nimodipine	60–120
Flunarizine	5–10

for effects on headache. The plasma peak level is obtained at 3 hours, and the elimination half-life is usually 3 to 7 hours. This level increases significantly during chronic administration and in patients with liver or renal insufficiency. Despite nearly complete absorption with oral doses, bioavailability is only 10 to 20%, due to high first-pass liver metabolism.

Verapamil can dilate previously constricted arteries and thus improve cerebral blood flow. Furthermore, platelet-induced vasospasm can also be reversed (51). Interestingly, verapamil also has β_2 and α_2 adrenoreceptor blocking potency. α-Adrenergic effects are also responsible for modulation of neurotransmitters in brain synaptic cells, with ultimate increase of norepinephrine release in the hypothalamus (52).

Verapamil also competitively inhibits binding to D-2 dopamine receptors, similar to the ergot alkaloids. By blocking dopamine receptors, varapamil treatment may elevate prolactin levels, which we have often observed in our patients. Verapamil also has effects on serotonin by decreasing serotonin release from brain tissue and blocking platelet serotonin uptake and release.

The average dose of verapamil is 240 to 360 mg per day. Higher doses may be more effective. Studies comparing verapamil 240 mg/day with 320 mg/day showed the mean monthly migraine frequency to be 3.4 on the dosage of 320 mg/day as opposed to 5.7 mean migraine frequency on lower dosage (53). Jansdottir and his associates (54) reported benefits in 81% of 26 patients with migraine without aura and 72% of 25 patients with migraine with aura who were treated prophylactically with verapamil. When compared with placebo, the differences in both frequency and headache unit index (the number of headaches over the number of days in a visit period) were significant. However, the differences in response between migraine with and without aura was not significant (40).

Therapy with verapamil should continue for at least 8 weeks before assessing significant improvement. Verapamil is contraindicated in patients with congested heart failure and AV conduction disturbances. This drug may be used in patients with asthma or insulin-dependent diabetes.

Side effects are quite common, occurring in about 30% of those treated. The most common complaints are constipation, GI disturbances, numbness of the limbs, and gynecomastia. Coadministration of β-blockers and calcium antagonists is possible, but one must be aware of the risk of hypotension. Verapamil may also lower serum lithium levels and increase sensitivity to lithium.

Diltiazem

Diltiazem is a benzothiazepine, which has not been used widely in the treatment of migraine. Research and therapeutic trials with diltiazem have been limited. The results, although promising, need to be confirmed in controlled studies before the efficacy of the drug can be assessed (28). Doses range from 60 to 90 mg, four times daily. This drug is considered to be well tolerated with infrequent adverse reactions such as GI upset, rash, edema, and headache.

Nifedipine

Nifedipine is a dihydropyridine used at doses of 30 to 120 mg per day in three divided daily doses. Kahan et al. (55) studied nifedipine in a double-blind, placebo-controlled crossover study in patients diagnosed with migraine associated with Raynaud's phenomenon. After a 1-month trial at doses of 10 mg three times a day, both the frequency and severity of the migraine attacks were significantly reduced. In a different group (54), decreases in both the frequency and severity of headache were reported by 65% of patients. Patients diagnosed with migraine with aura had the best response (77%), compared with 65% of patients with migraine without aura, and 41% of mixed headache patients. Side effects are relatively frequent. The most common complaints are postural hypotension, flushing, edema, GI upset, and headache. Results at the Diamond Headache Clinic with nifedipine have been poor to equivocal.

Nimodipine

Nimodipine is also a dihydropyridine. It is more selective for cerebral blood vessels, selectively reducing cerebral vascular tonus and increasing cerebral blood flow. Nimodipine blocks both voltage-dependent and ligand-gated channels. The plasma half-life is about 3 hours, and peak concentration is achieved 1 to 2 hours after administration. The daily dosage is 20 to 40 mg three times daily.

Several studies have evaluated the efficacy of the drug. In the study by Gelmers (56), significant reduction in the frequency and intensity of attacks was achieved. Duration of the attacks was not affected. In other study groups, the patients with migraine without aura had the best response (84%). Seventy-three percent of patients with migraine with aura and 33% of those with mixed headache reported benefit (53). Other sources reported no significant differences between nimodipine and placebo (43, 57). Adverse effects from nimodipine included GI complaints, postural hypotension, muscular cramps, and behavioral changes.

Nicardipine

Nicardipine is also a dihydropyridine. The usual dose is 20 to 40 mg three times a day. Nicardipine has a greater affinity than most other dihydropyridines for the binding site of the calcium channel in vascular smooth muscle. Nicardipine reduces the level of the prostaglandin PGE_2 and thromboxane A2 in the saliva of migraine suffers (58).

The study of Leandri and his associates (45) documented significant and marked improvement after nicardipine treatment in comparison with placebo. The drug was very well tolerated, with occasional reports of dizziness and gastralgia. No effects on weight, blood test, or attention were documented.

Flunarizine

Flunarizine, a difluorinated piperazine derivate, has undergone extensive laboratory testing in experimental conditions and several clinical trials, primarily in Europe. In the U.S., this promising antimigrainous drug has not yet been marketed and has had difficulty obtaining approval by the FDA because of some adverse reactions.

Flunarizine is highly lipophilic, facilitating easy passage through the blood-brain barrier and producing high blood levels in the CNS. Its antimigraine action is complex and not limited to a vasodilator mechanism. Notably, the clinical effectiveness of calcium antagonists in migraine does not correlate with their vasodilator potency (59). Flunarizine also seems to have a direct action on the calcium channels by inhibiting intracellular calcium overload. In experimental animal models, this drug inhibits spreading depression (47). It modulates some neurotransmitters, namely reducing the release of dopamine and metenkephalins in the corpus striatum. Flunarizine therapy can induce extrapyramidal side effects, depression, and an increase in prolactin levels by increasing the pituitary reserve of the hormone. This neuroendocrine effect supports the hypothesis of an antidopaminergic action of flunarizine, at least at the tuberoinfundibular dopaminergic system level (49). The drug is administered in 5- or 10-mg single evening doses in prophylactic treatment. In the treatment of acute migraine attacks, 10 to 20 mg is given IV or sublingually.

Diamond and Schenbaum (60) studied 20 patients with migraine, with or without aura, for 2 to 6 months with a single nighttime dose of 10 mg of flunarizine, in a single-blind crossover study. Seventeen of 20 patients obtained a statistically significant favorable response, with a greater than 50% average reduction in migraine symptoms. Reported side effects were mild, including fatigue or lethargy, difficulty sleeping, weight gain, mild muscle aches, and dry mouth. Most of the side effects resolved as treatment continued.

The latest double-blind, placebo-controlled study of Diamond and Freitag (61) demonstrated a 50% reduction of headaches in 50% of 101 patients treated with flunarizine. These results were similar to those of patients treated with verapamil, oxygen, or nimodipine.

It remains uncertain whether flunarizine is equally efficient in both migraine with and without aura. Amery et al. (62) compiled the data from seven studies, with 202 subjects included, and 85.7% of patients reported benefit. The benefit was seen in a progressive fashion over the first 3 months, and the improvement was observed as reducing the frequency of the migraine attacks. Furthermore, better response was noted in those with a shorter history of migraine and in patients younger than 35 years old. No difference was noted in sex or type of migraine.

Flunarizine has also been evaluated in a group of pediatric patients with migraine. The response was similar, and the drug was more effective after 3 months of therapy. The most common side effects were somnolence and weight gain (63). Less common but more dramatic side effects have been observed, including tardive dyskinesia, parkinsonism, and depression (Table 12.9).

Clonidine

Clonidine, an antihypertensive drug, acts centrally by inhibiting sympathetic outflow from the vasomotor center in the medulla. It also acts peripherally by reducing the response of blood vessels to both vasoconstrictors and vasodilators. This drug has also been recommended for prophylaxis of migraine, although the results of controlled studies are controversial.

A statistically significant study by Stensrud and Sjaastad (64) found clonidine to be effective in 62% of their patients in a short-term study. Only 40% of the patients reported efficacy in a long-term study. These results have been confirmed in several subsequent studies.

Clonidine has been used successfully in opiate withdrawal. It suppresses the autonomic signs and symptoms observed during withdrawal. This drug should be considered for those migraineurs habituated to opiates.

The usual dose is 0.1 mg twice daily orally or 0.1 mg transdermally once weekly. Rebound hypertension has been observed when clonidine had been discontinued abruptly. The drug should be reduced gradually over 2 to 4 days. Side effects are frequent but mild, including orthostatic hypotension, drowsiness, dry mouth, constipation, and occasional disturbances of ejaculation.

Papaverine

Papaverine is a vasodilator that has not gained popular acceptance in the prophylactic treatment of migraine. The vasodilator properties of papaverine are probably mediated by inhibition of the cyclic nucleotide phosphodiesterase, resulting in elevated levels of intracellular cAMP.

Papaverine has been used primarily in complicated migraine patients in whom neurological symptoms preceded the onset of headache. A hypothesis explaining therapeutic action is that the intracerebral vasoconstrictive phase of a migraine attack is a constant part of the migraine mechanism. Blocking this vasoconstrictive phase by a vasodilator (papaverine) may abort the development of attacks. Papaverine can indeed increase the cerebral blood flow, presumably by reduction in cerebrovascular resistance (65).

Papaverine is administered at daily doses of 300 to 600 mg, is very well absorbed, and its peak plasma level is reduced in 1 to 2 hours. Because of its short biologic half-life, a sustained-release preparation has been used. The most common side effects are constipation, nausea, drowsiness, vertigo, hypotension, and tachycardia.

ANTIINFLAMMATORY DRUGS AND PLATELET ANTAGONISTS

There has been considerable interest in the use of nonsteroidal antiinflammatory drugs (NSAIDs) in the treatment of migraine. Since the late 1960s, several studies have been conducted to evaluate the efficacy of the NSAIDs. These drugs may be used either as abortive agents for their analgesic properties or as prophylactic agents. The NSAIDs suppress inflammation through their effects on chemotaxis, lysosomal enzyme release, phagocytosis, complement and kinin generation, and formation of prostaglandins (Table 12.10).

One of the possible mechanisms of action of the mi-

Table 12.9.
Side Effects during 4 Months of Treatment with Flunarizine 5–10 MG/Daily[a]

Weight gain	70%
Sleepiness	20%
Depression	12.5%
Appetite gain	15%
Essential tremor	2.5%

[a]Adapted from Centonze V, Magrone D, Vino M, Caporaleti P, Attolini E, et al. Flunarizine in migraine prophylaxis efficacy and tolerability of 5 mg and 10 mg dose levels. Cephalalgia 1990;10:17–24.

Table 12.10.
NSAIDs

Drugs Generic/Trade Name	Plasma Half-Life (hours)	Dosage (mg)
Salicylates		
Aspirin		
Diflunisal/Dolobid	8–12	500–1000
Other salicylates/Disalcid, Salflex	4–16	1000–3000
Indoles		
Indomethacin/Indocin	2–3	75–150
Sulindac/Clinoril	18	200–400
Tolmetin/Tolectin	1–3	600–1800
Pyrazoles		
Phenylbutazone/ Butazolidine	55–100	400
Fenamates		
Mefenamic acid/Ponstel	3–4	1500
Meclofenamate sodium/ Meclomen	2–3	200–400
Propionic acid derivatives		
Ibuprofen/Motrin	2	1200–2400
Naproxen/Anaprox, Naprosyn	12–15	1000–1500
Fenoprofen calcium/ Nalfon	3	1800
Flurbiprofen/Ansaid	4	200–300
Ketoprofen/Orudis	2–4	150–300
Phenylacetic acid derivatives		
Diclofenac/Voltaren	2	100–150
Oxicams		
Piroxican/Feldene	45	20

graine drugs is a modulation of serotonergic neurotransmission and inhibition of prostaglandin synthesis. Prostaglandin production responds to numerous stimuli by the release to the blood stream directly from the site of production. Prostaglandins inhibit or activate adenylate cyclase, an enzyme converting ATP to cAMP, thus affecting postsynaptic production of neurotransmitters, including serotonin (Fig. 12.5). NSAIDs also prevent platelet aggregation, the abnormal reaction associated with the release of vasoactive substances observed in migraine (34). The role of prostaglandins in migraine is summarized in Table 12.11. The NSAIDs affect prostaglandin synthesis in the initial enzymatic step by inhibiting cyclooxygenase, the

enzyme converting arachidonic acid to the prostaglandin precursor (Fig. 12.5).

By their antiinflammatory properties, the NSAIDs reduce or suppress the consequences of the inflammatory changes (sterile inflammation) occurring in the late phase of a migraine attack. The NSAIDs are a chemically heterogenous group. However common characteristics, such as a variable degree of inhibition of prostaglandin formation, analgesia, antipyretic action, and liposolubility, distinguish these agents. Some common properties have been identified for specific drugs. Aspirin, tolfenamic acid, and naproxen have platelet antiaggregant action. Indomethacin has demonstrated vasoconstrictive action. Finally, aspirin and ketoprofen have central analgesic activity.

Naproxen

Naproxen is a propionic acid derivate, completely absorbed after oral administration. It achieves therapeutic serum concentration after 20 to 30 minutes and maximum concentration after 2 hours. Its half-life is 12 to 15 hours. Naproxen sodium achieves earlier and higher plasma levels and, therefore, may also be used as an abortive agent. Twice-daily dosing results in steady-state plasma levels within 2 to 3 days.

A study by Lindegaard and his associates (66) showed significant reduction in frequency, but no significant difference in duration of attack. The dose of naproxen in a double-blind, placebo-controlled crossover study was 250 mg twice daily. In another study (67), naproxen sodium

Table 12.11.
Role of Prostaglandins in Migraine[a]

Intravenous infusion of PGE_1 in nonmigrainous individuals produces a vascular type of headache

Infusion of serotonin into the pulmonary artery releases prostaglandin into the pulmonary vein and the response can be antagonized by ergotamine and methysergide

Infusion of serotonin into the cerebral ventricles results in a release of PGE into CSF

Intracarotid PGE_1 produces extracranial vasodilatation and loss of cerebral vasomotor autoregulation

Elevated salivary PGE_2 levels during migraine attacks, although no alterations of PGE levels have been observed in blood during migraine

Biphasic effects upon vascular beds; profound dilation of extracranial arterial circulation

[a]Modified from Raskin NH. Headache. 2nd ed. New York: Churchill Livingstone, 1988:135–213.

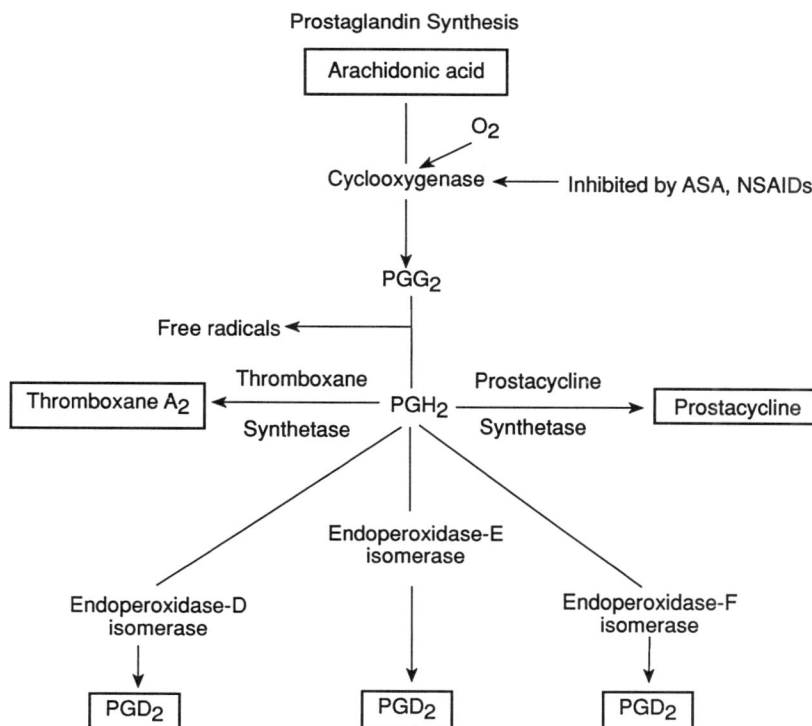

Figure 12.5. Prostaglandin synthesis from arachidonic acid, and level of cycle where NSAIDs and ASA inhibit the system.

Table 12.12.
Risk Factors of NSAID Nephrotoxicity[a]

Age >60 years, atherosclerotic cardiovascular disease, receiving concurrent diuretics
Renal insufficiency, usually serum creatinine level >2.0 mg/dl
States of renal hypoperfusion
  Sodium depletion
  Diuretic use
  Hypotension
  Sodium avid states—hepatic cirrhosis, nephrotic sy, CHF

[a]Adapted from Welch KMA, Ellis DJ, Keenan PA. Successful migraine prophylaxis with naproxen sodium. Neurology 1985;35:1304–1310.

was given at 550 mg twice daily for 8 weeks. Significant differences were noted in duration of the attack and the need for relief medication.

The most common side effects are related to the gastrointestinal tract. Other symptoms include dizziness, tinnitus, fluid retention, and skin reactions. Naproxen, as a prostaglandin inhibitor, exerts a direct effect on the renal tubule. In patients with diabetes mellitus, CHF, or cirrhosis, this agent may cause acute renal failure, nephrotic syndrome, or interstitial nephritis. Also, the NSAIDs as a group may cause electrolyte imbalance, such as dilutional hyponatremia due to fluid retention, hyperkalemia due to hyporeninemia, hypoaldosteronemia, and edema caused by sodium retention (Table 12.12). Although diarrhea occurs in up to 2% of patients taking NSAIDs, serious lower gastrointestinal complications are rare. Nevertheless, idiopathic inflammatory bowel disease, ulceration of the colon, and acute eosinophilic colitis were attributed to naproxen therapy (68).

Fenoprofen

Fenoprofen calcium, a derivative of propionic acid, is rapidly absorbed. This NSAID achieves a peak plasma level within 2 hours. Its plasma half-life is about 3 hours, and 99% is bound to albumin.

A double-blind, placebo-controlled study by Diamond's group (69) evaluated 110 migraine patients treated three times daily with 200 or 600 mg or fenoprofen or placebo. More than 50% improvement in headache unit index was observed in 22% of patients on fenoprofen 200 mg and 35% of patients on fenoprofen 600 mg. The difference was statistically significant, demonstrating that the 600-mg dose of fenoprofen is more effective in reducing headache intensity and duration than the 200-mg dose of the drug or placebo. Most of the reported side effects were from the gastrointestinal tract, such as nausea, abdominal pain, dyspepsia, and flatulence. Although no reports of renal failure occurred in this group, fenoprofen generally accounts for more than one-half of all renal failure cases associated with NSAID use.

Ketoprofen

Ketoprofen is a propionic acid derivative, exhibiting inhibitory effects on prostaglandin and leukotriene synthesis as well as antibradykinin activity and lysosomal membrane-stabilizing action. It is rapidly and completely absorbed from the gastrointestinal tract (GIT) and reaches the peak plasma levels in 0.5 to 2 hours. The mean plasma half-life ranges from 2 to 4 hours. Steady-state concentrations are attained within 24 hours after commencing treatment.

The dosage ranges from 150 to 300 mg in three to four divided doses. The dose should be reduced by 1/2 to 1/3 in patients with impaired renal function, including the elderly, who normally have decreased renal function.

Piroxicam

Piroxicam, a member of the oxicam family, is also used in the prophylactic management of migraine. The drug is well absorbed from the GIT, achieves the peak within 3 to 5 hours after consuming medication, and subsequently declines with a mean half-life of 50 hours. Steady-state plasma levels are achieved within 7 to 12 days. The dosage is 20 mg in a single daily dose. Piroxicam is well tolerated, with side effects similar to those of other NSAIDs.

Aspirin

Aspirin is one of the oldest known drugs with analgesic, antiinflammatory, and antipyretic actions. It is also a platelet antagonist, which provides aspirin a new role in cardiovascular medicine. The Physicians' Health Study, a double-blind, placebo-controlled trial that included 22,071 male physicians demonstrating decreased cardiovascular mortality with low-dose aspirin (325 mg every other day), was analyzed in morbidity follow-up. Of those randomized to aspirin, 6% reported migraine at some time after randomization, compared with 7.4% of those allocated to the placebo group. These data represent a statistically significant 20% reduction in recurrence rate (70).

As mentioned previously, platelets contain virtually all of the plasma serotonin. Therefore, it is likely that changes in platelet aggregability, found in migraine patients, lead to changes in levels of plasma serotonin. Although the platelet inhibition is a presumable mode of action of aspirin in migraine, the role of aspirin in prophylactic treatment is questionable (71). The Physicians' Health Study was a retrospective study that did not consider all aspects of migraine, such as sex distribution (study included only males), frequency, intensity, and duration of migraine attacks. Furthermore, self-diagnosis of migraine (done by these physicians) is at least debatable. More studies evaluating the efficacy of aspirin in migraine prophylaxis are needed.

ANTIDEPRESSANTS

The introduction of antidepressants to the treatment of migraine was based on two observations. In the early 1960s, an anticonvulsant, carbamazepine, an analogue of the tricyclic antidepressant (TCA) imipramine, was found effective in the treatment of trigeminal neuralgia and chronic pain. This observation empirically led to use of the tricyclic antidepressants in a variety of painful states including chronic headache. Furthermore, because one of the symptoms of depression is headache and many migraineurs become depressed, it was thought that an antidepressant would be effective in alleviating the pain of migraine. The efficacy of antidepressants in migraine therapy however, does not only depend on their antidepressant effects (72). Other mechanisms of action may help control the headaches.

Amitriptyline can serve as a model for understanding the TCA's mechanism of action. Amitriptyline blocks the amine (norepinephrine or serotonin) reuptake pump, causing a higher intrasynaptic concentration of neurotransmitters at the receptor site, and in turn, decreasing the firing

rate. Amitriptyline binds to the serotonin S_2 receptors more readily than to the S_1 receptors.

Fluoxetine inhibits CNS neuronal uptake of serotonin as well as uptake of serotonin into human platelets. Animal studies also suggest that fluoxetine is a more potent uptake inhibitor of serotonin than norepinephrine. Binding to muscarinic, histaminic, and α_1-adrenergic receptors is less avid than with TCAs. This action explains the lower side effect profile associated with anticholinergic, sedative, and cardiovascular effects.

Although neurotransmitters' uptake blockade may not be directly related to antidepressant effects, this property may be associated with certain side effects of antidepressants (73). (Table 12.13). Specifically, histamine interacts with two different types of receptors, H_1 and H_2. Some TCAs, such as doxepin, trimipramine, and amitriptyline, have a greater affinity to H_1 receptors. These drugs are likely responsible for the adverse reactions of drowsiness, sedation, and weight gain. However, the low affinity of trazodone for the H_1 receptor suggests that another mechanism may be responsible for the sedation (Table 12.14).

Cholinergic receptors, namely nicotinic and muscarinic, outside the brain are associated with contraction of smooth muscle, i.e. in the GIT. Because nicotinic receptors are involved mainly with locomotion, the term anticholinergic generally refers (for our purposes) to blockade of antimuscarinic receptors. Muscarinic blockade by the antidepressants, mainly amitriptyline, protriptyline, and trimipramine, causes blurred vision, dry mouth, constipation, urinary retention, impaired cognition, and sinus tachycardia. Trazadone is the least potent in blocking muscarinic receptors (Table 12.14).

Blockade of the α_1-adrenergic receptors is responsible for side effects such as postural hypotension, dizziness, and reflex tachycardia. The most potent α_1-blockers are doxepin, trimipramine, amitriptyline, and trazodone. The least potent of this class is protriptyline.

Antidepressants are only weak blockers of α_2 receptors and do not cause any adverse effects. This may explain the blunting of the antihypertensive effects of clonidine and methyldopa, which stimulate the α_2-receptors. Antide-

Table 12.13.
Adverse Effects of Antidepressants

Type	Minor, Early	Major
Sedation	Lassitude, fatigue	Sleepiness, impaired, consciousness with alcohol and other drugs
Sympathomimetic	Tachycardia, tremor, sweating	Agitation, insomnia, aggravation of psychosis
Antimuscarinic	Blurred vision, constipation, urinary hesitancy, furry thinking	Aggravation of glaucoma, paralytic ileus, urinary retention, delirium
Cardiovascular	Orthostatic hypotension, ECG abnormalities	Delayed cardiac conduction, arrhythmias, cardiomyopathy, sudden death
Psychiatric	Confusion	Central antimuscarinic syndrome, withdrawal
Neurological	Tremor, paresthesia, EEG alterations	Seizures, neuropathy
Allergic/toxic		Cholestatic jaundice, agranulocytosis
Metabolic/endocrine	Weight gain, sexual disturbance	Gynecomastia, amenorrhea
Birth defects		Uncertain
Hematologic		Hemolytic anemia

Table 12.14.
Effects of Antidepressants

Drug	Serotonin Inhibition	Norepinephrine Inhibition	Dopamine Inhibition	Sedative Effects	Anticholinergic Effects
Amitriptyline	Moderate	Weak	Inactive	Strong	Strong
Desipramine	Weak	Potent	Inactive	Mild	Moderate
Doxepin	Moderate	Moderate	Inactive	Strong	Strong
Imipramine	Fairly potent	Moderate	Inactive	Moderate	Strong
Nortriptyline	Weak	Fairly potent	Inactive	Mild	Moderate
Protriptyline	Weak	Fairly potent	Inactive	None	Strong
Trimipramine	Weak	Weak	Inactive	Moderate	Moderate
Amoxapine	Weak	Potent	Moderate	Mild	Mild
Trazodone	Fairly potent	Weak	Inactive	Strong	Mild
Fluoxetine	Potent	Weak	Inactive	None	Mild–none
Bupropion HCl	Weak	Weak	Weak	None	None
Maprotiline	Weak	Moderate	Inactive	Moderate	Moderate

pressants that antagonize the dopamine D_2 receptors, although weakly, may cause exrapyramidal movement disorders and endocrine changes, i.e., prolactin elevation. This relatively high affinity is observed with amoxapine and trimipramine (Table 12.14).

Some recent research findings (74) indicate additional pharmacological actions of TCAs. The TCAs also exhibit a direct membrane action and act as potent local anesthetics and membrane-stabilizing agents. Furthermore, they inhibit Na^+, K^+, and ATPase activity, and possibly influence prostaglandin synthesis.

The efficacy of amitriptyline in the prophylactic treatment of migraine was demonstrated by Couch et al (72). Migraine improvement was reported at more than 50% in 72% of the patients, and more than 80% in 57% of the patients. Two-thirds of patients who benefit from amitriptyline therapy show improvement within the first week. However, initial improvement may range up to 6 weeks. The doses and side effect profiles are summarized in Tables 12.13, 12.14, and 12.15.

MONOAMINE OXIDASE INHIBITORS (MAOIs)

In 1969, Anthony and Lance (75) published a study of 25 patients with migraine who had been unsuccessfully treated with conventional antimigrainous agents. These patients subsequently underwent treatment with the MAOI phenelzine, for a period ranging from 5 to 24 months. Twenty-eight percent of the patients completed the study headache-free, 28% demonstrated 75% improvement, 24% improved by 50%, and only 20% were unimproved. The study was based on the hypothesis that the serotonin released from the platelets during a migraine attack results in arterial dilation. Since serotonin is catabolized to a monoamine, 5-hydroxyindolacetic acid, by monoamine oxidase, the MAOIs block this degradation step, resulting in the elevation of plasma and tissue levels, thus preventing uncontrolled vasodilation (Fig. 12.3).

Chronic MAOI administration results in the down-regulation of brain serotonin and β-adrenoreceptors.

The MAOIs are underutilized in the treatment of migraine. As the study of Anthony and Lance (75) and our own long-term experience with MAOIs have demonstrated, the MAOIs have a definitive role in the prophylactic treatment of migraine that has failed to respond to conventional therapy. The MAOIs, however, are not a first-line drug. Because of the potential risk of drug and food interactions, these agents should only be used in carefully selected individuals.

Combination therapy with MAOI and TCA compounds has been long considered taboo, or at least a poor or dangerous practice. The severe reactions and deaths that have occurred during dual therapy were overstated, as indicated in the reviews of the case reports of these fatalities (76, 77). There is evidence that amitriptyline may actually be safely used with phenelzine. Amitriptyline, by inhibiting the uptake of tyramine, prevents the pressor response to tyramine in subjects receiving MAOIs (78).

Phenelzine is well absorbed, achieving a peak blood level in 2 to 4 hours after ingestion. The maximum inhibition and efficacy occur within 1 to 3 weeks after initiation of therapy. This is the critical period when the patient needs to be encouraged not to lose faith in the treatment. Phenelzine metabolism is dose-dependent, meaning a longer eliminating half-life with high doses. The maintenance doses range from 30 to 75 mg, although higher doses may be used if tolerated. Isocarboxazid, another MAOI, is given in the usual starting dose of 30 mg daily and may be increased to 40 to 50 mg, with subsequent reduction to a maintenance dose.

Patients on MAOIs must be warned about possible reactions from interaction of MAOIs and certain foods containing tyramine (Table 12.16). In this interaction, hypertensive crisis may occur, caused by the facilitation of norepinephrine release from its binding sites by tyramine that escaped oxidative deamination in the GIT. Also, nasal decongestants, including over-the-counter medications, pseudoephedrine, epinephrine, and meperidine, should be avoided during treatment with an MAOI or for 2 weeks after cessation of the therapy.

Side effects include increased appetite, weight gain, fluid retention, and constipation. Orthostatic hypotension may occur primarily in conjunction with β-blockers,

Table 12.15.
Usual Starting and Maintenance Dose

Drug	Starting Dose	Maintainence Dose (mg)
Tricyclics		
Amitriptyline/Elavil, Endep	50	75–200
Desipramine/Norpramin	50	75–200
Doxepin/Sinequan, Adapin	50	75–300
Nortriptyline/Pamelor	50	75–150
Protriptyline/Vivactil	10	20–40
Trimipramine/Surmontil	50	75–200
Second-generation		
Fluoxetine/Prozac	20	20–80
Trazodone/Desyrel	50	50–600
Bupropion/Wellbutrin	200	300
MAOI		
Isocarboxazide/Marplan	20	30–60
Phenelzine/Nardil	30	30–75

Table 12.16.
Common Food Items Containing High Concentration of Tyramine

Liquor, wine (esp. red), beer
Ripened cheeses
Excessive amount of chocolate or caffeine
Nuts
Fresh baked breads
Sour cream
Broad beans
Anything marinated or fermented

which can block sympathetic response to hypotension and mask its symptoms. Other side effects include insomnia, loss of libido, inhibition of ejaculation, perspiration, and CNS overstimulation with anxiety, jitter, and muscle jerks (Table 12.16).

OTHER PHARMACOLOGICAL AGENTS
Methysergide

Methysergide, a lysergic acid derivate, was developed for migraine prophylaxis, as one of the semisynthetic ergot alkaloids derived from the naturally occurring ergonovine. Approved by the FDA and used since 1959, methysergide became a hope for millions of migraineurs and an impetus for researchers working on migraine agents. The introduction of methysergide as a powerful antimigraine drug led investigators to a better understanding of the processes occurring during a migraine attack.

The mechanism of action is uncertain. There are several blood vessel responses to migraine. Methysergide is capable of producing a permanent state of vasoconstriction, primarily noted as a side effect. It potentiates the pressor effects of catecholamine and other vasoconstrictor agents. This drug may reduce the pain-producing effect of serotonin when released from the platelets. Methysergide may reduce the vasoconstrictor activity of serotonin on small arteries. Also, it may maintain tonic vasoconstriction of larger arteries once the serotonin level has fallen (79).

The drug also affects unstable vasomotor functions, as it tends to dampen the activity of the conjunctival blood vessels when these vessels are stimulated during oliguria and diuresis. Furthermore, methysergide has mild antiinflammatory effects and is capable of reducing cutaneous inflammation produced by a variety of irritants.

Methysergide is absorbed rapidly, achieving peak plasma levels in 1 hour. The drug should be started at 2 mg daily and gradually increased, to lessen some unpleasant side effects. The maintenance dosage is 4 to 6 mg daily in two to three divided doses. The beneficial effect becomes evident within 7 to 10 days. The treatment should not exceed 6 consecutive months. If the patient must continue on methysergide, a drug hiatus of 6 to 8 weeks is indicated after 6 months of therapy. Prolonged therapy with methysergide is known to cause cardiopulmonary and retroperitoneal fibrosis.

The efficacy of methysergide has been shown in a study by Curran et al. (80) in which substantial improvement resulted in about 60% of patients. The side effects, predominately nausea, abdominal discomfort, and muscle cramps may be reported in about 30 to 40% of patients. These symptoms will usually subside over a period of days to weeks. Other, less common side effects include drowsiness, insomnia, anxiety, weight gain, nasal congestion, flushing, and limb claudication. Unlike lysergic acid, methysergide has little effect on the nervous system.

The incidence of the more serious problem of fibrotic disorders is about 1:500 (81). The disorders probably develop idiosyncratically. Fibrosis will recede upon the cessation of the drug. Endocardial fibrosis is manifested by the development of new murmurs, reflecting vascular involvement, ultimately resulting in CHF. Auscultation of the heart and ECG should be performed on a regular basis. Pleuropulmonary fibrosis can be identified by dyspnea, chest pain, pleural friction rubs with pleural effusions, and fibrotic changes on chest x-ray. Retroperitoneal fibrosis is the most common fibrotic complication of this therapy. It may present with flank pain, fever, urinary problems, or elevation of ESR. However, it usually remains clinically silent. Patients on prolonged methysergide therapy should undergo IVP or abdominal MRI at 6-month intervals.

Methysergide is contraindicated in patients with peripheral vascular disease, coronary artery disease, thrombophlebitis, peptic ulcer disease, and pregnancy. Because of the serious problems with fibrotic disorders, methysergide should only be prescribed in carefully selected patients.

Cyproheptadine

Cyproheptadine is an antihistamine with mild to moderate antiserotonin activity, similar to that of methysergide. It resembles the phenothiazine antihistaminic and the ergot alkaloids in chemical structure.

The possible mode of action is similar to that of methysergide and ergot alkaloids. Cyproheptadine is a presynaptic serotonin receptor agonist with the net functional effect of depressing the firing rate of serotonergic neurons via presynaptic autoreceptors (17). The drug also has calcium channel blocking properties (82). However, the peripheral effects on the cranial vasculature are less pronounced than those of methysergide.

The overall effect in patients with migraine is less beneficial. However, cyproheptadine is still considered the drug of choice in children with migraine (83). Younger patients tolerate this medicine well. The usual dosage for children is 8 to 16 mg in two to four divided doses daily. The most troublesome and common side effects are increased appetite, weight gain, sedation, and dry mouth. Cyproheptadine has not been approved by the FDA for indication in the treatment of migraine.

Lithium

Occasionally, a patient will present with migraine attacks occurring in cycles or clusters. The headaches occur every few days for several weeks, then become less frequent, and eventually completely disappear for several weeks or a few months. The headache attacks, although reoccurring in clusters, are not typical cluster headaches. There is a female predominance. These cyclic migraines (84) may be successfully treated with lithium carbonate. In median and Diamond's study (84), 19 of 22 patients treated with lithium had a good response. Lithium has no effect on cerebral hemodynamics, but there is evidence that lithium stabilizes and facilitates serotonergic neurotransmission at the site of the hypothalamic pacemaker regulating circadian rhythms (85).

Lithium is well absorbed from the GIT, and peak plasma levels are reached within 2 to 4 hours. The average dose is 900 mg daily in three divided doses. Plasma levels should be carefully monitored weekly during the first few weeks of treatment. Therapeutic levels should be maintained to prevent lithium toxicity.

The side effects include tremor, nausea, diarrhea, and polyuria. Dysarthria, myoclonic jerks, fasciculations, convulsions, and renal failure may be observed with high plasma levels. Lithium intoxication can be caused by interaction with other drugs, particularly indomethacin, phenytoin, carbamazepine, thioridazine, methyldopa, haloperidol, and thiazide diuretics.

Lithium may impair urinary concentrating ability and induce nephrogenic diabetes insipidus. It also increases renal tubular resorption of calcium and causes hypercalcemia. Because lithium blunts the calcium feedback inhibition of parathyroid hormone release, hyperparathyroidism may develop. Other disturbances caused by lithium include weight gain, thyroid dysfunction, gonadal function abnormalities, and cutaneous lesions. Lithium should not be used during the first trimester of pregnancy.

Anticonvulsants

Anticonvulsants are not considered routine antimigraine therapy. However, some of these agents may be beneficial in the treatment of a small population of migraineurs who fail to respond to established migraine prophylactic agents. An adequately large controlled study has never been published, but there are a few studies comprising small populations. Phenytoin, a commonly used anticonvulsant, has been found beneficial in certain refractory cases of migraine. The mechanism of action is unknown, but the drug affects ion-conduction membrane potentials and the concentrations of amine acids and the neurotransmitters norepinephrine, acetylcholine, and GABA. At high concentrations, it also inhibits the release of serotonin and norepinephrine, promotes the uptake of dopamine, and inhibits monoamine oxidase activity. Furthermore, it reduces calcium permeability and inhibits the calcium influx across the cell membrane. It is difficult to determine which mechanism could be implicated in its efficacy in migraine treatment. However, the mechanism of phenytoin's action probably involves a combination of actions at several levels. Phenytoin has been effective in treating migraine in children (86) and adults (87).

Valproic Acid

Another anticonvulsant, valproate, was pragmatically introduced recently into the armamentarium of migraine treatment. The mechanism of action of valproate is not fully explained; however, it is hypothesized that the drug mainly involves the GABA system or has a neurogenic effect on the vascular system.

Sørenson conducted a prospective open trial of valproate in 22 patients with migraine, with and without aura (88). Fifty percent of the patients achieved complete cessation of migraine attacks; 26% had a significant reduction of the frequency. The starting dose was 600 mg twice a day. The onset of action was reported within the first and second week of treatment. Its effect seems to be dose-related, with optimal serum level about 700 μmol/p. Reported side effects were slight weight gain and drowsiness. It is necessary to monitor liver enzymes and bleeding time to avoid hepatic toxicity, which is reversible after withdrawal of the drug.

REFERENCES

1. Diamond S, Dalessio D. The practicing physician's approach to headache. 4th ed. Baltimore: Williams & Wilkins, 1986.
2. Olsen TS, Friberg L, Lassen NA. Ischemia may be the primary cause of the neurologic deficits in classic migraine. Arch Neurol 1987;44:156–161.
3. Olesen J, Lauritzen M, Tfelt-Hansen P, Henriksen L, Larsen B. Spreading cerebral oligemia in classical - and normal cerebral blood flow in common migraine. Headache 1982;22:242–248.
4. Sacks H, Wolf A, Russell JAG, Christman DR. Effect of reserpine on regional cerebral glucose metabolism in control and migraine subjects. Arch Neurol 1986;43:1117–1123.
5. Anthony M, Hinterberger H, Lance JW. The possible relationship of serotonin to the migraine syndrome. Res Clin Stud Headache 1969;2:29–59.
6. Malmgren R. The central serotoninergic system. Cephalalgia 1990;10:199–204.
7. Anselmi B, Baldi E, Cassaci F, Salmon S. Endogenous opiates in cerebrospinal fluid and blood in idiopathic headache sufferers. Headache 1980;20:294–299.
8. Solomon GD, Kunkel RS, Frame J, Procaccino E, Senenayake P. Plasma vasoactive peptide levels in migraine. Headache 1990;30:294.
9. Nicolodi M, Del Bianco E. Sensory neuropeptides (substance P_1 calcitonin gene-related peptide) and vasoactive intestinal polypeptide in human saliva; their pattern in migraine and cluster headache. Cephalalgia 1990;10:39–50.
10. Snyder SH. Brain receptors. the emergence of a new pharmacology. Trends Neurosci 1986;9:455–459.
11. Worley PF, Barban JM, Snyder SH. Beyond receptors; multiple second messenger systems in brain. Ann Neurol 1987;21:217–229.
12. Raskin NH. Headache. 2nd ed. New York: Churchill Livingstone, 1988:135–213.
13. Hamon M, Bourgoin S, El Mestikawy S, Goetz C. Central serotonin receptors. In: Lajtha A, ed. Handbook of neurochemistry. 2nd ed. Receptors in the neuro system. New York: Plenum, 1984:107–143.
14. Berge OG. Regulation of pain sensitivity, influence of prostaglandin. Cephalalgia 1986;6:21–31.
15. Appenzeller O. Pathogenesis of migraine. Med Clin North Am 1991;75:763–789.
16. Dahlstrøøm A, Fuxe K. Evidence for the existence of monoamine-containing neurons in the CNS. I. Demonstration of monoamine in cell bodies of brain neurons. Acta Physiol Scand 1964;62:1–55.
17. Nanopoulos D, Belin MF, Maitre M, Vincendou G, Pujol JF. Immunocytochemical evidence for the existence of GABA-ergic neurons in the nucleus raphe dorsalis. Possible existence of neurons containing serotonin and GABA. Brain Res 1982;232:375–389.
18. Haigler HJ, and Aghajanian GK. Serotonin receptors in the brain. Fed Proc 1977;36:2159–2164.

19. Riblet LA, Taylor DP. Pharmacology and neurochemistry of trazodone. J Clin Psychopharmacol 1981;1:175–225.

20. Aghajanian GK. Influence of drugs on the firing of serotonin-containing neurons in brain. Fed Proc 1972;31:91–96.

21. Fuller RW, Wong DT. Inhibition of serotonin re-uptake. Fed Proc 1977;36:2154–2158.

22. Berkowitz BA, Spector S. The effect of caffeine and theophylline on the disposition of brain serotonin in the rat. Eur J Pharmacol 1971;16:322–325.

23. Palmer GC. Significance of phosphodiesterase in the brain. Life Sci 1981;28:2785–2798.

24. Costa E, Meek J. Regulation of biosynthesis of catecholamine and serotonin in the CNS. Annu Rev Pharmacol 1974;14:491–511.

25. Middlemiss DN. Blockade of the central 5-HT autoreceptor by beta-adrenoceptor antagonists. Eur J Pharmacol 1986;120:51–56.

26. Middlemiss DM. Stereo-selective blockage at [³H] 5-HT binding sites and at the 5-HT autoreceptor by propranolol. Eur J Pharmacol 1984;101:289–293.

27. Rabkin R, Stables DP, Levin NW, Suzman M. The prophylactic value of propranolol in angina pectoris. Am J Cardiol 1966;18:370–383.

28. Andersson KE, Vigre E. β-Adrenoceptor blockers and calcium antagonists in the prophylaxis and treatment of migraine. Drugs 1990;39:355–373.

29. Freitag FG, Diamond S. Nadolol and placebo comparison study in the treatment of migraine. J Am Osteopath Assoc 1984;84:343–347.

30. Stellar S, Ahrens SP, Meibohn AR, Reines SA. Migraine prevention with timolol. JAMA 1984;252:2576–2580.

31. Strensrud P, Sjaastad O. Comparative trial of Tenormin (atenolol) and Inderal (propranolol) in migraine. Headache 1980;20:204–207.

32. Vilming S, Stendnes B, Hedman C. Metoprolol and pizotifen in the prophylactic treatment of classical and common migraine: a double-blind investigation. Cephalalgia 1985;5:17–23.

33. Olesen J. Beta-adrenergic effects on cerebral circulation. Cephalalgia 1986;6:41–46.

34. Deshmukk SV, Meyer JS. Cyclic changes in platelet dynamics and the pathogenesis and prophylaxis of migraine. Headache 1977;17:101–108.

35. Opie LH, Sonnenblick EH, Kaplan NM, Thodoni U. Drugs for the Heart. 2nd ed. Orlando: Grune & Stratton, 1987:1–18.

36. Diamond S, Medina JL. Double-blind study of propranolol for migraine prophylaxis. Headache 1976;16:238–245.

37. Diamond S, Kudrow L, Stevens J, Shapiro DB. Long-term study of propranolol in the treatment of migraine. Headache 1982;22:268–271.

38. Venter CP, Joubert PH. Severe peripheral ischemia during concomitant use of beta blockers and ergot alkolids. Br Med J 1984;289:288–289.

39. Webster J. Interactions of NSAIDs with diuretics and β-blockers. Mechanisms and clinical implications. Drug 1985;30:32–41.

40. Greenberg DA. Calcium channels and calcium channel antagonists. Ann Neurol 1987;21:317–330.

41. Solomon GD, Spaccavento LJ. Verapamil prophylaxis of migraine: A double-blind, placebo-controlled trial. JAMA 1983;250:2500–2502.

42. Amery WK, Wauquier A, Van Nueten JM, De Clerck F, Van Reempts JV, Janssen PAJ. The antimigrainous pharmacology of flunarizine, a calcium antagonists. Drug Exp Clin Res 1981;7:1–10.

43. Olesen J. Calcium antagonists in migraine and vertigo. Possible mechanisms of action and review of clinical trials. Eur Neurol 30:31–34.

44. Solomon GD. The action and uses of calcium channel blockers in migraine and cluster headache. Headache Quart 1990;1:152–159.

45. Leandri M, Rigardo S, Schizzi R, Parodi CI. Migraine treatment with nicardipine. Cephalalgia 1990;10:111–116.

46. Amery WK. Migraine and cerebral hypoxia: a hypothesis with pharmacotherapeutic implications Cephalalgia 1985;2:131–133.

47. Marrannes R, Wauquier A. Influence of flunarizine on spreading depression. Cephalalgia 1985;5:208.

48. Lauritzen M. Spreading cortical depression in migraine. In: Amery WK, Van Nueten JM, Wauquier A, eds. The pharmacological basis of migraine therapy. London: Pitman, 1984 149–160.

49. Piccini P, Nuti A, Paoletti AM, Napolitano A, Melis GB, Bonncelli U. Possible involvement of dopaminergic mechanisms in the antimigraine action of flunarizine. Cephalalgia 1990;10:3–8.

50. Centonze V, Magrone D, Vino M, Caporaleti P, Attolini E, et al. Flunarizine in migraine prophylaxis efficacy and tolerability of 5 mg and 10 mg dose levels. Cephalalgia 1990;10:17–24.

51. Leblanc R, Fiedel W, Yamamoto LY, Milton JG, Frojmovic MM, Hodge CP. The effects of calcium antagonism on the epicerebral circulation in early vasospasm. Stroke 1984;15:1017–1020.

52. Glazin AM, Langer SZ. Presynaptic alpha 2-adrenoceptor antagonism by verapamil, but not by diltiazem in rabbit hypothalamic slices. Br J Pharmacol 1983;78:571–577.

53. Solomon GD, Diamond S. Verapamil in migraine prophylaxis in comparison of dosages. Clin Pharmacol The⁻ 1987;41:202.

54. Jonsdottir M, Meyer JS, Rogers RL. Efficacy, side effects and tolerance compared during headache treatment with three different calcium blockers. Headache 1987;27:364–369.

55. Kahan A, Weber S, Amor B, Guerin F, Degeorges M. Nifedipine in the treatment of migraine inpatients with Raynaud's phenomenon. N Engl J Med 1983;308:1102–1103.

56. Gelmers NJ. Nimodipine, a new calcium antagonist in the prophylactic treatment of migraine. Headache 1983:23:106–109.

57. Migraine-Nimodipine European Study Group: European Multicenter. Trial of nimodipine in the prophylaxis of classic and common migraine. Headache 1983;29:633–642.

58. Oback Tuca J, Planas, JM, Puig Parellada P. Increase in PgE₂ and TXA₂ in the saliva of common migraine patents. Action of calcium channel blockers. Headache 1989;29:498–50⁻.

59. Peroutka SJ, Banghart SD, Allen GS. Relative potency and selectivity of calcium antagoists used in the treatment of migraine. Headache 1984;24:55–58.

60. Diamond S, Schenbaum H. Flunarizine, a calcium channel blocker, in the prophylactic treatment of migraine. Headache 1983;23:39–42.

61. Diamond S, Freitag FG. Flunarizine and migraine therapy. In: New Advances in Headache Research: 2. London: Smith-Gordon, 1991.

62. Amery WK, Caers LI, Aerts TJL. Flunarizine, a calcium entry blocker in migraine prophylaxis. Headache 1985;25:249–254.

63. Caers LI, De Beukelaar F, Amery WK. Flunarizine a calcium-entry blocker in childhood migraine, epilepsy, and alternating hemiplegia. Clin Neuropharmacol 1987;10:162–168.

64. Stensrud P, Sjaastad O. Clonidine (Catapress); double-blind study after long term treatment with the drug in migraine. Acta Neurol Scand 1976;53:233–236.

65. Poser CM. Papaverine in prophylactic treatment of migraine. Lancet 1974;1:1290.

66. Lindegard KF, Ovrelid L, Sjaastad O. Naproxen in the prevention of migraine attacks. A double-blind placebo-controlled cross-over study. Headache 1980;20:96.

67. Welch KMA, Ellis DJ, Keenan PA. Successful migraine prophylaxis with naproxen sodium. Neurology 1985;35:1304–1310.

68. Bridges AJ, Marshall JB, Diaz-Arias AA. Acute eosinophilic colitis and hypersensitivity reaction associated with naproxen therapy. Am J Med 1990;89:526–527.

69. Diamond S, Solomon GD, Freitag FG, Mehta ND. Fenoprofen in the prophylaxis of migraine: a double-blind, placebo controlled study. Headache 1987;27:246–249.

70. Buring JE, Peto R, Hennekens CH. Low-dose aspirin for migraine prophylaxis. JAMA 1990;264:1711–1713.

71. Hosman-Benjaminse SL, Bolhuis PA. Migraine and platelet aggregation in patients treated with low dose acetylsalicylic acid. Headache 1986;26:282–284.

72. Couch JR, Ziegler DK, Hassanein R. Amitriptyline in the prophy-

laxis of migraine. Effectiveness and relationship of migraine and antidepressant effects. Neurology 1976;26:121–127.

73. Richelson E. Pharmacology of antidepressants. Desyrel—a compendium of three years of clinical use. Proceedings of a symposium held September 14, 1989 in Chicago, Illinois.

74. Preskorn SH, and Hartman BK. Tricyclic antidepressants: new sites of action. Behav Med 1979;5:30–33.

75. Anthony M, Lance JW. Monoamine oxidase inhibition in the treatment of migraine. Arch Neurol 1969;21:263–268.

76. Schuckit M, Robins E, Feighner J. Tricyclic antidepressants and monoamine oxidase inhibitors. Arch Gen Psychiatry 1971;24:509–514.

77. White K, and Simpson G. Combined MAOI-tricyclic antidepressant treatment: a reevaluation. J Clin Psychopharmacal 1981;5:264–282.

78. Pare CM, Kline N, Hallstrom C, Cooper TB. Will amitriptyline prevent the "cheese" reaction of monoamine oxidase inhibitors. Lancet 1982;2:183–186.

79. Lance JW. Mechanism and management of headache. 4th ed. London: Butterworth, 1982:178–204.

80. Curran DA, Hinterberger H, Lance JW. Methysergide. Res Clin Stud Headache 1967;1:74–122.

81. Graham J. Cardiac and pulmonary fibrosis during methysergide therapy for headache. Am J Med Sci, 1967;254:1–12.

82. Peroutka SJ, Allen GS. The calcium antagonist properties of cyproheptadine: implications for antimigraine action. Neurology 1984;34:304–309.

83. Bille B. Migraine in childhood. Panminerva Med., 1982;24:57–62.

84. Medina JL, Diamond S. Cyclical migraine Arch Neurol 1981;38:341–344.

85. Blier P, DeMontigny C. Short-term lithium administration enhances serotonergic neurotransmission: electrophysiological evidence in the rate of CNS. Eur J Pharmacol 1985;113:69–77.

86. Millichap JG. Recurrent headaches in 100 children. Childs Brain 1978;4:95–105.

87. Swanson JW, Vick NA. Basilar artery migraine: 12 patients with an attack recorded electroencephalographically. Neurology 1978;28:782–786.

88. Sørensen KV. Valproate: a new drug in migraine prophylaxis. Acta Neurol Scand 1988;78:346–348.

13

Nonpharmacological Treatment of Migraine

STEVEN M. BASKIN and RANDALL E. WEEKS

Biobehavioral considerations in the diagnosis and treatment of headache have become more broad-based in order to more fully examine issues related to diagnosis, pathophysiology, and therapeutic agents of change. As a result, there is a wide body of literature with contributions from many different disciplines. The present discussion focuses on nonpharmacological approaches to migraine.

Physical therapy approaches have been shown to reduce and control head pain, but most have combined tension-type headache patients with migraine patients. For example, physical therapy approaches (with and without TENS units) have been found to be effective in the treatment of the chronic daily headache patient (1, 2). The controlled application of cold and heat has also been shown to reduce head pain (3).

Acupuncture, one of the earliest forms of stimulation-produced analgesia, has been practiced in the Orient for thousands of years. Most of the research in acupuncture has been with chronic pain syndromes without clearly delineating the number of headache sufferers in their population. There have been four studies suggesting moderate improvement in migraine with acupuncture (4–7). Acupuncture decreases the number of days of migraine headache (7) and is possibly effective in the prophylaxis of migraine (5). Some of these data suggest that acupuncture reduces the frequency and duration of headache, if successful, rather than the severity of pain (5–7). In spite of this, the National Council Against Health Fraud fails to find any scientific literature to indicate that acupuncture is more effective than placebo and suggests that health practitioners remind patients that acupuncture is an experimental treatment and has some risk of complications (8).

There is a controversial and inconsistent literature on treatment for craniomandibular dysfunction and its effect on migrainous events (9–13). Two recent articles suggest that migraine frequency was significantly reduced with nighttime use of a soft occlusal splint (14, 15). In one of these studies (15), the likelihood of migraine improvement was not related to the presence or absence of craniomandibular dysfunction signs or symptoms at the beginning of therapy. In this study, the splint therapy was significantly more effective in migraine subjects than in patients with chronic tension-type headache.

Self-hypnosis has been shown to be effective in decreasing headache frequency in children with migraine with aura, compared with propranolol and placebo (16). Finally, variable-frequency photo-stimulation goggles have been shown to decrease the duration and frequency of migraine attacks (17).

Comprehensive multidiscipline treatment programs have emerged to address the diverse factors affecting the clinical picture of migraine. The present review describes such an integrated approach to a self-regulation and skill-training model to help control migraine.

The first phase of this model includes a thorough assessment with multiple types of data collection (clinical interview, questionnaires, and psychophysiological evaluation) to set observable and measurable treatment goals. The second phase of this model involves intervention. The patient becomes an active participant in treatment and learns coping skills targeting different dimensions of the headache problem (physiological, affective, cognitive, and behavioral factors). The treatment phase involves education, skills acquisition, and generalization of therapeutic effects.

ASSESSMENT

Clinical Interview

The first phase of the behavioral assessment is an in-depth clinical interview (18). This interview must be done by a practitioner with an in-depth knowledge of headache pathogenesis and treatment. Even though all our patients are medically referred, many have a fear of significant brain pathology and/or are terrified that the clinician thinks that their problem is psychogenic. These patients may distort the history in relation to their own "naive" conceptualization of headache and may omit or distort certain key points. Patients have often consulted with many other professionals and nonprofessionals (family, friends, etc.) and have many misconceptions about head pain as well as the various therapeutic alternatives. Some are taking many medications, either self-prescribed or prescribed by a physician, that may paradoxically have a negative effect on their headache frequency and response to treatment (19). Often these patients report "daily" migraine headaches that are, in actuality, rebound headaches secondary to analgesics, ergotamine, and/or caffeine.

It is important during this interview to assess whether the patient is having more than one type of headache. Patients often refer to their problem as "my headache," without accurately differentiating two different headache types. These patients typically have had episodic migraine attacks over the years, which have become complicated by a daily constant headache between attacks, as well as by chronic, often excessive, analgesic usage. We find it very helpful to question the patient along a four-point intensity scale. For example, the following questions are often helpful: What is the frequency of headache that will either incapacitate you or dramatically decrease your ability to function? How often do you have a headache that is moderate to severe in intensity but doesn't significantly affect your functional capacity? How often do you have a dull headache? How often are you completely clear-headed?

It is important to establish the ages and circumstances (menarche, physical/psychological trauma, etc.) of onset, if known, for each headache type. Some patients recognize various environmental factors that may trigger a headache attack. Psychological events may play a role in headache onset, and careful questioning about the number and types of recent life changes may explain an increase in headache frequency. Some migraineurs may notice that their headaches increase during a poststress let-down period and, often, on weekends or vacations. Some patients notice increased headache in association with biological rhythm changes, such as change in sleep patterns or travel. Other patients notice dietary triggers. It is also important to assess the role of hormonal factors in migraine exacerbation and the possibility of improvement during pregnancy. Characteristics of pain for each headache type are recorded including location, pain quality, and duration. The typical time of onset for migraine and any prodromal symptoms (even if they are vague) should be noted. It has been our impression, clinically, that close observation of migraine prodromes improves outcome.

It is important to assess alcohol, nicotine, and recreational drug usage. The amount of caffeine ingested daily should be noted, as many patients believe that because caffeine is contained in many abortive migraine medications, increased consumption of it will have an antimigraine effect. It must be explained to them that significant daily caffeine consumption increases the frequency of headache, because of caffeine withdrawal.

It is very helpful to get a family history of headache, psychiatric disorder, and alcoholism. The clinician must thoroughly but, subtly, evaluate the symptoms of major depression. Often, it is helpful to ask about psychological problems as secondary to the headache problem. It is

helpful to determine the psychological background of the headache sufferer. Careful questioning about family and marital relationships, occupational history, social/environmental stressors, and recent life changes, both positive and negative, should be undertaken. It is helpful to gather information on activity level, coping skills, disability issues, responses to pain, and perceptions (often misperceptions) about headache.

Patients complete a battery of self-administered psychological questionnaires. These typically include the Minnesota Multiphasic Personality Inventory, a depression inventory, an anxiety inventory, and an index of recent life changes. Interpretations of test results must take into account that chronic pain can affect performance on these scales and that issues of depression and anxiety may be primary or secondary phenomena. These questionnaires are helpful screening instruments and, for some patients, help to tailor the treatment plan.

Psychophysiological Evaluation

Psychophysiological evaluation is the second phase of the assessment. This typically involves a physiological stress profile, a diagnostic muscle scan, and sometimes, a dynamic movement assessment to help identify certain physiological/sensory targets for intervention. A stress profile (20–21) assesses generalized arousal (some combination of electrodermal response, heart rate, and respiration dynamics), skeletal muscle changes (trapezius, frontotemporal), and smooth muscle/vascular changes (peripheral blood flow, temporal pulse amplitude) in response to a variety of stimulus conditions. These include adaptation, baseline, mental and physical stressors, recovery, and relaxation. This profile is a clinical measure of autonomic reactivity.

A static muscle scan uses surface electrode electromyography to scan different skeletal muscles in two positions, sitting and standing (22, 23). Muscles assessed include frontalis, temporalis, masseter, sternocleidomastoid, cervical paraspinals, upper trapezius, and T1 paraspinals. These are compared with normative data. It is also helpful to assess muscular response patterns with dynamic movements of the neck and shoulders as well as other postural changes (24). There is much inconsistency and controversy in the literature about psychophysiological profiling in headache (21). However, we feel it is clinically useful for an "individual" patient to help identify certain sensory targets for intervention.

TREATMENT

Intervention is based on the detailed behavioral assessment. This program is built on the premise that if one increases coping skills and self-regulation ability, one will increase a patient's sense of mastery and control. Even in strictly pharmacological interventions, these skills are of paramount importance.

Much of the time, we combine behavioral and medical treatments to provide a comprehensive multifaceted treatment program for headache. The program is composed of (*a*) education about the causes, triggers, and treatments of headache; (*b*) dietary modification and behavioral and biological rhythm interventions that help alter certain lifestyle patterns that can trigger headache; and (*c*) self-regulation skills that incorporate a sensory component and a reactive component. The sensory component teaches the patient to control various physiological responses, to help abort and prevent headaches. The reactive component is a combination of cognitive-behavioral interventions that examine and help change certain actions, thoughts, attitudes, expectations, and emotional states that often heighten the level of sympathetic arousal and participation, on the premise that it is important for the patient to take some responsibility for headache improvement. The patient actively participates in the acquisition of certain skills. This program exists as a series of appointments following the initial evaluation. The absolute number of sessions is determined by clinical considerations and is typically under 15 appointments.

Education

A detailed educational program is undertaken noting that headache is determined by a complex group of factors. This may include explanations of pathophysiology to better understand nonpharmacological and pharmacological treatment rationale. These explanations may include biological predispositions, biochemical changes, the physiology and psychology of the stress response, dietary factors, biological rhythm factors, and relevant cognitive, emotional, and behavioral issues. It is often important to reinforce information about the various classes of headache medications, including mechanisms of action and potential side effects. Traditionally accepted myths regarding personality factors in headache are examined and exposed as unfounded. Questions about biofeedback and behavioral treatments are answered. Goals of treatment are explained, giving the rationales for the often combined pharmacological and nonpharmacological approaches. The anticipated "time lag" is explained with respect to withdrawal of certain abortive medications and the onset of therapeutic effect of preventative pharmacological and behavioral treatments.

Finally, patients are taught to keep a headache calendar that is brought to each treatment session. The patient is taught how to self-monitor the frequency, intensity, and duration of each headache. The patient also monitors the type and amount of medication taken, (both prescription and over-the-counter), degree of relief from medical or nonmedical interventions, menstrual days (for menstruating women), and environmental triggers (if known). These calendars generate important data and are easy and efficient to use, given an adequate format (see Fig. 13.1).

Skills Acquisition

Numerous factors have been implicated as headache triggers. They certainly vary between patients. Some individ-

uals are affected by diet, sleep rhythm changes, acute stress, chronic stress, exertional factors, fasting and skipping meals, as well as other factors.

When appropriate, patients are put on an elimination diet to limit foods that have been shown, in the research literature, to trigger headaches (Fig. 13.2). Much has been written about dietary factors in relation to migraine (25–34). However, there are few well-designed research protocols and these studies indicate that dietary modification may be of some benefit for some patients, although, in our opinion, widespread efficacy has not been established. Some recent controlled investigations have yielded promising results (30–34).

Patients are taught that a variety of factors may act as headache triggers (Fig. 13.3). They are taught some general "hints" to help with headache control. They are encouraged to maintain consistent biological rhythms such as keeping to normal sleep patterns, even on weekends. They are encouraged to go to bed and awaken at approximately the same time every night and to avoid oversleeping. They are advised not to skip meals and to eat nutritional meals at regular intervals. They are encouraged to reduce their intake of caffeine and alcoholic beverages, if indicated. We encourage patients to set behavioral goals such as increasing pleasurable activities, decreasing "down" time, and modifying their schedule in an adaptive fashion. We assess "Type A" behavior patterns, which often place excessive demands on the patient.

Patients are instructed in ways to better self-manage medication compliance. Studies suggest that about 50% of chronic headache sufferers fail to adhere properly to drug regimens (35). Ergotamine tartrate is often not optimally used (36). As stated previously, recent evidence (37–39) suggests that nonadherence to abortive medications creates "rebound" phenomena limiting the effectiveness of preventative pharmacological interventions. Brief educational interventions using a self-management model will dramatically increase compliance to abortive medications (36, 40). These time-limited interventions help patients better manage side effects, teach them how to use an experimental approach to assessing outcome, and set specific limits to prevent rebound from overuse. We have found that these brief self-management interventions are also very helpful in increasing compliance to preventative pharmacotherapy. The forementioned headache calendar as a self-monitoring index is of great importance in assessing medication effect.

In self-regulation, patients learn to intervene on two components; sensory and reactive (41). The sensory component consists of the precursors to, and the sensations of, pain, determined by both central and peripheral factors. The reactive component is cognitive and affective and consists of thoughts and feelings that often precede or accompany headache attacks. In many of these chronic patients the disorder has acquired a life of its own. We find that situational antecedents become less important as the

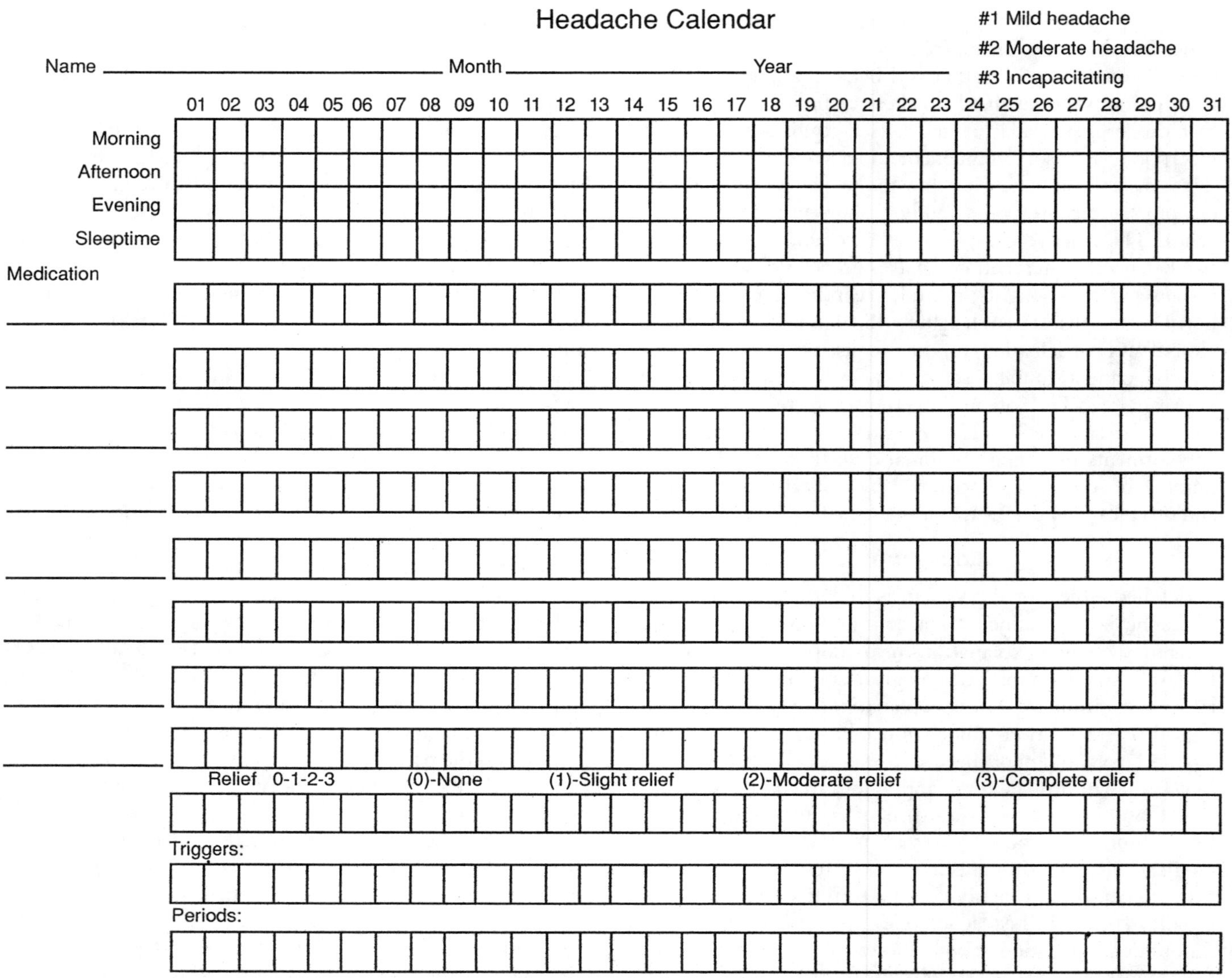

Headache Calendar

#1 Mild headache
#2 Moderate headache
#3 Incapacitating

Name _____ Month _____ Year _____

	01	02	03	04	05	06	07	08	09	10	11	12	13	14	15	16	17	18	19	20	21	22	23	24	25	26	27	28	29	30	31
Morning																															
Afternoon																															
Evening																															
Sleeptime																															

Medication

Relief 0-1-2-3   (0)-None   (1)-Slight relief   (2)-Moderate relief   (3)-Complete relief

Triggers:

Periods:

Figure 13.1. Headache calendar. (Reprinted with permission of the New England Center for Headache.)

frequency of migraine increases. It is almost as if they have a lowered threshold for attack, which makes it more difficult to discriminate triggers.

The initial sessions of treatment are directed toward the sensory component, using relaxation and biofeedback training to learn physiological self-regulation. Later sessions focus on the thoughts and feelings that accompany migraine attacks and also contribute to headache susceptibility.

Biofeedback facilitates self-regulation. Instrumentation provides immediate objective information about the patient's physiological response system. This feedback may be visual and/or auditory, and this allows responses to be "shaped" in the most adaptive direction (e.g., decreased muscle tension and increased peripheral blood flow). The type of training and sites used are based on the forementioned psychophysiological evaluation.

The biofeedback program is a step-by-step skill-building approach over a series of sessions. Each session must be mastered before moving to the next one. Audiocassettes are given to the patient for each step, and home records are kept to help monitor progress. Generalization strategies are discussed to encourage the patient to practice self-regulation on an ongoing basis. Patients use "mini-exercises" throughout the day to heighten body awareness and reduce physiological arousal. Booster sessions are held (infrequently) to insure continued maintenance of acquired responses. While a review of the literature on biofeedback and the treatment of migraine is beyond the scope of this chapter, excellent reviews have been published elsewhere (42).

In the second part of the program, patients learn to identify and modify maladaptive styles of thinking (40–45). Distress-related cognitions and negative self-talk ("Why me? I can't believe I'm getting another migraine! It's no use.") mediate poor outcome via a variety of mecha-

Avoid the following:

CHOCOLATE	ONIONS	HERRING
CANNED FIGS	PIZZA	CHICKEN LIVERS
NUTS	SOUR CREAM	AVOCADO
PEANUT BUTTER	YOGURT	NUTRASWEET

*RIPENED CHEESES (CHEDDAR, GRUYERE, BRIE, CAMEMBERT, ETC.)—CHEESES THAT ARE PERMISSIBLE ARE: AMERICAN, COTTAGE, CREAM, AND VELVEETA

*VINEGAR—(HOWEVER, WHITE VINEGAR IS PERMISSIBLE)

*ANYTHING THAT IS FERMENTED, PICKLED, OR MARINATED

*HOT FRESH BREADS, RAISED COFFEECAKES AND DOUGHNUTS (DUE TO ACTIVATED YEAST)

*PODS OF BROAD BEANS (LIMA, NAVY, AND PEA PODS)

*MONOSODIUM GLUTAMATE—ANY FOODS CONTAINING LARGE AMOUNTS (CHINESE FOODS)

*CITRUS FRUITS (EXAMPLE: NO MORE THAN ONE ORANGE PER DAY)

*BANANAS (NO MORE THAN ½ BANANA PER DAY)

*PORK—LIMIT INTAKE

*TEA, COFFEE, COLA BEVERAGES (AVOID EXCESSIVE AMOUNTS)

*FERMENTED SAUSAGE (BOLOGNA, SALAMI, PEPPERONI, SUMMER, AND HOT DOGS)

*ALCOHOLIC BEVERAGES—AVOID IF POSSIBLE. OF ALL POSSIBLE FOOD TRIGGERS FOR MIGRAINE, ALCOHOL IS MOST FREQUENTLY CITED.

We recommend that you begin with a total elimination of the above for one month. If you observe a decrease in frequency or severity of headache, slowly reintroduce foods one at a time and observe the effect. If headache increases, eliminate that food and go on.

Figure 13.2.   Elimination diet hand-out sheet.

nisms, such as increased anxiety and distress, increased depression, overuse of analgesics, ergotamines, and benzodiazapines. Patients are taught that this "reactive" component can be treated with coping strategies to help actively "challenge" counterproductive automatic thinking. Self-statements are used to help develop alternative cognitive responses to the experience of recurrent severe pain. These self-instructions help the patients rehearse adaptive cognitive and behavioral responses to the development of a migraine. This involves preparation for an attack, initial symptoms, critical moments, and postheadache (41).

We feel that migraine is significantly influenced by the patient's cognitive actions and reactions in dealing with the symptoms themselves. We train patients to become keen observers and to be "prepared" to cope adaptively with a migraine without being hypervigilant to pain sensations. Many headache patients exhibit irrational ideation about loss of control or perceived threat of a future event and underestimate their coping skills. They frequently misinterpret bodily sensations and "catastrophize." The key to cognitive treatment of these anxiety-related factors is to help the patient accurately interpret and react to perceived danger signals with rational self-statements. Patients use the following sequence of self-statements:

What is it I have to do? What does the situation require? What strategies can I use? One step at a time, I can handle the attack, use many strategies, and take appropriate medicines at the appropriate amount and time. Just focus on what the situation requires. I can use my relaxation skills and can keep things under control without creating a catastrophe. I won't make this worse; worrying will not help anything. Remember, I have many strategies to use if I stay focused. I did well, used my skills, and only had a small amount of time that I could not function.

Hormones
1. Menses
2. Ovulation
3. Hormone replacement (Progesterone)

Diet
4. Alcohol
5. Chocolate
6. Aged cheese
7. Monosodium glutamate (MSG)
8. Aspartame (Nutrasweet)
9. Caffeine
10. Nuts
11. Nitrites, nitrates
12. Other

Biology

Changes
13. Weather
14. Seasons
15. Travel (crossing time zones)
16. Altitude
17. Schedule changes
18. Sleeping patterns
19. Diet
20. Skipping meals

Sensory Stimuli
21. Strong light
22. Flickering lights
23. Odors

"Stress"
24. Let-down periods
25. Times of intense activity
26. Loss (death, separation, divorce)
27. Moving
28. Job loss/change
29. Crisis
30. Other

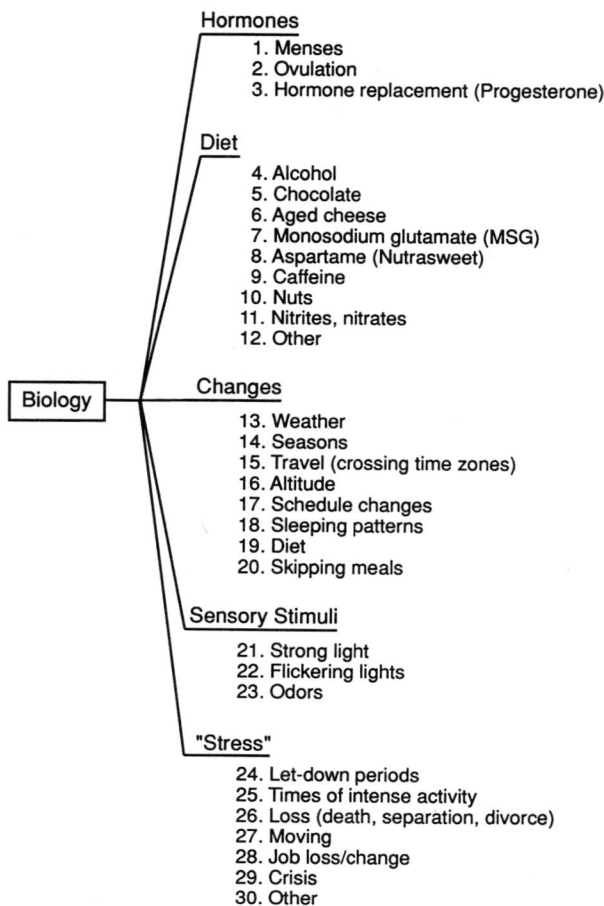

Figure 13.3. Headache triggers.

As patients with chronic daily headache begin to have more and more clearheaded periods, we find it essential that they learn this cognitive behavioral approach to aid relapse prevention.

Some patients require cognitive therapy for depression (47). This involves modifying a patient's automatic internal dialogue that predisposes the patient to helplessness and self-blame with an expectation that he or she cannot control future events. It is a time-limited psychotherapeutic approach.

These cognitive behavioral therapies use a self-management model that helps the headache patient incorporate a variety of skills to become an "active" collaborator with the health professional. These techniques are invaluable for patients with complex headache problems, and they interact well with traditional pharmacotherapy.

REFERENCES

1. Jay GW, Brunson J, Branson SJ. The effectiveness of physical therapy in the treatment of chronic daily headaches. Headache 1989;29:156–162.
2. Solomon S, Guglielmo KM. Treatment of headache by transcutaneous electrical stimulation. Headache 1985;25:12–15.
3. Lance JW. The controlled application of cold and heat by a new device (Migra-lief apparatus) in the treatment of headache. Headache 1988;28:458–461.
4. Lenhard L, Waite PME. Acupuncture in the prophylactic treatment of migraine headaches; pilot study. NZ Med J 1983;96:663–666.
5. Loh L, Nathan PW, Schott GD, Zilkha KJ. Acupuncture versus medical treatment for migraine and muscle tension headache. J Neurol Neurosurg 1984;47:333–337.
6. Dowson DI, Lewith GT, Machin D. The effects of acupuncture vs. placebo in the treatment of headache. Pain 1985;21:35–42.
7. Boivie J, Brattberg G. Are there long lasting effects on migraine headache after one series of acupuncture treatments? Am J Chin Med 1987;15:69–75.
8. The National Council against Health Fraud. Acupuncture. Clin J Pain 1991;7(2):162–166.
9. Forssell H, Kirveskari P, Kangasnjemi P. Response to occlusal treatment in headache patients previously treated by mock occlusal adjustment. Acta Odontol Scand 1987;45:77–80.
10. Moss RA. Oral behaviour patterns in common migraine. J Craniomandibular Pract 1987;5:196–202.
11. Reik L. Unnecessary dental treatment of headache patients for temporomandibular joint disorders. Headache 1985;25:246–248.
12. Reik L, Hale M. The temporomandibular joint pain dysfunction syndrome. A frequent cause of headache. Headache 1981;21:151–156.
13. Watts PG, Peet KM, Juniper RP. Migraine and the temporomandibular joint: the final answer. Br Dent J 1986;161:170–173.
14. Lamay PJ, Barclay SC. Clinical effectiveness of occlusal splint therapy in patients with classical migraine. Scot Med J 1987;32:12–14.
15. Quayle AA, Gray RJM, Metcalfe RJ, Guthrie E, Wastell D. Soft occlusal splint therapy in the treatment of migraine and other headaches. J Dent 1990;18:123–129.
16. Olness K, MacDonald JT, Uden DL. Comparison of self-hypnosis and propranolol in the treatment of classic migraine. Pediatrics 1987;79(4):593–597.
17. Anderson DJ. The treatment of migraine with variable frequency photo-stimulation. Headache 1989;29(3), 154–155.
18. Baskin SM. The headache history. In: A. M. Rapoport, Sheftell FD, eds. Headache. New York: PMA Publishing, in press.
19. Diener HC, Wilkinson M. Drug induced headache. Berlin: Springer-Verlag, 1988.
20. Cram JR. Clinical EMG: muscle scanning and diagnostic manual for surface recordings. Seattle: Clinical Resources, 1986.
21. Flor H, Turk DC. Psychophysiology of chronic pain: do chronic pain patients exhibit symptom-specific psychophysiological responses? Psychol Bull 1989;105:215–259.
22. Cram JR. EMG muscle scanning and diagnostic manual for surface recordings. In: Cram JR, ed. Clinical EMG for surface recordings: vol 2. Seattle: Clinical Resources, 1990:1–141.
23. Scloenen J, Gerard P, DePasqua V, Sianard-Gainko J. Multiple clinical and paraclinical analyses of chronic tension-type headache associated or unassociated with disorder of pericranial muscles. Cephalolgia 1991;11:135–139.
24. Taylor W. Dynamic EMG biofeedback in assessment and treatment using a neuromuscular re-education model. In: Cram JR, ed. Clinical EMG for surface recordings: vol 2. Seattle: Clinical Resources, 1990:175–196.
25. Hanington E. Diet and migraine. J Human Nutr 1980;34:175–180.
26. Medina JL, Diamond S. The role of diet in migraine. Headache 1978;18:31–34.
27. Selzer S. Foods, and food and drug combinations, responsible for head and neck pain. Cephalalgia 1982;2:111–124.
28. Zeigler DK, Stewart R. Failure of tyramine to induce migraine. Neurology 1977;27(7):25–27.
29. Salfield SA, Wardley BL, Houlsby WT, Turner SI, Spalton AP, Beckless-Wilson NR, Herber SM. Controlled study of exclusion of dietary vasoactive amines in migraine. Arch Dis Child 1987;62:458–460.

30. Cornwell N, Clarke L. Dietary modification in patients with migraine and tension-type headache [abstract]. Cephalalgia 1991;(supplement 2):143–144.
31. Hasselmark L, Malmgren R, Hannerz J. Effect of a carbohydrate-rich diet, low in protein-trytophan, in classic and common migraine. Cephalalgia 1987;7:87–92.
32. Radnitz CL, Blanchard EB. Assessment and treatment of dietary factors in refractory vascular headache. Headache Quart 1991;3:214–220.
33. Radnitz CL. Food triggered migraine: a critical review. Ann Behav Med 1990;12:51–65.
34. Egger J, Carter CM, Soothil JF, Wilson J. Oligoantigenic diet treatment of children with epilepsy and migraine. J Pediatr 1989;114:51–58.
35. Packard RC, O'Connel P. Medication compliance among headache patients. Headache 1986;26:416–419.
36. Holroyd KA, Holm JE, Hursey KG, Penzien DB, Cordingley GE, Theofanous AG. Recurrent vascular headache: home-based behavioral treatment versus abortive pharmacological treatment. J Consult Clin Psychol 1988;56:218–223.
37. Kudrow L. Paradoxical effects of chronic analgesic use. In: Critchley M, Friedman A, Gorini S, Sicuteri F, eds. Headache: physiopathological and clinical concepts (Advances in neurology, vol 33). New York: Raven Press, 1982.
38. Saper JR. Ergotamine dependency: a review. Headache 1987;27:435–438.
39. Mathew NT, Kurman R, Perez F. Drug induced refractory headache: clinical features and management. Headache 1990;30:634–638.
40. Holroyd KA, Cordingley GE, Pingel JD, Jerome A, Theofanous AG, Jackson DK, Leard L. Enhancing the effectiveness of abortive therapy: a controlled evaluation of self-management training. Headache 1989;29:148–153.
41. Bakal DA. The psychobiology of chronic headache. New York: Springer, 1982.
42. Blanchard EB, Andraskik F. Biofeedback treatment of vascular headache. In: Hatch JP, Fisher JG, Rugh JD, eds. Biofeedback: studies in clinical efficacy. New York: Plenum, 1987.
43. Andrasik F. Psychological and behavioral aspects of chronic headache. In: Mathew NT, ed. Neurologic clinics. Philadelphia: Saunders, 1990.
44. Holroyd KA, Andrasik F. A cognitive behavioral approach to recurrent tension and migraine headache. In: Kendall PC, ed. Advances in cognitive-behavioral research and therapy. New York: Academic Press, 1982.
45. Blanchard EB, Andrasik F. Management of chronic headaches: A psychological approach. New York: Pergamon Press, 1985.
46. Sorbi M, Tellegen B. Differential effects of training in relaxation and stress—coping in patients with migraine. Headache 1986;26:473–481.
47. Beck AT. Cognitive therapy and the emotional disorders. New York: International Universities Press, 1976.

14

Biofeedback and Psychological Management of Migraine

ANTHONY IEZZI, HENRY E. ADAMS, and CLAREN SHECK

DIAGNOSIS OF MIGRAINE

Without an accurate headache classification system, headache treatment studies are likely to be fraught with conceptual, methodological, and clinical pitfalls. As headache diagnosis is relatively in its infancy, this has been a problem throughout the migraine headache literature.

For the past 30 years, the Ad Hoc Committee on the Classification of Headache (AHCCH) (1) has determined the types of headache disorders. Fifteen headache types were identified and organized primarily on the basis of pain mechanisms and on the presence or absence of prodromal symptoms. Four types of headache in the AHCCH scheme appear to have psychological factors involved in the etiology, exacerbation, and maintenance of headache (2): migraine (with 5 subtypes), muscle contraction, combined migraine and muscle contraction, and delusional, conversion, or hypochondriacal headache. Unfortunately, the AHCCH classification scheme has been used extensively with little empirical evidence demonstrating its reliability and validity (3, 4). One of the major factors contributing to the equivocal findings of biofeedback treatment for migraine over other techniques is related to inaccurate and poorly defined headache diagnoses provided by the AHCCH classification system.

A major effort has been put forth by members of the International Headache Society (IHS) to improve headache classification. Collaboration by these experts in the headache field has produced a new hierarchically organized classification system (5). Compared with the two-page article by the AHCCH, the new classification system is comprehensively outlined in a 96-page document. It is readily acknowledged in the preface of the IHS document that the newly proposed classification system is based on the experience of experts rather than empirical data. However, the IHS classification system is a heuristic research tool that attempts to increase the nosographic and epidemiologic foundation for the study of headache. It is only a question of time before all headache clinicians become influenced by the new classification system. A second edition is tentatively planned for release in 1993.

With the new classification system, headache typology is not only classified according to pain mechanisms and the presence and absence of prodromal symptoms but also according to frequency, location, and duration. Unlike the prior headache classification system, the IHS classification system allows multiple headache diagnoses in the same headache patient. For instance, patients who would have been diagnosed as having combined migraine and muscle contraction headache are now given a dual diagnosis of migraine headache and tension-type headache and coded in order of importance. The terms *classic migraine* and *common migraine* have now been, respectively, replaced by *migraine with aura* and *migraine without aura*. Delusional, conversion, or hypochondriacal headache has been reclassified to a subcategory of tension-type headache. The reader is referred to Chapter 2 of this book for more information on the new classification system and detailed definitions of migraine and other types of headache.

DEFINITION OF BIOFEEDBACK

Biofeedback essentially arose from studies examining whether autonomic nervous system responses could be controlled by reinforcement. Traditionally, it was presumed that the behavior of skeletal muscles, but not visceral responses, could be conditioned (6). Miller and Dicara (7) used an ingenious design to challenge this assumption. While controlling for skeletal muscle activity by curare anesthesia, they showed that rats' heart rates could be conditioned using electrical stimulation of brain structures, associated with reinforcement. Using this procedure, they could shape heart rate to both increase and decrease. Further studies (8) in this area demonstrated the conditionability of other visceral responses (i.e., dilation or constriction of blood vessels in the skin, increased or decreased intestinal motility). There has been some controversy regarding these findings. No one, including Miller himself, has been able to consistently replicate the initial results with cardiovascular responses (9). Nevertheless, these findings sparked interest in the therapeutic application of visceral conditioning to health problems, and the development of biofeedback.

Biofeedback represents an operant learning process (10) in which an individual or organism is provided with continuous feedback on a specified physiological response (e.g., polygraph or self-contained portable units). Feedback is provided to assist the individual in learning how to self-regulate or voluntarily control a targeted physiological response system producing a change in the target response usually associated with a pathophysiological condition such as migraines. With the aid of an auditory signal or visual display reflecting a proportional change in the targeted physiological response, the individual learns, usually by trial and error, to modify the target response. There are two types of central illustrating learning. In biofeedback control, the person learns to modify a physiological response with the assistance of a cue. In instructional control, the individual produces the desired physiological changes without the aid of an external feedback system. This is the goal of training. Cognitive aids (e.g., relaxing mental images) are also used in combination with biofeedback to obtain the desired physiological change. It is then assumed that biofeedback will be associated with concomitant decreases in the target condition such as headache.

To properly evaluate the effectiveness of biofeedback of any type, it must be demonstrated that the individual can voluntarily control the targeted physiological response within and across sessions, that baseline level of the response decreases over time, that the individual can generalize the self-regulation to other environments, that self-regulation can be maintained over time, and (last but not least) that this learning is associated with a reduction or change in symptoms (i.e., headaches).

BIOFEEDBACK TECHNIQUES FOR MIGRAINE

There are three major biofeedback treatment approaches to migraine headache management: temporal artery, thermal, and electromyographic biofeedback.

Temporal Artery Biofeedback

A rationale for the use of temporal artery biofeedback is based largely upon Wolff's work. His initial studies demonstrated that the vasoconstrictor ergotamine tartrate reduced temporal artery pulse amplitude by 16 to 84% and produced concomitant reductions in reported migraine head pain (11). Later studies lead Wolff and colleagues to propose an etiological model of classic migraine headache involving initial vasoconstriction of extracranial arteries followed by a dilatation of these arteries and inflammation of surrounding tissues. The later dilation stage presumably is associated with head pain.

With temporal artery biofeedback, a photoelectric transducer is placed on an extracranial artery (usually the zygomaticofacial branch). This allows frequency and amplitude monitoring of a blood volume pulse. To decrease head pain associated with increased blood flow to the extracranial arteries, the goal of temporal artery biofeedback is for the patient to learn how to reduce pulse amplitude. In other terms, by teaching the patient to remain in a vasoconstrictive state and to avoid vasodilation of the tem-

poral artery, the head pain will be eliminated altogether. At the least, the intensity and duration of head pain can be significantly reduced.

Much of the early research on the effectiveness of temporal artery biofeedback in the treatment of migraine headache came from the University of Georgia laboratory under the direction of Henry E. Adams (12–15). To learn voluntary control of blood volume pulse and depending on the individual case, some 8 to 12 one-hour sessions are required; however, 50 to 60 sessions have been conducted with more refractory cases (10). The temporal artery biofeedback protocol can be complicated by tranducer placement difficulties, movement artifacts, eye blinks, clenching of the jaw, and ambient light.

Thermal Biofeedback

Body temperature, particularly from a finger, has been used as an indirect measure of peripheral blood volume. Higher temperatures indicate more blood volume; lower temperatures indicate less blood volume. Thermal biofeedback requires attaching a temperature-sensitive thermistor to a finger and training the patient to increase the finger temperature. The rationale for thermal biofeedback has traditionally been that by increasing peripheral blood flow, a decrease in sympathetic tone and an increase in relaxation occur. Thus, it was assumed that by increasing blood flow to the periphery, blood flow to the extracranial vasculature is decreased, reducing cephalic dilatation, throbbing, and pain. However, Sovak and colleagues (16) have argued that the mode of action of thermal biofeedback is not hemodynamic, but rather a general decrease in sympathetic tone, an idea supported by other investigators (17, 18).

Regardless of its mechanism, thermal biofeedback is an effective therapeutic approach to the treatment of migraine headaches. The first reports to attract attention to thermal biofeedback came from the Menninger Foundation Clinic (19, 20). In addition to thermal biofeedback, these investigators included autogenic phrases (e.g., "My hands are warm, I feel quiet, and the beach is hot") in their treatment protocol. The subjects were trained once or twice weekly until they acquired the hand-warming response and were followed-up from 1 to 3 years at 3-month intervals (20). Seventy-four percent of 62 migraine headache patients were considered "improved" by the authors at the end of follow-up (20). Portable temperature units that can be taken home by the patient for practice significantly reduce the time it takes to "control" finger temperature. As a word of caution, finger temperature measurement can be compromised by sensitivity to ambient temperature and movement artifacts as well as tight clothes, exercise, and smoking.

Electromyographic Biofeedback

Although electromyographic biofeedback was originally used to treat tension headache (21, 22), it has also been used to treat migraine headache. With electromyographic biofeedback, three surface electrodes placed equidistant from each other on the frontalis muscle are required. Electromyographic electrodes can also be placed on nuchal, sternocleidomastoid, and trapezoid muscles. The rationale for electromyographic biofeedback is to reduce elevated levels of muscle tension and, thereby, indirectly reduce sympathetic arousal. Not surprisingly, it typically takes fewer training sessions to learn how to voluntarily control muscle sites than temporal artery blood volume pulse or hand temperature. The effectiveness of electromyographic biofeedback can also be increased by portable units for home practice and training in relaxation strategies. Interelectrode impedance, improper electrode placement, type of electrodes used, bandpass setting, and size of contact surface are some of the factors that may complicate the electromyographic assessment and treatment protocol.

PSYCHOLOGICAL MANAGEMENT TECHNIQUES

Relaxation and cognitive techniques are often used alone or in combination with biofeedback approaches to manage patients with migraines. There are several different versions of relaxation techniques, with progressive relaxation training being one of the most popular (23). This technique requires the individual to alternatively tense and relax a number of muscle groups throughout the whole body. The progressive relaxation training sequence involves 8 to 12 training sessions. The procedure eventually is shortened in terms of the number of muscle groups and length of time involved, with no apparent loss in the treatment effect. By the end of training, the individual should be able to obtain the same physical and mental relaxation through deep breathing and counting from one to ten as in the initial training session. The sessions usually take 30 to 40 minutes to complete. Home practice between sessions is crucial and is recommended about twice daily.

Commercially available relaxation tapes assist the patient in learning how to relax, and significantly reduce the clinician's time with the patient. Other, more passive relaxation training techniques including transcendental meditation (24) and autogenic training (suggestions of warmth and heaviness, passive concentration, and attention to breathing and imagery) are also useful (25).

The goal of relaxation techniques is to reduce elevated levels of muscle tension or stress that may initiate or increase head pain. Relaxation techniques also help the individual learn to identify subtle changes in muscular activity and, like EMG biofeedback, indirectly reduce sympathetic overarousal. Crucial to the successive implementation of relaxation skills is the ultimate use of the relaxation response as an active coping skill with everyday stressors. Relaxation techniques have been used in combination with self-hypnosis (26), psychotherapy (27), and frontalis electromyographic biofeedback (28) in managing migraine headache.

Cognitive techniques (e.g., stress-inoculation, cognitive reappraisal, rational thinking, and desensitization) are aimed at providing the individual with a general set of problem-solving skills as well as coping strategies that can be used in a wide range of situations that trigger and maintain headache episodes (29). The rationale for cognitive techniques is that headaches can result from maladaptive cognitions (e.g., "I should be a perfect parent or spouse"). Such cognitions lead to disturbed emotional and behavioral responses that, in turn, increase the level of sympathetic arousal. The aims of cognitive techniques are to teach the patient to identify maladaptive distressing thoughts, increase the patient's understanding of how thoughts contribute to emotional distress, and to provide more adaptive modes of thinking. In various forms, early applications of cognitive techniques have been used successfully to treat migraine headache (30–32).

SELECTIVE REVIEW OF THE BIOFEEDBACK OUTCOME LITERATURE OF MIGRAINE

Over the past decade, several reviews of the biofeedback literature of migraine have appeared (33–37). We shall provide a summary of the findings contained in some of them and discuss the use of home-based, minimal therapist contact versus clinic-based treatment of migraine. In addition, we shall attempt to evaluate the cost-effectiveness of biofeedback outcome. An evaluation of the cost-effectiveness of biofeedback interventions can be conducted along several dimensions (37): (a) efficacy (Does treatment achieve the desired results?); (b) relative efficacy (Is one treatment approach better than another?); (c) generality (What proportion of a patient sample benefits from treatment?); (d) relative efficiency (Which treatment works faster?); (e) convenience (Which treatment is easier to give and easier to comply with?); and (f) cost. The clinician's selection of interventions should be guided by these dimensions.

Because the biofeedback literature contains many contradictory findings, it is difficult to arrive at any conclusions about the efficacy of different treatment approaches. As one solution to this difficulty, Blanchard and his colleagues have used "meta-analysis" to evaluate treatment effects across a number of empirical studies. The goal of meta-analysis is to calculate mean changes in headache parameters across studies, and these mean changes represent the actual unit of analysis. The analysis yields an estimation of the average magnitude of improvement in headache density (i.e., the product of duration and intensity of head pain) from baseline. The improvement from baseline is often summarized as a percentage score. Although meta-analysis has intuitive appeal, it can be compromised by differential dependent measures, sample sizes, treatment protocols, and methodological rigor that vary across studies. This makes it very difficult to compare studies. Meta-analysis also has been criticized for obscuring individual responses to treatment. With this caveat in mind, the meta-analyses by Blanchard and associates (34–36) of biofeedback management of migraine are discussed below. The reader is referred to the original sources for a list of the studies included in this meta-analysis and in other review articles cited in this section.

The original meta-analysis by Blanchard and associates (34) examined treatment effectiveness for both migraine and tension headaches. Only the results pertinent to migraine headache are discussed here. Twenty-three studies were included in the analysis, with each study presenting data on a minimum of five subjects per treatment group. Thermal biofeedback plus autogenic training, thermal biofeedback alone, relaxation training, and medication placebo were compared. All three active treatments were shown to be superior to the placebo but not different from one another in improving headache parameters (65.1%, 51.8%, 52.7%, and 16.5% mean improvement, respectively).

At the time of the original meta-analysis, few studies examining temporal artery biofeedback had been completed. Following the appearance of additional reports in this and other migraine treatment methods, another meta-analysis was conducted (35). From this analysis, thermal biofeedback plus autogenic training emerged as the most effective treatment for migraine, yielding a mean of 64.9% improvement in headache parameters. In addition, thermal biofeedback, temporal artery biofeedback, and relaxation led to mean improvements over baseline of 34.6%, 42.3%, and 47.9%, respectively. These improvements were not statistically different from one another. All active treatments were significantly superior to headache monitoring (17.2% improvement). Of the active treatments, only thermal biofeedback plus autogenic training was significantly superior to psychological placebo (27.6%). However, the authors note that half of the studies in the placebo condition used training to decrease hand temperature, a procedure that has subsequently been shown to be an active treatment (38).

The most recent meta-analysis (36) included 22 controlled outcome studies. Inclusion in the analyses required at least 9 subjects per treatment group. Comparisons of the controlled studies revealed the following (mean headache parameter improvement scores in parenthesis): temporal artery biofeedback (43.2%), relaxation training (48.3%), and thermal biofeedback plus autogenic training (48.5%) were not different but were superior to EMG biofeedback (29%), thermal biofeedback alone (27.2%), attention placebo (25.8%), and headache monitoring (13.3%).

In summary, various forms of biofeedback and relaxation training have consistently been shown to be superior to headache monitoring and placebo for the treatment of migraine headaches. Autogenic training likely adds to improvements that can be gained from thermal biofeedback. Temporal artery biofeedback, thermal biofeedback plus

autogenic training, and relaxation training may be equally superior means of treating migraine headache.

With this in mind, cost-effectiveness becomes important in evaluating these three treatments. Relaxation training requires neither the equipment nor the greater number of sessions that biofeedback entails. Thus, it would appear to be the more cost-effective treatment. However, there is some evidence that the "machines may be necessary some of the time for some patients" (39, p. 480). Blanchard and associates demonstrated further improvements in reducing headache parameters with subsequent thermal biofeedback training for migraineurs who had not benefited from initial relaxation training. However, this finding must be viewed tentatively, as length of treatments was not controlled in the experimental design. What appears to be most needed at this point is a method to predict which individual migraine patient will benefit most from what type of treatment. Research that will begin to answer this question is being conducted.

Chapman (37) has conducted a comprehensive review of electromyographic biofeedback and thermal biofeedback treatment of chronic headaches. For the purposes of this chapter, we are concerned only with conclusions pertaining to migraine headache. Though Chapman's review was not a meta-analysis, his conclusions were based on a greater number of treatment studies. In 8 of 10 studies examining differences between groups of migraine and mixed headache patients receiving thermal biofeedback, relaxation training, or combinations of the two, no significant differences were found, and these findings continued at 3-months to 1-year posttreatment. No significant differences were observed in 7 of 8 studies evaluating the effectiveness of electromyographic biofeedback versus thermal biofeedback in the management of migraine. Chapman states that 3 to 24 sessions of either biofeedback or relaxation, or both, with volunteers and clinical referrals who had a wide range of initial headache severity produce essentially the same results. He attributes the equivocal findings to the fact that both biofeedback and relaxation focus on repetitive quiet concentration and psychological and physical passivity (i.e., a relaxation response).

Chapman cites a host of reasons why biofeedback in general has fallen in estimation among headache clinicians. First, there are no high correlations between the target physiological response (e.g., finger temperature) and measures of headache parameters. Second, there has been a lack of convincing control conditions demonstrating that biofeedback is responsible for decreases in head pain. Third, there are few data about how biofeedback causes headache reduction. Finally, it is hard to measure head pain objectively without relying on self-report. As most clinicians know, the report of pain can be altered by a number of factors, including attention from the clinician, expectancy, medication intake, and the social context of pain.

Another meta-analysis (40) compared pharmacological (propranolol) and nonpharmacological (relaxation/thermal biofeedback) interventions of recurrent migraine headache. Twenty-five clinical trials of propranolol and 35 trials of relaxation/thermal biofeedback were compared, for a total of 2445 patients, and similar rates of improvement in headache parameters were found. Both resulted in a 43% reduction in migraine headache activity. There was 20% more improvement for both types of interventions when studies using less stringent outcome measures were included. In both cases, improvements were significantly greater than placebo medication (14%) and untreated patients (no reduction), but they were not significantly different from each other. Based on their findings, Holroyd and Penzien list several hypotheses worth evaluating: Does either intervention result in similar rates of improvement in the quality of life? Do these two interventions differ in short-term versus long-term benefits? Does the combination of both yield better results than either used alone?

Because of increasing attention on cost-effectiveness of health care delivery, an interest in home-based, minimal therapist contact treatment of headache has emerged (41–43). The original self-help treatment for headache was conducted by Kohlenberg and Cahn (44). Of 117 migraine subjects who started the study, 51 subjects completed all headache records at 3- and 6-months follow-up. Subjects were randomly assigned either a treatment book or a control book. The treatment book contained instructions on thermal biofeedback, relaxation, and cognitive-behavioral strategies. In addition, subjects in the treatment condition received a liquid crystal device for measuring finger temperature. The control book was a popular paperback presenting information on headache treatment, diagnosis, and case presentations. No therapist was involved in this study. Remarkably, there was a 62% decrease in headache frequency at 6 months in the treatment condition, compared with 14% decrease in the control condition. Significant decreases in headache duration and intensity as well as medication intake was noted in the treatment group. While the treatment condition appeared to be highly effective, the number of dropouts from both groups was significant (about 50%). This study may best indicate what very motivated migraine patients can do for themselves with proper instructions.

In a more elaborate investigation (41), 87 vascular headache subjects (39 migraine and 48 combined migraine and muscle contraction) were assigned to either a clinic-based or home-based treatment protocol. The clinic-based protocol required subjects to come in for 16 sessions (progressive relaxation training and thermal biofeedback) spread over 8 weeks. Clinic-based subjects were given a relaxation audiocassette and an alcohol-in-glass thermometer for home practice. The home-based relaxation and thermal biofeedback group was seen once a month, with two 10- to 15-minute telephone consultations between office visits,

over an 8-week period. Subjects in this group also were given relaxation audiocassettes and an alcohol-in-glass thermometer for home practice. The total therapist time required to conduct the clinic-based protocol was 11.4 hours, on average, compared with 2.5 hours for the home-based treatment.

Both treatments resulted in equivalent decreases in headache parameters for the two groups of migraine subjects. The authors calculated the cost-effectiveness for each treatment protocol by dividing the percentage improvement by the total therapist contact time. Home-based treatment for migraine and mixed headache, respectively, was four and six times more cost-effective than the clinic-based treatment.

Approximately 75% of vascular patients who were initially improved at posttreatment, remained improved at 2-year follow-up (42). Adding 2 hours of cognitive stress-coping strategies to the clinic-based relaxation and thermal biofeedback protocol did not have a significant effect over the home-based relaxation and thermal biofeedback protocol (43).

SUMMARY

Although many different biofeedback psychological techniques are used in the management of migraine, no single intervention emerges as clearly more efficacious. As a whole, thermal biofeedback, relaxation training, and cognitive strategies appear easiest to implement and the simplest for patients. Studies also show that thermal biofeedback and relaxation are as effective as propranolol in reducing migraine headache symptomatology. Home-based, minimal therapist contact treatment seems to be the most cost-effective psychological intervention for migraine. Further studies are needed to evaluate the stability of this finding.

Biofeedback has lost a great deal of its initial glamour, and some clinicians appear ready to abandon this type of treatment for headache. We contend that this would be premature since this procedure has not been adequately evaluated or developed. For example, very few biofeedback studies have actually included a voluntary control phase in their design, making it questionable whether learning has occurred (2). The assumption in these studies seems to have been that self-regulation or "learned control" of a targeted physiological system should be an "automatic" consequence of 10 sessions of any biofeedback technique. That assumption is questionable, particularly with temporal artery feedback. If no evaluation of voluntary control is conducted, so that it is uncertain whether learning occurred, then it must be assumed that biofeedback is, at best, a nonspecific or placebo effect.

It is also likely that an unclear and unfocused headache classification system (1) has contributed to the equivocal findings on the effectiveness of biofeedback. It is anticipated that the new headache classification system (5) will produce a better match between homogenous headache groups and specific biofeedback techniques. However, for this to happen, the new classification criteria need to undergo multiple tests of validity and reliability. Future research should examine the relationship between multiple physiological sites and headache parameters, influential subject characteristics, specificity of feedback parameters, etiologic models of migraine, and factors (e.g., secondary gain) contributing to the experience of head pain. Consequently, increased understanding of the nature and the parameters of effective intervention strategies can be elucidated. The ultimate goal should be to develop a better match between the headache patient and treatment procedure.

REFERENCES

1. Friedman AP. Ad Hoc Committee on the Classification of Headache. Neurology 1962;12:378–380.
2. Iezzi A, Adams HE, Pilon R, Averitt S. Psychological management of headache pain. In: Tollison CD, ed. Handbook of chronic pain management. Baltimore: Williams & Wilkins, 1989.
3. Turkat I, Brantley PJ, Orton K, Adams HE. Reliability of headache diagnosis. J Behav Assess 1981;3:1–4.
4. Thompson JK. Diagnosis of head pain: an idiographic approach to assessment and classification. Headache 1982;22:221–232.
5. Headache Classification Committee of the International Headache Society. Classification and diagnostic criteria for headache disorders, cranial neuralgias and facial pain. Cephalagia 1988;8(suppl 7):1–96.
6. Mowrer, OH. On the dual nature of learning—a reinterpretation of "conditioning" and "problem solving." Harv Educ Rev 1947;17:102–148.
7. Miller NE, And DiCara L. Instrumental learning of heart rate changes in curarized rats: shaping and specificity to discriminative stimulus. J Comp Physiol Psychol 1967;63:12–19.
8. DiCara LV. Learning in the autonomic nervous system. Sci Am 1970;222:30–39.
9. Miller NE, Dworkin BR. Visceral learning: recent difficulties with curarized rats and significant problems for human research. In: Obrist PA, Black AH, Brener BJ, DiCara LV, eds. Cardiovascular psychophysiology. Chicago: Aldine, 1974.
10. Adams HE, Brantley PJ, and Thompson K. Biofeedback and headache: methodological issues. In: White L, Tursky B, eds. Clinical biofeedback: efficacy and mechanisms. New York: Guilford Press, 1982.
11. Graham JR, Wolff HG. Mechanisms of migraine headache and action of ergotamine tartarate. Arch Neurol Psychiatry 1938;39:737–763.
12. Feuerstein M, Adams HE, Beiman I. Cephalic vasomotor and electromyographic feedback in the treatment of combined muscle contraction and migraine headaches in a geriatric case. Headache 1976;16:232–237.
13. Feuerstein M, Adams HE. Cephalic vasomotor feedback in the modification of migraine headache. Headache 1977;2:241–254.
14. Sturgis ET, Tollison CD, Adams HE. Modification of combined migraine-muscle contraction headaches using BVP and EMG biofeedback. J Appl Behav Anal 1978;11:215–223.
15. Bild R, Adams HE. Modification of migraine headache by cephalic blood volume pulse and EMG biofeedback. J Consult Clin Psychol 1980;48:51–57.
16. Sovak M, Kunzel M, Stemback RA, Dalessio DJ. Is volitional manipulation of hemodynamics a valid rationale for biofeedback therapy of migraine? Headache 1978;18:197–202.
17. Merrill B, Blanchard EB. Two studies of the potential mechanisms of action in thermal biofeedback of vascular headache. Headache 1989;29:169–176.
18. Largen JW, Mathew RJ, Dobbins K, Claghorn JL. Specific and nonspecific effects on skin temperature control in migraine management. Headache 1981;21:36–44.
19. Sargent JD, Green EE, Walters ED. The use of autogenic training in a pilot study of migraine and tension headaches. Headache 1972;12:120–124.
20. Sargent JD, Green EE, Walters ED. Preliminary report on the use of autogenic training in the treatment of migraine and tension headaches. Psychosom Med 1973;35:129–135.
21. Budzynski TH, Stoyva JM, Adler CS. Feedback-induced muscle relaxation: an application to tension headache. J Behav Ther Exp Psychiatry 1970;1:205–211.
22. Budzynski TH, Stoyva JM, Adler CS, Mullaney DJ. EMG biofeedback and tension headache: a controlled outcome study. Psychosom Med 1973;35:484–496.
23. Bernstein DA, Borkovec TD. Progressive relaxation training. Il; Research Press, 1973.
24. Benson H. The relaxation response. New York: William Morrow, 1975.
25. Schultz J, Luthe W. Autogenic therapy. New York: Grune & Stratton, 1969.
26. Andreychuk T, Skriver C. Hypnosis and biofeedback in the treatment of migraine headache. Int J Clin Exp Hypn 1975;23:172–183.
27. Paulley JW, Haskell DAL. The treatment of migraine without drugs. Psychosom Res 1975;19:367–374.
28. Werbach MR, Sandweiss JH. Peripheral temperatures of migraineurs undergoing relaxation training. Headache 1978;18:211–214.
29. Meichenbaum D. Cognitive behavior modification: an integrative approach. New York: Plenum Press, 1977.
30. Mitchell KR, Mitchell DM. Migraine: an exploratory treatment application of programmed behavior therapy techniques. J Psychosom Res 1971;15:137–157.
31. Bakal DA, Demjen S, Kaganov JA. Cognitive behavioral treatment of chronic headache. Headache 1981;21:81–86.
32. Knapp TW, Florin I. The treatment of migraine headache by training in vasoconstriction of the temporal artery and a cognitive stress-coping training. Behav Anal Modif 1981;4:267–274.
33. Adams HE, Feuerstein M, Fowler JL. Migraine headache: review of parameters, etiology, and intervention. Psychol Bull 1980;87:217–237.
34. Blanchard EB, Andrasik F, Ahles TA, et al. Migraine and tension headaches: a meta-analytic review. Behav Ther 1980;11:613–631.
35. Blanchard EB, Andrasik F. Psychological assessment and treatment of headache: recent developments and emerging issues. J Consult Clin Psychol 1982;50:859–879.
36. Blanchard EB, Andrasik F. Biofeedback treatment of vascular headache. In: Hatch JP, Fisher JG, Rugh J, eds. Biofeedback: studies in clinical efficacy. New York: Plenum Press, 1987.
37. Chapman SL. A review and clinical perspective on the use of EMG and thermal biofeedback for chronic headaches. Pain 1986;27:1–43.
38. Gauthier J, Bois R, Allaire D, Drolet M. Evaluation of skin temperature biofeedback training at two different sites for migraine. J Behav Med 1981;4:407–419.
39. Blanchard EB, Andrasik F, Neff DF, Teders SJ, Pallmeyer, et al. Sequential comparisons of relaxation training and biofeedback in the treatment of three kinds of chronic headache, or the machines may be necessary some of the time. Behav Res Ther 1982;20:469–481.
40. Holroyd KA, Penzien DB. Pharmacological versus nonpharmacological prophylaxis of recurrent migraine headache: a meta-analytic review of clinical trials. Pain 1990;42:1–13.
41. Blanchard EB, Andrasik F, Appelbaum KA, et al. The efficacy and cost-effectiveness of minimal-therapist-contact, non-drug treatments

of chronic migraine and tension headache. Headache 1985;25:214–220.

42. Blanchard EB, Appelbaum KA, Guanieri P, et al. Two studies of the long-term follow-up of minimal therapist contact treatments of vascular and tension headache. J Consult Clin Psychol 1988;56:427–432.

43. Blanchard EB, Appelbaum KA, Nicholson NL, et al. A controlled evaluation of cognitive therapy to a home-based biofeedback and relaxation treatment of vascular headache. Headache 1990;30:371–376.

44. Kohlenburg RJ, Cahn T. Self-help treatment for migraine headaches. Headache 1981;21:196–200.

15

Clinical Symptomatology and Differential Diagnosis of Tension-Type Headaches

SEYMOUR SOLOMON, RICHARD B. LIPTON, and LAWRENCE C. NEWMAN

Tension-type headaches may be the most common of all headaches, a phenomenon that almost everyone has experienced at one time or another. People who get an occasional, mild, nondescript tension-type headache may take a simple over-the-counter analgesic or often just wait for the headache to spontaneously disappear. Since most people with tension-type headache never consult a doctor, most of these headaches remain below the clinical horizon (1). Medical help may be sought if the headache recurs with increasing frequency or severity.

What does the term *tension* mean when used with reference to headaches? Some believe that it refers to inner tension, a psychological phenomena, though these patients do not have distinctive psychological profiles. Others assert that it indicates tension of the muscles of the head, especially of the scalp; hence the term *muscle contraction headache.* However, study samples derived from subspecialty clinics suggest that scalp muscle contraction is no greater in patients with tension-type headache than in those with migraine; pericranial muscle involvement, as measured by the degree of tenderness or by the level of electromyographic (EMG) activity, is not necessarily present during "tension" headache (2–4). For this reason, the new headache classification of the International Headache Society (IHS) uses the term *tension-type headache*, since it is by no means clear what, if anything, is tense (5).

There are many difficulties in diagnosing and classifying tension-type headache. Migraine without aura and episodic tension-type headache share many clinical symptoms, therapeutic responses, and physiological profiles. No single feature or combination of features unequivocally differentiates migraine without aura from episodic tension-type headache (6–12). Medications and other therapies that benefit migraineurs may similarly benefit patients with tension-type headache (13–15). Psychophysiological comparisons of migraine and tension-type headache fail to reveal consistent differences (2, 16–18). Biochemical changes, such as depletion of beta endorphin in the serum and cerebrospinal fluid, alterations in serotonin and platelet physiology, and sympathetic hypofunction have been found during both migraine

and tension-type headache (19–27). Because of this overlap, many believe that both migraine and tension-type headaches have similar central nervous system mechanisms with considerable variation in clinical manifestations (28, 29). Some advocate the term *essential* or *idiopathic* headache to suggest that tension-type headache and migraine represent polar expressions of a single disorder. The authors consider the relationship between tension-type headache and migraine to be an open question.

In the widely used, older headache classification, often referred to as the NIH consensus criteria, muscle contraction headache (a synonym for tension headache) was defined as "an ache or sensation of tightness, pressure or constriction, widely varied in intensity, frequency and duration, sometimes long-lasting and commonly suboccipital" (30). While the quality of pain is adequately described, this definition is vague; apparently, any level of pain intensity, duration, and frequency and any combination of associated features is acceptable. In the quarter-century since these criteria were proposed, the controversies about the pathophysiology (and hence the legitimacy) of the diagnosis of tension-type headache have not been resolved.

In an effort to improve classification, the IHS subclassified tension-type headache, based on temporal frequency and evidence of pericranial involvement (5). With frequency as a parameter, tension-type headaches are considered "episodic" if they occur less than 15 days per month and "chronic" if they occur at least 15 days per month. To better define the role of muscle tension in this disorder, the headaches are subdivided into those with and those without disorder of pericranial muscles. Involvement of pericranial muscles is assumed when there is increased tenderness (by palpation or algometer) or increased electromyographic activity of muscles, or both.

The relationship of pericranial muscles to tension-type headache is uncertain. According to the traditional concept, scalp or neck muscle contraction is evoked by obvious or covert stress. In predisposed individuals, the muscle contraction, as a response to stress or other factors, is excessive or prolonged with resultant pain, headache. The pain in turn increases emotional tension, which evokes muscle tension, and a self-perpetuating cycle may develop. Unfortunately, little evidence supports this simple concept.

Scientific documentation of the presence or absence of pericranial muscle tenderness in patients with tension-type headache and in normal controls has occurred only recently (3, 31, 32). Tenderness of muscles to palpation is difficult to assess objectively; every muscle can be made tender if the "palpation" is sufficiently vigorous. Quantitation of muscle tenderness by palpation or algometry requires a consistent systematic technique, and for research purposes, the examiner must be "blinded" to the headache diagnosis. Recent studies have shown that patients with tension-type headache have significantly more pericranial muscle tenderness than controls, when palpation was performed by blinded examiners (3, 31, 32). There was a correlation between pressure pain thresholds as determined by algometer measurements and degree of tenderness by palpation. That muscle tenderness is not the sole cause of pain was emphasized by the discrepancy between degrees of pain and tenderness in some patients. As already noted, excessive tenderness is also a feature of migraine, suggesting that this finding is not specific for tension headache (7, 32).

The relationship of trigger points to tension-type headache is controversial. Trigger points are knots of muscle tissue that when palpated are either locally tender or evoke (trigger) pain at a distant site (33, 34). The evoked pain is sometimes reported to be typical of the patient's spontaneous pain. But, "the distribution of referred trigger point pain rarely coincides with the entire distribution of a peripheral nerve or dermatome" (34). The distribution of these trigger points by insertion of a needle (with or without local anesthetic) is said to break up the pathophysiological local contraction and ameliorate the associated pain. This subject has been studied even less well by scientific methods than that of muscle tenderness.

EPISODIC TENSION-TYPE HEADACHE

Episodic tension-type headache is described by the Headache Classification Committee of the IHS as "Recurrent episodes of headache lasting minutes to days. The pain is typically pressing/tightening in quality, of mild or moderate intensity, bilateral in location and does not worsen with routine physical activity. Nausea is absent, but photophobia *or* phonophobia may be present" (5). The IHS provides operational diagnostic criteria for the selection of homogenous patient groups in research studies; the criteria for episodic tension-type headache are listed in Table 15.1 (5).

In practice, the diagnosis of episodic tension-type headache is often made by negative factors. If an intermittent headache is not migraine, cluster headache, or another primary headache disorder, and it is not due to organic disease, it usually falls into the category of episodic ten-

Table 15.1.
Diagnostic Criteria of Episodic Tension-type Headache[a]

A. At least 10 previous headache episodes fulfilling criteria B–D listed below; number of days with such headache <180/year (<15/month)
B. Headache lasting from 30 minutes to 7 days
C. At least 2 of the following pain characteristics:
   1. Pressing/tightening (nonpulsating) quality
   2. Mild or moderate intensity (may inhibit, but does not prohibit activities)
   3. Bilateral location
   4. No aggravation by walking stairs or similar routine physical activity
D. Both of the following:
   1. No nausea or vomiting (anorexia may occur)
   2. Photophobia and phonophobia are absent, or one but not the other is present
In addition, organic disorder is ruled out by the initial evaluation or by imaging studies; if disease is present, the headaches should not have started in close temporal relationship to the disorder.

[a]Adapted from Headache Classification Committee of the International Headache Society. Classification and diagnostic criteria for headache disorders, cranial neuralgias and facial pain. Cephalalgia 1988;8(suppl 7):1–96.

sion-type headache. In the IHS classification, the pain features and associated symptoms are often described in negative terms and deliberately contrasted to migraine. While the pain of migraine is pulsatile, severe, unilateral, and increased by routine activity, the pain of tension-type headache should *not* have these features. There are few, if any, associated features. They should not include nausea or vomiting, and if photophobia occurs, it should not be accompanied by phonophobia and vice versa.

In terms of positive attributes, the pain may be a dull ache or have a pressure or tight quality. It may be described as a band-like sensation around the head or a tight cap over the top of the head. There is no consistent site; the pain is usually bilateral and often occipitonuchal, bifrontal, bitemporal, or scattered. Sometimes, the pain extends into the shoulders. These headaches are usually of short duration, most commonly lasting hours to 1 day. By IHS criteria, they should occur less than 15 times per month (5). In our experience, even this number suggests evolution to daily/chronic tension-type headache. Most people with episodic tension-type headache have no more than 2 headaches per week, but exceptionally, a series of headaches may occur more often. It has been said that tension-type headaches occur mainly toward the end of the day, as the stresses of the day build up, but this has not been scientifically validated.

As in migraine, episodic tension-type headaches tend to begin in adolescence and young adult life, but they are not uncommon in children. They affect women more often than men. In contrast with migraine, there are few precipitating factors other than emotional stress. Whereas the attack of migraine most commonly occurs after stress, episodic tension-type headache occurs in anticipation of or during the stress. When emotional factors are not obvious, it has been postulated that the headaches are a physiological reaction to the stresses of everyday life.

Ameliorating factors are less distinct in patients with episodic tension-type headache than in migraineurs. Most patients with these headaches do not lie down in a quiet dark room and apply cold compresses during a headache. Rather, they carry on their usual activities with or without taking an analgesic.

There may be evidence of excessive muscle contraction besides that of the pericranial muscles. Some patients with episodic tension-type headache appear tense and anxious. They may sit rigidly on the edge of their chairs rather than in a relaxed manner. Difficulty in relaxation may be manifested by passively elevating the patient's arms and then quickly withdrawing support. Many people with episodic tension-type headache will maintain their arms extended rather than allow them to loosely drop to their sides (35).

The IHS has placed oromandibular dysfunction under the category of tension-type headache (5). Under this rubric are listed temporomandibular joint (TMJ) dysfunction, myofascial pain dysfunction (MPD), and craniomandibular dysfunction. Many dentists and other specialists believe that TMJ dysfunction and MPD are separate entities. The mechanism of oromandibular dysfunction (in contrast to organic disease of the TMJ) is still in dispute.

The IHS criteria require 3 of 6 features for the diagnosis of oromandibular dysfunction: TMJ noise on jaw movements, limited or jerky jaw movements, pain on jaw function, locking of jaw on opening, clenching or grinding of teeth, or other parafunctions (tongue, lips, or cheek biting or pressing) (5). Tenderness is not listed as a feature because it already is a subheading. We believe these criteria are not sufficiently precise. Joint noise is a common symptom in otherwise asymptomatic adults and, in our opinion, is not specific for any disorder. Clenching teeth and oral parafunctions may be mechanisms of oromandibular dysfunction but need not be criteria for diagnosis. In our opinion, the criteria for TMJ dysfunction or MPD should be pain and tenderness in the area of the TMJ and/or muscles of mastication, increase in pain with jaw function, and limitation of jaw movement.

Episodic tension-type headaches often occur in patients with migraine. They may occur between attacks of migraine (interval headaches) or may be mixed with the features of migraine (mixed headache). In addition, some people with migraine develop an increased frequency of attacks and begin to lose the features usually associated with migraine (10, 36). For example, nausea and photophobia may remit. The headaches begin to resemble tension-type headache and begin to recur daily or almost every day (37, 38). This evolution is cited as additional evidence that migraine and tension-type headache have a common mechanism. While we have frequently observed this phenomenon in our subspecialty practice, the relationship between episodic tension-type headache and chronic daily headache evolving from migraine remains uncertain.

CHRONIC (DAILY) TENSION-TYPE HEADACHE

Many people who seek treatment in headache centers experience the symptoms of tension-type headaches every day for months or years; these headaches are termed chronic tension-type headaches. The IHS criteria require a frequency of at least 15 days per month for at least 6 months (5). In subspecialty clinics, most patients report daily or near-daily headaches. They may last for several hours, but more often are continuous from awakening in the morning to sleep at night. Many patients who report daily headaches that last only a few hours also have an additional persistent, nagging ache that may not be noticed when they are distracted by work or other attention-focused activity.

The pain characteristics, paucity of associated symptoms, and absence of organic disease form the other criteria for chronic tension-type headache and are the same as for episodic tension-type headache (Table 15.1). Like episodic tension-type headache, chronic tension-type headaches have been subdivided into those associated with disorder of pericranial muscles (former term—chronic muscle-contraction headache) and those without disorder of pericranial muscles (former terms—chronic idiopathic headache or chronic psychogenic headache) (5). The latter term was an old assumption and is no longer appropriate.

Many studies have compared patients with tension-type headache and migraineurs. Differences, if any, have not been striking, with one exception. Electrical stimulation of the labial commissure during teeth clenching normally evokes early and late exteroceptive periods of electromyographic suppression in the temporalis muscle. In patients with chronic tension-type headache, but not in those with migraine nor in a control group, the late exteroceptive suppression period is shortened or abolished (39).

Several mechanisms have been proposed for chronic tension-type headache; they are discussed in detail in Chapter 18. In a minority of cases, chronic tension-type headache may evolve from episodic tension-type headache or occur de novo. Usually, however, chronic tension-type headaches evolve from migraine, occur as a rebound phenomenon associated with overuse of medication, or both (37). (The IHS classification would assign the latter headaches to the category "headache associated with substances or their withdrawal" and then note chronic tension-type headache as a subgroup (5).). A history of migraine in the past may not be obvious unless the patient is specifically queried about past headaches. Years earlier, patients may have reported unilateral, pulsating headaches associated with nausea and photophobia, which may not have been recognized as migraine. Similarly, patients may not report a history of medication overuse. They are often ashamed of the many pills they take each day or fear the doctor's advice to discontinue the pills. Some don't regard over-the-counter pills (often bought at the supermarket) as "medicine." The doctor must determine the type and the quantity of medication the patient is using, since many patients use several different kinds of headache remedies. It may help to ask such questions as "How long does a bottle of 100 tablets of brand X last?" The agents that perpetuate chronic tension-type headache on a rebound basis are caffeine, barbiturates, benzodiazepines or ergotamines, and most often, common analgesics. The most common offending analgesics are acetaminophen and aspirin in combination with other agents and narcotics (40). The nonsteroidal antiinflammatory agents and tricyclic antidepressants-analgesics are not associated with the rebound phenomena that perpetuate chronic tension-type headache and are the preferred pharmacological agents for this condition.

Psychological factors are an invariable aspect of chronic pain in general and chronic tension-type headache in particular. Depression and anxiety are most common. Often, the depression is viewed as a consequence of chronic headache. Patients are sure they would be fine if only their headaches would disappear. Depression lowers pain threshold, and pain evokes depression; it is usually difficult or impossible to determine whether the depression is a cause or a consequence of headache. However, it is not fruitful to attempt to resolve this dilemma; from the practical point of view, it doesn't matter which came first. It is more important for the patient to understand and acknowledge that pain and the psychological response to pain cannot be separated. Both must be addressed if the quality of life is to be improved.

Most patients who experience chronic, frequent headaches have overt or covert signs of depression (41, 42). The depression may not be obvious to the patient, family, or friends. Some patients may deny feelings of sadness, but depression may be manifested by change in sleep pattern or in appetite; constipation; loss of libido; loss of interest in family, friends, and occupation; and withdrawal from social activities. There may be difficulty in concentration, with loss of work efficiency or memory impairment. These symptoms, in mid or late life, may simulate Alzheimer's disease. Occasionally, the headache may be the chief manifestation of depression and may "mask" depression. Rarely, the headache may be part of a delusional system.

Stressful situations are a fact of life, but no two people react to stress in the same way. A particularly stressful situation might not evoke any obvious reaction in one person; another might experience indigestion; a third, anxiety; and a fourth, headache. Many patients with chronic tension-type headache are understandably frustrated by persistent pain. They are often angry at unsympathetic family and friends and hostile to doctors who have failed to "cure" their headache. Recognition of these factors by physicians and patients enhances the understanding of some of the headache's mechanisms and leads to proper treatment.

DIFFERENTIAL DIAGNOSIS

The differential diagnosis of tension-type headache is basically the same as the differential diagnosis of headache per se (see Chapter 4). These headaches were once thought to be predominantly psychogenic, with or without muscle contraction as the physical mechanism. Primary psychogenic headaches may enter the differential diagnosis of tension-type headache, particularly in its chronic forms. When headache is a manifestation of depression, there are usually other somatic symptoms or symptoms of altered mood. Rarely, headache is a symptom of a conversion reaction. When this is the case, the patient's affect is usually inconsistent with the "severe" symptom, and other hysterical features may be present. Headache is rarely a delusional manifestation. When headache is a delusional symptom, some other evidence of serious psychopathology is often present. Simply asking patients about the cause of their headache may elicit the delusion.

Episodic tension-type headache may be confused with a number of other headache disorders. The differential features of migraine without aura and tension-type headache have been discussed earlier. Disease and dysfunction of the cervical spine may cause headaches that are similar to episodic or chronic tension-type headache. Some European specialists attribute many headaches to a cervicogenic mechanism, but most physicians in North America discount this as an important type of headache (43).

The other pathophysiological headache, cluster headache, is easily differentiated from episodic tension-type headache by the focal nature, great severity, daily recurrence, and associated ipsilateral autonomic symptoms. Almost any organic disease may cause headaches that simulate episodic tension-type headaches. The episodic headaches evoked by an intracranial mass usually increase in frequency and duration just as other associated focal or generalized neurological symptoms progress. Cerebrovascular disease may be heralded by episodic headaches (44). These most often simulate migraine and begin at a later age than tension-type headache. Posttraumatic/postconcussion headaches may have qualities indistinguishable from episodic or chronic tension-type headaches.

A small leak ("sentinal hemorrhage"), rather than rupture, of an intracranial vascular anomaly may cause a headache that is similar to an episodic tension-type headache. This disease must be considered with the sudden onset of any new headache. The intermittent headache of giant cell arteritis almost always begins after the age of 55. The headaches of infectious diseases are usually associated with fever and other systemic symptoms. The headaches associated with systemic illness or with local disease of the head, neck, or face will usually be accompanied by other evidence of these illnesses.

Chronic tension-type headache, as noted earlier, often evolves from migraine, but the most important consideration is daily abuse or overuse of headache medication. Other daily headaches (such as chronic cluster headache) are clearly differentiated by their very specific criteria (5). The continuous dull aching pain of hemicrania continua might be mistaken for chronic tension-type headache, but as the name implies, the headache of hemicrania continua is almost exclusively unilateral and recurs on the same side; this condition is remarkably responsive to indomethacin (45). Virtually all of the organic diseases of the head and systemic diseases discussed in the differential diagnosis of episodic tension-type headache are also applicable to chronic tension-type headache. Often, headache caused by these illnesses begins with intermittent episodic headaches and evolves into chronic daily headaches as the underlying disease progresses. Because there is no laboratory test or biological marker for tension-type headaches, one must always recognize that an initial diagnosis of tension-type headache may be wrong. In following these patients, always continue to consider the possibility of underlying organic disease.

REFERENCES

1. Linet MS, Stewart WF, Celentano DD, Ziegler D, Sprecker M. An epidemiologic study of headache among adolescents and young adults. JAMA 1989;261:2211–2216.
2. Bakal DA, Kaganov JA. Muscle contraction and migraine headache: psychophysiologic comparison. Headache 1977;17:208–215.
3. Langemark M, Olesen J. Pericranial tenderness in tension headache—a blind controlled study. Cephalalgia 1987;7:249–255.
4. Jensen K, Tuxen C, Olesen J. Pericranial muscle tenderness and pressure-pain threshold in the temporal region during common migraine. Pain 1988;35:65–70.
5. Headache Classification Committee of the International Headache Society. Classification and diagnostic criteria for headache disorders, cranial neuralgias and facial pain. Cephalalgia 1988;8(suppl 7):1–96.
6. Bakal DA, Kaganov JA. Symptom characteristics of chronic and non-chronic headache sufferers. Headache 1979;19:285–289.
7. Tfelt-Hansen P, Lous I, Olesen J. Prevalence and significance of muscle tenderness during common migraine attacks. Headache 1981;21:49–54.
8. Nikiforow R. Features of migraine: comparison of a questionnaire study and a neurologist-examined random sample. Cephalalgia 1981;1:157–166.
9. Ziegler DK, Hassanein RS, Couch JR. Headache syndromes suggested by statistical analysis of headache symptoms. Cephalalgia 1982;2:125–134.
10. Drummond PD, Lance JW. Clinical diagnoses and computer analyses of headache symptoms. J Neurol Neurosurg Psychiatry 1984;47:128–133.
11. Drummond PD. A quantitative assessment of photophobia in migraine and tension headache. Headache 1986;26:465–469.
12. Solomon S, Guglielmo-Cappa K, Smith CR. Common migraine: criteria for diagnosis. Headache 1988;28:124–129.
13. Chapman SL. A review and clinical perspective on the use of EMG and thermal biofeedback for chronic headache. Pain 1986;27:1–43.
14. Barrie MA, Fox WR, Weatherall M, Wilkinson MIP. Analysis of symptoms of patients with headaches and their response to treatment with ergot derivatives. Q J Med 1968;37:319–336.
15. Bono G, Micieli G, Sances G, Calvani M, Nappi G. L-5HTP treatment in primary headaches: an attempt at clinical identification of responsive patients. Cephalalgia 1984;4:159–165.
16. Anderson CD, Frank RD. Migraine and tension headache: is there a difference? Headache 1981;21:63–71.
17. Arena JG, Blanchard EB, Andrasik F, Appelbaum K, Myers PE. Psychophysiologic comparisons of three kinds of headache subjects during and between headache states: analysis of post-stress adaptation periods. J Psychosom Res 1985;29:427–441.
18. Merskey H, Brown J, Brown A, Malhotra L, Morrison D, Ripley C. Psychological normality and abnormality in persistent headache patients. Pain 1985;23:35–47.
19. Facchinetti F, Nappi G, Savoldi F, Genazzani AR. Primary headaches: reduced circulating β-lipoprotein and B-endorphin levels with impaired reactivity to acupuncture. Cephalalgia 1981;1:195–201.
20. Genazzani AR, Nappi G, Facchinetti F, et al. Progressive impairment of CSF β-EP levels in migraine sufferers. Pain 1984;18:127–133.
21. Rolf LH, Wiele G, Brune GG. 5-Hydroxytryptamine in platelets of patients with muscle contraction headache. Headache 1981;21:10–11.
22. Takeshima T, Shimomura T, Takahashi K. Platelet activation in muscle contraction headache and migraine. Cephalalgia 1987;7:239–243.
23. Shukla R, Shanker K, Nag D, Verma M, Bhargava KP. Serotonin in tension headache. J Neurol Neurosurg Psychiatry 1987;50:1682–1684.
24. Anthony M, Lance JW. Plasma serotonin in patients with chronic tension headaches. J Neuro Neurosurg Psychiatry 1989;52:182–184.
25. Giacovazzo M, Bernoni RM, Di Sobato F, Martelletti P. Impairment of 5HT binding to lymphocytes and monocytes from tension-type headache patients. Headache 1990;30:220–223.
26. Takeshima T, Takao Y, Takahashi K. Pupillary sympathetic hypofunction and asymmetry in muscle contraction headache and migraine. Cephalalgia 1987;7:257–262.
27. Mikamo K, Takeshima T, Takahashi K. Cardiovascular sympathetic hypofunction in muscle contraction headache and migraine. Headache 1989;29:86–89.
28. Featherstone HJ. Migraine and muscle contraction headaches: a continuum. Headache 1985;25:194–198.
29. Raskin NH. Headache. 2nd ed. Philadelphia: WB Saunders, 1988:215–224.
30. Committee on Classification of Headache of the National Institute of Neurological Diseases and Blindness. Classification of headache. JAMA 1962;179:717–718.
31. Langemark M, Jensen K, Jensen TS, Olesen J. Pressure pain thresholds and thermal nociceptive thresholds in chronic tension-type headache. Pain 1989;38:203–210.
32. Drummond PD. Scalp tenderness and sensitivity to pain in migraine and tension headache. Headache 1987;27:45–50.
33. Malzack R, Stillwell DM, Fox EJ. Trigger points and acupuncture points for pain: correlations and implications. Pain 1977;3:3–23.
34. Travell JG, Simons DG. Myofascial pain and dysfunction. The trigger point manual. Baltimore: Williams & Wilkins, 1983:4.
35. Lance JW. Mechanism and management of headache. 4th ed. Boston: Butterworth Scientific, 1982:105.
36. Ostfeld A. The natural history and epidemiology of migraine and muscle contraction headache. Neurology 1953;13:11–15.
37. Mathew NT, Stubits E, Nigam MP. Transformation of episodic migraine into daily headache: analysis of factors. Headache 1982;22:66–68.
38. Baldrati A, Bini L, D'Alessandro R, et al. Analysis of outcome predictors of migraine toward chronicity. Cephalalgia 1985;5(suppl 2):195–199.
39. Schoenen J, Jamart B, Gerard P, Lenarduzzi P, Delwaide PJ. Exteroceptive suppression of temporalis muscle activity in chronic headache. Neurology 1987;37:1834–1836.
40. Saper JR. Headache disorders. Current concepts and treatment strategies. Boston: John Wright PSG, 1983:263–278.
41. Dalessio DJ, ed. Wolff's headache. 5th ed. New York: Oxford University Press, 1987:174–181.
42. Andrasik F. Psychologic and behavioral aspects of chronic headache. Neurol Clin 1990;8:961–976.
43. Edmeads, J. The cervical spine and headache. Neurology 1988;38:1874–1878.
44. Portenoy RK, Abissi CJ, Lipton RB, et al. Headache and cerebrovascular disease. Stroke 1984;15:1009–1012.
45. Sjaastad O, Spierings ELH. "Hemicrania continua": another headache absolutely responsive to indomethacin. Cephalalgia 1984;4:65–70.

16

Pathophysiology of Tension-Type Headache

In 1988, the International Headache Society developed a new classification of headache (1). What had been called muscle-contraction headache or tension headache was now classified as tension-type headache. The new nomenclature was most probably in deference to the still-questioned etiology of this entity: physical, emotional, or a combination of both aspects and/or other pathophysiological aspects as yet unidentified.

The burgeoning medical literature was also beginning to look at tension-type headache in other ways. The thought that migraine and tension-type headache were actually two aspects of the same disorder has been heavily investigated. Some authors feel that a continuum exists between these two entities and that simple migraine may evolve or transform into coexisting tension-type headache.

The central nervous system changes that accompany both types of headache are just beginning to come into pathophysiological focus. Pain-related systems are being recognized and some aspects of the endogenous opiate system changes as well as feasibly related bioaminergic system interactions are being charted. Each new-found piece of the pathogenetic puzzle brings more questions, possibly, than answers to the clinical understanding of the problem. Instead of a continuum of headache, we may be dealing with different aspects of a primary central nociceptive disorder presenting as headache.

Another possible etiologic aspect of tension-type headache may begin with the musculoskeletal system, particularly with changes in muscle. Pain induced by pathological changes in muscle may initiate central nervous system changes that may modulate and even perpetuate the clinical problem of tension-type headache. It should not be surprising that tension-type headache has been identified and recognized as a part of several muscle-induced pain syndromes, the myofascial pain syndrome and fibromyalgia.

TENSION-TYPE HEADACHE: SPECIFIC PATHOPHYSIOLOGY

The clinical aspects of tension-type headache are described elsewhere in this volume. The specific pathogenetic mechanisms of tension-type headache are not obvious. Some

researchers have suggested that the muscle contraction attributed to tension-type headache is not the cause but rather the epiphenomenon of headache (2–4).

The role of the central nervous system in the maintenance of muscle tone is one logical place to begin any mechanistic consideration. Muscle tone is determined, in part, by the state of activity of the gamma efferent neurons located in the anterior horn cells of the spinal cord. These act on the alpha motor neuron supplying the muscle spindles. This synaptic system is influenced by inhibitory cells such as the Renshaw cells, possibly via inhibitory transmitters such as γ-aminobutyric acid (GABA). There is then supraspinal control via cortical, subcortical, and limbic afferent and efferent systems. Interaction between all of these pathways allows both physiological and emotional input into the stable maintenance or flux in the established muscle tone. Adverse influences via pathological local stimulation, with or without limbic or affective stimulation, may produce significant muscle spasm and, if prolonged, tonic muscle contraction with the introduction of an anxiety-increased or maintained muscle contraction-pain cycle (5, 6).

Continued or tonic muscle contraction may produce hypoxia via compression of small blood vessels. The production of ischemia may be more accurately associated with an accumulation of pain-producing metabolites that may increase and also potentiate muscle pain and reactive spasm (7, 8).

Pathophysiological changes secondary to ischemia may stimulate nociceptors in muscle through the production of bradykinin, lactic acid, serotonin, and prostoglandins (9). The production of these nociceptive-enhancing chemicals may stimulate central mechanisms that, through continued stimulation, may induce further contraction and therefore maintenance of pain.

There has been no concordance concerning the relationship between increased muscle tension or spasm and headache in the literature. While researchers have confirmed the causal relationship between muscle spasm and headache (10–12), other authors felt that muscle contraction is a consequence rather than a cause of headache (13–15). While some authors have granted that increased muscle tension and headache are linked on some occasions in some people (16), other researchers felt that muscle activity may be less pronounced during muscle-contraction headache than in other types of headaches, such as migraine (17, 18). Much of this information was derived from electromyographic (EMG) studies, which evaluated different muscle groups in different types of patients with both clearly and poorly defined diagnoses (11, 17, 19, 20).

A different pain threshold to muscle tension has been postulated in chronic tension-type headache patients, as compared with normal volunteers (21).

Pericranial muscle tenderness was noted to be generally increased in patients with tension-type headache, compared with nonheadache controls. A positive correlation was found between headache intensity and tenderness. The authors felt that the tenderness in tension-type headache patients was pathological and was the source of nociception (22).

In another study, Langemark et al. (23) found that in chronic tension-type headache patients, pressure-pain thresholds were highly dependent on myofascial factors. They felt that the generally lower pain thresholds in these patients might suggest a central dysmodulation of nociceptive impulses and that sensitized nociceptors might also be part of this process.

In a study measuring scalp muscle tenderness and sensitivity to pain in both migraine and tension-type headache patients, Drummond (24) also felt that the pathophysiology of episodic tension-type headache might involve a diffuse disruption of central pain-modulating systems.

Patients with diagnosed myofascial pain syndromes, including low back pain, also have lower pain thresholds (25, 26). Patients diagnosed with fibromyalgia were also found to have lowered thresholds of tenderness (27).

Pericranial muscle tenderness is possibly characteristic of both episodic and chronic tension-type headache. Several of the functions of these muscles may relate to their possible role in tension-type headache: (a) the maintenance of posture and their effective stabilization of the head and (b) withdrawal and protection of the head (28).

Chronic tension-type headache patients may have a stereotypic posture, with their shoulders raised and their heads held in forward flexion. This tightly held posture is effective in preventing nonconscious head movement that can cause increased pain.

The pericranial muscles are innervated by sensory fibers running in nerves from the second or third cranial roots and in the trigeminal nerve divisions (28).

Tenderness in the paravertebral muscles of the neck and back has a positive correlation with pericranial tenderness (29). It was also noted in this study that environmental stress increased tenderness. Murphy and Lehrer (30) found that both contraction of shoulder and neck muscles, and emotional arousal contribute to tension-type headache.

Langemark and Jensen (28) consider three mechanisms of muscle pain to possibly be relevant to headache: (a)

low-grade inflammation associated with the release of pain-producing substances rather than signs of acute inflammation, (b) long-lasting relative ischemia, and (c) tearing of ligaments and tendons due to abnormal muscle tension. These theoretical mechanisms are also felt to be of etiological importance to other muscle-pain syndromes.

Four distinct muscle-pain syndromes often overlap and may make differential diagnosis difficult: (a) localized myofascial pain syndrome (MPS) caused by trigger points in muscles; (b) fibromyalgia (FMG), probably a systemic disorder; (c) a non-rapid-eye-movement (REM) sleep disturbance, and (d) articular dysfunction (31).

Tension-type headache is possibly interrelated to at least three of these muscle-pain syndromes, raising the possibility of a different pathogenetic continuum.

MYOFASCIAL PAIN SYNDROME

The contribution of muscle to the etiology of tension-type headache is given more support by the discovery of trigger points, small zones of hypersensitivity in muscle of the head, neck, and upper back of headache patients (14, 16). When a trigger point is palpated, pain may spread or be referred to adjacent or even distant sites on the head. Palpation may also elicit tinnitus, vertigo, and lacrimation.

The diagnosis of "myofascial pain due to trigger points was first advanced by Travell (32). She reported patterns of pain referral from trigger points in muscles throughout the body and also identified many perpetuating factors that may be important in converting an acute myofascial pain syndrome (MPS) to a chronic pain syndrome (33).

Myofascial trigger points are an extremely important and common source of musculoskeletal pain (34). A study by Fishbain et al. (35) found myofascial trigger points to be the primary cause of pain in 85% of 283 consecutive admissions to a comprehensive pain-management program. Other reports have also demonstrated the frequency of MPS with associated myofascial trigger points in the diagnosis of nonselected patients with a presenting complaint of pain (36, 37).

Clinically, MPS characteristically involves a localized or regional pain complaint associated with tender trigger points located in taut bands of skeletal muscle. The trigger point may be distant from the pain, but palpation may reproduce the patient's pain.

Trigger points may be active, with reproducible pain on palpation, or latent, without clinically associated complaints of pain. Latent trigger points may produce muscle dysfunction but not pain. Because of the occasional variation of patient pain complaints, it seems possible that trigger points may shift between active and latent.

Muscles in which trigger points are found may display increased stiffness, fatigability, and weakness and a restricted range of motion. These muscles may be shortened, with increased pain on stretching. Patients may therefore protect the muscle by adapting poor posture and sustained contraction (37). These muscle restrictions may perpetuate existing trigger points and aid in the development of others in the same muscle.

The local tenderness associated with trigger points may be due to sensitization of afferent nerve endings in the muscle (38). These sensitizing chemicals are thought to include prostaglandins, bradykinin, histamine, and others.

Histological evidence of a disturbance of the energy metabolism of trigger points was demonstrated (39). This energy crisis was also indicated by a decrease in high-energy phosphates and an increase in low-energy phosphates (40). Evidence of local vascular disturbance with hypoxia was also found (41).

Myofascial structures refer pain in reproducible patterns that do not follow dermatomal or even myotomal patterns but are specific for a particular myofascial trigger point (33). Several commonly referred muscular pain patterns associated with myofascial syndromes of the head and neck include (33, 38):

1. Myofascial trigger points in the masseter muscle may refer pain deep in the ear.
2. Temporalis muscle trigger points may refer pain to normal teeth of the upper jaw and may cause unilateral temporal headache.
3. Referred pain from trigger points in the lateral pterygoid muscle may draw attention to the temporomandibular joint. Trigger points in the upper trapezius, sternocleidomastoid, splenii, and suboccipital muscles characteristically refer pain to the head. Trigger points in these muscles were the most common cause of pain in a group of chronic headache patients (42).
4. Trigger points in the upper trapezius muscles commonly refer pain ipsilaterally over the back of the neck, often including the temporal region.
5. Referred from the sternocleidomastoid muscle (sternal division), pain may be found surrounding the eye, at the vertex and occiput. Autonomic dysfunction including lacrimation and ipsilateral scleral injection may be associated with myofascial trigger points in this muscle.
6. One of the most common sources of "muscle contraction" headache are trigger points in the clavicular division of the sternocleidomastoid muscle. These trigger points may also cause postural dizziness (43).

The referred pain patterns from these myofascial trigger points may provide the clinical picture of tension-type headache. What may be confusing is the frame of reference a clinician may take: are these headaches a primary problem with a secondary myofascial component? or are they manifestations of a primary muscle-pain syndrome? Of possibly equal importance is whether these two types of problems may be functionally correlated to a possible central dysfunction, possibly of pain modulation.

There are at least four mechanisms by which the nervous system may mediate referred pain (31, 38): 1. Convergence-projection, by which pain may be initiated by muscle nociceptors but then referred to an area served by other somatic receptors that may converge on the same spinothalamic tract cell; 2. Convergence-facilitation, where impulses from one somatic region (reference zone) are facilitated, or amplified in the spinal cord by other activity originating in nociceptors from a trigger point in another area of the body; 3. peripheral branching of primary afferent nociceptors, where the brain may misinterpret activity from nociceptors in one part of the body as coming from nerve branches originating in another part of the body; 4. sympathetic modulation of peripheral nociceptors, where increased sympathetic activity may induce an increase in substances that sensitize primary afferent nerve receptors in the area of referred pain. While the definitive mechanism for referred pain is still in question, these experimental models appear to demonstrate that referred pain from myofascial trigger points can occur.

MPS of the head and neck may also be associated with other clinical problems, some noted above in relation to myofascial trigger point referred pain. Many of these and other signs and symptoms of MPS may mimic other conditions, including migraine headaches, TMJ disorders, sinusitis, cervical neuralgias, and various otological problems including tinnitus, vertigo, ear pain, and dizziness (37).

A study of Fricton et al. (36) found a large percentage of patients with MPS of the head and neck had significant postural problems, including forward head tilt, rounded shoulders, and poor sitting and standing posture, findings also noted in tension-type headache patients.

The prevalence of headache in patients with MPS of the head and neck was 73% (44). Other studies of the prevalence of tension-type headache gave statistics between 35 and 41% of patients with headache (45–47). Unfortunately, no diagnostic criteria distinguished between the two groups.

The onset of acute single-muscle MPS may be associated with an acute event such as a motor vehicle accident or slip and fall. It may also come on more insidiously. In many patients, the syndrome may show a spontaneous regression to a latent status, with residual muscular dysfunction but resolution of the initial pain complaint. In other patients, the syndrome may "metastasize" and involve the associated musculature and become regional. There is some question as to whether the regional MPS may continue to spread to involve multiple regions or become systemic, i.e. fibromyalgia.

This progression may occur in patients with an autosomal dominant hereditary disposition to develop trigger points (48). Other mechanical factors (such as skeletal or muscular asymmetries) or psychological factors (such as anxiety or stress, which act as perpetuating factors) may encourage involvement of functionally related muscle groups and prevent recovery of muscles already involved.

NEUROANATOMY

Pain from headache, including the muscular factors of headache, appears to enter the central nervous system through cervical roots two and three (49) and is routed through the trigeminal brainstem sensory nuclear complex (50). The latter acts as the major brainstem relay center for orofacial sensory information. Other nuclei appear to be involved in the transmission of acute myofascial pain in the craniofacial region. Moskowitz (51) identified the trigeminovascular system through which, he suggests, nociceptive information is transmitted through unmyelinated C fibers associated with the arteries projecting mostly from trigeminal and cervical primary sensory neurons. These neurons are thought to then release vasoactive substances from peripheral axons into the vascular wall (such as substance P), which may then promote pain and local inflammation.

Central modulation of pain appears to originate in the brainstem and involve at least two systems. The "descending" analgesia system is inhibitory and appears to regulate the spinal cord "gating" mechanism. It comprises the midbrain periaquiductal grey region, the medial medullary raphe nuclei and its adjacent reticular formation, and the dorsal horn neurons of the spinal cord (52). An "ascending" pain modulation system originates in the midbrain and projects to the thalamus (53). The major neurotransmitters in both systems include biogenic amines, opiod peptides, and nonopiod peptides (52–54).

The ascending system may be of more relevance to headache disorders (54), but this would possibly not be true for aspects of myofascial involvement. This system has a brainstem to medial thalamus projection that includes a large number of both opiate and serotonergic receptors.

The midbrain dorsal raphe nucleus (DRN), a serotonergic nucleus, projects to the medial thalamus. This projection has been associated with central pain modulation (53). Raskin (55) reviews literature that implicates serotonergic projections to the forebrain in sleep cycle regulation, mood change, hypothalamic regulation of hormone release, and pain perception.

The neuroanatomic systems give a reasonable mechanism for linking pathological myofascial stimulation to the central pain modulating systems that also would subserve nonmyofascial and nonanatomic, or central chemical mechanisms associated with the etiology of headache pain. The neurochemical modulating systems are discussed in greater detail below.

TENSION-TYPE HEADACHE: OTHER CLINICAL ASPECTS

Most authors agree that psychological/emotional factors are important in the genesis and possibly the maintenance of tension-type headaches. The exact role of emotional problems such as stress, anxiety, and depression is uncertain; the literature is equivocal.

Olesen (56) stated that he felt that almost any psychiatric disorder, except psychoses, would predispose patients to tension-type headache. Elsewhere, Olesen and Langemark (57) note that tension-type headaches may signal to pa-

tients that they are anxious, stressed, or depressed, and cause them to make appropriate lifestyle changes.

Anxiety has been thought to contribute directly (58) or to initiate a psychophysiological reaction leading to tension-type headaches. Somatization of anxiety, poorly repressed anger, or hostility has been suggested as an initiating factor (59, 60).

While several authors have associated tension-type headaches with environmental stress (29, 61), others have found a poor correlation between stress and tension-type headache (62).

Depression has been definitely linked to the initiation of tension-type headaches by some researchers (6, 63); others remain uncertain (64). It might be more appropriate to evaluate the onset of tension-type headaches in depressed patients versus those patients who develop tension-type headache and then become depressed. Obviously, without premorbid psychological evaluations, this would be difficult. If, however, neurochemical changes associated with tension-type headache, such as a possible central serotonergic dysfunction, also initiated depression as a response to these changes, these data would need to be interpreted in a different manner.

Several authors felt that the triad of increased responses on hypochondriasis, depression, and hysteria scales of the Minnesota multiphasic personality inventory (MMPI) was characteristic of the tension-type headache population (65, 66). Similar responses, however, were found in chronic nonheadache pain patients (67).

Evidence of vasomotor instability has been seen in patients with tension-type headache (11, 68–70). (See below for further details.)

Sleep disturbance has been noted to accompany tension-type headache (6). The interrelationships between sleep, central nervous system levels of serotonin, and headache, particularly migraine, have been studied (71, 72). The latter authors (72) note that chronic headache patients have more problems secondary to a more disturbed sleep cycle than intermittent migraineurs. The sleep disorder in tension-type headache patients was similar to that of the sleep disorder associated with fibromyalgia.

The relationship between electromyographic (EMG) results and tension-type headache are confusing. The putative relationship between EMG levels and pain have been investigated using biofeedback to alleviate the headache pain (73, 74). Other authors concluded that EMG activity did not correlate well with headache intensity (75).

Several studies found a positive correlation between resting frontalis EMG levels and frequency of headache (76, 77). Van Boxten and van der Ven (78) found EMG levels to be consistently higher in tension-type headache subjects than in controls. Several other authors found that EMG levels were higher in the neck muscles than the frontalis muscles in tension-type headache patients (17, 20).

The relationship between tension-type headache symptoms and EMG was found to be equivocal in one review (79). Anderson and Franks (80) found a negative correlation between frontalis EMG and tension-type headache pain.

Two possible mechanical etiologies of tension-type headache must also be mentioned. Cervical spondylosis is defined as a degenerative disease affecting intervertebral discs and apophyseal joints of the cervical spine. Several authors have noted the correlation between cervical spondylosis and tension-type headache (5, 6, 14). Iansek et al. (81), however, conclude that the incidence of tension-type headache is low in cervical spondylosis and suggest that the basis of existing headache is secondary muscle contraction.

A possible correlation between temporamandibular joint (TMJ) dysfunction and tension headache has been reported, mainly in the dental literature (82, 83). The existing relationship appears to depend mainly on masticatory muscle tenderness, which may have other causes (29, 84, 85).

TENSION-TYPE HEADACHE AND MIGRAINE: A CONTINUUM?

Over the last decade and a half, research has looked at the possible interrelationship between tension-type headache and migraine. Two main concepts have been recognized. The first is the headache severity model, which states that the difference between tension-type headache and migraine is quantitative rather than qualitative. This model states that tension-type headache is really mild migraine (86–88).

The second concept is that tension-type headache and migraine are two aspects of one headache continuum (88, 89). Simple episodic migraine headache attacks may eventually transform into daily, or tension-type headache (90). This hypothesis is based on the reported similarities between the two headache entities. Clinically, these patients, who may have started with occasional migraine attacks, develop daily pain seemingly of muscular origin and then daily headache, considered tension-type, with fewer or more interspersed vascular headaches. These patients commonly develop a sleep disorder as well as elements of anxiety and depression (89, 91). This might represent the natural evolution of migraine headache (89), or it might be secondary to a central nervous system dysfunction (92).

Bakal and Kaganov (17) have suggested that both muscle contraction (tension-type) and migraine patients have a similar physiological predisposition for headaches. Electroencephalographic (EEG) abnormalities have been found in both migraine and tension-type headache patients, with more frequent abnormalities seen in the vascular headache patients (93). Basser's (94) data agreed that epilepsy was more prevalent in a migrainous population than in tension-type headache patients. Lance and Anthony (95) found slightly more epilepsy within the tension-type headache group. Jay (96) found more evidence of EEG abnormalities in a pediatric migraine population.

Psychophysiological Comparisons

General Autonomic Changes. Patients with common migraine, who do not experience visual aura or the neurological symptoms of complicated migraine, often have more nonspecific autonomic-mediated changes before a headache, including depression, euphoria, hyper- or hyposexuality, and appetite changes. A minority of tension-type headache patients complain of mild associated symptoms such as lack of appetite, hyperirritability, dizziness, and increased sensitivity to light (56). It is notable that some of these symptoms can be secondary to autonomic changes associated with active myofascial trigger points located in the head and neck.

Muscle Spasm. EMG studies have shown that neck muscles are more contracted than temporal muscles during headache attacks, with migraine headache patients developing more intense contractions than tension-type headache patients (17). Pozniak-Patewicz (20) also found that neck and temporal muscle activity was greater for migraine than tension-type headache patients during both the headache attack and in headache-free periods. Cervical muscle contraction has been reported to be a prodomal symptom in migraine (97) as well as in tension-type headache. Frontalis muscle EMG could not discriminate between tension-type headache and migraine patients (61). Finally, tension-type headache patients with the lowest frontalis EMG values were also the patients who appeared to experience the most diffuse and nonspecific pain (17).

While muscle contraction and tenderness may be the primary symptoms of tension-type headache, EMG activity and muscle tenderness increase more often during migraine than during tension-type headache (70, 98, 99).

Autonomically Mediated Cardiovascular Responses. Psychophysiological testing has produced evidence of vasoconstrictive and pulse changes in the different headache entities. In a study comparing tension-type headache patients with common migraine patients exposed to auditory stimulation, tension-type headache patients exhibited a lower heart rate reactivity than migraine patients. Temporal artery pulse response showed migraine patients to exhibit stronger pulse amplitude decrease than controls, while tension-type headache patients showed pulse amplitude increases (100).

Haynes (101) found that tension-type headache patients evidenced the greatest cardiovascular arousal, especially during headache. Bakal and Kaganov (17) found both migraine and tension-type headache patients decreased pulse velocity in response to noise, while controls increased pulse velocity.

Cohen (70), in a psychophysiological comparison of migraine and muscle contraction headache, found temporal artery vasoconstriction to be a differentiating factor. He found that migraine patients are vasodilated and tension-type headache patients are vasoconstricted both during and between headache attacks. In a study on the vasoconstrictive aspects of tension-type headache, administration of vasoconstrictive agents such as ergotamine tartrate increased the pain of muscle contraction headache, while amyl nitrite, a vasodilator, yielded transient pain relief (102).

Migraine patients have been thought to have an unstable autonomic nervous system (103). Murphy and Lehrer's data (30) suggest greater sympathetic arousal during a tension-type headache attack (versus controls).

Mikamo et al. (104) reported both tension-type headache and migraine patients to have evidence of cardiovascular sympathetic hypofunction, demonstrated by low basal levels of norepinephrine and orthostatic hypotension. Data from another study (105) suggests that tension-type headache patients have phasic hypersympathetic activity, while migraineurs do not differ from controls during psychogalvanic response testing.

Havanka-Kanniainen et al. (106) report both mild parasympathetic hypofunction as well as sympathetic hypofunction in adult migraine patients during headache-free intervals.

Takeshima et al. (107) showed evidence of pupillary sympathetic hypofunction and subtle anisocoria in both tension-type headache patients and migraineurs. They suggested that this may reflect a central aminergic system dysfunction or imbalance.

Another report (108) also suggested a pupillary sympathetic system imbalance, as tension-type headache patients showed asymmetric mydriasis after tyramine instillation and in the physiologic pupillary tests.

Carlsson and Rosenhall (109) also noted that tension-type headache experienced oculomotor dysfunction in the amplitude and number of corrective saccades during testing. They suggest that increased tension in neck muscles of tension-type headache patients may induce abnormal eye motor function.

Drummond (110) found more photophobia in tension-type headache patients than in controls, but possibly less than in migraine patients. He hypothesized that the photophobia may be secondary to general sensitivity or hyperexcitability of the special senses, possibly from changes in central modulation.

Platelet and Serotonin Studies. Platelet abnormalities with associated serotonergic dysfunction has been well documented in migraine (111, 112). Decreased platelet serotonin in tension-type headache patients has also been identified (113).

Psychological Data. There does not appear to be any clinically distinguished difference between migraine and tension-type headache patients (114).

Hereditary Data. The hereditary aspects of migraine headache are well documented. There does not seem to be a similar positive correlation to tension-type headache, although some families include both migraine and tension-type headache patients (115).

Conclusion. While these data show clinical and psychophysiological correlations between tension-type headache and migraine, they do not necessarily demonstrate a primary mechanistic or definitive continuum between the two. Other explanations may also provide insight as to how these entities may have either a primary or secondary etiologic relationship to each other.

ENDOGENOUS CENTRAL PAIN-MODULATING SYSTEMS

In general, our understanding of the endogenous opiate systems (EOS) is probably incomplete. In the central nervous system, the EOS may act as a nociceptive rheostat, setting our pain modulation capacity at a certain level. As this level changes, an individual's pain tolerance may also change. Pathological conditions may cause excessive production or deficiency, which may cause clinical sequelae. Fluctuations in the intensity of pain may be interpreted as being caused by fluctuations in the function of antinociceptive pathways (116, 117).

Patients diagnosed with chronic neuropathic pain are characterized by low β-endorphin levels, possibly indicating a low tolerance for pain (118). These patients have lower pain thresholds and lower tolerance to experimental pain (119). Terenius (118) suggested that these patients may be more prone to develop a pain syndrome not caused by excessive nociceptive stimulation but by a deficiency in the EOS control mechanisms.

Failure of the antinociceptive systems presents clinically with spontaneous pain. The rostral section of the analgesic system subserves the head, neck, and shoulders, which may explain the preferential localization of headache and pain to this area. It is possibly more susceptible to inducing pain because of its close neuroanatomical affiliation with the affective areas of the brain. Headache and other "non-organic" central pain problems are felt to be the most common expression of impairment of the antinociceptive system (120).

Endogenous opioids have been implicated as the primary protagonists in idiopathic headache, including migraine (121). They also modulate the neurovegetative triad of spontaneous pain, depression, and autonomic disturbances which is thought to be found in only two conditions, headache and morphine abstinence (120). The impairment of vegetative functions in idiopathic headache suggests that the endorphin system, if imbalanced, may be involved in the pathogenesis of the disorder. Endogenous opioid concentrations in the cerebrospinal fluid (CSF) collected from headache patients during a headache attack was lower than the level found in pain-free periods (122). Similar results were found in a study by Von Knorring et al. (119).

β-Endorphin has been found to bind mainly to the μ-receptors (123), which are closely related to analgesia, hedonia, and autonomic stability (121). An inverse relationship between β-endorphin and pain was noted in tension-type headache patients (124). Published studies differ in assay methods used and nomenclature, and many don't indicate whether the subjects were taking medication, which may alter interpretation of the published data.

Most studies find that headache is accompanied by changes in circulating endorphin and enkephalin levels (125, 126). Reduced plasma concentration of β-endorphin was found in idiopathic headache sufferers including tension-type headache (126–129). Gawal et al. (130) found normal plasma levels of immunoreactive β-endorphin in chronic tension-type headache patients. Bella et al. (122) found increased levels of β-endorphin at the end of a headache attack, possibly associated with the stress provoked by the headache pain.

An increased level of plasma enkephalin has been found during migraine attacks (121). Ferrari et al. (131) found that in tension-type headache, there is low platelet methionine enkephalin and high plasma methionine enkephalin. In migraine, there is a high platelet level of methionine enkephalin and decreased plasma levels. They note that a rise in plasma methionine enkephalin during headache may be directly related to increased serotonin levels. Methionine enkephalin appears to be costored with serotonin and other monoamines, and its concomitant release may make it a natural antagonist to serotonin (131). Amitriptyline is known to increase platelet methionine enkephalin (132), which may explain its effectiveness in tension-type headache. Some authors hypothesize that the CSF content of methionine enkephalin is poorly related to opiate-mediated antinociceptive systems (128).

Interestingly, moderate dose levels of naloxone do not ameliorate chronic tension-type headache pain (133). Naloxone does reverse the analgesia induced by a myofascial trigger point injection (134).

Substance P, an excitatory neuropeptide that may increase nociception in primary afferents (135), is found at all levels of the neuroaxis (136). Almay et al. (136) found lower substance P levels in chronic pain patients with either neurogenic or idiopathic pain than in normal volunteers. Patients with central pain or pain of the head or face had higher levels, although not as high as the controls. In other studies (137), after stepwise multiple-regression analysis, pain was found to be most related to levels of substance P, methionine enkephalin, and β-endorphin.

Clinical and pharmacological information indicates that perturbed serotonergic neurotransmission probably generates headache and head pain (54). In the same paper, Raskin hypothesizes that ordinary periodic headache may be the "noise" of serotonergic neurotransmission.

Serotonergic uptake mechanisms in the platelet are similar to those of neurons (138). Platelet serotonin levels were found to be lower in patients with chronic tension-type headache than in controls (113); low levels of plasma serotonin were also described in similar patients (139). Shimomura and Takahashi (140) also found decreased levels of serotonin in the platelets of tension-type headache patients and felt that it indicated a central serotonergic disturbance

in these patients. Giacovazzo et al. (139) found that during tension-type headache, there was a disappearance of specific serotonergic binding sites on lymphocytes and monocytes, which they felt could be secondary to a high rate of serotonin turnover. They felt their study supported other observations indicating an impairment of serotonergic metabolism in tension-type headache.

Low levels of plasma norepinephrine were found in patients with tension-type headache or migraine who submitted to a cold pressor test, suggesting possible peripheral sympathetic hypofunction (141). Another study suggested a failure of central noradrenergic activity in chronic tension-type headache patients (125). Other data implies that noradrenergic pathways could participate in central opiod dysfunction (129).

Opiod receptor mechanisms are apparently extremely susceptible to desensitization or the development of tolerance (142). For significant tolerance to develop, exposure over days is necessary.

In migraine, receptor supersensitivity is marked, probably induced by chronically diminished secretion of neurotransmitters, which Sicuteri has termed "empty neurons" (143). The empty neuron hypothesis may be extended to the nociceptive system, in a deafferentation pattern. Sicuteri also states that the empty neuron syndrome may be latent, subpathological, or pathological, with spontaneous manifestations; this problem may involve both autonomic and nociceptive afferent systems.

Langemark et al. (23) concluded that tension-type headache may result from a dysmodulation of nociceptive impulses, but sensitized receptors probably also are involved.

The endogenous opiate system modulates monoaminergic neurons. Chronic endogenous opiate system deficiency would be expected to provoke transmitter leakage, leading to neuronal exhaustion and emptying. A compensatory effector cell hyperactivity would then be expected. The most important phenomena of the hypoendorphin syndromes, including headache, would appear to be the poor release of transmitter and cell hypersensitivity (120).

Idiopathic headache could be considered a "pain disease" linked to central dysmodulation of the nociceptive and antinociceptive systems, either latent or pathological in nature.

Research indicates that one of the main endogenous antinociceptive systems, the endogenous opiate system is impaired in chronic tension-type headache. This problem is progressive, but it is uncertain whether the opiod dysfunction results from a genetic deficiency or neuronal exhaustion secondary to continuous activation of the system (124, 128).

Many of the clinical phenomena of tension-type headache may be explained by centrally related phenomena. There may be other, unidentified, triggering factors. Chronic central stimulation from the periphery via myofascial mechanisms (trigger points) in the MPS and in fibromyalgia may be part of the pathogenesis. These may be reinforced or complemented by other central dysfunctions, such as those found in associated sleep disorders.

FIBROMYALGIA

Fibromyalgia is a systemic disorder that is clinically associated with a generalized increase in tenderness in susceptible areas over the entire body. These sites may have a particular vulnerability to central nociceptive pathways, such as the local areas where myofascial trigger points are commonly found (31). This disorder was also known as fibrositis, a term introduced by Gowers in 1904 (144). In 1990, the American College of Rheumatology published diagnostic criteria for fibromyalgia, further establishing it as a clinical entity and not a "waste basket" diagnosis (145).

Typically, patients with fibromyalgia are diagnosed between 30 and 50 years of age. Women are more likely than men to have the disorder, possibly between 5 to 10:1. Fibromyalgia patients may have complaints of generalized pain, with bilateral, symmetric tenderness for at least 3 months. On physical examination, at least 11 of 18 symmetric tender points must be found to confirm the diagnosis (146). Anxiety and depression are common in patients with fibromyalgia. Historically, the most common complaints found in these patients include morning stiffness, fatigue, sleep disturbances with nonrestorative sleep, chronic tension-type headaches, and the irritable bowel syndrome.

Fibromyalgia and the myofascial pain syndrome have many similarities. Bennett (147) concludes that they are two distinct disorders that may have the same underlying pathophysiology. He notes that many patients with fibromyalgia have myofascial trigger points, and many of the tender points associated with fibromyalgia (which do not have associated referred pain on palpation) are latent trigger points that become active or symptomatic as a result of depressed pain modulation. A subset of patients with MPS go on to develop fibromyalgia.

Langemark and Jensen (28) noted the frequency with which trigger points with local and referred pain are found on palpation in headache patients. Table 3 in Olesen's paper (56), comparing headache-free with headache-prone patients in Denmark, showed that women with headache had more frequent complaints of symptoms associated with fibromyalgia, including fatigue, colic, and large bowel and intermittent stomach pain; a history of low back pain was found in men and women.

The energy crisis in localized trigger points found in MPS (described above) is felt to also occur in fibromyalgia, involving the muscles in general (31). The energy crisis involves a depletion of high-energy phosphates. Martucci et al. ((148) note that plasma levels of cyclic AMP (which increase during migraine attacks) may be considered to be an index of catecholamine system function. This has not been specifically elucidated in the muscle-pain syndromes.

EMG findings in fibromyalgia are similar to those found in tension-type headache, i.e., they are generally negative or equivocal about correlating muscle tension with pain (147, 149).

There are no specific psychological findings on psychometric testing of fibromyalgia patients (147).

The nonrestorative sleep disorder found in fibromyalgia, alpha intrusion in stage 4 sleep, may be linked to a deficiency of serotonin (150).

Severely disturbed oculomotor function has been found in patients with fibromyalgia (151). A similar but milder form of oculomotor disturbance occurs in tension-type headache (109).

Sympathetic blockade will alleviate pain and decrease tender points in fibromyalgic patients, implying that sympathetic overactivity and a related microcirculation disturbance are involved (149, 152, 153).

Preliminary studies of serum β-endorphin in fibromyalgia patients showed no abnormalities (154). Moldofsky reported that administration of 1 mg naloxone at bedtime was associated with a dramatic increase in pain the next morning as well as an increase in stage 1 sleep and decreases in sleep stages 2, 3, and 4 (155). This would seem to suggest that endorphins affect sleep and the symptoms of fibromyalgia.

Increased levels of substance P in the CSF have been reported in fibromyalgia (156).

Abnormalities of serotonin binding to platelets, a marker of central nervous system serotonergic efficacy, have been reported in fibromyalgia (156, 157).

Epidural opiods produced analgesia in fibromyalgia patients, leading the authors of this study to conclude that the pain of fibromyalgia is of peripheral nociceptive or spinal origin (158).

Jay (159) analyzed patients seen with a chief complaint of chronic tension-type headache. Three groups of 20 patients were gathered with final diagnoses of tension-type headache, myofascial pain syndrome, or fibromyalgia, on the basis of physical examination and published diagnostic criteria. A continuum of symptom severity in the three groups was seen, as well as progressively increasing affective and physical problems as age, time in pain, and severity increased. A progression of findings, less to more severe, was noted from tension-type headache patients to MPS and finally to the fibromyalgia group. The signs and symptoms of tension-type headache were identified in the MPS and fibromyalgia groups; localized trigger points were found in patients with simple tension-type headache.

ASSOCIATED DISORDERS OF SLEEP

The relationship between sleep and headache and muscle-pain syndromes appears to be important. Gans (160) mentioned the possible association between migraine and sleep disturbance 40 years ago. Collected data imply that central biogenic amines, particularly serotonin and norepinephrine, both of which are important to sleep physiology, are also important to the central pain modulation systems.

The brainstem locus ceruleus is important to the initiation of sleep. Stimulation of this center produces vascular changes similar to those seen in migraine (161). The relationship between serotonin and migraine is also well established. Serotonergic systems are known to influence the endogenous opiate system as well as the activity of the trigeminal system (162). Human and animal research has shown that central serotonin metabolism plays a role in pain modulation, affective states, and the regulation of non-REM sleep (156).

A high incidence of sleep disturbance has been suggested in chronic headache patients (163). Different sleep disorders may be associated with different headache problems. Migraine has been noted to occur in association with REM sleep; excessive stage 3, 4, and REM sleep is also seen (71). Tension-type headache has been found to be associated with frequent awakenings and decreased slow wave sleep, similar to the sleep changes in fibromyalgia (72).

Moldofsky et al. (164) reported the first laboratory-based abnormality of fibromyalgia, a disturbance in stage 4 sleep. A similar alpha non-REM pattern of alpha intrusion in delta sleep was produced in normals via stage 4 sleep deprivation. Their subjects developed temporary musculoskeletal pain and mood changes comparable to those of fibromyalgia patients. Small doses of serotonergic tricyclic antidepressant medications, which reduce alpha intrusions into stage 4 sleep, were found to ameliorate the symptoms.

Alpha wave intrusion into deep sleep has also been found in patients with rheumatoid arthritis and other chronic pain syndromes (157). Nonrestorative sleep, a hallmark of fibromyalgia, has also been reported in patients with depression and posttraumatic pain syndromes (166, 167). The alpha non-REM sleep disturbance has also been found in asymptomatic people and in people who experience severe emotional stress, such as combat during war (156). In the latter group, the veterans with the sleep abnormality also complained of headaches, diffuse pain, and emotional distress.

Sleep disturbance is associated with increased pain severity. Chronic headache patients appear to have a higher incidence of sleep abnormalities than normal, pain-free subjects. The mechanistic aspects of chronic headache may be linked to sleep abnormalities as an initiating factor or as a result of the underlying pathological neurochemical factors inducing the sleep disturbance.

The interrelationship between sleep, headache, and pain and central neuropeptides and biogenic amines seems to be extremely important in both pathogenesis and treatment. The research on sleep and central biogenic amine metabolism and their relationship to the modulation of headache and myofascial pain appears to be consistent with a central neurochemical dysfunction associated with one or more antinociceptive systems.

CONCLUSIONS

Perhaps continuous peripheral stimulation can effectively trigger a change in the central pain "rheostat" that modu-

lates nociceptive input. The longer the peripheral stimulation persists, the greater the possibility that the central modulating mechanisms will assume a primary (rather than secondary or reactive) role in pain perception, causing the actuating mechanism for pain perception to shift from the periphery to the central nervous system. Such a shift may make typically innocuous stimuli more aggravating to the pain-modulating systems. Internal feedback mechanisms, already "dysmodulated," may overreact, until or unless central neurochemical mechanisms take ascendance, with such aspects as neurotransmitter exhaustion, abnormal biogenic amine metabolism, and receptor hypersensitivity assuming primary roles in the perpetuation of nociception.

From neurophysiological data, it is not unlikely that peripheral pathology (such as myofascial trigger points, which for reasons previously stated may produce continuous nociceptive stimulation) (138) may initiate or contribute to this abnormal or pathological resetting of the central controls of antinociception.

The relationship between tension-type headache and the myofascial pain syndrome and fibromyalgia is complex. There are definite clinical similarities in the clinical description of headache and physical findings. Most neurochemical data indicate similar pathological changes in the biogenic amine systems, particularly the serotonergic system, in all three entities. The intrinsic nature, as far as we understand it, of the relationship between serotonin and pain, affective states and sleep is acknowledged, although the entire story is probably not yet known. The similarities between the sleep disorder found in fibromyalgia and sleep abnormalities in tension-type headache may reflect the same pathophysiological substrate. It is so far problematic whether these nociceptive and antinociceptive changes have a genetic predisposition or are a reaction to continuous peripheral stimulation, with affective input acting as an initiating or reinforcing factor, or both.

Many of the studies reviewed suggest that central neurochemical dysmodulation is found in tension-type headache. Conversely, tension-type headache may be a primary expression of the impairment of antinociceptive systems.

Myofascial nociception is possible and may in fact be found in tension-type headache patients. Abnormal central modulation of this nociceptive information is possibly more important, making tension-type headache a central rather than peripheral disorder. This would explain some of the divergent clinical information, such as the lack of positive EMG correlations between muscle tension and pain. This may also, at least in part, explain why pericranial muscle tenderness is not typically associated with significant degrees of active muscle spasm.

Figure 16.1 demonstrates a possible mechanistic explanation of the pathophysiology of tension-type headache. Myofascial nociceptive input to the central nervous system via ascending spinal, brainstem, thalamic, and cortical

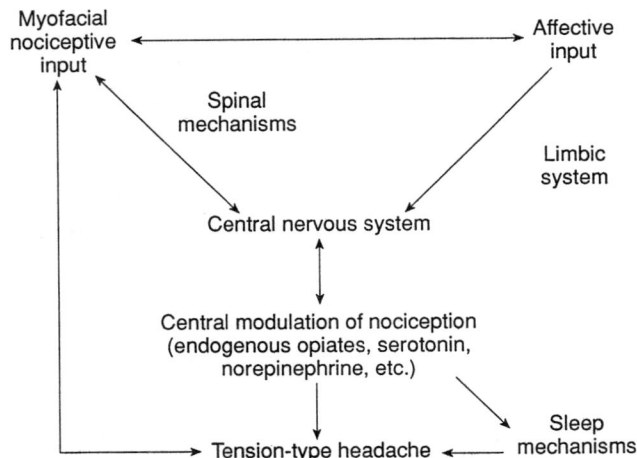

Figure 16.1. Possible pathophysiology of tension-type headache. Refer to discussion in body of paper.

pathways is also reinforced by affective stimulation mediated through the limbic system. As noted above, there are close anatomical and neurochemical correlations between the primary cortical pain pathways and the limbic system. Stimulated "hard-wired" pain pathways would induce initial changes in the chemical pain-modulating systems. With continued peripheral nociceptive stimulation, these systems may become exhausted, with secondary hyperstimulation of receptors. Intrinsic modulatory feedback systems might then become reset or "dysmodulated," creating a new primary source of pain in the initially painful area, thus perpetuating tension-type headache (possibly reinforced by continued peripheral stimulation). Tension-type headache may also occur initially or solely through local muscle spasm and/or myofascial trigger points and referred pain mechanisms, causing more infrequent or episodic headaches. Bioaminergic changes appear to affect sleep physiology, which may then perpetuate or reinforce tension-type headache and other muscle-pain syndromes.

Chronic tension-type headaches may then be a disorder of perception rather than of muscle, while infrequent or episodic tension-type headache is probably secondary to myofascial mechanisms.

The proposed tension-type headache–migraine continuum may be secondary to different aspects of the effects of central nociceptive dysmodulation, making the central nervous system primarily responsible for transformational headache.

As reviewed above, there are many reasons to consider tension-type headache, at least initially, a myofascially related entity, similar in many ways, clinically and pathophysiologically, to the myofascial pain syndrome and possibly also fibromyalgia. When two disorders, such as tension-type headache and the muscle-pain syndromes, are so frequent in the general population, it would make good clinical sense to evaluate a patient with tension-type headache for the other entities.

As we learn more about the myogenic aspects of pain and the central pain-modulating systems, this pathophysiological formulation will probably take more explicit or different form. For the sake of the many patients with tension-type headache, this is something to strive for, as knowledge of pathogenesis contributes mightily to treatment.

REFERENCES

1. Headache Classification Committee of the International Headache Society. Classification and diagnostic criteria for headache disorders, cranial neuralgias and facial pain. Cephalalgia 1988;8(suppl 7).
2. Riley TL. Muscle-contraction headache. Neurol Clin 1983;1:489–500.
3. Philips C. Tension headache: theoretical problems. Behav Res Ther 1978;16:249–261.
4. Philips C, Hunter MS. A psychophysiological investigation of tension headache. Headache 1982;22:173–179.
5. Speed WG. Muscle contraction headaches. In: Saper JR, ed. Headache disorders. Boston: John Wright, 1983:115–124.
6. Diamond S, Dalessio DJ. The Practicing Physician's Approach to Headache. 3rd ed. Baltimore: Williams & Wilkins, 1980:99–108.
7. Dorpat TL, Holmes TH. Mechanisms of skeletal muscle pain and fatigue. Arch Neurol Psychiatry 1955;74:628–640.
8. Perl S, Markle P, Katz LN. Factors involved in the production of skeletal muscle pain. Arch Intern Med 1934;53:814–824.
9. Hong S, Kniffki K, Schmidt R. Pain abstracts. Vol 1. Montreal: Second World Congress on Pain, 1978:58.
10. Rodbard S. Pain associated with muscle contraction. Headache 1970;10:105–115.
11. Martin PR, Mathews AM. Tension headaches: psychophysiological investigation and treatment. J Psychosom Res 1978;22:389–399.
12. Sakuta M. Significance of flexed posture and neck instability as a cause of chronic muscle contraction headache. Rinsho Shinkeigato 1990;30(3):254–261.
13. Simons DJ, Day E, Goodell H, Wolff HG. Experimental studies on headache: muscles of the scalp and neck as sources of pain. Assoc Res Nerv Ment Dis Proc 1943;23:228–244.
14. Robinson CA. Cervical spondylosis and muscle contraction headaches. In: Dalessio DJ, ed. Wolff's headache and other head pain. 4th ed. New York: Oxford University Press, 1980:362–380.
15. Haynes SN, Cuevas J, Gannon LR. The psychophysiological etiology of muscle-contraction headache. Headache 1982;22:122–132.
16. Pikoff H. Is the muscular model of headache still viable? A review of conflicting data. Headache 1984;24:186–198.
17. Bakal DA, Kaganov JA. Muscle contraction and migraine headache: psychophysiologic comparison. Headache 1977;17:208–215.
18. Cohen MJ. Psychological studies of headache: is there a similarity between migraine and muscle contraction headaches? Headache 1978;18:189–196.
19. Anderson CD, Franks RD. Migraine and tension headache: is there a physiological difference? Headache 1981;21:63–71.
20. Pozniak-Patewicz E. "Cephalgic" spasm of head and neck muscles. Headache 1976;15:261–266.
21. Borgeat F, Hade B, Elie R, Larouche LM. Effects of voluntary muscle tension increases in tension headache. Headache 1984;24:199–202.
22. Langemark M, Olesen J. Pericranial tenderness in tension headache. A blind, controlled study. Cephalalgia 1987;7(4):249–255.
23. Langemark M, Jensen K, Jensen TS, Olesen J. Pressure pain thresholds and thermal nociceptive thresholds in chronic tension-type headache. Pain 1989;38(2):203–210.
24. Drummond PD. Scalp tenderness and sensitivity to pain in migraine and tension headache. Headache 1987;27:45–50.
25. Yang JC, Richlin D, Brand L, Wagner J, Clark WC. Thermal

sensory decision theory indices and pain threshold in chronic pain patients and healthy volunteers. Psychosom Med 1985;47:461–468.

26. Malow RM, Grimm L, Olsen RE. Differences in pain perception between myofascial pain dysfunction and normal subjects: a signal detection analysis. J Psychosom Res 1980;24:303–309.

27. Quimby LG, Block SR, Gratwick G. Fibromyalgia: generalized pain intolerance and manifold symptom reporting. J Rheumatol 1988;15:1264–1270.

28. Langemark M, Jensen K. Myofascial mechanisms of pain. In: Olesen J, Edvinsson L, eds. Basic mechanisms of headache. Amsterdam: Elsevier Science Publishers B.V. 1988:321–341.

29. Langemark M, Olesen J, Poulsen DP, Bech P. Clinical characterization of patients with chronic tension headache. Headache 1988;28:590–596.

30. Murphy AI, Lehrer PM. Headache versus nonheadache state: a study of electrophysiological and affective changes during muscle contraction headache. Behav Med 1990;16(1):23–30.

31. Simons D. Muscular pain syndromes. In: Fricton JR, Awad E, eds. Advances in pain research and therapy. Vol 17. New York: Raven Press, 1990:1–41.

32. Travell J, Rinzler SH. The myofascial genesis of pain. Postgrad Med 1952;11:425–434.

33. Travell JG, Simons DG. Myofascial pain and dysfunction: the trigger point manual. Baltimore: Williams & Wilkins, 1983.

34. Simons DG. Myofascial pain syndromes: where are we? where are we going? Arch Phys Med Rehabil 1988;69:207–212.

35. Fishbain DA, Goldberg M, Meagher BR, Steele R, Rosomoff H. Male and female chronic pain patients categorized by DSM-III diagnostic criteria. Pain 1986;26:181–197.

36. Fricton JR, Kroening R, Haley D, Siegart R. Myofascial pain syndrome of the head and neck: a review of clinical characteristics of 164 patients. Oral Surg 1985;60:615–623.

37. Fricton JR. Myofascial pain syndrome. In: Fricton JR, Awad E, eds. Advances in pain research and therapy. Vol 17. New York: Raven Press, 1990:107–127.

38. Simons DG. Myofascial pain syndromes of head, neck and low back. In: Dubner R, Gebhart GF, Bond MR, eds. Proceedings of the Vth World Congress on Pain. Amsterdam: Elsevier Science Publisher BV, 1988:186–200.

39. Bengtsson A, Henriksson KG, Larsson J. Muscle biopsy in primary fibromyalgia. Scand J Rheumatol 1986;15:1–6.

40. Bengtsson A, Henriksson KG, Larsson J. Reduced high-energy phosphate levels in painful muscle in patients with primary fibromyalgia. Arthritis Rheum 1986;29:817–821.

41. Lund N, Bengtsson A, Thorborg P. Muscle tissue oxygen pressure in primary fibromyalgia. Scand J Rheumatol 1986;15:165–173.

42. Graff-Radford SB, Reeves JL, Jaeger B. Management of chronic head and neck pain: the effectiveness of altering factors perpetuating myofascial pain. Headache 1987;27:186–190.

43. Weeks VD, Travell J. Postural vertigo due to trigger areas in the sternocleidomastoid muscle. J Pediatr 1955;47:315–327.

44. Sternbach RA. Survey of pain in the United States: the Nuprin pain report. Clin J Pain 1986;2:49–53.

45. Nikiforow RC. Headache in a random sample of 200 persons. A clinical study of a population in northern Finland. Cephalalgia 1981;1:99–107.

46. Lance JW, Curran DA, Anthony M. Investigations into the mechanism and treatment of chronic headache. Med J Aust 1965;2:909–914.

47. Nikiforow R, Hokkanen E. An epidemiological study of headache in an urban and a rural population in northern Finland. Headache 1978;18:137–145.

48. Pellegrino MJ, Waylonis GW, Sommer A. Familial occurance of primary fibromyalgia. Arch Phys Med Rehabil 1989;70:61–63.

49. Langemark M, Jensen K. Myofascial mechanisms of pain. In: Olesen J, Edvinsson L, eds. Basic mechanisms of headache. Amsterdam: Elsevier Science Publisher BV, 1988:321–341.

50. Sessle BJ. Central nervous system mechanisms of muscular pain. In: Fricton JR, Awad E, eds. Advances in pain research and therapy. Vol 17. New York: Raven Press, 1990;87–105.

51. Moskowitz MA. The neurobiology of vascular head pain. Ann Neurol 1984;16:157–168.

52. Basbaum AI, Fields HL. Endogenous pain control systems: brainstem spinal pathways and endorphin circuitry. Annu Rev Neurosci 1984;7:309–338.

53. Andersen E, Dafny N. An ascending serotonergic pain modulation pathway from the dorsal raphe nucleus to the parafascicularis nucleus of the thalamus. Brain Res 1983;269:57–67.

54. Raskin NH. On the origin of head pain. Headache 1988;28:254–257.

55. Raskin NH. Headache. 2nd ed. New York: Churchill Livingstone 1988.

56. Olesen J. Clinical characterization of tension headache. In: Olesen J, Edvinsson L, eds. Basic mechanisms of headache. Amsterdam: Elsevier Science Publishers B.V., 1988:9–14.

57. Olesen J, Langemark M. Mechanisms of tension headache. In: Olesen J, Edvinsson L, eds. Basic mechanisms of headache. Amsterdam: Elsevier Science Publishers B.V., 1988:457–461.

58. Friedman AP, von Storch TJC, Merritt HH. Migraine and tension headaches. A clinical study of 2000 cases. Neurology 1954;22:773–788.

59. Martin MJ. Psychogenic factors in headache. Med Clin North Am 1978;62:559–570.

60. Martin MJ, Rome HP, Swenson WM. Muscle contraction headache: a psychiatric review. Res Clin Stud Headache 1967;1:184–204.

61. Gannon LR, Haynes SN, Cuevas J, Chavez R. Psychophysiological correlates of induced headaches. J Behav Med 1987;10:411–423.

62. Ziegler DK, Hassanein R, Hassanein K. Headache syndromes suggested by factor analysis of symptom variables in a headache prone population. J Chron Dis 1972;25:353–363.

63. Blumer D, Heilbrohn M. Chronic muscle contraction headache and pain-prone disorder. Headache 1982;22:180–183.

64. Philips C, Hunter M. Headache in a psychiatric population. J Nerv Ment Dis 1982;170:34–40.

65. Kudrow L. Muscle contraction headaches. In: Amsterdam: Rose FC, ed. Handbook of clinical neurology. Vol 48. Amsterdam: Elsevier Science Publishing, 1986:343–352.

66. Martin MJ, Rome HP. Muscle-contraction headache: therapeutic aspects. Res Clin Stud Headache 1967;1:205–217.

67. Jay GW, Grove RN, Grove KS. Differentiation of chronic headache from non-headache pain patients using the Millon clinical multiaxial inventory (MCMI). Headache 1987;27:124–129.

68. Krabbe AA, Olesen J. Headache provocation by continuous intravenous infusion of histamine. Clinical results and receptor mechanisms. Pain 1980;8:253–259.

69. Drummond PD, Lance JW. Extracranial vascular reactivity in migraine and tension headache. Cephalalgia 1981;1:149–155.

70. Cohen MJ. Psychophysiological studies of headache: is there similarity between migraine and muscle contraction headaches? Headache 1978;18:189–196.

71. Sahota PK, Dexter JD. Sleep and headache syndromes: a clinical review. Headache 1990;30:80–84.

72. Drake ME, Pakalnis A, Andrews JM, Bogner JE. Nocturnal sleep recording with cassette EEG in chronic headaches. Headache 1990;30:600–603.

73. Budzynski TH, Stoyva JM, Adler CS. Feedback induced muscle relaxation: application to tension headache. Behav Ther Exp Psychiatry 1970;1:205–211.

74. Blanchard EB, Young LD. Clinical applications of biofeedback training. Arch Gen Psychiatry 1974;30:573–589.

75. Harper RG, Steger JC. Psychological correlates of frontalis EMG and pain in tension headache. Headache 1978;18:215–218.

76. Budzynski TH, Stoyva JM, Adler CS, Mullaney PJ. EMG biofeedback and tension headache: a controlled outcome study. Psychosom Med 1973;35:484–496.

77. Haynes SM, Griffin P, Mooney O, Parise M. Electromyographic feedback and relaxation instruction in the treatment of muscle contraction headaches. Behav Ther 1975;6:672–678.

78. van Boxten A, van der Ven R. Differential EMG activity in subjects with muscle contraction headaches related to mental effort. Headache 1978;17:233–237.

79. Yates AJ. Biofeedback and the modification of behavior. New York: Plenum Press, 1980:90–92.

80. Anderson CD, Franks RD. Migraine and tension headache: is there a physiological difference? Headache 1981;21:63–71.

81. Iansek R, Heywood J, Karnaghan J, Balla JI. Cervical spondylosis and headaches. Clin Exp Neurol 1987;23e:175–178.

82. Forsell H. Mandibular dysfunction and headache. Proc Finn Dent Soc 1985;81(suppl II):591.

83. Mikail M, Rosen H. History and etiology of myofascial pain-dysfunction syndrome. J Prosthet Dent 1980;44:438–444.

84. Magnusson T, Carlsson GE. Comparison between two groups of patients in respect to headache and mandibular dysfunction. Swed Dent J 1978;2:85–92.

85. Magnusson T, Carlsson GE. Recurrent headaches in relation to temporomandibular joint pain-dysfunction. Acta Odontol Scand 1978;36:333–338.

86. Takeshima T, Takahashi K. The relationship between muscle contraction headache and migraine: a multivariate analysis study. Headache 1988;28:272–277.

87. Takeshima T, Shimomura T, Takahashi K. Platelet activation in muscle contraction headache and migraine. Cephalalgia 1987;7:239–243.

88. Featherstone HJ. Migraine and muscle contraction headaches: a continuum. Headache 1985;25:194–198.

89. Saper JR. Headache disorders. Boston: John Wright, 1983:125–130.

90. Mathew NT, Stubits E, Nigam MP. Transformation of episodic migraine into daily headache. Headache 1982;22:66–68.

91. Saper JR, Winters M. Chronic "mixed" headaches: profile and analysis of 100 consecutive patients experiencing daily headache. Headache 1982;22:145–146.

92. Sicuteri F. The nature of pain and central analgesia. In: Beers RF, Bassett EG, eds. Mechanisms of pain and analgesic compounds. New York: Raven Press, 1979:295–307.

93. Friedman AP, Rowan AJ, Wood EH. Recent observation on migraine with particular reference to thermography and electroencephalography. In: Bonica JJ, ed. Advances in neurology. Vol 4. International Symposium on Pain. New York: Raven Press, 1976:403–409.

94. Basser LS. The relation of migraine and epilepsy. Brain 1969;92:285–300.

95. Lance JW, Anthony M. Some clinical aspects of migraine. Arch Neurol 1966;15:356–361.

96. Jay GW. Epilepsy, migraine and EEG abnormalities in children: a review and hypothesis. Headache 1982;22:110–114.

97. Pearce J. Migraine: a psychosomatic disorder. Headache 1977;17:125–128.

98. Tfelt-Hansen P, Lous I, Olesen J. Prevalence and significance of muscle tenderness during common migraine attacks. Headache 1981;21:49–54.

99. Olesen J. Some clinical features of the acute migraine attack. An analysis of 750 patients. Headache 1978;18:268–271.

100. Ellertsen B, Norby H, Sjaastad O. Psychophysiological response patterns in tension headache: effects of tricyclic antidepressants. Cephalalgia 1987;7:55–63.

101. Haynes SN. Muscle contraction headache—a psychophysiological perspective. In: Haynes SN, Gannon LR, eds. Psychosomatic disorders: a psychophysiological approach to etiology and treatment. New York: Praeger Press, 1981.

102. Tunis MM, Wolff HG. Studies on headache: cranial artery vasoconstriction and muscle contraction headache. Arch Neurol Psychiatry 1954;71:425–434.

103. Selby G, Lance JW. Observations on 500 cases of migraine and allied vascular headache. J Neurol Neurosurg Psychiatry 1960;23:23–32.

104. Mikamo K, Takeshima T, Takahashi K. Cardiovascular sympathetic hypofunction in muscle contraction headache and migraine. Headache 1989;29:86–89.

105. Covelli V, Ferrannini E. Neurophysiological findings in headache patients. Psychogalvanic reflex investigation in migraineurs and tension headache patients. Acta Neurol 1987;9:354–358.

106. Havanka-Kanniainen H, Tolonen U, Myllyla VV. Autonomic dysfunction in adult migraineurs. Headache 1986;26:425–430.

107. Takeshima T, Takao Y, Takahashi K. Pupillary sympathetic hypofunction and asymmetry in muscle contraction headache and migraine. Cephalalgia 1987;7:257–262.

108. Shimomura T, Takahashi K. Pupillary functional asymmetry in patients with muscle contraction headache. Cephalalgia 1986;6:141–145.

109. Carlsson J, Rosenhall U. Oculomotor disturbances in patients with tension headaches. Acta Otolaryngol 1988;106:354–360.

110. Drummond PD. A quantitative assessment of photophobia in migraine and tension headache. Headache 1986;26:465–469.

111. Hanington E, Jones RJ, Amess JAL, Wachowicz B. Migraine: a platelet disorder. Lancet 1981;ii:720–723.

112. D'Andrea G, Toldo M, Cortelazzo S, Milone FF. Platelet activity in migraine. Headache 1982;22:207–212.

113. Rolf LH, Wiele G, Brune GG. 5-Hydroxytryptamine in platelets of patients with muscle contraction headache. Headache 1981;21:10–11.

114. Raskin NH. Headache. 2nd ed. New York: Churchill Livingstone, 1988:215–227.

115. Shimomura T, Nishikawa S, Takahashi K. Hereditary dysrhythmic headache. Headache 1986;26:33–36.

116. Fields HL. Sources of variability in the sensation of pain. Pain 1988;33:195–200.

117. Wall PD. Stability and instability of central pain mechanisms. In: Dubner R, Bond MR, eds. Proceedings of the Vth World Congress on Pain. Amsterdam: Elsevier Science Publishers BV, 1988:13–24.

118. Terenius L. Endorphins and modulation of pain. In: Critchley M, Friedman AP, Gorini S, Sicuteri F, et al. eds. Advances in neurology. Vol 33. New York: Raven Press, 1982:59–64.

119. von Knorring L, Almay BGL, Johansson F, Terenius L. Pain perception and endorphin levels in cerebrospinal fluid. Pain 1978;5:359–365.

120. Sicuteri F. Natural opiods in migraine. In: Critchley M, Friedman AP, Gorini S, Sicuteri F, et al. eds. Advances in neurology. Vol 33. New York: Raven Press, 1982:65–74.

121. Sicuteri F, Spillantini MG, Fanciullacci M. 'Enkephalinase' in migraine and opiate addiction. In: Rose C, ed. Migraine. Proceedings of the 5th International Migraine Symposium, London, 1984. Basel: Karger, 1985:86–94.

122. Bella DD, Carenzi A, Casacci F, et al. Endorphins in the pathogenesis of headache. In: Critchley M, Friedman AP, Gorini S, Sicuteri F, et al. eds. Advances in neurology. Vol 33. New York: Raven Press, 1982:75–79.

123. Martin WR. Pharmacology of opiods. Pharmacol Rev 1984;4:283–323.

124. Martignoni E, Facchinetti F, Rossi F, et al. Neuroendocrine evidence of deranged noradrenergic activity in chronic migraine. Psychoneuroendocrinology 1989;14:357–363.

125. Ansalmi B, Baldi E, Casacci F, Salmon S. Endogenous opiods in cerebrospinal fluid and blood in idiopathic headache sufferers. Headache 1980;20:294–299.

126. Mosnaim AD, Diamond S, Wolf ME, et al. Endogenous opiod-like peptides in headache. An overview. Headache 1989;29:368–372.

127. Genazzani AR, Nappi G, Facchinetti F, et al. Progressive impairment of CSF B-EP levels in migraine sufferers. Pain 1984;18:127–133.

128. Facchinetti F, Genazzani AR. Opiods in cerebrospinal fluid and blood of headache sufferers. In: Olesen J, Edvinsson L, eds. Basic mechanisms of headache. Amsterdam: Elsevier Science Publishers, BV, 1988:261–269.

129. Nappi G, Gacchinetti F, Legnante G, et al. Impairment of the central and peripheral opiod system in headache. 4th Int Symp of Migraine Trust, Lond. England, 1982.

130. Gawel M, Fettes I, Kuzniak S, Edmeada J. Endorphin levels in headache syndromes. In: Rose C, ed. Migraine. Proceedings of the 5th International Migraine Symposium, London, 1984. Karger, Basel, 1985:66–71.

131. Ferrrari MD, Odink J, Frolich M, et al. Methionine-enkephalin in migraine and tension headache. Differences between classic migraine, common migraine and tension headache, and changes during attacks. Headache 1990;30:160–164.

132. Boiardi A, Picotti GB, Di Giulio AM, et al. Platelet met-enkephalin immunoreactivity and 5-hydroxytryptamine concentrations in migraine patients: effects of 5-hydroxytryptophan, amitriptyline and chlorimipramine treatment. Cephalalgia 1984;4:81–84.

133. Langemark M. Naloxone in moderate doses does not aggravate chronic tension headache. Pain 1989;39:85–93.

134. Fine PG, Milano R, Hare BD. The effects of myofascial trigger point injections are naloxone reversible. Pain 1988;32:15–20.

135. Pernow B. Substance P. Pharmacol Rev 1983;35:85–141.

136. Almay BGL, Johansson F, von Knorring L, et al. Substance P in CSF of patients with chronic pain syndromes. Pain 1988;33:3–9.

137. von Knorring L. Affect and pain: neurochemical mediators and therapeutic approaches. In: Dubner R, Gebhart GF, Bond MR, eds. Proceedings of the Vth World Congress on Pain. Amsterdam: Elsevier Science Publishers BV, 1988:276–285.

138. Pletsher A, Affolter H, Cesuro AM, Ezne P, Muller K. Blood platelets as a model for neurons: similarities of the 5-hydroxytryptamione system. In: Schlessberger HG, Kocheau W, Linzen B, Steinbast H, eds. Berlin: Walter de Gzuyter, 1984:231–239.

139. Giacovazzo M, Bernoni RM, Di Sabato F, Martelletti P. Impairment of 5HT binding to lymphocytes and monocytes from tension-type headache patients. Headache 1990;30:220–223.

140. Shimomura T, Takahashi K. Alteration of platelet serotonin in patients with chronic tension-type headache during cold pressor test. Headache 1990;30:581–583.

141. Takeshima T, Takao Y, Urakami K, et al. Muscle contraction headache and migraine. Platelet activation and plasma norepinephrine during the cold pressor test. Cephalalgia 1989;9:7–13.

142. Sharma SK, Nirenberg M, Klee WA: Morphine receptors as regulators of adenylate cyclase activity. Proc Natl Acad Sci USA 1975;72:590–594.

143. Sicuteri F, Nicolodi M, Fusco BM. Abnormal sensitivity to neurotransmitter agonists, antagonists and neurotransmitter releasers. In: Olesen J, Edvinsson L, eds. Basic mechanisms of headache. Amsterdam: Elsevier Science Publishers BV, 1988:275–286.

144. Gowers WR. Lumbago: its lesson and analogues. Br Med J 1904;1:117–121.

145. Wolfe F, Smythe HA, Yunus MB, et al. The American College of Rheumatology 1990 criteria for the classification of fibromyalgia: a report of the Multicenter Committee. Arthritis Rheum 1990;33:160–172.

146. Campbell SM, Clark S, Tindall EA, Forehand ME, Bennett RM. Clinical characteristics of fibrositis. 1. A "blinded" controlled study of symptoms and tender points. Arthritis Rheum 1983;26:817–824.

147. Bennett RM. Myofascial pain syndromes and the fibromyalgia syndrome: a comparative analysis. In: Fricton JR, Awad E, eds. Advances in pain research and therapy. Vol 17. New York, Raven Press, 1990:43–65.

148. Martucci N, Manna V, Porto C, Agncli A. Migraine and the noradrenergic control of vasomotricity: a study with alpha-2 stimulant and alpha-2 blocker drugs. Headache 1985;25:95–100.

149. Zidar J, Backman E, Bengtsson A, Henriksson KG. Quantitative EMG and muscle tension and painful muscles in fibromyalgia. Pain 1990;40:249–254.

150. Semble EL, Wise CM. The fibrositis syndrome, part 1. Pain Management 1988;Sept/Oct:202–214.

151. Rosenhall U, Johansson G, Orndahl G. Eye motility dysfunction in patients with chronic muscular pain and dysesthesia. Scand J Rehab Med 1987;19:139–145.

152. Henriksson KG, Bengtsson A. Muscle pain with special reference to primary fibromyalgia (PF). In: Dubner R, Gebhart GF, Bond MR, eds. Proceedings of the Vth World Congress on Pain. Amsterdam: Elsevier Science Publishers BV, 1988:232–237.

153. Vaeroy H, Zhi-Gai Q, Morkrid L, et al. Altered sympathetic nervous system response in patients with fibromyalgia (fibrositis syndrome). J Rheumatol 1989;16:1460–1465.

154. Yunis MB, Denko CW, Masi AT. Serum B-endorphin in primary fibromyalgia syndrome: a controlled study. J Rheumatol 1986;13:183–186.

155. Moldofsky H. The contribution of sleep-wake physiology to fibromyalgia. In: Fricton JR, Awad E, eds. Advances in pain research and therapy. Vol 17. New York: Raven Press, 1990:227–240.

156. Goldenberg DL. Fibromyalgia and chronic fatigue syndrome: are they the same? J Musculoskel Med 1990;7:19–28.

157. Goldenberg DL. Diagnostic and therapeutic challenges of fibromyalgia. Hosp Pract 1989;9:39–52.

158. Bengtsson M, Bengtsson A, Jorfeldt L. Diagnostic epidural opiod blockade in primary fibromyalgia at rest and during exercise. Pain 1989;39:171–180.

159. Jay GW. Myofascial mechanisms in the etiology of chronic daily headache: two syndromes, one entity? Presented at the 32d Annual meeting of the American Association for the Study of Headache, Los Angeles, June, 1990.

160. Gans M. Migraine as a form of neurasthenia. J Nerv Ment Dis 1951;113:315–331.

161. Lance JW, Lambert GA, Goadsby PJ, Duckworth B. Brainstem influences on the cephalic circulation: experimental data from cat and monkey of relevance to the mechanisms of migraine. Headache 1983;23:258–265.

162. Yaksh TL. Direct evidence that spinal serotonin and noradrenalin terminals mediate the spinal antinociceptive effects of morphine in the periaquaductal gray. Brain Res 1979;160:180–185.

163. Mathew NT, Glaze D, Frost J. Sleep apnea and other sleep abnormalities in primary headache disorders. In: Rose C, ed. Migraine. Proceedings of the 5th International Migraine Symposium, London, 1984. Basel: Karger, 1985:40–49.

164. Moldofsky H, Scariabrick P, England R, et al. Musculoskeletal symptoms and non-REM sleep disturbances in patients with fibrositis syndrome and healthy subjects. Psychosom Med 1975;37:341–351.

165. Moldofsky H, Scariabrick P. Inducton of neurasthenic musculoskeletal pain syndrome by selective sleep stage deprivation. Psychosom Med 1976;38:35–44.

166. Wittig R, Zorick FJ, Blumer D, et al. Disturbed sleep in patients complaining of chronic pain. J Nerv Ment Dis 1982;170:429–431.

167. Saskin P, Moldofsky H, Lue FA. Sleep and posttraumatic rheumatic pain modulation disorder (fibrositis syndrome). Psychosom Med 1986;48:319–323.

17

Medical Management of Acute Tension-Type Headache Episodes

R. MICHAEL GALLAGHER

The treatment of acute muscle contraction headache can present a formidable challenge to the physician. Usually referred to as "tension headache," this is probably the most common type of headache, accounting for 70 to 80% of all nonorganic types. Up to 90% of the American population experiences tension headache at some time, usually during periods of increased emotional stress.

Tension headache is characterized by intermittent or persisting pain in various areas of the scalp. It is often described as a tightness or "hatband-like" sensation around the head. The pain, which can vary from mild to severe and is usually not incapacitating, may be preceded by a stiffness of the shoulders and neck. The pain is produced by the sustained contraction of muscles in the scalp, neck, or both, which may not always be apparent to the patient.

The precise mechanism for the pain has not been clearly delineated, but it has been suggested that the metabolic products of sustained contraction produce chemical stimulation of pain nerve endings. It is clear, though, that some patients experience discomfort that is out of proportion to the degree of muscle contraction that is evident. This may indicate the role of other complexities, including changes in pain receptors and subtle organic pathology (1–3).

Some headaches may be secondary to certain underlying disorders, including eye disturbances, arthritis, and inflammation. Most, however, are associated with stress, anxiety, depression, and unresolved dependency needs. Often complicating the problem is a self-sustaining circle of events: muscle contraction leads to pain, which leads to anxiety, which reinforces muscle contraction, and so on (4). Ideally, the patient with frequent or severe muscle contraction headaches should be assisted in recognizing the precipitating events with the goal of reducing the severity and duration of attacks. This is a most difficult task, however, and is completely successful in only a few patients, making adequate treatment of the pain that much more important.

It is not unusual for patients to seek treatment while suffering the severe pain of an acute attack. Unfortunately, this is the most inopportune time for evaluation and diagnosis. A more productive evaluation is possible when the patient is headache-free and not incapacitated. Only then is it possible to take a complete history, do a thorough physical examination, and develop a realistic, achievable treatment plan.

The medical treatment of headache has two primary elements:

1. Prophylactic treatment. Assuming the patient has experienced headaches with some frequency, an attempt should be made to reduce that frequency. When headaches are frequent or abortive therapy has been ineffective, prophylactic treatment is indicated.
2. Abortive or reversal treatment. When headaches are relatively infrequent or when pain breaks through an otherwise successful prophylactic regimen, abortive treatment should be instituted.

Whether treatment is prophylactic or abortive, it should follow a definite plan in which the patient and physician form a team whose goal is to reduce the frequency and severity of the headaches. Once such a plan is developed, follow-up and continuing care are the keys to a successful outcome.

Treatment of muscle contraction headache pain is complicated by the array of therapeutic choices available and idiosyncratic differences in individual patients' responses to them. Among the drugs available are various types of nonnarcotic over-the-counter or prescription analgesic preparations, nonsteroidal antiinflammatory drugs (NSAIDs), muscle relaxants, anxiolytics, and other stronger or potentially addicting drugs. Many of these drugs may be used either alone or in combination with other drugs. In addition, nonpharmacological therapies such as manipulation and relaxation may be appropriate for certain patients. The wide diversity of choices in part reflects the fact that no single medication or treatment regimen has yet proven satisfactory for all patients.

It is recommended, therefore, that physicians be familiar with medications from the various categories that have shown efficacy in treating patients with the acute variety of muscle contraction headache. The remainder of this chap-

143

ter is devoted to a discussion of these pharmacological treatment options. The medical management of recurrent and chronic tension headaches is covered in Chapter 18 in this volume.

SIMPLE ANALGESICS

The simple, nonnarcotic analgesics, such as aspirin, acetaminophen, or ibuprofen, either alone or in combination with other agents, are often helpful for relieving the pain of acute muscle contraction headache. Generally classified as nonsteroidal antiinflammatory drugs, they act at peripheral sites and are most effective against pain of low-to-moderate intensity. Their maximal effects are much less than those of the opioids. At the same time, they do not cause dependence or the unwanted central nervous system side effects associated with opioids. For example, except for the reduction in pain, the simple analgesics do not alter sensory perception (5). They do have other important side effects that are discussed below.

The primary mode of action of the simple analgesics, as well as of all NSAIDs, is thought to lie in their ability to inhibit the synthesis of prostaglandin by blocking the action of cyclooxygenase. This enzyme mediates the conversion of arachidonic acid to prostaglandin. Prostaglandins are synthesized from cellular membrane phospholipids following activation or injury and play a role sensitizing pain receptors (5, 6).

Aspirin

Aspirin, a nonsteroidal antiinflammatory drug, is the prototype and most widely prescribed member of the class of drugs known as the salicylates. In addition to its analgesic effects, aspirin is a potent antiinflammatory and antipyretic, capable of lowering body temperature rapidly and effectively (5). Ingestion of aspirin also prolongs bleeding time, even at very low doses. A dose of 0.65 gm of aspirin doubles bleeding time for 4 to 7 days. The recommended adult dose for treatment of acute muscle contraction headache is 650 mg q6h (5). Larger doses rarely result in greater pain relief and may cause adverse gastrointestinal (GI) effects. Aspirin should be administered orally, preferably with food and a large quantity (240 ml) of water or milk to minimize gastric irritation. The use of enteric-coated aspirin reduces GI distress but may also decrease potency. Peak levels of aspirin are attained within 0.75 hours, and the drug has a plasma half-life of 2 to 30 hours.

Acetaminophen

Use of acetaminophen for treating acute muscle contraction headache has become increasingly common. In addition to producing about the same degree of analgesia as aspirin, this drug is well tolerated, lacks many of the GI side effects of aspirin, and is available without a prescription. Acetaminophen's precise mode of action is unclear, although inhibition of prostaglandin synthesis in the cen-

tral nervous system (CNS) has been suggested (5, 6). However, acetaminophen, which is the active metabolite of phenacetin, is a relatively poor inhibitor of this enzyme, which probably accounts for its weaker antiinflammatory action and fewer NSAID-like side effects. The drug is rapidly absorbed from the GI tract, attaining peak levels in 30 to 60 minutes. Its plasma half-life is 2 to 4 hours. Acetaminophen is widely marketed under a large number of brand names (e.g., Tylenol, Anacin-3, Panadol). The maximum recommended dosage is 1000 mg q6h.

Ibuprofen

Ibuprofen, a member of the class of NSAIDs known as proprionic acid derivatives, is the most recent addition to the group of drugs that offer aspirin-like analgesia without a prescription. (Higher-dose preparations are available by prescription only.) Like other NSAIDs, though, ibuprofen can cause significant GI distress, although it is probably less active than aspirin. Ibuprofen has a half-life of 2 to 4 hours, with peak levels attained at 1 to 2 hours. The recommended adult dosage is 200 to 400 mg every 4 to 6 hours, with a maximum of 1200 mg per 24 hours. Patients should use the smallest effective dose. Ibuprofen is marketed as an over-the-counter analgesic under many brand names (e.g., Advil, Motrin IB, Nuprin, Mediprin).

Simple Analgesic Combinations

Several simple analgesic preparations are combinations of either aspirin or acetaminophen with caffeine. Although caffeine exerts no intrinsic analgesic activity, some data suggest that it potentiates the analgesic effects of aspirin and acetaminophen. Patients taking combinations that include caffeine should be aware that high intake of caffeine may result in tolerance, habituation, and psychological dependence. Abrupt cessation of the drug after prolonged use has been associated with analgesic rebound, including dizziness, irritability, and paradoxically, headache.

Aspirin-caffeine combinations include Anacin (aspirin 400 mg, caffeine 32 mg) and Maximum Strength Anacin (aspirin 500 mg, caffeine 32 mg). Aspirin, acetaminophen, and caffeine have been combined in products such as Excedrin Extra-Strength Analgesic (aspirin 250 mg, acetaminophen 250 mg, caffeine 65 mg) and Vanquish (aspirin 227 mg, acetaminophen 194 mg, caffeine 33 mg). The recommended dose for each combination is two tablets with water q6h.

NONSTEROIDAL ANTIINFLAMMATORY DRUGS

NSAIDs are useful for many acute muscle contraction headache sufferers with mild-to-moderate pain, especially those who have underlying organic contributing factors such as degenerative joint disease of the cervical spine or temporomandibular joint dysfunction (TMJ), also known as myofascial pain dysfunction. As described above, these drugs act peripherally, producing analgesia and reducing the inflammatory process by interfering with the action of the enzyme cyclooxygenase in synthesizing prostaglandins. There are several classes of NSAIDs. Table 17.1 lists the common drugs in each class.

Because of variability in the efficacy, pharmacokinetics, and side effect profiles of these drugs, patients who do not benefit from treatment with one class may benefit from a comparable agent and dose from another class. The choice of an agent is often determined by idiosyncratic differences in the way the individual patient responds to these drugs, as well as other factors such as allergies and concomitant medications and medical conditions.

Frequently Prescribed NSAIDs

The most frequently prescribed class of NSAIDs for treatment of acute muscle contraction headache is the propionic acid derivatives. All drugs in this class have useful antiinflammatory, analgesic, and antipyretic activity. There are considerable differences in their relative potency in inhibiting cyclooxygenase, however. For example, naproxen is 20 times more potent than aspirin, while ibuprofen and fenoprofen are about equal to aspirin (5). Like aspirin, all propionic acid derivatives alter platelet function and prolong bleeding time. It should be assumed that patients who are intolerant to aspirin will also be intolerant to these drugs.

GI side effects are common with propionic acid derivatives and all NSAIDs, occurring in as many as 15% of patients. Symptoms include epigastric pain, nausea, heartburn, abdominal discomfort, and sensations of "fullness." In the most serious cases, GI bleeding and peptic ulcers have been seen. These drugs should be used with caution in patients who have a history of GI bleeding or ulceration.

Table 17.1.
Nonsteroidal Antiinflammatory Drugs

Class	Brand Name	Generic Name
Nonacetylated salicylates	Trilisate	Choline magnesium trisalicylate
	Dolobid	Difunisal
	Magan	Magnesium salicylate
	Disalcid	Salsalate
Pyrrole acetic acids	Indocin	Indomethacin
	Clinoril	Sulindac
	Tolectin	Tolmetin
Propionic acids	Nalfon	Fenoprofen
	Ansaid	Flurbiprofen
	Motrin	Ibuprofen
	Rufen	Ibuprofen
	Orudis	Ketoprofen
	Naprosyn	Naproxen
	Anaprox	Naproxen sodium
Fenamates	Meclomen	Meclofenamate
	Ponstel	Mefenamic acid
Oxicams	Feldene	Piroxicam
Quinazolinone	Biarsan	Proquazone[a]
Pyrrolo-pyrroles	Toradol	Keterolac tromethamine

[a]Not yet available in the United States.

Naproxen Sodium (Anaprox). Naproxen sodium is rapidly absorbed, reaching peak levels in 1 to 2 hours with a mean half-life of 13 hours. The drug is available in 275-mg tablets and 550-mg tablets (Anaprox DS). The recommended adult starting dosage is 550 mg followed by 275 mg q6–8h. The total daily dose should not exceed 1375 mg.

Ibuprofen (Motrin, Rufen). Ibuprofen is rapidly absorbed from the GI tract, reaching peak plasma concentration in 1 to 2 hours. It is available in 300-, 400-, 600-, and 800-mg tablets. A 200-mg dose is available without a prescription (see above). Suggested dosage for mild-to-moderate pain is 400 mg q4–6h.

Flurbiprofen (Ansaid). Flurbiprofen is the newest member of the propionic acid class. It reaches peak plasma concentration in about 1.5 hours. It is available in 50- and 100-mg tablets and can be taken every 4 hours as needed, not to exceed 300 mg per day.

Meclofenamate (Meclomen). Meclofenamate, a member of the fenamate class, is rapidly absorbed from the GI tract, reaching peak plasma concentration in 0.5 to 1 hour. The drug is available in 50- and 100-mg tablets, and the recommended dose for mild-to-moderate pain is 50 mg q4h as needed. For some patients, the dose may need to be increased to 100 mg to produce optimal pain relief. Therapy should be initiated at the lower dose and then increased if necessary to increase the clinical response. Daily dosage should not exceed 400 mg.

Difunisal (Dolobid). Difunisal is a member of the nonacetylated salicylate class of NSAIDs. It is rapidly absorbed from the GI tract, reaching peak plasma concentrations within 2 to 3 hours. Significant analgesia for mild-to-moderate pain has been reported within 1 hour, with maximum effects at 2 to 3 hours. Dolobid is available in 250- and 500-mg tablets. An initial dose of 1000 mg is recommended for most patients, followed by 500 mg q12h, although some patients may require 500 mg q8h. Maximum daily dosage should not exceed 1500 mg.

Keterolac Tromethamine (Toradol). Keterolac tromethamine is an injectable NSAID that can be administered to patients with moderate-to-severe acute headache pain in emergency situations. Peak plasma levels are reached about 50 minutes after a single 30-mg intramuscular injection. Its analgesic effects are roughly equivalent to a 10-mg IM dose of morphine.

MUSCLE RELAXANTS

Significant stiffness and discomfort, including headache, can result from sustained abnormal muscle contraction. The muscles of the neck are especially prone to spasm from many causes, especially injury such as motor vehicle accidents, falls, work and athletic injuries, or overstretching. Other causes include prolonged anxiety or stress and inflammatory diseases. The problem is further complicated by a self-perpetuating cycle of muscle spasm→pain→ anxiety→ muscle spasm.

Centrally acting skeletal muscle relaxant drugs are frequently effective in breaking this cycle and relieving moderate acute muscle-contraction headache. Although their exact mechanism of action is unclear, these drugs do not directly affect muscle tissue, the myoneuronal junction, or motor nerves. Instead, they produce relaxation by depressing the central nerve pathways, possibly through their effect on higher centers. This action modifies the central perception of pain without interfering with peripheral pain reflexes or motor activity. Many clinicians prefer this group of drugs, because they are generally well tolerated and have a low toxicity profile.

Carisoprodol (Soma)

Carisoprodol is a CNS depressant with analgesic properties (7). It has been reported to reduce local muscle spasm without interfering significantly with muscular or neuromuscular function. Carisoprodol is thought to depress polysynaptic transmission in interneuronal pools at the supraspinal level in the brainstem reticular formation. Its muscle-relaxing effect may also be due in part to its sedative qualities.

Carisoprodol has a relatively short-lived action with minimal cumulative effect. Peak blood levels are attained within 1 to 2 hours following oral administration. Its duration of effect is about 4 to 6 hours. The drug is generally well tolerated with extremely low potential for organ toxicity. An additive sedating effect occurs when the drug is taken with other CNS depressants such as alcohol or antihistamines. The adult oral dosage of carisoprodol is 350 mg q6–8h.

Carisoprodol plus Aspirin (Soma Compound)

The combination of carisoprodol 200 mg with aspirin 325 mg (Soma Compound) adds the antiinflammatory and analgesic effects of aspirin to the muscle-relaxing effect of carisoprodol. The drug is intended for the treatment of patients suffering from significant pain. The recommended dosage for Soma Compound is one to two tablets q6h.

Soma Compound with Codeine

The addition of codeine 16 mg to Soma Compound is intended to provide additional analgesic activity. Recommended dosage is one to two tablets q6h. The usual aspirin and codeine prescribing precautions should be followed.

Adverse reactions to any of the carisoprodol-containing agents usually occur within the first few days of use and tend to be transient. Side effects include drowsiness, vertigo, dizziness, ataxia, tremor, agitation, irritability, headache, depression, syncope, and insomnia. If side effects do not resolve within 48 to 72 hours, a reduction in dose should provide relief. Allergic or idiosyncratic reactions are rare and tend to occur within the first several doses.

Chlorzoxazone (Parafon Forte)

Chlorzoxazone is a centrally acting muscle relaxant with sedative qualities. While its mode of action has not been clearly explained, it is known to act at the level of the spinal cord and subcortical areas of the brain, where it inhibits the reflex arcs involved in producing and maintaining muscle spasm.

Chlorzoxazone is rapidly absorbed, reaching peak blood levels in 3 to 4 hours. Onset of action occurs about 1 hour after oral administration, with a duration of action of 3 to 4 hours.

Chlorzoxazone is available in 250-mg and 500-mg tablets. The recommended initial dose is 750 mg to 2000 mg in three to four equal doses. If a patient is unresponsive, the daily dosage may be increased to 3000 mg and then reduced as improvement occurs.

Chlorzoxazone is generally well tolerated, and undesirable side effects, including GI disturbances, drowsiness, dizziness, lightheadedness, overstimulation, and allergic rash, are uncommon. Serious reactions, such as angioneurotic edema or anaphylaxis are extremely rare.

Metaxalone (Skelaxin)

Metaxalone is a centrally acting skeletal muscle relaxant that is chemically related to the mild tranquilizer mephenoxalone. Its mode of action is not well understood, although it is thought to induce muscle relaxation via CNS depression. Metaxalone has been used clinically for many years as adjunctive therapy in acute musculoskeletal disorders.

Absorption of metaxalone after oral administration is rapid, with onset of action about 1 hour later. Peak blood levels are attained in about 2 hours, and the duration of action is 4 to 6 hours.

Metaxalone is available in 400-mg tablets. The recommended daily dosage is 2400 mg to 3200 mg in divided doses. The drug should be administered with caution in patients with impaired liver function and is contraindicated in those with significant renal or liver disease and in those with a history of drug-induced anemias.

Metaxalone is generally well tolerated. Adverse reactions include nausea, vomiting, GI upset, drowsiness, dizziness, headache, nervousness and irritability, and rash and pruritis. Jaundice or hemolytic anemia are extremely rare.

Orphenedrine Citrate (Norflex, Norgesic, Orphengesic)

Orphenedrine is a centrally acting skeletal muscle relaxant with anticholinergic properties. It is thought to relax skeletal muscle by blocking neuronal circuits, the hyperactivity of which may be implicated in hypertonia and spasm.

Peak orphenedrine blood levels are attained within 2 hours of oral administration, with a duration of action of 4 to 6 hours. In its sustained-release form, absorption occurs over 8 to 10 hours, with peak blood levels being attained about 8 hours after administration.

Orphenedrine is available in both injectable and oral formulations. The parenteral formulation (Norflex) contains 30 mg/ml in aqueous solution. The daily intramuscular or intravenous dosage is 2 ml (60 mg). The oral formulation is available in 100-mg sustained-release tablets (Norflex) and in combination with caffeine and aspirin (Norgesic: orphenedrine 25 mg, caffeine 30 mg, aspirin 385 mg; Norgesic Forte: orphenedrine 50 mg, caffeine 60 mg, aspirin 770 mg). Recommended dosing is as follows: Norflex tablets—one tablet q12h; Norgesic—one or two tablets q6–8h; Norgesic Forte—one-half to one tablet q6–8h.

Because of its anticholinergic effects, patients with glaucoma, achalasia, prostatic enlargement, or bladder outlet obstruction should not take orphenedrine. In addition, the usual guidelines associated with aspirin should be followed for patients taking Norgesic or Norgesic Forte.

Orphenedrine's anticholinergic properties are responsible for many of its side effects, which are typically dose-related. Among these are tachycardia, palpitations, urinary retention, dry mouth, blurred vision, increased intraocular tension, weakness, nausea, vomiting, headache, dizziness, constipation, and drowsiness. Rare side effects include confusion, excitation, hallucinations, and syncope.

Methocarbamol (Robaxin, Robaxisal)

Methocarbamol is a centrally acting skeletal muscle relaxant that has been used successfully in the United States for more than 30 years. The drug's mechanism of action is still not understood. It does not directly affect striated muscle or the myoneuronal junction. Animal studies have shown that it inhibits nerve transmission in the internuncial neurons of the spinal cord and blocks polysynaptic reflexes.

Methocarbamol's onset of action occurs 30 minutes after oral administration. Peak blood levels are attained in about 2 hours, and its duration of action is 4 to 6 hours.

Methocarbamol is available in two oral formulations— 500 mg and 750 mg. Tablets containing both methocarbamol 400 mg and aspirin 325 mg (Robaxisal) are also available. The recommended starting dose of Robaxin is 1000–1500 mg followed by 500–1000 mg q6h as needed. The dosage for Robaxisal is two tablets q6h.

Most patients tolerate methocarbamol quite well. Many reported side effects occur early in treatment and resolve with time. These include lightheadedness, dizziness, vertigo, headache, mild muscular incoordination, blurred vision, urticaria, rash, flushing, GI upset, nasal congestion, and fever.

THERAPEUTIC COMBINATIONS

Among the most effective treatments for severe tension headache are those aimed at the multiple components of the problem. The pain of tension headache is but one link in the muscle contraction–pain–anxiety–muscle contraction chain. Many medical treatments are aimed at just one of these components, but those therapeutic combinations that attack two or three are often more effective. One researcher has noted that "an agent combining both a sedative and one or more analgesics appears to be an ideal choice for relieving tension headache" (8).

Among the most commonly used of these combination drugs are those containing the barbiturate butalbital, which has both sedative and muscle-relaxant properties. Other drugs contain the anxiolytic agent meprobamate. These drugs are intended to neutralize two links in the tension-headache chain: tight muscles and anxiety. Both butalbital and meprobamate are available in combination with various analgesic agents in order to provide coverage of all major symptoms. Clinical experience has shown these drugs to be generally safe and effective for treating tension headache.

The addition of the centrally acting narcotic codeine to several of these combinations has been shown to provide enhanced relief (9) and a more rapid onset of analgesic activity (10). In one randomized, placebo-controlled, double-blind study, the addition of codeine to the combination of butalbital, aspirin, and caffeine (Fiorinal with codeine) made it significantly superior to the butalbital combination alone in decreasing pain and muscle stiffness associated with tension headache. The largest differences occurred at the 1- and 2-hour evaluations (9).

Other drugs, including those combining a form of codeine or propoxyphene and aspirin or acetaminophen, have also been used in patients with tension headache, but many clinicians find them to be less appropriate. The compositions of the combination drugs commonly used to treat acute muscle contraction headache are summarized in Table 17.2.

Physicians should be aware that these are very powerful drugs—especially those that include a habit-forming narcotic or barbiturate. They should be used with caution and only in patients who have shown no propensity for taking excessive quantities of drugs. Unfortunately, patients who have a history of excessive drug use are common.

Because of the possibility of their developing a dependence on the drug, patients should be cautioned not to use it too frequently. There is no hard-and-fast rule for developing an effective, yet safe, regimen, but a useful starting point might be as follows: Drug should be taken no more than 2 days per week. If the patient requires more frequent analgesia than this, a nonaddicting, caffeine-free drug, such as a NSAID or nonaddicting muscle relaxant, should be prescribed. If headaches are frequent and nonresponsive to treatment, the physician should begin thinking in terms of prophylactic therapy.

By the same token, because these drugs are often so effective, physicians should take care not to overprescribe them. While most tension-headache patients could benefit from them, many would gain equal benefit from other drugs that carry less risk.

Table 17.2.
Composition of Combination Analgesics for Muscle Tension Headache[a]

Drug/Components	Quantity (mg)	Recommended Dosage	Drug/Components	Quantity (mg)	Recommended Dosage
Butalbital combinations			Empirin with Codeine		1–2 tablets q4h; ≤8
Fiorinal		1–2 tablets q4h as need-	#3 Codeine	30	tablets/day
Butalbital	50	ed; no more than 6/day	Aspirin	325	
Aspirin	325		#4 Codeine	60	1–2 tablets q4h; ≤4
Caffeine	40		Aspirin	325	tablets/day
Fiorinal with Codeine		1–2 tablets q4h as need-	*Propoxyphene combinations*		
Butalbital	50	ed; no more than 6/day	Darvon Compound		1 tablet q4h; as needed
Aspirin	325		Propoxyphene	32	≤4 tablets/day
Caffeine	40		Aspirin	389	
Codeine	30		Caffeine	32.4	
Fioricet		1–2 tablets q4h as need-	Darvon Compound-65		1 tablet q4h; as needed
Butalbital	50	ed; no more than 6/day	Propoxyphene	65	≤4 tablets/day
Acetaminophen	325		Aspirin	389	
Caffeine	40		Caffeine	32.4	
Fioricet with Codeine		1–2 tablets q4h as need-	Darvocet-N 50		1–2 tablet q4h; as
Butalbital	50	ed; no more than 6/day	Propoxyphene	50	needed ≤8 tablets/day
Acetaminophen	325		Acetaminophen	325	
Caffeine	40		Darvocet-N 100		1 tablet q4h; as needed
Codeine	30		Propoxyphene	100	≤4 tablets/day
Esgic		1–2 tablets q4h as need-	Acetaminophen	650	
Butalbital	50	ed; no more than 6/day	*Hydrocodone*		
Acetaminophen	325		*combinations*		
Caffeine	40		Hydrocet		1–2 tablets q4h; as
Phrenilin		1–2 tablets q4h as need-	Hydrocodone	5	needed ≤6 tablets/day
Butalbital	50	ed; no more than 6/day	Acetaminophen	500	
Acetaminophen	325		Vicodin		1–2 tablets q4h; as
Axotol		1–2 tablets q4h as need-	Hydrocodone	5	needed ≤6 tablets/day
Butalbital	50	ed; no more than 6/day	Acetaminophen	500	
Aspirin	650		*Oxycodone*		
Meprobamate combinations			*combinations*		
Equagesic		1–2 tablets q4h; ≤8	Percodan		1 tablet q6h; as needed
Meprobamate	200	tablets/day	Oxycodone	4.5	≤4 tablets/day
Aspirin	325		hydrochloride		
Micrainin		1–2 tablets q4h; ≤8	Oxycodone	0.38	
Meprobamate	200	tablets/day	terephthalate		
Aspirin	325		Aspirin	325	
Codeine combinations			Percocet		1 tablet q6h; as needed
Tylenol with Codeine		1–2 tablets q4h; ≤8	Oxycodone	5	≤4 tablets/day
#3 Codeine	30	tablets/day	hydrochloride		
Acetaminophen	300		Acetaminophen	325	
#4 Codeine	60	1–2 tablets q4h; ≤4	Tylox		1 tablet q6h; as needed
Acetaminophen	300	tablets/day	Oxycodone	5	≤4 tablets/day
Synalgos			hydrochloride		
Dihydrocodeine	16	2 capsules q4h; ≤8	Acetaminophen	500	
Aspirin	356.4	capsules/day			
Caffeine	30				

[a]Data from Physician's desk reference. Oradell, NJ, 1990.

NARCOTIC DRUGS

Narcotic drugs are usually contraindicated in the management of patients with muscle contraction headache because of the risk of dependence on these agents. If prescribed for an occasional case of tension headache that is unresponsive to other treatments, these drugs must be used with extreme care.

CONCLUSION

Patients with muscle contraction headache require treatment for acute pain. Certainly, not every drug is appropriate for every patient or every headache. The choice of an appropriate agent should be based on the physician's knowledge of the many choices available as well as on his or her experience with each drug and each patient.

Analgesics, whether used alone or in combination with a muscle relaxant, are often the best choice for most patients. Many analgesics, including aspirin, acetaminophen, and ibuprofen, are available without a prescription and will often suffice for treatment of patients with acute episodic muscle contraction headache. Should patients be unresponsive to these, other choices include the NSAIDs, muscle relaxants, or combination agents that include a muscle relaxant, sedative, or anxiolytic plus an analgesic. Drugs that may cause dependency should be used with great care and only in those patients who have shown no propensity for taking excessive quantities of drugs.

Whichever agent is selected, it should be sufficient to relieve the patient's symptoms, but should be appropriate to the degree of pain. Physicians should always resist the temptation to overtreat a minor headache because of the risk of dependency on the drug or other negative consequences.

REFERENCES

1. Diamond S. Muscle contraction headache. In: Dalessio DJ, ed. Wolff's headache and other head pain. New York: Oxford University Press, 1987.
2. Speed WG. Treatment of muscle contraction headache. In: Gallagher RM, ed. Drug therapy for headache. New York: Marcel Dekker, 1990.
3. Bakal DA. Muscle contraction and migraine headache: psychophysiologic comparison. Headache 1977;17:208–215.
4. Dalessio DJ. Mechanisms of headache. Med Clin North Am 1978;2:429–442.
5. Flower RJ, Moncada S, Vane JR. Analgesic-antipyretics and anti-inflammatory agents; drugs employed in the treatment of gout. In: Gilman AG, Goodman LS, Rall TW, Murad F, eds. Goodman and Gilman's the pharmacological basis of therapeutics. New York: Macmillan, 1985:674–715.
6. Mochan E. Analgesics in the treatment of headaches. In: Gallagher RM, ed. Drug therapy for headache. New York: Marcel Dekker, 1990.
7. Bergen FM, Kletztein M, Ludwig BJ, Margolin S. History, chemistry and pharmacology of carisoprodol. Ann NY Acad Sci 1960;86:90–107.
8. Friedman AP. Assessment of Fiorinal with Codeine in the treatment of tension headache. Clin Therapeut 1986;8:703–721.
9. Friedman AP. Fiorinal with Codeine in the treatment of tension headache—the contribution of components to the combination drug. Clin Therapeut 1988;10:303–315.
10. Sunshine A, Roure C, Olson N, et al. Analgesic activity of two ibuprofen-codeine combinations for the treatment of postepisiotomy and postoperative pain. Clin Pharmacol Ther 1987;42:374–380.

18

Medical Management of Recurrent Tension-Type Headache

JAMES R. COUCH, JR.

WHAT IS A TENSION HEADACHE?

Definition and Epidemiologic Studies

In any discipline in medicine it is always necessary to determine the correct diagnosis prior to proceeding with therapy. For this reason it is necessary to review briefly problems associated with diagnosing tension headache by focusing on associated practical implications.

The concept of muscle tension headache was formulated early in this century (1). In the report of the ad hoc Committee on Classification of Headache (2), a definition of tension headache was formulated as follows: "Ache, or sensation of tightness, pressure or constriction widely varied in intensity, frequency and duration, sometimes long lasting and commonly suboccipital. It is associated with contraction of skeletal muscles in the absence of permanent structural change, usually as part of the individual's reaction during life stress." This definition was refined and reformulated in the International Headache Society classification presented in 1988 as follows: "Recurrent episodes of headache lasting minutes to days. The pain is typically pressing/tightening in quality, of mild or moderate intensity, bilateral in location and does not worsen with routine physical activity. Nausea is absent, but photophobia or phonophobia may be present" (3).

Despite these efforts, the definition of tension headache remains somewhat vague. In more or less practical terms, a tension headache is defined as a functional headache that (a) is not associated with a definable neurological disease or other medical disease, (b) is not associated with progressive neurological deterioration over time, and (c) does not manifest features that would classify it as a migraine or cluster headache, the other two major categories of functional headache. The tension headache, then, is defined more or less as follows: a headache that is widely varying in occurrence and intensity, which may be unilateral or bilateral; may be frontal, vertex, or suboccipital in location, and may be associated with pain in the jaw, neck, or shoulder muscles. The tension headache is not associated with the gastrointestinal symptoms of nausea, vomiting, or diarrhea

and is not associated with transient visual or neurological symptoms (4). Greater refinement of the definition encroaches upon and merges into the migraine syndrome, allowing degrees of photophobia, phonophobia, mild nausea, or anorexia (5).

Because of this latter problem, Ziegler has proposed that migraine and tension headache are a continuum of the same syndrome (6–8). This has produced a great deal of controversy which has not yet been resolved. Certainly the usual patient seeking medical help at the neurologist's office often manifests elements of both migraine and tension headache. From the work published, it is unclear whether this association may be in part artifactual or whether coexistence of these types of headache imply a single syndrome with a broad spectrum of clinical manifestations as Ziegler proposed.

One approach to the problem is to look at epidemiologic studies on headache, which clearly indicate that headache is a very common problem and that tension headache is a major part of this pattern. In the Pontypridd study, Waters surveyed 2000 subjects and obtained adequate responses from 1718 (773 males, 945 females), giving response rates of 94% for men and 93% for women (9). He found that 63.5% of men and 78.4% of women had a headache in the prior year. Using unilaterality, nausea, and aura as markers for migraine, Waters found that only 187/491 (38%) of men with headache and 198/741 (27%) of women with headache did not have at least one of these features, while for subjects with at least one of these features, of those with one symptom of migraine, only 32% of men and 19% of women did not have a second feature. Summarizing the data for 491 men with headache, 38% had no migrainous features, 19% had one, and 43% had 2 or more features suggesting migraine. For 741 women with headache, the corresponding figures were 27% none, 30% one, and 44% two or more migrainous features. Considering the entire population of 1718 subjects, 704 (40%) had a pure tension or a "borderline" (only one migrainous feature) tension headache. The figures indicate that tension headache is a common problem and seen in approximately

40% of the population. The study of Ziegler et al. suggests a similar proportion (10).

Another approach to tension headache is to look at the medical resources needed to manage the problem; however, this approach may be misleading. Obtaining medical help for a headache is expensive and time consuming. In societies with a fee-for-service medical system such as the United States, the expense of seeing a physician likely limits the headache population that comes for medical attention to only those with more severe headaches or to those with a more troubling aspect to the headache such as periodic neurological or gastrointestinal symptoms that cause patient concern. Under a socialized medicine system, expense is not a factor but waiting time required to obtain medical care is. In these societies, such as in the English system, the time invested in obtaining medical consultation regarding headache may be significant enough to discourage any but the more severe headache patients from seeking medical help. For these reasons, only studies such as those of Waters (9) and Ziegler (10) allow a reasonable estimate of the number of individuals who may have occasional mild or even moderate headaches that cause some discomfort but do not interfere with the subjects' daily activities.

Are Tension and Migraine Headaches Separable?

The population studies cited above (9, 10) demonstrate the difficulty with isolating the "pure tension headache" as a diagnostic entity. Clinically, tension headache appears to start as a definable syndrome and then merge gradually into the migraine syndrome. Likewise, therapy of the tension headache has many overlaps with migraine therapy.

Data presented by Ziegler (6, 7) from factor analysis of large numbers of patients suggested that tension headache and migraine headache could not be differentiated clinically. Ziegler went on to suggest that migraine and tension headache are part of the same syndrome, which has a spectrum of manifestations ranging from the pure "tension" to the pure "migraine" headache. The data of Waters (9), reviewed above, agree. He found a relationship between headache severity and migrainous symptoms, and the number of migrainous symptoms increased with increasing headache severity. Drummond and Lance (11), in their analysis of 537 patients, found they could separate cluster headache but could not separate migraine and tension headaches in a factor analysis study. Pikoff (12) reviewed this area extensively and summarized the data for and against a distinction between migraine and tension headache. Generally, only a weak case can be made for a distinction.

The above material notwithstanding, two observations suggest a difference. The first comes from Olesen's work in which spreading oligemia was seen in subjects with classic migraine but not in those with common migraine (13, 14). Common migraine often has features of a tension headache. Findings such as these suggest that perhaps common migraine and tension headache needs to be combined into one entity with classic migraine remaining separate. Secondly, Olesen reported on a feature of tension headache that physicians who treat headache have been aware of for many years. Most patients with classic or common migraine headache want to lie down and be very still. Movement exacerbates their headaches (5). Patients with pure tension headache generally are neutral about activity and indicate that walking or running may actually relieve the headache. The issue of separation into two syndromes of migraine and tension headache or combination into a spectrum of functional headache as suggested by Ziegler (7) remains unresolved but certainly deserves further research.

ETIOLOGY OF TENSION HEADACHE

Perhaps the simplest "tension headache" can be illustrated by the individuals who have presbyopia and have recently had their eyeglasses changed. These individuals often find that reading requires extra concentration and probably more intense contraction of the muscles controlling eye movement. Patients in this situation frequently report that when they attempt to read, they develop pain around the eyes (headache) after 5 to 15 minutes. Taking off the glasses and stopping the reading produces relief from the headache in a short time. A similar experiment can be carried out by simply raising the eyebrows and corrugating the forehead and then maintaining this muscle contraction for a period of 1 to 5 minutes. This will produce a pain over the forehead, which will be relieved as soon as the muscle contraction ceases. It is from observations of this type that the chronic muscle contraction theory of tension headache evolved, and indeed, the term *chronic muscle contraction headache* was applied to this entity for a number of years. As reviewed by Pikoff, however, attempts to identify elements of chronic muscle contraction or to show excess muscle contraction in patients with tension headache have generally been unsuccessful (12). Clearly, patients with definable muscle spasm (for whatever reason) will have pain in those muscles, and if the muscles involve the head or have some pathway or pain referral to the head, the patient may develop a head pain related to the muscle tension. The question to be resolved is whether this represents the same entity as the tension headache for which individuals seek medical help.

The temporomandibular joint syndrome represents another situation where muscle tension can cause pain (15, 16). The secondary muscle spasm related to temporomandibular joint dysfunction may produce pain in the area of the temporalis or masseter muscles. At times, referral pathways in the brainstem or spinal cord may produce spreading of the pain to the head, neck, or shoulder. Patients with cervical fracture or a herniated cervical disc may have associated muscle spasm in the muscles at the segment involved, and pain may be referred to the C-2 or even retroorbital region. In the above situations, definable prolonged muscle contraction produces pain. This observation has been extrapolated to the "universe" of tension headache and used to develop a theory for the physiopathology of the condition. As reviewed by Pikoff, some support exists for this theory but most evidence is negative (12).

It appears that the patients who have definable muscle contraction and pain on that basis constitute a small minority of patients who can be defined as having pure tension headache or mixed tension migraine headache. Perhaps this group of patients with definable muscle contraction and pain on that basis should be separated and given a different classification. There is, however, still evidence that the tension headache patient demonstrates differences in central processing of reflex loops. Schoenen et al. (17) and Wallasch et al. (18) have shown delay in the late exteroceptive suppression period of temporalis muscle following a painful stimulus in subjects with tension headache.

In addition to the headaches with definable muscle tension, a number of other headaches have been referred to as tension or tension-like headaches. These include headaches associated with endocrine problems such as hypothyroidism, hyperthyroidism, hypoparathyroidism, and pituitary problems (19); headaches associated with certain types of intoxications; and headaches associated with habituation withdrawal due to ergot compounds, barbiturates, or narcotics (20). Because these have a definable cause, they should be termed "tension-like" headaches. These headaches should respond to specific therapy directed at a particular cause.

After these entities are removed, there remains a large body of patients who have headaches that vary widely in frequency and intensity and which fit the definition of the tension headache. These tend to become more frequent as patients age (8, 12). Depression appears to be a concomitant of the increasing frequency of tension headache (21). Emotional and psychological stress often, but not always, appear to be related to significant headache. Evaluation of these latter factors is usually important in designing a therapeutic plan. A unifying theory of etiology and pathogenesis for tension headache is still not enunciated.

MEASUREMENT OF PAIN

In discussion of therapy and evaluation of studies of various medications, it is necessary to review the means of measurement used. Pain is a subjective symptom and therefore difficult to quantitate. The methods developed for pain measurement include digital and analog scales (22–25). These scales are applied to quantitate pain intensity initially and at various points in time after administration of the test agent, and also to measure the degree of pain relief.

The digital scale for pain intensity usually consists of 4 to 8 categories based on descriptors of none, mild, moderate, and severe (23–25). They may be expanded by interpolating points between the above-noted categories. Pain relief is usually categorized as none, minimal, "a great deal" or "lots", and complete. Occasionally, a category of "worse" is added. This is usually termed the categorical scale (CS). The analog method usually employs a 10-cm line with descriptors of "no pain" at the one end and "worst pain ever" at the other. This is termed the visual analog scale (VAS).

Numerous studies have been done to validate use of these scales (22–26) and generally have demonstrated their validity in pain measurement. Validity exists only when the patient is able to understand the scale, the purpose of the study, and the reason for use of the scale.

In general, the analog method (VAS) is found to be somewhat more sensitive to pain measurement than the categorical one (CS) (22, 25). There is good agreement between CS and VAS for the most part, with a high correlation of relative pain intensity measurements (23). The actual relationship between the two scales was found to be semilogarithmic, with a logarithmic scale for CS versus linear for VAS in cancer pain patients (24). Where minor variations in pain make little clinical difference, either method may be used. The CS is usually easier to understand and use and may be superior where >50% reduction in pain may be the only clinically meaningful measure.

In addition to measurement of pain intensity at various points, the degree of pain relief can also be measured by categorical and analog scales (23–25). For the categorical scale, the terms "no relief," "minimal relief," "marked relief," and "total relief" may be used. For the analog scale, a 20-cm line with a mark at the center may be used. The 10 cm to the left represent worsening of the pain and the 10 cm to the right represent improvement with total relief at 10 cm. The patient is asked to mark the degree of relief relative to the initial level of pain represented by the center point.

The usual measures of pain relief are pain intensity difference (PID), sums of pain intensity difference over time (SPID), pain relief score (PAR), and total pain relief (TOT PAR) (23). Table 18.1 summarizes calculation of these scores.

These scores and derived scores can be subjected to statistical analysis. It is still necessary, however, to decide before analysis the degree of change that is clinically meaningful. It is quite possible to have a statistically significant change in score that is clinically insignificant. This is particularly true in headache, where a change in pain intensity ≥50% is usually needed for demonstration of clinical significance. von Graffenried et al. used these scores in a study of headache to demonstrate their applicability to this area (26). In studies of tension headache done since 1975, the usual method of reporting results has involved use of CS or VAS to develop the derived calculations of PID, SPID, PAR, and TOT PAR.

PLACEBO EFFECT

When dealing with therapy for any disease, it is always worthwhile to have some idea of the overall baseline against which therapeutic efforts can be measured. In diseases such as Huntington's chorea or Parkinson's disease, a stable baseline is readily available; patients serve as their own controls. Once therapeutic intervention is terminated, return to baseline status is essentially guaranteed. In other diseases, such as stroke or multiple sclerosis, variability of the patient's course is much more likely. In these conditions, it is much more difficult to determine whether treatment has had any specific effect or whether one is simply measuring the natural course of the disease.

The placebo effect is well known to researchers involved in clinical trials of headache. Some individuals have excellent response to placebo, while others do not, and many promising therapeutic modalities have been found to be no different from placebo. Before discussing therapeutic efficacy, it is worthwhile to look at the placebo effect in studies of treatment of tension headache. Table 18.2 presents results from patients treated with placebo from 12 well-designed and well-executed studies in which the extent of placebo effect could be readily ascertained. It can be seen that the extent of placebo effect is quite variable. The extent of relief with placebo ranged from 4% in the study of Schachtel (36) to 55% in Friedman's study (34). In all these studies, patients in the drug treatment track had greater relief than those in the placebo track. Nevertheless, it would appear that a placebo effect of 20 to 30% can be expected in the usual well-designed and well-executed study. This provides a benchmark against which the effectiveness of a particular drug should be measured. If the study does not demonstrate a placebo effect of at least this magnitude, validity of results of comparison of drug and placebo must be seriously questioned. These results would have to be carefully scrutinized before the drug treatment regimen could be recommended and would become part of the standard therapeutic armamentarium.

THERAPY OF TENSION HEADACHE
Subdivision of Tension Headache

In the literature prior to 1985, research tended to divide tension headache into two categories-tension headache without vascular manifestation (5) and the so-called tension-vascular headache. In the pure tension headache, the patient had pain and muscle tension, but no associated gastrointestinal neurological symptoms. In the tension-vascular headache, the patient had mild nausea, throbbing pain, and possibly photophobia or phonophobia. This was considered a somewhat intermediate syndrome between tension headache and a classic, or at least easily defined migraine headache. The tension-vascular headache usually represented a more severe and chronic headache syndrome. This nomenclature has evolved into the terms mixed tension-migraine headache, chronic daily headache, or chronic almost-daily headache. The suggestion of a lack of a clear distinction between tension, tension-vascular, and migraine headaches provided the background for Ziegler and others to suggest that migraine and tension headaches were part of a continuum (6, 7). Earlier researchers such as Friedman (38) and Lance (1) noted the tendency toward a furrowed brow, increased muscle tone in the neck, and scalp tenderness and suggested that these were major features of the tension headache as a separate syndrome. The work of Olesen's group (4, 5) has confirmed and extended these earlier studies. Nevertheless, the significant difficulty in separating these syndromes is underscored by the fact that tension headache patients, as their headache problems progress, may evolve a pattern of typical migraine for their more severe headaches. In addition, patients with pure intermittent migraine often develop tension-type headaches as the frequency of their headaches increase or as they come under greater psychological or emotional stress.

The above considerations notwithstanding, there are

Table 18.1
Calculation of Derived Measures of Pain Intensity and Relief

Measure
1. Pain intensity difference (PID)
2. Sum of pain intensity differences (SPID)
3. Pain relief score (PAR)
4. Total pain relief score (TOT PAR)

Definitions
P_o = pain score at baseline, time 0
$P_a, P_b, P_c \ldots$ etc. = pain scores at various intervals after time 0
R_a, R_b, R_c = pain relief scores at various intervals after time 0

Calculations
PID = $P_o - P_x$ (x = any observation)
SPID = $(P_o - P_a) + (P_o - P_b) + \ldots + (P_o - P_x)$ (Where x = the final observation)
PAR = R_x Where x = any time interval selected
TOT PAR = $R_a + R_b + R_c + \ldots + R_x$ Where x = the final observation

Table 18.2.
Extent of Placebo Response in Studies of Therapy of Tension Headache

	Type of Measurement and Percentage Improvement Based on Percentage Change Relative to Measurement Scale			
	Pain Intensity Difference (PID)		Pain Relief	
First Author & Year	by VAS	by CS	SPID	PAR
Ryan, 1977 (27)	—	—	30%	—
von Graffenried, 1980 (26)	13%	17%	—	43%
Diamond, 1981 (28)	—	—	—	25%
Diamond, 1983 (29)	—	18%	—	—
Peters, 1983 (30)	—	—	50–60%	—
Friedman, 1987 (31)	—	33%	—	—
Langemark, 1987 (32)	12–15%	—	—	—
Miller, 1987 (33)	19%	—	—	40%
Friedman, 1988 (34)	—	55%	—	70%
Sargent, 1988 (35)	—	17%	—	—
Schachtel, 1988 (36)	4%	—	—	—
Langemark, 1990 (37)	—	—	—	47%

significant differences in the extent to which migraine headaches will respond to therapy for tension headache and vice-versa. While there is a significant crossover in therapy, there are still medications that work better at different ends of the spectrum.

In dealing with treatment options, the format used by "older" investigators of dividing tension and tension-vascular type headache is useful. Table 18.3 lists the medications usually considered, the doses recommended, and the major side effects (39).

Evaluation of the Patient and Identification of Factors Related to the Headache

The first step toward therapy for headache patients is accurate diagnosis and identification of factors associated with the headache. At times, treatment of associated factors may be more important than treatment of the headache.

Simple tension headache is a problem that "headache specialists" or "pain specialists" are seldom called upon to treat. This headache usually lies in the domain of the primary care physician and even then, often is mentioned only as a secondary complaint. The usual individuals consulted by sufferers of this headache are neighbors, co-workers, or pharmacists. Physicians are usually consulted only when the headache occurs very frequently, such as daily or almost-daily, or if the sufferer becomes concerned that something medically serious such as cancer, vascular disease, or major organ failure is producing the headache. When evaluating the patient with tension or tension vascular headache, it is always necessary to be certain about the diagnosis and be sure there are no other associated medical or psychiatric problems. A thorough history and physical examination should be performed and include the elements outlined in Table 18.4. The history and physical examination should be followed by a thorough neurological examination. Often a screening laboratory panel (CBC and Chemistry-20) and antinuclear antibody and thyroid function studies help to rule out occult causes of headache.

Once the diagnosis of tension headache without other medical complications has been established, the possibility of therapeutic options should be discussed frankly with the patient. For those patients whose primary concern is the presence of other medical conditions, drug therapy or other therapeutic modalities may not be desired. The reassurance that the patient does not have any serious medical problem may produce a major degree of relief from the headache. The presence of major psychological or emotional stress factors related to marriage, family, or job should be explored. If a major psychological stressor is instrumental in the occurrence of the headache, the potential contribution of this stressor to the headache should be discussed with the patient. At times, avoidance of a stress situation may be the major aspect of the patient's treatment. Occasionally the job situation is such that a change in job is necessary to bring about relief of the headache.

Often, resolution of the psychological stress produces relief from the headache and may be the only way to obtain lasting relief.

Depression is often a major factor in headache problems severe enough to cause a patient to visit the physician (21, 40). Frequently, this is a masked depression in which the major outward symptoms are agitation, anxiety, increased irritability, poor concentration, sleep loss, loss of interest in usual activities, anhedonia, decreased libido, poor appetite, and poor job performance. Often the patients do not appear depressed, nor will they admit to feeling depressed or crying easily. If the patient admits to decreased appetite or interest in food, insomnia, anhedonia, diminished libido, and increased irritability, depression should be suspected. If an agitated depression exists, then discussion of this with the patient as a factor in the headache will often be helpful. It is necessary to reassure the patient that agitated depression is a common syndrome that will remit over time and can be treated successfully. Patients should also be reassured that they are not "crazy." If however, the patient admits to thoughts of self-harm or suicide or if there are symptoms of frank psychosis, referral to a psychiatrist may be needed.

The patient's use of, and reason for use of, medication should be explored thoroughly. Patients frequently will indicate they take a particular symptomatic medication only when they need it and only when they have a headache. When frequency of use is explored further, however, the physician may find the patient using the medication very frequently or daily, which may lead to a habituation withdrawal-type pattern (20, 21). This pattern usually develops insidiously, and it is often difficult for the patient to admit to frequent medication use. In the situation of frequent use of medication leading to habituation or abuse, the reason for use of the medication should be explored. Patients in this situation commonly take the medication because of a transient euphoria or "high" that the medication produces. Butalbitol, for instance, may produce a brief euphoria in small doses. Patients addicted to ergot usually feel mentally more clear and more energetic upon dosing and find themselves mentally slowed and much less energetic without the ergot effect. This effect is also seen in patients showing habituation to narcotics such as propoxyphene or codeine compounds.

The problem of depression again must be explored in this context. Patients may take barbiturates in the butalbitol-analgesic combination drugs because of the brief euphoria and transient relief from depression felt shortly after the medication is taken. Sedative-tranquilizer medications usually enhance depression over the longer term. Patients taking frequent barbiturates or benzodiazepines as well as alcohol are particularly good candidates for this type of depression syndrome. The same type of process may be seen with analgesic and minor narcotic abuse. It is always necessary to define and determine the reason for medication abuse and treat that problem as well. If the

Table 18.3.
Medications for Tension Headache

I. Simple tension headache
A. Nonsteroidal antiinflammatory drugs (NSAID)

Drug	Individual Dose	Maximum Dose/Day	Toxic/Side Effects of NSAIDs[a]
Aspirin	650–1000 mg	4000–5000 mg	Gastric distress and abdominal pain
Ibuprofen	400–800 mg	2400 mg	GI bleeding, diarrhea, hepatitis, abnormal liver function tests
Naproxen	250–500 mg	1100 mg	Renal failure, papillary necrosis
Fenoprofen	200–600 mg	2400 mg	Vesiculobullous eruption, urticaria
Tolectin	400 mg	2000 mg	Neutropenia, agranulocytosis, aplastic anemia
Miancerin	10 mg	60 mg	Depression, insomnia, confusion, paresthesia, hallucination, aseptic meningitis, tinnitus, hearing loss dry mucous membrane

B. Muscle relaxants

Drug	Individual Dose	Maximum Dose/Day	Toxic/Side Effects of Muscle Relaxants[a]
Orphenadrine	50–100 mg	200 mg	CNS—sedation, dizziness, drowsiness, confusion
Carisoprodol	350 mg	1400 mg	GI—nausea, vomiting, constipation, gastric irritation; transient weakness, quadriplegia, visual loss (rarely reported)
Methocarbamol	400–800 mg	3200 mg	Hematologic—aplastic anemia (rare), venous thrombosis
Diazepam[b]	2–5 mg	10–60 mg	Dermatologic—urticaria dermatoses, erythemamultiforme
Cyclobenzaprine	10 mg	20–40 mg	Same as tricyclic antidepressant category (II.A.) GI—urinary retention, impotence, psychiatric dependence, habituation with chronic use

C. Other agents

Drug	Individual Dose	Maximum Dose/Day	Toxic/Side Effects[a]
Acetaminophen	650–1050 mg	5000 mg	Dizziness, sedation nausea, vomiting, hepatic necrosis in acute doses of >15 gm
Butalbital[b] (usually formulated with analgesic or NSAID—(i.e., Fiorinal, Esgic))	50 mg	300 mg	Drowsiness, dizziness, nausea, vomiting, confusion; chronic use may lead to habituation and dependence

D. Minor narcotics

Drug	Individual Dose	Maximum Dose/Day	Toxic/Side Effects of Minor Narcotics[a]
Codeine[b] (usually formulated with analgesic or NSAID)	15–60 mg	300 mg	Drowsiness, dizziness, nausea, vomiting, constipation, rash, abdominal pain; overdose may produce respiratory depression and coma
Propoxyphene[b] (usually formulated with analgesic or NSAID)	60–100 mg	600 mg	Chronic use may lead to habituation and dependence

Table 18.3.—*continued*
Medications for Tension Headache

II. Tension-vascular headaches
A. Antidepressants and tricyclic compounds

Drug	Individual Dose	Maximum Dose/Day	Toxic/Side Effects of Tricyclics[a]
Amitriptyline	10–50 mg	150–350 mg	CV—hypotension, orthostatic hypotension, hypertension, MI, stroke, arrhythmia, heart block
Imipramine	10–50 mg	150–250 mg	GI—ileus obstipation, nausea, vomiting, epigastric distress, diarrhea
Doxepin	10–50 mg	150–350 mg	Hematologic—bone marrow depression, agranulocytosis, leukopenia, thrombocytopenia, eosinophilia
Cyproheptadine	4 mg	16–40 mg	CNS—confusion, poor concentration, hallucination anxiety, insomnia, nightmares, paresthesia, incoordination, ataxia, tremor, seizure, parkinsonism, akathisia, dyskinesia Anticholinergic—dry mouth, constipation, urinary retention Endocrine—testicular swelling, gynecomastia, galactorrhea, changes in libido Allergic—rash Withdrawal syndromes—sudden withdrawal may produce malaise, headache nausea

B. β-Adrenergic blocking agents

Drug	Individual Dose	Maximum Dose/Day	Toxic/Side Effects of β-Blockers[a]
Propranolol	10–40 mg	120–130 mg	CV—bradycardia, heart block, decreased cardiac output
Nadolol	20–40 mg	80–160 mg	GI—nausea, vomiting, constipation, diarrhea, ischemic colitis
Atenolol	25–50 mg	100 mg	Hematologic—agranulocytosis, nonthrombocytopenic
Metoprolol	25–50 mg	100–200 mg	purpura, thrombocytopenia purpura; Respiratory—bronchospasm CNS—giddiness, lassitude, depression Allergic—pharyngitis, fever, rash Other—elevated SGOT, alkaline phosphatase, and lactate dehydrogenase

C. Less commonly used agents

Drug	Individual Dose	Maximum Dose/Day	Toxic/Side Effects Methysergide[a]
Methysergide	2 mg	6–12 mg	Nausea, vomiting, diarrhea, abdominal pain, paresthesia, edema, weight gain, retroperitoneal, pleural and cardiac value fibrosis

Drug	Individual Dose	Maximum Dose/Day	Toxic/Side Effects Phenelzine[a]
MAO inhibitor—Phenelzine	15 mg	90 mg	Dizziness, headache, drowsiness, postural hypotension, hypernatremia, sexual disturbances, elevated transaminase; rare—hepatic necrosis, hypertensive if exposed to amines[a]

[a]See reference 39 for more complete information on toxic effects and side effects.
[b]Significant potential for habituation and dependence.

Table 18.4.
Evaluation of the Tension Headache Patient: Factors Assessed to Determine Diagnosis and Help with Choice of Therapy

Age, sex, age of onset of headache
Severity of headache or severity of each type of headache if more than one type (e.g., mild and severe)
Location of headache pain for each type of headache
Duration of usual headache
Duration of longest headache
Frequency of each type headache
Symptoms associated with each type headache (i.e., gastrointestinal, visual, neurological)
Precipitating factors
Psychological stressors (e.g., job, family, financial)
Other medical conditions
Psychiatric conditions such as depression, anxiety compulsion psychosis
Present medications—type and frequency of use (including use of potentially habituating medications)
Past medications—type, frequency of use, and effectiveness
Physical and neurological examination
Basic laboratory tests—complete blood count, laboratory panel (Chem-20, or SMAC panel), thyroid function tests, antinuclear antibody.

patient is depressed and is using barbiturates, benzodiazepines, or minor narcotics frequently, these medications often will enhance the depression. It is also important to recognize the syndrome of agitated depression and the anxiety associated with the condition. Use of medications for anxiety, such as benzodiazepines, may create further habituation problems and will not relieve the depression. Use of antidepressants is appropriate, and doxepin, with its antidepressant and antianxiety effects, may be particularly effective.

A pattern of habituation or abuse of an analgesic, minor narcotic, or ergot compound must be discontinued. Work by Rapoport et al. (20) suggests that as long as the abused medication is continued, a rebound headache will continue to occur. The rebound headache is usually holocranial, dull and aching, and may be somewhat different from the original headache.

MEDICAL THERAPY OF SIMPLE TENSION HEADACHE

Following accurate diagnosis and discussion of stress factors relating to the headache, then further specific therapeutic measures may be in order. The most common treatment for the pure tension headache is a nonsteroidal antiinflammatory agent (NSAID). A number of papers demonstrate that aspirin is effective in treating pure tension headache (26, 27, 29, 30, 32). Most of these papers demonstrate a significant placebo effect of 15 to 35% improvement, as outlined in Table 18.2. Studies have generally shown aspirin to be significantly better than placebo, with 50 to 70% overall improvement in tension headache. These studies have included use of a visual analog scale and/or a categorical scale to report pain intensity and degree of pain relief. The most common method of

reporting results are those of von Graffenried, who used scales of pain intensity and pain relief (26). The data generated allowed calculation of pain intensity difference (SPID) scores as well as pain relief (PAR) and summed pain relief (SPAR) scores. Various studies have compared other NSAIDs with aspirin for treatment of tension headache. The NSAIDs evaluated include ibuprofen (27, 29, 36), naproxen (33, 35), zomepirac (28), and mianserin (37) (another ibuprofen analogue). Studies have generally shown these drugs to be equivalent to aspirin in their degree of relief of tension headache and, in some cases, the mean pain relief is somewhat better than that with aspirin. None of the studies has shown a statistically significant difference between the relief produced by aspirin and that produced by the other nonsteroidal antiinflammatory agent.

In general, then, with regard to nonsteroidal antiinflammatory drugs (NSAIDs), use of aspirin is recommended if the patient tolerates it. Generally, a patient who cannot tolerate aspirin will have difficulty with the other NSAIDs. It may, however, be worthwhile to try another NSAID to achieve the psychological effect of giving the patient a "new drug." The usual effective dose of aspirin is 650 to 1000 mg taken every 4 to 6 hours; naproxen, 250 to 375 mg taken every 6 hours; ibuprofen, 400 mg taken every 4 to 6 hours. Other medications to be considered include fenoprofen, 300 to 600 mg; tolectin 400 mg; mecolmen, 100 mg taken every 8 hours. It is unclear whether there may be a significant difference in the overall results from one NSAID to another, but there may be some idiosyncratic difference in patient response from one to another.

Acetaminophen is an analgesic without antiinflammatory effects. It was compared with aspirin in the studies of Miller et al. (33) and Peters et al. (30) and was found to be somewhat less effective than aspirin, but the difference was not significant.

The muscle relaxant medications used in treatment of tension headache include orphenadrine and orphenadrine-aspirin combinations (Norgesic), as well as carisoprodol and carisoprodol-aspirin combinations (Soma and Soma Compound) and methocarbamol. There are relatively fewer studies of these medications and more anecdotal data. Studies available suggest that these medications are probably no more effective than the nonsteroidal antiinflammatory medications. The butalbitol-analgesic combinations (Fiorinal, Esgic) were originally introduced for treatment of migraine headache. Studies on these medications or combinations of these with codeine have demonstrated that they provide effective pain relief for tension headache (31, 34). These medications are, however, habituating and must be used with care. Frequent use can be associated with development of a habituation withdrawal headache related to the medication.

Minor narcotic or narcotic analgesic preparations such as codeine in combination with aspirin or acetaminophen, or propoxyphene in combination with aspirin or acetaminophen have become popular in treatment of pain disorders. These can also be used for symptomatic relief of tension headache; they are potentially habituating and the usual precautions apply.

MEDICAL THERAPY OF CHRONIC TENSION OR TENSION-VASCULAR HEADACHE

The tension-vascular headache with its chronicity and lack of clear-cut identifying factors was largely ignored until the 1960s. This entity came to be recognized during the 1960s and then better defined in the 1970s, culminating in the work of Saper (41), Mathew (42), and Olesen (44, 45), who brought better definition to the concept of the mixed migraine-tension headache. This type of headache constitutes a major problem for the physician who deals with a significant number of headache patients. These are generally the patients who respond poorly to easily-applied headache therapies and who require extensive evaluation of history, psychiatric factors, medical factors, and factors of possible medication abuse to define their condition fully. The patient usually manifests a mixture of headaches, some of which fit the definition of migraine headache, while others are more tension-type, with somewhat less specific pain and not associated with the gastrointestinal, visual, or neurological symptoms that help define the migraine syndrome. These patients usually have frequent headaches, which may range from daily to four times a week. The patient often indicates that the more severe headaches are those with the characteristics of migraine and the less severe headaches are those with characteristics more like tension headache. Usually, the tension component is the more frequent, with clearly defined and migraine-like headache occurring significantly less frequent.

The mixed migraine-tension headache is difficult to study because it requires measurement of more than one type of headache and the interaction of factors that may produce the different types of headaches. As reported by Mathew (42) and Saper (41), these patients often are depressed or quite anxious. A number of studies have suggested that these patients have hysterical tendencies, but even removal of these factors from the picture does not always result in significant improvement in the patient's headache pattern. Not infrequently, there is no significant identifiable stressor or indication of depression whose initiation coincides with the onset of the tension-migraine syndrome.

The first study approaching therapy of this entity was that of Lance in 1964 (43). In that study, Lance looked at most of the medications that are still being used for treatment of this entity, including simple sedatives, vasodilators, methysergide, orphenadrine, ergotamine, benzodiazepines, imipramine, and amitriptyline, and compared these with placebo. He found a significant improvement in

the headache only with amitriptyline, although imipramine, benzodiazepines, and ergotamine also showed some effectiveness. Lance did not find a relationship between depression and response of headache to amitriptyline.

In 1971, Diamond and Baltes (46) carried out a 4-week study using amitriptyline as a 10-mg or a 25-mg tablet and placebo. In patients with chronic tension headache, they found improvement only in patients who received amitriptyline as a 10-mg tablet, taking between 10 and 60 mg daily. The 25-mg tablet was not significantly different from placebo. In 1976, Couch et al. (47) looked at amitriptyline in the prophylaxis of migraine and tension headache. Amitriptyline produced a significant improvement in both types of headache (P<.01). A weak correlation was found between the change in the depression score and the change in headache score: r = .33 for the most severe headache patients, and r = .26 for those with moderate headache. For those with mild headache, there was no correlation between change in depression score and change in headache score.

Mathew looked at the treatment of mixed headache by using amitriptyline and propranolol (48). He found propranolol to be more effective for pure intermittent migraine and amitriptyline more effective for mixed headache. Propranolol was also effective in treating mixed headache. In combination with amitriptyline, propranolol produced the greatest improvement, with a 66% improvement in headache score in the 4th through 6th months of therapy.

Subsequently, most of the medications that can be used for intermittent migraine headaches have been tried in the patient with chronic tension headaches. There are not controlled studies to show overall effectiveness in tension headache. These medications are outlined in Table 18.3, which provides information on dosing and side effects.

In treating tension-vascular headache, the most effective medication is usually amitriptyline, which may be given in doses of 50 to 300 mg per day. If the dose is to be raised above 200 mg per day, this should be done only in conjunction with use of amitriptyline levels. Likewise, patients should be followed carefully for development of toxicity. In patients over the age of 50, an electrocardiogram should be obtained, and if there is any indication of cardiac problems, amitriptyline should not be used, as it has been associated with sudden cardiac death. Other tricyclics that have been found effective in treating mixed tension migraine include imipramine, doxepin, protriptyline, and cyproheptadine.

As indicated above, propranolol, a β-adrenergic agent without intrinsic sympathomimetic activity, has been found effective for tension-vascular headache. Other β-blocking agents without intrinsic sympathomimetic activity may also be effective, including nadolol, atenolol, and metoprolol. Anecdotally, methysergide and the monoamine oxidase (MAO) inhibitors have been effective in occasional cases. Valproic acid may also be used in this syndrome, although relatively few data exist on this particular aspect of the chronic headache (49).

Finally, combinations of the above agents may be used. Mathew's study suggests the use of amitriptyline and propranolol (48). Either of these drugs may also be combined with a nonsteroidal antiinflammatory agent such as ibuprofen, fenoprofen, or naproxen. At times, addition of muscle relaxants such as orphenadrine or cyclobenzaprine may be useful in treating the tension component of the headache (50, 51). Unfortunately, the patients find that they adapt to the adjuvant effect of the muscle relaxant fairly quickly, and its enhancement of therapeutic effect is frequently short-lived. Benzodiazepines should not be used in these patients because of the high habituation potential and because the therapeutic effect of muscle relaxation is usually short-lived and accommodation occurs rapidly.

NONDRUG THERAPEUTIC MODALITIES

It is relatively easy for the physician to simply prescribe some type of medication for a patient sitting in the office; however, as noted above, there are many other facets to patient evaluation and treatment. The strategies of nondrug therapy evolved from a recognition that types of physical treatment other than drugs could be useful in handling the headache patient. The major therapeutic modalities employed have included biofeedback, relaxation therapy, and physical therapy.

In most instances, a combination of relaxation therapy and biofeedback is used. Diamond has reviewed this area, and the theoretical background for these techniques (52–54). Briefly, the chronic pain situation is viewed as having a "learned" component that helps to reinforce and intensify the pain. This "learned" component of pain can be approached by another learning process or counterprocess that modifies the pain. The counterprocess is usually biofeedback or relaxation therapy.

The most common form of biofeedback involves temperature and muscle contraction. In the former, the subject learns to increase the skin temperature of the hand (HST biofeedback). In the latter, the subject has surface electrodes placed over a muscle and learns to decrease muscle activity measured electromyographically (EMG biofeedback). These models of biofeedback were developed to mesh with the presumed pathophysiological bases of headache. Consequently, HST biofeedback would cause vasodilatation with hand warming, and vasodilatation fits loosely with a vascular theory of migraine. EMG biofeedback would represent lowering muscle tension and fits much more closely with a myogenic theory of tension headache.

Relaxation training is a technique in which certain phrases are used to help induce muscle relaxation and lower psychological tension (55, 56). Patients are taught the techniques of relaxation and told to use them whenever the headache begins to increase.

Diamond et al. reported two uncontrolled biofeedback studies with the largest numbers of patients. In these studies, patients were identified retrospectively from a headache clinic practice over 5-year (53) and 4-year (54) periods, respectively. Questionnaires were mailed to the patients; 73% of 556 subjects responded for the first study (53) and only 57% of 693 subjects responded for the second (53, 54). Of the respondents, 70 to 80% found that biofeedback produced moderate or better improvement. Diamond found that young females under age 40 without habituation problems to the headache medication were the best subjects.

While these studies had large numbers, the study design prevents reliance on the results, and the study must be viewed with caution. Patients were identified retrospectively, and the data were generated by a mailed questionnaire without the authors seeing the patients. The data do not account for subjects who did not answer the questionnaire. These nonresponders constituted 27% of the earlier (53) and 43% of the later (54) study populations. Finally, the study was uncontrolled. For these reasons, the studies can be considered as pilot studies but not as definitive research in the area.

A number of other studies have addressed biofeedback. In general, these studies are of two types. The first type includes studies that are retrospective or uncontrolled, with patients generated from a headache clinic and treated with biofeedback if interested (57–60). In the second type, a prospective protocol is developed, and patients are recruited and followed through a study period (55, 56, 61–63).

In general, well-controlled studies of biofeedback or relaxation therapy are very difficult, because the process is therapist-intensive, and a large placebo effect can be generated by such contact. In addition, a large element of bias is generated by the self-selection of patients. Those patients who are inclined to believe that self-control of pain is possible and are willing to submit themselves to the discipline required for biofeedback or relaxation therapy are the ones who will volunteer for a study, or who will agree to biofeedback as a therapy in the clinic situation. These patients constitute a biased group who are going to be more susceptible to a placebo effect of high therapist contact. For these reasons, truly double-blind studies are virtually impossible, and the initial self-selection bias probably will not allow testing on a "normal" population.

Despite the theoretical problems associated with proof of efficacy of these modalities, they appear to be effective in a population of patients. For this reason, biofeedback and relaxation therapy appear to be effective treatment modalities for tension headache for a group of patients interested in self-control and nondrug therapy. They may be used as primary therapies in some patients, but more often are effective only as adjunctive treatments. Work by several authors suggest this mode of treatment is particularly effective in children (54, 57).

CONCLUSION

Therapy of tension headache is somewhat complex and is based on good physician-patient relationships. First and foremost, there must be a thorough evaluation and establishment of the diagnosis. Next, associated factors of stress, depression, anxiety, or other medical disease must be ruled out. Often these factors are identified, and appropriate specific therapies must be considered before treatment of the tension headache can be undertaken. For the patient with simple tension headache, simple analgesics may be adequate. For the most complex tension-vascular or mixed headache, preventive or prophylactic medication may be needed. Nondrug treatments may provide primary or adjuvant approaches that may be valuable in selected patients, especially children, adolescents, and women under age 40.

REFERENCES

1. Lance JW. Mechanism and management of headache. 3rd ed. London: Butterworths, 1978.
2. Ad Hoc Committee on Classification of Headache. Classification of headache. Arch Neurol 1962;6:173–176.
3. Committee of the International Headache Society. Classification and diagnostic criteria for headache disorders, cranial neuralgias and facial pain. Cephalalgia 1988;8(suppl 7):10–90.
4. Langemark M, Olesen J, Poulsen DL, Bech P. Clinical characterization of patients with chronic tension headache. Headache 1988;28:590–596.
5. Rassmussan BK, Jensen R, Olesen J. A population-based analysis of the diagnostic criteria of the International Headache Society. Cephalalgia 1991;11:129–134.
6. Ziegler DK, Hassanein RS, Couch JR. Headache syndromes suggested by factor analysis of symptom variables in a headache prone population. J Chron Dis 1972;25:353–363.
7. Ziegler DK, Hassanein RS, Couch JR. Headache syndromes suggested by statistical analysis of headache symptoms. Cephalalgia 1982;2:125–134.
8. Ziegler DK, Hassanein RS. Specific headache phenomena: their frequency and coincidence. Headache 1990;30:152–156.
9. Waters WE. The Pontypridd headache survey. Headache 1974;14:81–90.
10. Ziegler DK, Hassanein RS, Couch JR. Characteristics of life headache histories in a nonclinic population. Neurology 1977;27:265–269.
11. Drummond PD, Lance JW. Clinical diagnosis and computer analysis of headache symptoms. J Neurol Neurosurg Psychiatry 1984;47:128–133.
12. Pikoff H. Is the muscular model of headache still viable? A review of conflicting data. Headache 1984;24:186–198.
13. Olesen J, Larsen B, Lauritzen M. Focal hyperemia followed by spreading oligemia and impaired activation of rCBF in classic migraine. Ann Neurol 1981;9:344–352.
14. Olesen J, Friberg L, Olesen TS, et al. Timing and topography of cerebral blood flow, aura, and headache during migraine attacks. Ann Neurol 1990;28(6):791–798.
15. Heir GM. Facial pain of dental origin—a review for physicians. Headache 1987;27:540–547.
16. Schellhas KP, Wilkes CH, Baker CC. Facial pain, headache, and temporomandibular joint inflammation. Headache 1989;29:228–231.
17. Schoenen J, Jamart B, Gerard P, et al. Exteroceptive suppression of temporalis muscle activity in chronic headache. Neurology 1987;37:1834–1836.
18. Walasch TM, Reinecke M, Langohr HD. EMG analysis of the late exteroceptive suppression period of temporal muscle activity in episodic and chronic tension-type headaches. Cephalalgia 1991;11:109–112.
19. Couch JR. Toxic and metabolic headache. In: Rose FC, ed. Handbook of clinical neurology. Amsterdam: Elsevier, 1986;48:417–430.
20. Rapoport AM. Analgesic rebound headache. Headache 1988;28:662–665.
21. Diamond S, Dalessio DJ. Muscle contraction headache. In: The practicing physician's approach to headache, 4th ed. Baltimore: Williams & Wilkins, 1986.
22. Joyce CRB, Zutshi DE, Hrubes V, Mason RM. Comparison of fixed interval and visual analog scales for rating chronic pain. Eur J Clin Pharmacol 1975;8:415–420.
23. Littman GS, Walker BR, Schneider BE. Reassessment of verbal and visual analog ratings in analgesic studies. Clin Pharmacol Ther 1985;38:16–23.
24. Wallenstein SL, Heidrich G, Kaiko R, Houde RW. Clinical evaluation of analgesics: the measurement of clinical pain. Br J Clin Pharmacol 1980;10:319S–327S.
25. Carlsson AM. Assessment of chronic pain. I. Aspects of the reliability and validity of the visual analogue scale. Pain 1983;16:87–101.
26. von Graffenried B, Hill RC, Nuesch E. Headache as a model of assessing mild analgesic drugs. J Clin Pharmcol 1980;20:131–144.
27. Ryan RE. Motrin—a new agent for the symptomatic treatment of muscle contraction headache. Headache 1977;16:280–283.
28. Diamond S, Medina JL. A double-blind study of zomepirac sodium and placebo in the treatment of muscle contraction headache. Headache 1981;21:45–48.
29. Diamond S. Ibuprofen versus aspirin and placebo in the treatment of muscle contraction headache. Headache 1983;23:206–210.
30. Peters BH, Fraim CJ, Masel BE. Comparison of 650 mg aspirin and 1000 mg acetaminophen with each other, and with placebo in moderately severe headache. Am J Med 1983;74(6):36–42.
31. Friedman AP, DeSerio FJ. Symptomatic treatment of chronically recurring tension headache: a placebo-controlled, multicenter investigation of Fioricet and acetaminophen with codeine. Clin Ther 1987;10(1):69–81.
32. Langemark M, Olesen J. Effervescent ASA versus solid ASA in the treatment of tension headache. A double-blind, placebo controlled study. Headache 1987;27:90–95.
33. Miller DS, Talbot CA, Simpson W, Korey A. A comparison of naproxen sodium, acetaminophen and placebo in the treatment of muscle contraction headache. Headache 1987;27:392–396.
34. Friedman AP, Boyles WF, Elkind AH, et al. Fiorinal with codeine in the treatment of tension headache—the contribution of components to the combination drug. Clin Ther 1988;10(3):303–315.
35. Sargent JD, Peters K, Goldstein J, et al. Naproxen sodium for muscle contraction headache treatment. Headache 1988;28(3):180–182.
36. Schachtel BP, Thoden WR. Onset of action of ibuprofen in the treatment of muscle-contraction headache. Headache 1988;28:471–474.
37. Langemark M, Loldrup D, Bech P, Olesen J. Clomipramine and mianserin in the treatment of chronic tension headache. A double-blind, controlled study. Headache 1990;30:118–121.
38. Friedman AP, Von Storch TJC, Merritt HH. Migraine and tension headache: a clinical study of two thousand cases. Neurology 1954;4:773–787.
39. Gilman AG, Goodman LS, Gilman A. Goodman and Gilman's the pharmacological basis of therapeutics. 6th ed. New York: Macmillan, 1980.
40. Couch JR, Ziegler DK, Hassanein RS. Evaluation of the relationship between migraine headaches and depression. Headache 1975;15:41–50.

41. Saper JL. Chronic headache complex (CHC): the mixed syndrome. A new perspective? In: Headache disorders: current concepts and treatment strategies. Boston: John Wright, 1983.

42. Mathew NT, Stubits E, Nigam MP. Transformation of episodic migraine into daily headache: analysis of factors. Headache 1982;22:66–68.

43. Lance JW, Curran DA. Treatment of chronic tension headache. The Lancet 1964;i:1236–1239.

44. Olesen J, Edvinsson L. Basic mechanisms of headache. Amsterdam: Elsevier, 1988.

45. Langemark M, Olesen J. Pericranial tenderness in tension headache. Cephalalgia 1987;7:249–255.

46. Diamond S, Baltes BJ. Chronic tension headache—treated with amitriptyline—a double-blind study. Headache 1971;111:110–116.

47. Couch JR, Ziegler DK, Hassanein RS. Amitriptyline in the prophylaxis of migraine: effectiveness relation of anti-migraine and anti-depressant effects. Neurology 1976;26:121–127.

48. Mathew NT. Prophylaxis of migraine and mixed headache. A randomized controlled study. Headache 1981;21:105–109.

49. Mathew NT, Sabiha A. Valproate in the treatment of persistent chronic daily headache. An open label study. Headache 1991;31:71–74.

50. Friedman AP. The treatment of chronic headache with meprobamate. Ann NY Acad Sci 1957;67:822–827.

51. Friedman AP. Treatment of chronic headache. Int J Neurol 1962;3:388–397.

52. Diamond S. Biofeedback and headache. Headache 1979;19(3):180–184.

53. Diamond S, Medina J, Diamond-Falk J, DeVeno T. The value of biofeedback in the treatment of chronic headache: a five-year retrospective study. Headache 1979;19(2):90–96.

54. Diamond S, Montrose D. The value of biofeedback in the treatment of chronic headache: a four-year retrospective study. Headache 1984;24(1):5–18.

55. Blanchard EB, Andrasik F, Appelbaum KA, et al. The efficacy and cost-effectiveness of minimal-therapist-contact, non-drug treatments of chronic migraine and tension headache. Headache 1985;25:214–220.

56. Attanasio C, Andrasik F, Blanchard EB. Cognitive therapy and relaxation training in muscle contraction headache: efficacy and cost-effectiveness. Headache 1987;27:254–260.

57. Werder DS, Sargent JD. A study of childhood headache using biofeedback as a treatment alternative. Headache 1984;24(3):122–126.

58. Billings RF, Thomas MR, Rapp MS, et al. Differential efficacy of biofeedback in headache. Headache 1984;24(3):211–215.

59. Hudzinski LG, Levenson H. Biofeedback behavioral treatment of headache with locus of control pain analysis: a 20-month retrospective study. Headache 1985;25(7):380–386.

60. Grazzi L, Frediani F, Zappacosta A, et al. Psychological assessment in tension headache before and after biofeedback treatment. Headache 1988;28:337–338.

61. Passchier J, van der Helm-Hylkema H, Orlebeke JF. Lack of concordance between changes in headache activity and in psychophysiological and personality variables following treatment. Headache 1985;25:310–316.

62. Blanchard EB, Appelbaum KA, Nicholson NL, et al. A controlled evaluation of the addition of cognitive therapy to a home-based biofeedback and relaxation treatment of vascular headache. Headache 1990;30:371–376.

63. Bruhn P, Olesen J, Melgaard B. Controlled trial of EMG feed back in muscle contraction headache. Ann Neurol 1979;6:34–36.

19

Nonpharmacological Management
of Tension-Type Headache

JOSEPH D. SARGENT

My approach to medicine has been influenced by personal experiences not always connected with my practice of medicine. Such personal experiences have profoundly influenced my attitude toward nonpharmacological approaches to medical problems.

Our first two daughters were delivered by traditional methods with parenteral medications and nerve blocks, but my wife believed that there must be a better way to give birth. She decided she wanted to be free from the influence of drugs at delivery of our third daughter, so both of us began to learn the Lamaze method. This approach relies on breathing techniques and voluntary control of abdominal and perineal muscles to control pain during labor and delivery. With the sympathetic encouragement of her physician and the nursing staff, my wife delivered our third daughter without medication. Our experience was not an accident; many women were delivered by the Lamaze method in this same hospital. Two years later, my wife delivered our fourth daughter by the Lamaze method in a hospital in another community. These experiences in the late 1960s astonished me and helped open my mind to the potential of drugless medicine. The Lamaze method continues to be taught in prenatal classes and is widely used to reduce or eliminate the need for medications in deliveries.

I have related these experiences to frame the discussion about alternative approaches to tension headache. I believe that our minds must remain open to these approaches while we seek for objective evidence regarding their efficacy.

POSSIBLE UNDERLYING MECHANISMS

Spasm of the head and neck muscles occurs with all types of headaches during the attack as well as during the headache-free period and, as measured by the amplitude of EMG action potentials in temporal and neck muscles, is less severe in tension-type headache than in other types of head pain according to Pozniak-Patewicz (1). Borgeat, et al. (2) showed that, with similar amounts of muscle activity before, during, and after periods of voluntary frontal mus-

cle contractions, patients with chronic tension-type headache feel more pain than normal subjects. This finding suggests that something is different in the head and neck muscles of patients with tension-type headaches. Thus increased muscular tension alone does not explain the tension-type headache pattern.

Whether tension-type headaches can be distinguished from migraine remains debatable. Headaches that are intermittent or episodic cannot be easily distinguished as migraine and often are categorized as tension-type headaches. Tension-type headaches may have other mechanisms that produce this pattern of pain rather than being only a quantitatively different clinical expression of a single centrally mediated disordered mechanism, as proposed by Raskin (3). Forssell and Kangasniemi's (4) study found that patients with tension-type headaches may be indistinguishable from patients with mandibular dysfunction. Iansek et al. (5) concluded that the incidence of headache is low in cervical spondylosis, but when headache occurs, its pattern has no features that distinguish it from tension-type headache. They suggested that the basis of headache in patients with cervical spondylosis is secondary muscle contraction. Bogduk (6) outlined a set of criteria that he believes might reveal how frequently the cervical spine is a source of headache and to what extent headache originating in the cervical spine masquerades as tension-type headache. Furthermore, myofascial trigger points in the upper trapezius muscles, when involved bilaterally, can refer pain upward along the posterolateral aspect of the neck to the mastoid process, and when intense, the referred pain can extend to the side of the head, centering in the temple and back of the orbit (7). This pattern is quite similar to tension-type headache. In addition, myofascial trigger points in the sternocleidomastoid muscles can also produce a pattern of referred pain similar to tension-type headaches. Tension-type headaches have been called "psychogenic headaches," but Packard (8) discounts the validity of such a diagnostic category. I heartily agree. However, my practice includes patients with tension-type headaches who have obvious psychological stressors that correlate well with headache activity. Thus tension-type headache is a complex syndrome for which there is probably no single mechanism; these headaches may respond to many therapeutic modalities, depending on the underlying mechanism(s).

TREATMENT

Robinson, writing in the fourth edition of *Wolff's Headache and Other Head Pain* (9), addressed the use of physical modalities in the treatment of tension-type headaches. In some patients, the application of local heat (moist and dry) or ice packs can be extremely beneficial. If the posterior neck muscles are involved, a cervical pillow is helpful. The use of a cervical collar for short periods of time can be beneficial, but rigid immobilization of the cervical spine should be avoided.

Increasingly, newspapers and magazines report disorders of the head and neck that have been produced or aggravated by environmental factors in offices and factories, such as ambient noise, fluorescent lights, and pungent odors. Maintaining certain strained postures, such as bending over a typewriter, for prolonged periods of time can produce soreness in the posterior neck. Sturgis et al. (10) have suggested that in the evaluation and treatment of tension-type headache a more dynamic movement-oriented approach would provide more meaningful information than the previous static methods because most such headaches begin while people are active. They state that electromyographic activity of cervical and facial muscles is markedly affected by a number of factors that are typically overlooked and that measuring EMG potentials in frontalis muscles in a reclining, resting subject simply cannot detect tension-type headache produced by strained postures.

Little has been written in the physical therapy literature regarding the use of diathermy, ultraviolet therapy, and massage for treatment of tension headache, although these techniques are quite often prescribed for posterior neck pain with associated tension-type headache.

Acupuncture and its application to tension-type headache has received some attention in the medical literature. For acupuncture to effectively relieve pain, the nucleus raphe magnus and endogenous opiates must be involved (11). (Chapter 46 in this textbook is devoted solely to acupuncture and explains its theoretical concepts in greater depth.) Vincent (12), using a controlled single-case design with time series analysis, concluded that acupuncture was a potentially valuable treatment for tension headache.

Hansen and Hansen (13) found that traditional Chinese acupuncture in a cross-over design was significantly more effective than placebo acupuncture and concluded that acupuncture was, therefore, a reasonable treatment for chronic tension headache. Loh et al. (14) studied the effectiveness of acupuncture versus medical treatment for migraine and tension-type headaches. They did not classify migraine and tension-type headache separately because

they believed that acupuncture was an effective prophylactic treatment for both varieties of headache. Because patients frequently have both varieties of headache and find it difficult to distinguish them when reporting their progress, these researchers believe that it is artificial to assign an individual headache to one or the other of these two categories. Although the results were not examined for statistical significance, acupuncture was clearly more effective than medical treatment. These findings indicate that acupuncture has a potential role in the treatment of tension-type headache.

Extending the acupuncture concept, Kurland (15) has offered autoacupressure as another effective therapeutic control of headache and has used it with more than 200 headache patients. The most effective main pressure point for treatment of tension-type headache is located on the back of the neck just below the occipital bone in the depression between the sternocleidomastoid and trapezius muscles, at a midpoint between the posterior midline of the neck and the top of the mastoid process.

Solomon and Guglielmo (16) treated 62 headache patients with transcutaneous electrical nerve stimulation (TENS). Using TENS equipment of low amperage and high frequency, the patients were assigned at random to one of following three groups:

1. TENS applied just above the patient's ability to perceive the stimuli (perceived stimuli);
2. TENS applied just below the perception threshold (subliminal stimuli);
3. Electrodes applied without electrical stimuli (placebo).

In the group with perceived stimuli, 55% of the patients improved, compared with 18% in the placebo group; there was a significant difference ($P<.025$) between the groups. Subliminal TENS was not statistically better than placebo. One finding of interest was that 6 of 11 patients with tension-type headache who received perceived stimuli improved, while only 2 of 20 patients with tension-type headache in the subliminal-stimuli and placebo groups improved. Thus TENS was seemingly effective for alleviating tension headache.

Farina et al. (17) used TENS to obtain exceptionally favorable clinical results in 35 patients with tension-type and mixed headache. Unfortunately, their report failed to state exactly how many patients had tension-type headache.

One hundred patients with tension-type headache were enrolled in a multicenter double-blind study to evaluate the safety and effectiveness of cranial electrotherapy. Elkind et al. (18) explained that cranial electrotherapy is distinct from TENS because the former uses a high-frequency transcranial current for pain reduction. Half of the patients received active treatment; the other half received placebo. Statistically significant differences in the global evaluation of effectiveness and in the headache severity scores favored the active treatment group. Furthermore, electrical craniotherapy appeared to be quite safe.

As stated previously, myofascial trigger points in the upper trapezius and sternocleidomastoid muscles produce referred pain patterns similar to tension-type headaches (7). The areas of referred pain show no muscular tenderness, in contradistinction to the trigger points, which are quite tender.

A myofascial trigger point is a hyperirritable point within a taut band of skeletal muscle and is located in the muscular tissue or its fascia. This locus is painful on palpation and compression and can cause characteristic referred pain and autonomic phenomena such as sweating, coryza, salivation, and localized vasoconstriction. A myofascial trigger point must be distinguished from a trigger point in other tissues, such as skin, ligaments, and periosteum.

A number of the myofascial trigger points do overlap acupuncture points that produce pain; however, non-pain-producing acupuncture points do correspond to myofascial trigger points. Each set of points is derived from vastly different concepts.

Many different therapeutic techniques have been used to deactivate myofascial trigger points. One is the stretch-and-spray technique, using a vaporcoolant substance. The second technique is ischemic compression using pressure from the fingers on the trigger point. The same effect can be achieved with various forms of massage, using kneading, deep stroking, or vibration. The third technique is puncture of the trigger points by dry needling, injection with saline, or instillation of a local anesthetic. Finally, ultrasound of low intensity has proved effective.

Vernon (19) discussed the role of the cervical spine in headache and stated that such headache is often confused with tension-type headache as well as with common migraine. Practitioners of spinal manipulation have reported success in the treatment of tension-type headaches; however, the only randomized control study dealt with common migraine and did not show that spinal manipulation was helpful.

Therapeutic touch was introduced into nursing by Krieger (20) in 1975 and is considered to be a modern derivative of the laying on of hands, which involves touching with intent to soothe or heal. All persons are considered to be highly complex fields of various forms of life energy. Life energy flows through the hands of the therapist to the recipient, who then may internalize the energy, use it to restore balance, and thereby promote self-healing.

Many nurse researchers, including Keller and Bzdek (21), have investigated the clinical therapeutic touch. They divided 60 volunteers with tension-type headache into treatment and placebo groups. They used the McGill-Melzack pain questionnaire to measure headache intensity before each intervention, immediately afterward, and again, 4 hours later. Their results showed statistically significant differences in favor of the therapeutic touch

group. Thus the study results indicated that therapeutic touch may help to reduce the pain of tension-type headache beyond the placebo effect.

I am not aware of any scientific studies in which surgical techniques have been examined as a method of treatment for tension-type headache. In my opinion, invasive techniques have at best a very limited role in the treatment of these headaches.

CONCLUSION

Writing this chapter presented a challenge that made me somewhat uneasy because there were two controversial problems involved. First, many physicians question the legitimacy of these alternative physical therapies, and second, many headache specialists believe that tension-type headache is not in itself a valid diagnostic entity. After reviewing articles for this chapter and considering these controversies, I believe that much more scientific investigation needs to be done before we dismiss these alternative therapies as ineffective. Meanwhile, we must remain open to the possibility of their efficacy, because many of our patients report that these therapies are helpful to them. Furthermore, the debate about the existence of tension-type headache will continue because we know more about what it is *not* than about what it is.

REFERENCES

1. Pozniak-Patewicz E. "Cephalgic" spasm of head and neck muscle. Headache 1976;15:261–266.
2. Borgeat F, Hade B, Elie R, Larouche LM. Effects of voluntary muscle tension increases in tension headache. Headache 1984;24:199–202.
3. Raskin NH. Headache. 2nd ed. New York: Churchill Livingstone, 1988:216.
4. Forssell H, Kangasniemi P. Mandibular dysfunction in patients with muscle contraction headache. Proc Finn Dent Soc 1984;80:211–216.
5. Iansek R, Heywood J, Karnaghan J, Balla JI. Cervical spondylosis and headaches. Clin Exp Neurol 1987;23:175–178.
6. Bogduk N. Headaches and the cervical spine (editorial). Cephalalgia 1984;4:7–8.
7. Travell JG, Simons DG. Myofascial pain and dysfunction: the trigger point manual. Baltimore: Williams & Wilkins, 1983:184–206.
8. Packard RC. What is psychogenic headache? Headache 1976;16:20–23.
9. Robinson CA. Cervical spondylosis and muscle contraction headaches. In: Dalessio DJ, ed. Wolff's headache and other head pain. 4th ed. New York: Oxford University Press, 1980:362–380.
10. Sturgis ET, Schaefer CA, Ahles TA, Sikora TL. Effect of movement and position in the evaluation of tension headache and nonheadache control subjects. Headache 1984;24:88–93.
11. Chung H, Dickenson A. Pain, enkephalin and acupuncture. Nature 1980;283:243–244.
12. Vincent CA. The treatment of tension headache by acupuncture: a controlled single case design with time series analysis. J Psychom Res 1990;34:553–561.
13. Hansen PE, Hansen JH. Acupuncture treatment of chronic tension headache: a controlled cross-over trial. Cephalgia 1985;5:137–142.
14. Loh L, Nathan PW, Schott GD, Zilkha KJ. Acupuncture versus medial treatment for migraine and muscle tension headaches. J Neurol Neurosurg Psychiatry 1984;47:333–337.

15. Kurland HD. Treatment of headache with auto-acupressure. Curr Psychiatr Ther 1977;17:271–274.
16. Solomon S, Guglielmo KM. Treatment of headache by transcutaneous electrical stimulation. Headache 1985;25:12–15.
17. Farina S, Granella F, Malferrari G, Manzoni GC. Headache and cervical spine disorders: classification and treatment with transcutaneous electrical nerve stimulation. Headache 1986;26:431–433.
18. Solomon S, Elkind A, Freitag F, et al. Safety and effectiveness of cranial electrotherapy in the treatment of tension headache. Headache 1989;29:445–450.
19. Vernon HT. Spinal manipulation and headaches of cervical origin. J Manipulative Physiol Ther 1989;12:455–468.
20. Krieger D. Therapeutic touch: the imprimatur of nursing. Am J Nurs 1975;75:784–787.
21. Keller E, Bzdek VM. Effects of therapeutic touch on tension headache pain. Nurs Res 1986;35:101–106.

20

Biofeedback and Psychotherapy in the Treatment of Muscle Contraction/Tension-Type Headache

BARRY A. REICH and MALCOLM GOTTESMAN

It is estimated that over 90% of all headaches that result in treatment by a physician fall into the category of tension-type or muscle contraction headache. Tension-type headache is responsible for the loss of approximately 156.9 million work days (in the United States alone) every year (1). Tension-type headache (previously referred to as tension headache or muscle contraction headache (2) is a ubiquitous disorder whose pathophysiological basis is controversial. Multiple factors have been implicated, including disordered autonomic function, vascular and humoral instability, central and peripheral pain threshold abnormalities, muscle ischemia, psychological stress, and psychiatric disorder. Ostfeld (3) and Wolff (4) postulated that muscle contraction (tension) headache was due to elevated tonus of neck and scalp muscles. The premise underlying muscle contraction headache is that pain is a function of excessive muscle activity. This muscle activity may even reflect a wider component of central neurophysiological hypersensitivity or pathology. Tension-type headache pain is usually bilateral and/or occipitofrontal and is usually manifested along the insertion mass of the suboccipital muscles. These muscles and others in the cephalic nuchal region used in postural positioning of the head are believed to be the prime instigators of muscle contraction headache pain (3–8).

Episodic tension-type headache usually responds quickly to intervention via use of minor analgesics and sedation. However daily or long-term use of such intervention creates a myriad of problems including tolerance, withdrawal, and addictive potential. Withdrawal of such medications can cause tension-type symptoms in patients who were previously headache free. Thus, the chronic tension-type headache poses a more complex problem that necessitates a multimodal approach including self-regulatory and insight techniques such as biofeedback and psychotherapy.

Electromyography (EMG) was introduced into the medical field by Adrian and Bonk (9) in 1929. But it was not until the late 1940s and 1950s that EMG was recognized as a diagnostic and rehabilitative procedure. Early studies using EMG biofeedback techniques for headache intervention (5, 10, 11) appeared to demonstrate that controlling or relaxing the frontalis or other scalp muscles could result in reduced headache distress. Budzinsky et al. (10) initially reported a 0.90 correlation between reduction in headache activity indicated by an individual and achieved reduction in frontalis EMG level. However, many studies indicate that recording activity of the frontalis muscle alone does not sufficiently reflect diffuse cranial/cervical muscular dysfunction. It is this diffuse dysfunctional muscle activity that correlates with most self-reported headache activity. It appears that the limited early protocols that examined singular muscles did not reliably discriminate headache sufferers from nonheadache subjects.

There is considerable disagreement about the correlation of the patient's perception of headache episode or pain and the degree of heightened EMG activity measured. Indeed, the most recent classification by the Headache Classification Committee of the International Headache Society: Classification and diagnostic criteria for headache disorders, cranial neuralgia and facial pain (2) even acknowledges that "tension" headaches may occur without hypersensitivity or contraction noted in the muscles.

PSYCHOPHYSIOLOGICAL CONCEPTS OF TENSION-TYPE HEADACHE

Muscular Findings

Arena et al. (12) investigated the relationship between muscle tension levels in the forehead and neck regions of headache sufferers. The researchers found that "headache sufferers had more clinically significant EMG abnormalities (60%) than controls (13%). Sherman et al. (13) investigated the relationship between continuous environmental recordings of "trunk muscle tension" and tension headaches. Patients wore a one-channel surface EMG recorder during waking hours for 4 to 5 days. A headache log was also kept. Tension headache sufferers showed a significant relationship between an increase in upper back muscle tension preceding increased headache activity and decreased muscle tension prior to reported decreases in pain.

Presently, clinicians using biofeedback intervention consider the specific examination site being measured, the EMG amplitude, and the pattern observed in determining the overall significance of the measurement. Testing or observing singular cranial muscles (e.g., frontalis, temporalis, occipitalis) does not seem beneficial in the treatment of muscle contraction headache. Cram (14) has been a major proponent of the neuromuscular scanning technique as being most appropriate for offering a diagnostic and rehabilitative framework for tension-type headache.

Hatch et al. (15) recently examined pericranial muscle tenderness and EMG activity in subjects with "episodic tension-type headache" and headache-free controls. Muscle tenderness was measured by a neurologist palpating suboccipital, posterior cervical, upper trapezius, sternocleidomastoid, masseter, and temporalis muscles (bilateral). The patient's tenderness was then recorded on a 4-point scale. EMG activity was measured from the frontal, posterior, cervical, and temporal (bilateral) regions. All readings and palpations were conducted while the patients were "headache-free." The results indicated a significant correlation between muscle tenderness and headache disorder. EMG amplitude was not correlated with headache disorder. There was no significance, but a weak association was observed between palpated muscle tenderness and EMG elevation. The authors concluded that "elevated pericranial EMG activity and muscle tenderness may index different aspects of abnormal muscle function."

The fact that abnormal tonus can be observed in one muscle site as a basic response to muscle overload in another area that has become inhibited must be taken into consideration. Training a patient to release or relax the elevated tonus in an individual muscle offers little knowledge of how this change would effect overall function in the surrounding musculature. Muscles that reveal high EMG recordings at rest may simply reflect adaptive lengthening, as a result of other dysfunctional muscles that have shortened. For instance, Headley (16) noted that a muscle stretched for prolonged periods has increased EMG activity. This observation makes clear that static and dynamic muscle EMG biofeedback must be involved, not only from a diagnostic point of view, but also with respect to selecting a training procedure to permit maximum rehabilitation. In the healthy body, muscles work by a pattern of complex interactions feeding back via a centralized loop. They do not work individually to accomplish movement or support.

Some researchers (17, 18) observed the relationship between hyperactivity of cranial muscles and reported pain during tension-type headache by having headache patients increase the muscle tonus via biofeedback techniques. An assessment of pain was made during and after the contraction, which was sustained for periods up to 5 minutes. Some patients showed a closer relationship than others

between head pain and muscle tension as measured by their responses to the voluntary muscle tonus increase.

The ability of the muscle to reveal normal characteristics after successive or sustained activity is most important. Almost all muscle contraction patients seem to complain of increased pain peaking after fatigue, stress, or overactivity. Inhibition of muscle activity following trauma may be a secondary cause of ischemia and cause cephalalgia (19). Increased pain works in a cyclical manner to increase reactive muscle tonus, which feeds back, causing additional vasoconstriction/ischemia and increased nociceptor sensitivity. Improper posture during the day can be a major contributor to excessive or overly sustained muscle activity. Additionally, there may be a relationship between time of day (circadian rhythmic pattern) and pain sensitivity of the pericranial musculature. Goebell and Cordes (20) noted significant differences in pain sensitivity correlated with time of day. Pain sensitivity was observed to be highest at 2 AM and lowest at 2 PM.

Blood Flow

Sustained contraction of muscles produces local ischemia and associated release of interstitial substances associated with increased nociception. Ischemia of scalp muscles, causing the accumulation of toxic metabolites, has long been considered a source of pain in tension-type headache (1). The occurrence of constricted conjunctival vessels during tension-type headache, the amelioration of pain with vasodilating agents (amyl nitrate, ethyl alcohol, and nicotinic acid), as well as diminished temporal artery pulse amplitude (21) have reinforced a vascular etiology of tension-type headaches.

Despite these observations, convincing evidence supporting muscle ischemia is lacking. Normal resting blood flow was recorded in 40 tension headache sufferers by injection of radioactive xenon-133 into the temporalis muscle (22). Most of the patients were experiencing headache at the time of the study. Interestingly, reactive hyperfusion after isometric contraction occurred in a greater percentage of tension headache patients than in controls. Onel (23) found increased Na^+-24 clearance. Xenon-133 inhalation studies indicate normal cerebral blood flow in tension headache sufferers (24, 25). Surface blood flow was measured in the face, temple, and neck regions of 21 tension headache sufferers (26). Results indicated that 52% of tension headache sufferers displayed vascular abnormalities as indicated by examination with video thermogram. In an experiment conducted by Chatman et al. (27), tension-type headache sufferers who learned to lower EMG levels did not exhibit an expected facilitation of skin temperature control. Diminished platelet serotonin levels have also been reported in tension-type headache patients (28–30).

The simple willful contraction of a muscle for a prolonged period of time may be followed by a period of reported discomfort far exceeding the time the muscle was in the contractile phase. Individual functional norms for muscle activity have been noted and may vary widely. There is recognition that both sustained muscle tonus and vascular anomalies are involved in the tension-type headache syndrome. However, the interrelationship and underlying cause has not been fully delineated.

Vascular/Tension-Type Headache Relationship

Traditionally, tension and migraine headaches were considered to be distinct entities. Many researchers now believe similar mechanisms are responsible for both. Saper (31) and Takashima (32) noted the frequent progression of intermittent migraine to daily chronic tension-type headache. Iacono and Koellner (33) conducted diagnostic EMG scanning of asymptomatic and then symptomatic migraineurs. Investigating the role of muscle contraction activity in this population, the authors found significant elevation of temporalis, masseter, trapezius, T6, and cervical paraspinal muscles during headache activity. The elevated EMG was not evident during nonmigraine state. The authors concluded that muscle tension may play a role in predisposing an individual to migraine activity and sustaining such activity. Langemark (34) studied 58 migraine patients. Of these, 15 eventually developed chronic tension-type headache. Sixteen migraineurs who initially experienced tension headache, later developed migraine. Other researchers have noted consistent increases in muscle activity as measured by EMG, and self-reported increases in muscle tenderness associated with migraine episodes (35–39).

Altered cardiac, vascular, and pupillary sympathetic functions have been observed in tension-type headache patients. Contrary to what occurs in a migraine attack, the scalp blood vessels constrict during an attack (40). This led Sargent et al. (41) to investigate the use of a temperature biofeedback device and relaxation procedures with tension-type headache patients. Patients who learned blood flow control were successful in moderating headache distress. Recent use of vasodilator medication has been shown to relieve accompanying pain (42). Additional studies found cardiovascular sympathetic hypofunction in tension-type headache patients by observing that systolic blood pressure readings were lower in headache sufferers after isometric activity. This same observation was made in migraine headache sufferers but not in control subjects. In addition, plasma norepinephrine levels were significantly reduced in both muscle contraction and migraine sufferers (compared with nonheadache controls) observed in orthostatic and isometric work tests. Such observations have given rise to the theory that a common central defective aminergic process may be present in muscle contraction and migraine patients.

Central and Autonomic Factors

Increased extracranial muscle sensitivity to pressure-induced pain has been demonstrated in tension headache

patients (43, 44). Langemark (43) found that tension-type headache sufferers had increased hand and scalp sensitivity to thermal pain, supporting the concept of a centrally mediated disorder of pain perception. Drummond (44), however, found no alteration in finger pain sensitivity.

Mikamo (45) found reduced supine plasma norepinephrine levels, lesser increases in norepinephrine concentration upon standing, and more pronounced drop in blood pressure in tension-type headache sufferers than in controls. Ellersten et al. (46) noted diminished changes in heart rate when tension headache patients were exposed to auditory stimuli. Additionally, augmented sympathetic activity has been found in tension-type headache sufferers. Gannon (47) exposed tension headache patients to a cognitive stressor and found increased heart rate. Pupillary sympathetic hypofunction has been observed in tension headache patients. Takeshima (48) found a reduced rate of pupillary dilation (sympathetically mediated), in addition to diminished pupillary size following dark adaption. Shimomara (49) demonstrated that darkness induced statistically significant asymmetric pupillary dilation (physiological pupillary test); however, immersion of the hand in cold water (Hines-Brown pressor test) produced normal pupillary responses. The direct instillation of tyramine (a sympathomimetic agent) into the eye caused more dilation of the pupil in tension headache patients than in controls. The authors concluded that the tyramine test indicated sympathetic hyperfunction; however an enhanced pupillary response would be expected if denervation hypersensitivity was present secondary to central sympathetic hypofunction. Abnormal smooth pursuit and saccadic eye movements have been noted in tension headache patients (50).

Electrical stimulation of the labial commissure during jaw clenching results in two brief periods of suppression of temporalis activity, the trigeminally mediated inhibitory jaw-closing reflex. Diminished amplitude of the second response (the late exteroceptive suppressor reflex) occurred in both tension-type headache and migraine patients, suggesting an abnormality of the trigeminal system (51). Somatosensory evoked potentials obtained by median nerve stimulation in tension headache patients have been reported to be normal (52). The psychogalvanic reflex response, a presumed indicator of sympathetic activity, was more reactive in tension-type headache patients than in controls or in migraine patients (53).

Psychological Features

Clinicians (54, 55) have long been aware of the high incidence of stress and depression in tension-type headache sufferers, at least from the time of Sigmund Freud, who postulated that unconscious conflict was evidenced as head pain (56). Friedman (57) reviewed 1000 cases and felt emotional factors were present 100% of the time. A retrospective review (58) of emergency room patients evaluated for tension headaches revealed that more than half of the patients were suffering from "anxiety or depression." Saper (59) studied 515 daily headache sufferers. Eighty-six percent were depressed; 50% had sleep disturbance. An increased incidence of alcoholism and depression was found in family members. Saper also reported that 26% of the 515 headache patients had abnormal dexamethasone suppression tests. The dexamethasone suppression test is a biological marker for major vegetative depression. Additionally, Saper reported diminished endorphin levels in patients with daily chronic headache. In contrast, Tuchman (60) found normal dexamethasone suppression test results in 20 outpatients who were diagnosed as "chronic muscle headache sufferers."

BIOFEEDBACK

Historical Relationship to Headache

Sainsbury and Gibson, in 1954, were the first in published literature to use EMG to detect the accompanying physiological change noted in "tension headache" sufferers (61). They found that the static baseline EMG activity was higher in headache sufferers than in the normal population. Since that time, the field has evolved to use sophisticated protocols that involve the surface scanning of numerous muscles via electromyograph. Currently, the recording of electrical activity displayed at rest and during and after voluntary activity is used to diagnose and treat tension-type headache.

Theoretical Basis and Physiological Observations

Biofeedback is the second most utilized method for the control of chronic headache (medication is the most widely used). Biofeedback intervention used for the tension-type headache patient can involve training the patient to be aware of muscle tonus and to voluntarily alter tonus and the contractile characteristics of the targeted muscle(s), or be used as a technique to enhance the overall relaxation response. Relaxation training and biofeedback produce physiological changes that include decreased oxygen consumption and diminished CO_2 elimination, decreased respiratory and heart rates, and lowered blood pressure. There is also an increased amount of alpha and theta activity on EEG (62).

Biofeedback probably induces a generalized relaxation response while specifically focusing on musculoskeletal training. Biofeedback breaks the maladaptive feedback cycle (Fig 20.1). In this paradigm, pain is the first feedback patients receive. At this point the pathological processes are well in motion and not easily corrected.

Biofeedback allows patients to diminish their arousal state and level of muscular activity with instrument-gained information rather than by relying on the perception of pain as the feedback modality, as depicted in Figure 20.2. Excessive muscular activity may not be the cause of muscle tension headache pain, but decreased muscular activity appears to be an essential component of successful biofeedback therapy.

Relationship of Headache to EMG Activity

EMG characteristics such as amplitude, number of spikes, rise time, and amplitude-rise time alter during changes in muscle tension. Basmajian (63) quite succinctly states "given visual and auditory cues through electronic amplification and feedback, subjects can be quickly trained to consciously activate motoneurons with great precision."

Although initial publications stressed a relationship between resting activity of the frontalis muscle and reported headache, a plethora of research has indicated that there is not a simple correlation. Haynes et al. (64) demonstrated little correlation between the observed EMG level of the frontalis muscle and patient-reported headache. Some individuals displaying high EMG levels reported no tension headaches, yet others reported many headaches. Contrasting results were also reported (65, 66) that demonstrated the amount of reduction in (muscle contraction) headache activity to be proportional to the degree of EMG change obtained. The early practice of solely observing the overall electrical activity (representing the motoneuron innervation) of frontalis or other pericranial muscles has been found to be inadequate to explain and treat muscle contraction headache (67–69). Shedivy and Kleinman (67) demon-

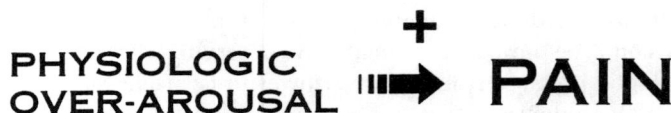

Figure 20.1.   Maladaptive pain feedback cycle.

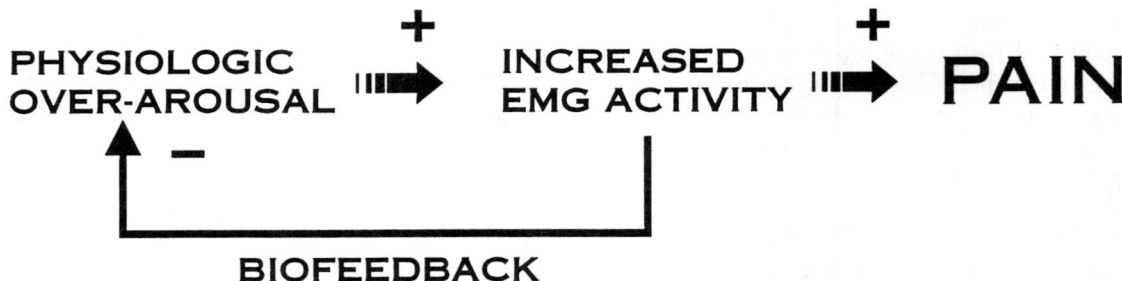

Figure 20.2.   Biofeedback modified pain cycle.

strated that having subjects voluntarily increase frontalis EMG tonus levels had no significant effect on the measurable variances in sternocleidomastoid and semispinalis/splenius EMG activity. This observation led the authors to conclude that "changes in frontalis EMG neither generalize to other somatic muscles nor correlate with verbal reports of cognitive tension or relaxation."

Additional research conducted by Cleary and Carlson (70) indicates that frontalis biofeedback alone is relatively ineffective in reducing peripheral and autonomic activity; however, multisite EMG training appears to be an effective mediator for producing a generalized decrease in arousal. Pozniak-Patewicz (35) proffered that muscle spasm noted in tension headache sufferers may be a "consequence rather than a cause of headache." Qualls and Sheehan (71) reviewed a number of studies that compared the degree of muscle relaxation attained via an EMG biofeedback technique with that attained using other training conditions. The dependent measure was frontalis EMG activity. The results indicate that EMG biofeedback was of equal or greater value in "reducing levels of muscle tension or alleviating tension-related behaviors." Two recent meta-analysis studies (72, 73) that observed the relationship of tension-type headache and EMG biofeedback treatment were limited in their scope to the use of the frontalis attachment; a testament to the original concept and assumed importance of this now-antiquated muscle measurement. Burg et al. (74) conducted a prospective study of 100 chronic tension-type headache patients. The research was concerned with documenting the frequency of pericranial muscle disorders noted in the tension-type patient population. The results indicated that 100% of the patients had significant pericranial muscle dysfunction.

Thus, to use EMG biofeedback as a training protocol, the clinician must possess a thorough knowledge of the muscle interrelationships that can reveal patterns amenable to intervention via such techniques. The lack of a direct positive relationship between resting muscle tonus level and reported headache activity may reflect the fact that the proper breadth of EMG measurements was not made. The main responsibility of the biofeedback clinician is to possess comprehensive knowledge of the field. Underlying the basic premise of biofeedback training is the ability of the patients to generalize the "learning" of physiological control so that they can generalize their response across the situations that they approach in everyday life. By using multichannel EMG equipment, patients can be taught to have a better understanding of the inner functioning of their bodies. The visual or audio feedback provides an additional sensory modality for the patient to enhance knowledge and ultimately gain control over dysfunctional physiological states. According to Bandura (75), individuals gain "self-efficacy" as they are placed in a control mode, no longer perceiving themselves simply as victims of their discomfort and pain. This process therefore allows in-creased physiological control and enhanced psychological feelings of well-being.

Research has demonstrated that for biofeedback training to be effective as a treatment intervention, "true" contingent learning of the physiological response appears efficacious. Reich (76–78), among others (71, 79, 80), has noted that the number of training sessions of biofeedback undertaken by the patient correlates positively with successful outcome. The appropriate generalization of learned physiological response across situations has been demonstrated in numerous studies (81).

Current Clinical Observations

BIOFEEDBACK COMPARED WITH OTHER NONINVASIVE TREATMENTS

Reich (76) studied biofeedback treatment for muscle contraction headache sufferers over a 3- to 4-year period. Five hundred twenty-two subjects (240 male, 282 female) were randomly assigned to one of four groups: (a) relaxation group—receiving cognitively oriented psychotherapy, hypnosis, autogenic training/progressive muscle relaxation, either singly or in combination; (b) electrical stimulation group—receiving traditional TENS or neurotransmitter modulation (electrical stimulation administered at subthreshold levels, which significantly elevates serotonin); (c) biofeedback group—receiving EMG biofeedback to trapezius, paracervical, and frontalis muscles; and (d) multimodal group—receiving any combination of two of the above treatment group modalities. Additionally, within each group, subjects were bifurcated into subgroups—those receiving over 15 treatment sessions and those receiving between 10 and 15 treatments. Each treatment was administered once per week. All the patients except the electrical stimulation group were instructed to follow practice schedules at home. Patients practiced three times per day for 10 minutes at a time. The electrical stimulation group participants were given home units and directed to administer stimulation/treatment once daily for 30 minutes according to the specific electrode placements.

Patients kept daily headache logs indicating frequency of headache and degree of pain over the course of treatment and the 36 months following discharge from treatment. A total of 311 (150 male and 161 female) patients returned sufficient data to be included in the repeated measures design. A copy of the headache treatment logs used for assessing patients is included in Appendix 20.1. Note that the patient is required to assess the degree of pain experienced during specific time blocks corresponding to a 24-hour day. The setting the patient was in, the associated activities, whether the patient was alone or with others (and whom), the patient's thoughts, mood, medication, and exercise involvement, and additional factors were included in the multivariate analysis. The logs were kept for 14 days in succession at each collection point in the study. In addition, a McGill-type log and the "Carnick Head/

Line" patient headache checklist were filled out during the same period.

Results indicated that the most effective treatment for reducing headache symptoms for tension-type headache patients was biofeedback. The subjects participating in this longitudinal study indicated an average of 31.1 hours of headache pain per week prior to intervention. At discharge, the patients indicated an average of only 1.25 hours of pain per week. Patients in the other groups indicated an average of 29.6 hours of headache at intake and 10.2 hours per week at discharge. These differences remained relatively consistent throughout the follow-up period. Patients in the biofeedback group reported an average of 1.5 hours per week of headache pain at 36 months after discharge from treatment. The patients in the other groups indicated an average of 14 hours of headache distress. All comparisons were statistically tested using Duncan's multiple range test and were significant at the .001 level.

Degree of pain revealed a similar pattern. There was no significant difference in reported degree of pain between the patients assigned to the treatment groups at intake. Patients who received biofeedback treatment reported the greatest reduction in degree of pain experienced during headache episodes, compared with patients in all the other treatment groups (P<.0001). This pattern also remained relatively consistent over time.

One of the most striking observations of this study was that within the biofeedback group the most important feature was the number of sessions attended by the patient. The patients who attended more than 15 sessions maintained both their decreased pain level and decreased frequency of headache better than those who attended fewer treatment sessions. Additionally, chronicity of tension-type headache was an important outcome variable. Patients who reported having headaches for more than 2 years demonstrated higher frequency of headache at discharge and throughout the follow-up, compared with patients who sought biofeedback treatment earlier. These findings were also observed by other researchers (82). Both groups, however, indicated comparable hours of reported headache at intake. Length of time of prior symptoms did not distinguish the treatment in terms of reduction of degree of reported headache pain for tension-type headache sufferers.

Since this study was published, in 1989, an additional 24 months of data have been collected on 297 of the original participants. The data reveal a continued significant beneficial effect of biofeedback, compared with all other treatment modalities. Specifically, significantly fewer episodes of headache and lessened intensity (when it does occur) were observed for the patients comprising the biofeedback group (P<.0001).

TRICYCLIC MEDICATION AND BIOFEEDBACK

Most recently, our center completed a longitudinal study of tension headache sufferers using interventions consisting of EMG biofeedback alone or EMG biofeedback combined with amitriptyline HCl. Tricyclic medications are one of the preferred pharmacological agents for tension-type headache prophylaxis (83). The benefits of this class of medications seem to be independent of their antidepressant action. Holroyd et al. (84) note that the effectiveness of antidepressant medication is unrelated to the presence or absence of depressive features, as tension headaches appear to respond more quickly (often within 1 week) and at a lower dose (often 25 to 75 mg/day) than does depression (21, 84–87).

While the precise mechanism of tricyclic medication tension-type headache prophylaxis is unknown, it has been widely presumed to depend upon its blockade of serotonin and norepinephrine reuptake (84, 87, 88).

The purpose of this study was to compare the effectiveness of a combined medication (amitriptyline)/biofeedback treatment group with a group being treated solely with biofeedback. The combined group was used, rather than a medication-alone group, to control for the number and type of clinician contact/interactions. Would the use of tricyclic medication facilitate biofeedback intervention for tension-type headache pain reduction?

Fifty (50) adult tension-type headache sufferers (26 male and 24 female), who were referred by their neurologists to the Nassau Pain and Stress Center, were studied over a 24-month period. All subjects had the diagnosis of muscle contraction/tension-type headache (according to the Ad Hoc Committee on the Classification of Headache—1962).

All subjects reported experiencing headache for over 36 months before entering the treatment program (range of 36 to 110 months, X = 58). None of the subjects had experienced intervention via biofeedback or tricyclic medication prior to entry into the treatment program. All subjects were off all prescription medication for at least 2 months prior to entry into the treatment program.

The subjects were randomly assigned to either of two groups:

Treatment group 1. Electromyograph biofeedback;
Treatment group 2. Electromyograph biofeedback & tricyclic medication.

Biofeedback consisted of a weekly 45-minute session, given for 30 weeks. Patients were taught to voluntarily control amplitude and hyperirritability in the suboccipital, posterior cervical, upper trapezius, sternocleidomastoid, and masseter muscle regions. By the time patients were discharged from the program, all had indicated significant EMG amplitude reductions in at least 3 of the measured muscle groups.

The tricyclic medication used was amytriptyline HCl. Medication was started at 25 mg h.s. for 5 days and then increased to 75 mg h.s. and continued for 15 months. The patients were then slowly titrated off all medication by the end of month 16.

Patients indicated frequency, intensity, and duration of

AVERAGE FREQUENCY OF HEADACHE OVER TIME

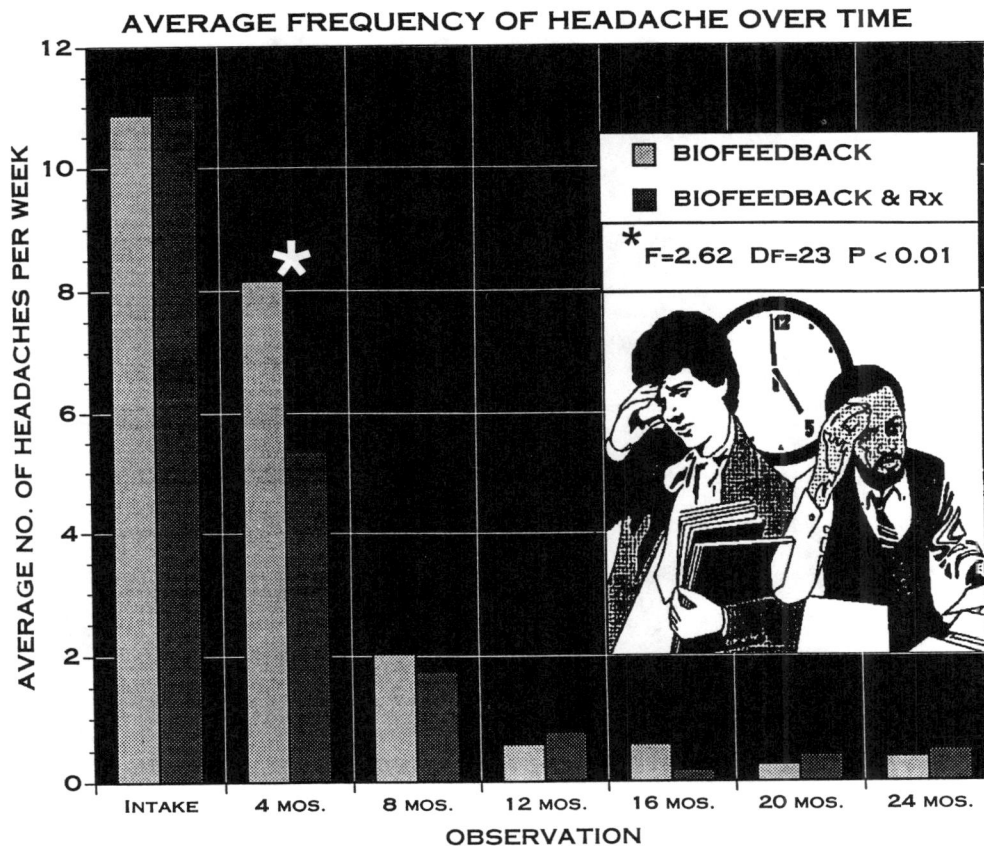

Figure 20.3. Average frequency of headache over time.

pain prior to entry into the program and at 4-month intervals thereafter, for a period of 24 months, via a "McGill-type" self-report questionnaire. In addition, the patients reported medication compliance, perceived psychological stress, and physical activity, and female patients tracked menses.

At intake, the two treatment groups did not differ statistically in gender or reported frequency, intensity, or duration of headache.

A significant reduction in the frequency, intensity, and duration of tension-type headache over the study period was observed, without regard to the grouping variable.

Frequency Results. The frequency of headache was reduced at a significantly faster rate for the patients in the combined biofeedback/medication group than for the patients in the biofeedback alone group. However, by the 8-month assessment, there was no longer a significant difference between the groups in frequency of headache episodes.

Intensity Results. Although a significant overall effect was found for reduction in intensity for both treatment groups, there were no differences observed between the treatment groups over time.

Duration Results. A significant difference was observed between the two treatment groups over time concerning the duration of headache. Patients in the biofeed-

back-alone group reported significantly less duration of headache at 4-, 20-, and 24-month assessment periods than patients in the combined biofeedback/medication group.

Male/Female Differences. No significant differences were found between the male patients of each group.

Female patients in the combined biofeedback/medication group reported a significantly lowered frequency of headache at the 4-month observation period than their counterparts in the biofeedback-alone group. This difference was not found during later observations.

The differences observed for female patients suggests that tricyclic medication provides a faster pathway of headache intervention for female tension-type sufferers. 5-Hydroxytryptamine (5-HT) levels have been documented to vary during menses. It is also known that 5-HT concentrations in platelets are significantly lower in patients with chronic tension-type headache than in controls and appear to play a role in the etiology of tension-type headache (30, 89, 90). A serotonergic-enhancing medication, such as amitriptyline, may act differentially upon female and male patients.

Consistency of Learned EMG Control. Just after the 24-month data-collection period, all patients were invited back to our center to have a free consultation and examination. As part of this examination, EMG readings were taken of all muscle groups originally measured in the

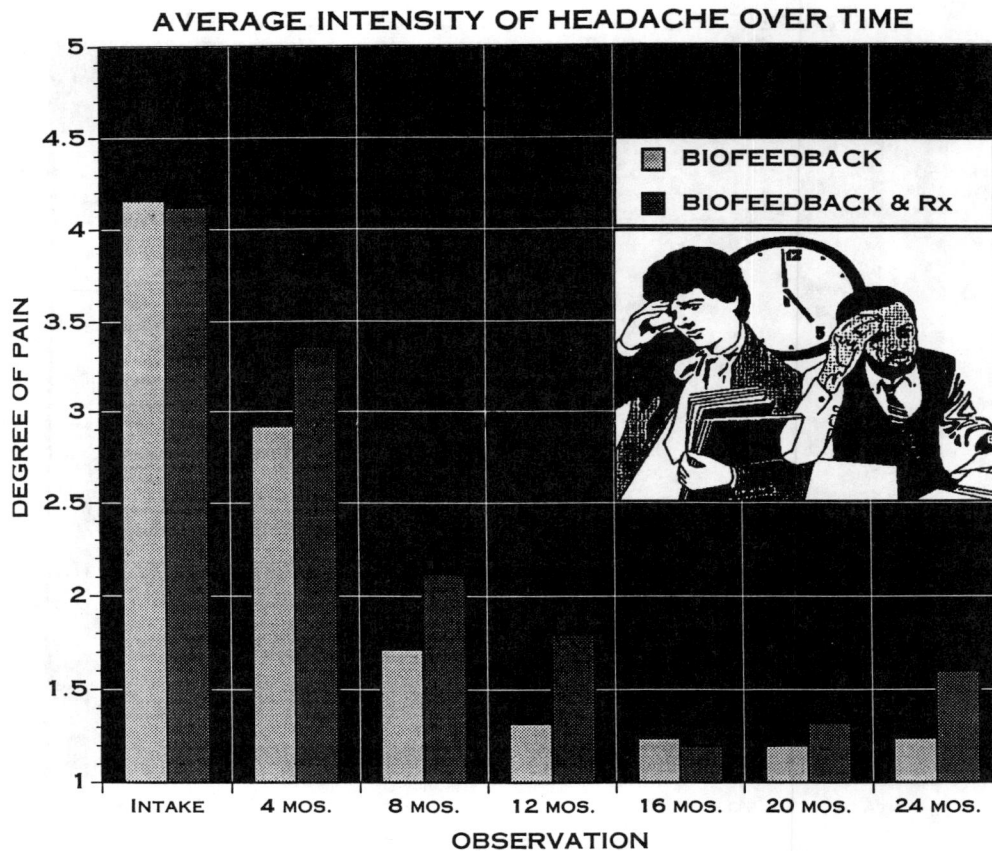

Figure 20.4. Average intensity of headache over time.

study. Thirteen female and 9 male patients agreed to participate in the follow-up. Thirteen subjects were from the biofeedback-alone group (8 female and 5 male) and 9 patients were from the combined biofeedback/medication group (5 female and 4 male). Systematic observation of electrode sites in sitting and standing positions, before and after isometric activity, indicated maintenance of significantly lowered EMG levels, compared with readings observed at initial intake. Furthermore, there was a significant difference observed between the two groups, with patients in the biofeedback-alone condition demonstrating a greater reduction in EMG measurements over time. No sex differences were observed.

Discussion. Both treatment groups displayed a significant reduction in dependent measures over time. However, differences observed between the groups indicate that specific mechanisms may be proffered as influencing the results.

Combined biofeedback/medication patients displayed a significantly greater reduction in the frequency of headache at the 4-month observation period. This may be because medication acted as a quicker mediator of headache, prior to any effect of physiological control being learned via biofeedback.

The fact that these differences were not observed for later time periods seems to reflect the finding that multi-

ple-site EMG biofeedback training typically takes more than 15 sessions to be mastered (76, 77, 80). At the 4-months observation, patients had had approximately 16 training sessions. As the biofeedback-group members had more sessions and became more proficient in their skills, the initial observed difference was no longer noticeable.

Interestingly, at the 16-month observation, a difference approaching significance was again noticed as the biofeedback/medication group demonstrated a trend toward a lower frequency of headache episodes. This may be ascribed to the finding that as individuals were phased off medication they became aware of the increased attention from the clinicians (Hawthorne effect). At the next two observation points, the trend actually reversed itself, with the biofeedback-alone group demonstrating less frequent tension-type episodes, at a level approaching statistical significance.

Although there was a significant reduction reported by both groups in the observed intensity of headache episodes over the assessment period, there were no between-treatment interactions noted.

Self-reported duration of headache showed marked, significant differences over time between the two treatment groups. Patients in the biofeedback-alone group reported headaches to be significantly shorter than those of patients in the combined biofeedback/medication group. This find-

AVERAGE NO. OF HOURS OF HEADACHE OVER TIME

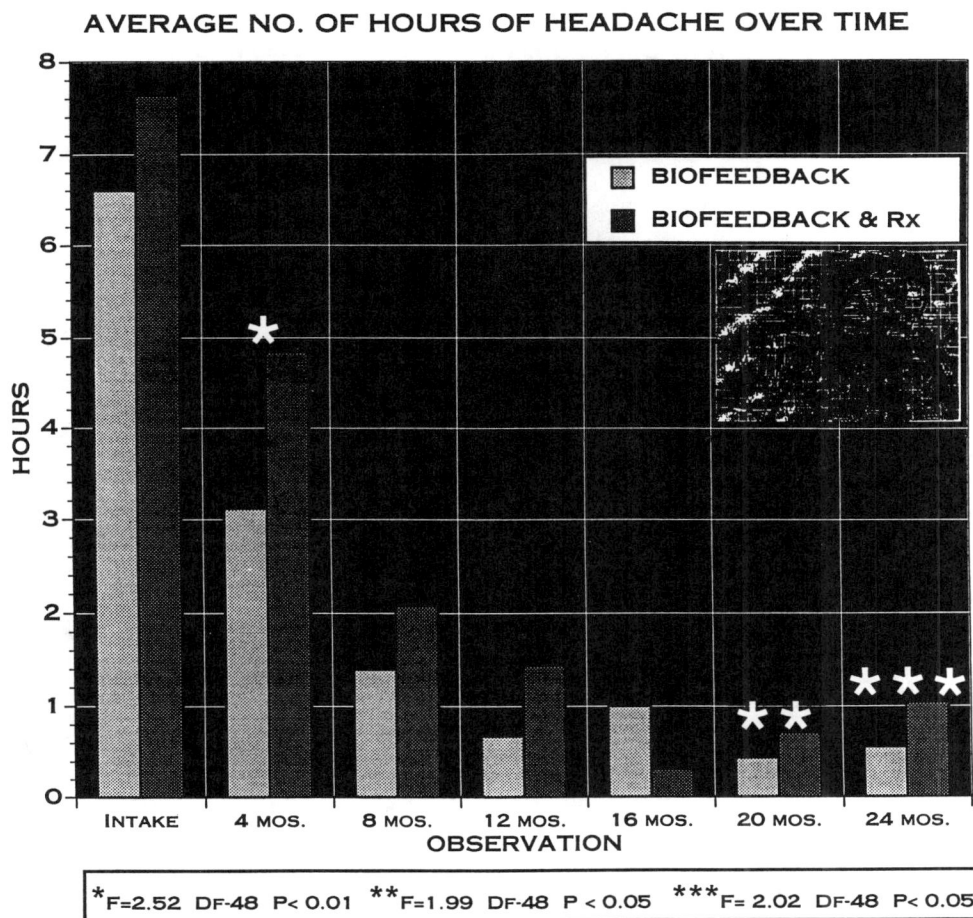

Figure 20.5. Average number of hours of headache over time.

ing may be attributed to the fact that the biofeedback alone group was less likely to look for outside (medication) intervention and took a more active involvement in the control of their headaches. This appears most noticeable at the 20- and 24-month observation periods, when the combined group was no longer taking any medication and displayed an increasing trend toward significantly longer headaches. Additional support for this concept is given by the finding that maintenance of lowered EMG levels was superior for the biofeedback group patients (versus the combined group) after the 24-month period.

Summary. Both treatment groups (biofeedback-alone and biofeedback coupled with tricyclic medication) displayed significant reduction in reported frequency, intensity, and duration of tension-type episodes over the 2-year observation period. The noninvasive, self-regulatory technique of EMG biofeedback appears to offer effective, reproducible, and consistent prophylactic treatment for tension-type headache attacks. These findings are similar to results by Bruhn et al. (91) that found biofeedback to be superior to standard pharmacological treatment in reducing tension-type headache symptomatology.

However, it appears that if quick reduction in the fre-

quency of headache is sought, the addition of tricyclic medication to a biofeedback regime may be used. This addition offers only a slight advantage, which may not outweigh the unwanted possibility of side effects associated with tricyclic medication (anticholinergic effects, weight gain, sluggishness, orthostatic hypotension, etc).

Additionally, the patient's dependence on or expectation of taking medication may actually undermine the intensity or effort applied to learning physiological control via the biofeedback training.

Although much is offered by this study to inspire additional follow-up research, we may conclude that if we have a motivated, diligent patient base, the noninvasive technique of biofeedback training offers effective, significant, consistent prophylaxis of chronic tension-type headache.

PSYCHOLOGICAL MANAGEMENT OF TENSION-TYPE HEADACHE

Relaxation training and various other behavioral interventions are the most commonly used nonpharmacological interventions for tension-type headache. Review studies indicate successful outcomes to range from 20 to over 60%. Holroyd et al. (84) recently found that 94% of tension-type

AVERAGE FREQUENCY OF HEADACHE OVER TIME
REPORTED BY FEMALE PATIENTS

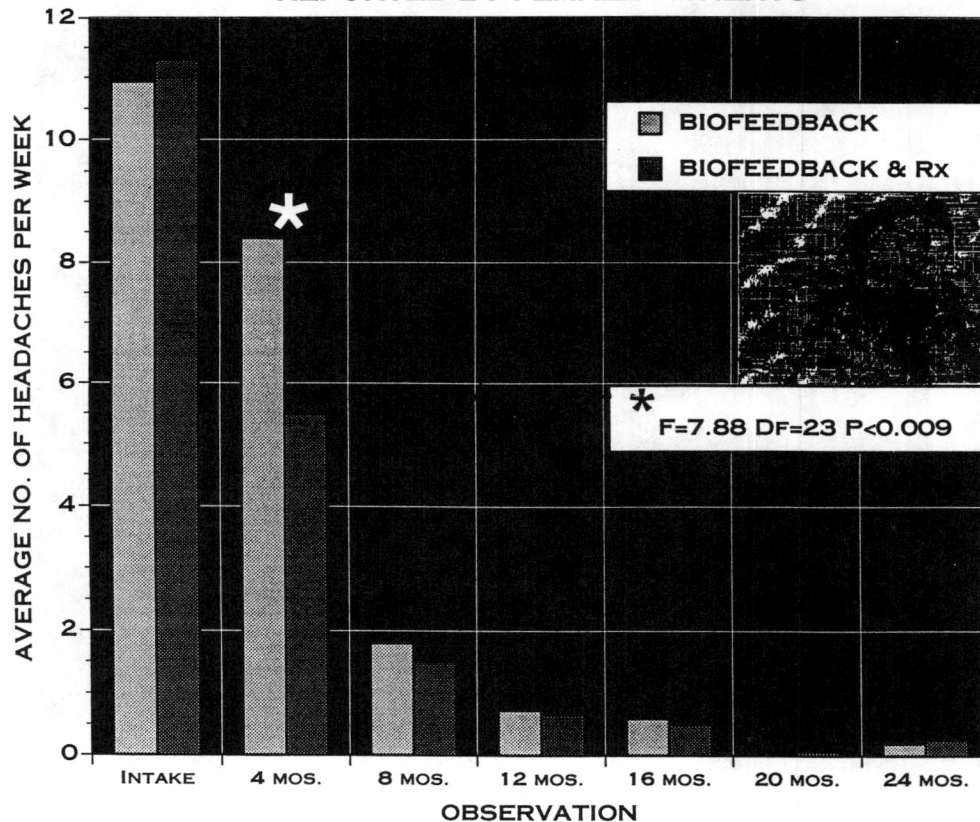

Figure 20.6.   Average frequency of headache over time reported by female patients.

headache patients who received cognitive behavior therapy were rated as "moderately improved" by neurologists conducting clinical evaluations. This success rate was higher than that found for patients receiving amitriptyline treatment (69% rated as "moderately improved"). Nicholson et al. (92) investigated psychophysiological symptoms and headache manifested by chronic tension-type headache sufferers. These patients were found to have a significantly higher number of different somatic symptoms, including backache and weakness along with higher Psychosomatic Symptom checklist scores (PSC) than vascular headache sufferers. Collet et al. (93) found an association between higher MMPI hypochondriasis, depression, hysteria, and psychasthenia scores and increased frontalis EMG activity. The researchers also noted that patients who reported greater intensity of headache pain tended to display significantly higher MMPI scores on the paranoia scale. Similarly, Andrasik et al. (94) noted that tension-type headache sufferers were more likely to evidence higher paranoia scores than other types of headache patients (migraine and "mixed headache"). Ziegler (95) conducted a community-based project comparing the prevalence of depression and anxiety in individuals with histories of headache with those without headache. Individuals who indicated "disabling or

severe" headaches had higher scores on the Zung Depression Scale and the Bendig-Taylor (anxiety test) than individuals reporting only mild headache or no headache. These results lend credence to an overall predisposing psychological component in tension-type headache patients. Additionally, these commonalities have led some to suggest that psychogenic headache (somatoform pain disorder DSM III 307.80) and tension-type headache may be indistinguishable (26).

Anxiety, stress, anger, frustration, and rage have all been associated with triggering tension-type headache episodes (96, 97). The psyche plays a predominant role in the etiology of tension-type headache. The mind/body interrelationship is well documented and linked by numerous biochemical/hormonal networks. Testament to this fact, many tension-type headache events are ameliorated by resolution of underlying psychological distress. This is not to say that the primary cause of tension-type headache is psychological pathology but rather that psychological factors often appear to provide a necessary but not sufficient condition giving rise, in the proper environmental circumstance, to headache events. According to a panel consensus of headache experts meeting at the 1989 American Association for the Study of Headache, "only rarely do psychological factors alone prove etiological in the pathogenesis of primary headache disorders" (98).

Thus, confrontation of underlying nervous/mental disorders along with psychotropic medication and psychotherapy/analysis can be instrumental in the resolution or moderation of tension-type cephalgia. We also know that underlying imbalances in biogenic amines and neurotransmitters responsible for psychological problems are implicated in the etiology and precipitation of physiological pain, particularly neurogenic and musculoskeletal disorders. Many primary psychiatric/psychological disturbances have their basis in biochemical and neurological disorders. Abnormal dexamethasone response test results have been observed in over 40% of tension-type headache patients (99).

Chronic tension-type headache has been described as a maladaptive response to environmental stimuli (100). Diamond has stated that chronic tension-type headache rarely presents without depression being involved as a precipitant or consequence (101) Patients who experience long-term chronic pain often present with psychological disorders that are secondary to unresolved disabling pain along with associated lifestyle changes. An assessment of underlying psychological dynamics and educational models for teaching pain-coping skills is paramount in reducing emotional overarousal and inappropriate reactive behaviors.

The clinician must not be afraid to tackle the psychological aspects of the headache etiology, proceeding in a manner that does not threaten, blame, or isolate the patient. Often, the patient's family and support structure must be incorporated into the overall treatment plan so that secondary gains and enabling behaviors can be identified and resolved within a nonthreatening framework. Without being consciously aware, the extended patient family may be primary contributors to the perpetuation of the pain behaviors manifested by the headache patient. The goal in such interactive psychotherapy is not to focus on the pain itself but on the function the pain plays in defining interactive roles of the family and significant others. If the patient is threatened with "taking the pain away," the therapist may isolate the trust and relationship necessary to explain the complex dynamics related to precipitation of the headache events. Reification of the patient's concerns and anxieties can often lower autonomic and sympathetic arousal states, offering a direct road to resolution of tension-type headache episodes.

One of the most important features to be assessed in the psychological intervention of tension-type headache is the extent to which symptoms may be used in an attempt to obtain prescription drugs. A detailed assessment of the type, length of use, and supply of drugs the patient presents with is important in designing an overall treatment plan for the resolution and remediation of pain. Many patients request specific medications and "doctor-shop" to support habits for narcotic and analgesic medications commonly prescribed for tension-type headache (butalbital,

codeine, Valium, Darvon, etc.). These behaviors must be adequately assessed with titration of medication, and replaced by proven nonpharmacological, self-regulatory interventions. Taking too many painkillers may possibly increase reported intensity and episodes of pain. Simple titration of such medications can often immediately result in significant lowering of tension-type headache frequency and distress. Intensive psychotherapy is usually the norm for patients with such drug behavior.

Prior to starting any intervention for chronic tension-type headache, all patients need a thorough assessment, including a behavioral analysis and medical evaluation. Psychiatric disorder, medical illness, medications, and the patient's physical environment, as well as all factors directly precipitating headache should be identified. The therapist must perform a comprehensive behavioral analysis prior to commencing treatment. We require our patients to complete a 2-week tracking sheet prior to starting therapy.

Patients with a major psychiatric disorder, such as depression or psychosis, should be treated for the underlying disorder. According to Diamond (1), a discriminant diagnosis can be made between patients with primary tension-type headache and those who manifest symptoms of the headache secondary to affective disorder. He suggests that pain consisting of a diurnal pattern (severe in the morning and evening), appearing at regular intervals, and located primarily in the temples, forehead, or neck is suggestive of depression. Psychotherapy, antidepressive medication, and biofeedback may be used in combination for these cases.

A number of researchers have found, via EMG measurements, that tension-type headache patients demonstrate a consistently higher muscle reactivity during perceived stress (102, 103). Many depressed patients have multiple somatic complaints, which abate with resolution of the depression. Cognitive behavioral therapy has been shown to be especially effective in reducing somatic complaints in depressed patients. Grazzi et al. (104) used the Zung anxiety and Zung depression tests, conducting a psychological assessment on 20 tension-type headache patients before and after treatment via EMG biofeedback. A significant reduction in frequency of headache attacks was observed. Additionally, a significant decrease was observed (pretreatment scores versus posttreatment scores) for both anxiety and depression, as measured by the Zung tests.

Reich (78) and Bell (105) studied the effects of treatment via biofeedback alone, biofeedback combined with psychotherapy, and psychotherapy on tension-type headache patients. All conditions consisted of the same number of hours of treatment. Self-reported information from headache/pain diaries demonstrated significant improvement in reduction of headache symptoms and reduced medication use associated with decline in EMG amplitude levels. Patients learning biofeedback were the most improved. Reich (78) noted greatest improvement in the biofeedback-alone group while Bell (105) noted no significant differences between the biofeedback-alone and the biofeedback combined with psychotherapy groups. He did note that the patients receiving biofeedback stated learning to relax, being able to relax at home, and increased ability to avoid stress more than those subjects receiving only psychotherapy.

Not all patients are psychologically suited for biofeedback. Borderline patients may find the experience too unstructured and have an exacerbation of their psychopathology, perhaps precipitated by the relative sensory deprivation of the biofeedback experience. These individuals may demand a relationship with the therapist and act out in some dramatic way to shift the focus of therapy from biofeedback to the patient-therapist relationship. Masochistic patients are also poor candidates, particularly if the pain is serving another psychological task such as retribution for real or imagined transgressions.

OTHER FACTORS

All patients should receive a medical assessment. Particular attention should be paid to ruling out the following disorders or conditions, which can mimic muscle tension headache: pseudotumor cerebri, subdural hematoma, temporal arteritis, temporomandibular joint dysfunction, and occupations that require maintenance of a fixed position for long periods, such as typist and computer operators. A thorough behavioral analysis can identify precipitating factors.

The relationship between the clinician and the patient is of extreme importance. Patients in our clinic range from those with serious psychiatric illness to individuals with maladaptive musculoskeletal responses to specific situations with little psychological component. Nonpsychologically minded or even alexothymic individuals may develop insights into psychological issues that cause increased EMG activity and physiological arousal. Many of these individuals would never seek out traditional psychotherapy, but they can use biofeedback in instrument-assisted psychotherapy. Tension-type headache patients treated with cognitive behavior psychotherapy have been shown to demonstrate significant reduction in pain episodes, especially when primary psychopathology has been identified.

The patient should not perceive biofeedback as a passive experience. The locus of control should be shifted from the therapist to the patient. Ultimately, patients should feel that they are in charge of their own treatment, with the therapist acting merely as a guide. Patients must practice the skills learned in biofeedback training sessions several times every day, both at home and work. The skills learned in the biofeedback session must become generalized, and not be limited solely to the biofeedback session. Most patients also require some assistance with stress management or other adjunctive psychotherapeutic interventions. Biofeedback should never be performed as an isolated

mechanical procedure but rather as the focal point of a comprehensive program of behavioral intervention.

REFERENCES

1. Diamond S. Tension headaches yield to multimodal therapy. Pain Topics 1990;4:1–6.
2. Headache Classification Committee of the International Headache Society. Classification and diagnostic criteria for headache disorders, cranial neuralgia and facial pain. Cephalalgia 1988;8(suppl 7):1–96.
3. Ostfeld AM. The common headache syndromes: biochemistry, pathophysiology, therapy. Springfield, IL: Charles C Thomas, 1962.
4. Wolff HG. Headache and other pain. 2nd ed. New York: Oxford University Press, 1963.
5. Budzynski TH, Stoyva JM, Adler C, Mullaney DJ. EMG and tension headache: a controlled outcome study. Psychosom Med 1973;35:484–496.
6. Travell J. Mechanical headache. Headache 1967;7:23–29.
7. Martin MJ. Tension headache: a psychiatric study. Headache 1966; 6:47–54.
8. Dixon H, Dickel HA. Tension headache. Northwest Med 1967;66: 817–820.
9. Adrian ED, Bonk DW. The discharge of impulses in motor nerve fibres. Part II. The frequency of discharge in reflex and voluntary contractions. J Physiol 1929;67:119–151.
10. Budzynski TH, Stoyva JM, Adler CS. Feedback induced muscle relaxation: application to tension headache. J Behav Ther Exp Psychiatry 1970;1:205–211.
11. Wickramasekera I. Electromyographic feedback training and tension headache: preliminary observations. Am J Clin Hypn 1972;2:83–85.
12. Arena JG, Hannah SL, Smith JD, Meador KJ. New evidence for EMG and vascular abnormalities in tension headache: implications for psychophysiological assessment and treatment. Biofeedback and Self-Regulation. Paper presented at the 21st Annual Meeting of the Association for Applied Psychophysiology, Washington, D.C., 1990.
13. Sherman RA, Sherman CJ. Relationship between continuous environmental recordings of posterior trunk muscle tension and patterns of low back pain and tension headaches. Paper presented at 20th Annual Meeting of the Association for Applied Psychophysiology and Biofeedback, March 17–22, San Diego, 1989.
14. Cram JR. Clinical EMG muscle scanning and diagnostic manual for surface EMG. Seattle: Clinical Resources, 1990.
15. Hatch JP, Moore PM, Cyr-Provost M, Boutros NN, Seleshi E, Borcherding S. The use of electromyograph and muscle palpation in the diagnosis of tension-type headache with and without pericranial muscle involvement. Biofeedback and Self-Regulation. Paper presented at the 21st Annual Meeting of the Association for Applied Psychophysiology, Washington, D.C., 1990.
16. Headley BJ. Muscle scanning : interpreting EMG scans. Pain Resources Ltd., St. Paul, Minnesota: 1987.
17. Borgeat F, Hadede B, Elie R. Larouche LM. Effects of voluntary muscle tension increases in tension headache. Headache 1984;24: 199–202.
18. Borgeat F, Elie R, Larouche LM. Pain response to voluntary muscle tension increases and biofeedback efficacy in tension headache. Headache 1985;25:387–391.
19. Bonica J. On pain management. Hosp Phys 1974;1:22–28.
20. Gobell H, Cordes P. Circadian variation of pain sensitivity in pericranial musculature. Headache 1990;30:423–427.
21. Raskin NH. Tension headache. In: Raskin NH, ed. Headache, 2nd ed. New York: Churchill Livingstone, 1988.
22. Langemark M, Jensen K, Olesen J. Temporal muscle blood flow in chronic tension type headache. Arch Neurol 1990;47:654–658.
23. Onel Y, Friedman AP, Grossman J. Muscle blood flow studies in muscle contraction headache. Neurology 1961;11:935–936.
24. Meyer JS, Zetusky W, Jonsdottir M, Mortel K. Cephalic hyperemia

during migraine headaches. A prospective study. Headache 1986;26:388–397.

25. Sakai F, Meyer JS. Regional cerebral hemodynamics during migraine and cluster headache measured by the 133Xe inhalation method. Headache 1978;18:122.

26. Haber JD, Kuczmierczk AR, Adams HE. Tension headache: muscle activity vs. psychogenic pain. Headache 1985;25:23–29.

27. Chatman JE, Barrett HR, Blalack JL, Pettaway GT. An exploratory study of the effects of clinical versus laboratory biofeedback training procedures on peripheral skin temperature control. (abstract) Biofeedback Self Regul 1988;13:60.

28. Lance JL. Tension headache. In: Lance JL. Mechanism and management of headache. 4th ed. London: Butterworth Scientific, 1982.

29. Rolf LH, Wiele G, Brune GG. 5-Hydroxytryptamine in platelets of patients with muscle contraction headache. Headache 1981;21:10–11.

30. Takeshima T, Shimomura T, Takahashi K. Platelet activation in muscle contraction headache and migraine. Cephalalgia 1987;7:239–243.

31. Saper JR. Daily chronic headache. In: NT Mathew, ed. Neurology Clinics. Philadelphia: WB Saunders, 1990.

32. Takashima T, Takahashi K. The relationship between muscle contraction headache and migraine: a multivariate analysis study. Headache 1988;28:272–277.

33. Iacono CU, Koellner KJ. Diagnostic EMG scanning of asymptomatic and then symptomatic migraine headache suffers. Paper presented at 20th Annual Meeting of the Association for Applied Psychophysiology and Biofeedback, March 17–22, 1989.

34. Langemark M, Oleson J, Poulesen DL. Clinical characterization of patients with chronic tension headache. Headache 1988;28:590–596.

35. Pozniak-Patewicz E. "Cephalic" spasm of head and neck muscles. Headache 1976;15:261–266.

36. Bakal DA, Kaganov JA. Muscle contraction and migraine headache: psychophysiologic comparison. Headache 1977;7:208–215.

37. Cohen MJ. Psychophysiological studies of headache: is there similarity between migraine and muscle contraction headaches? Headache 1978;20:189–196.

38. Olesen J. Some clinical features of the acute migraine attack: an analysis of 750 patients. Headache 1978;18:268–271.

39. Tfelt-Hansen P, Lous I, Olesen J. Prevalence and significance of muscle tenderness during common migraine attacks. Headache 1981;21:49–54.

40. Lous I, Olesen J. Evaluation of pericranial tenderness and oral function in patients with common migraine, muscle contraction headaches and "combination headache." Pain 1982;12:385–393.

41. Sargent J, Green E, Waltwers ED. Preliminary report on the use of feedback training in the treatment of migraine and tension headaches. Psychosom Med 1973;35:129–135.

42. Diamond S, Dalassio DJ. Classification and mechanisms of headache. In: Diamond S, Dalassio DJ, eds. The practicing physicians approach to headache. 4th ed. Baltimore: Williams & Wilkins, 1986:1–10.

43. Langemark M, Jensen K, Jensen TS, Olesen J. Pressure pain thresholds and thermal nociceptive thresholds in chronic tension type headache. Pain 1989;38:203–210.

44. Drummond PD. Scalp tenderness and sensitivity to pain in migraine and tension headache. Headache 1987;27:45–50.

45. Mikamo K, Takeshima T, Takahashi K. Cardiovascular sympathetic hypofunction in muscle contraction headache and migraine. Headache 1989;29:86–89.

46. Ellersten B, Norby H, Sjaastad O. Psychophysiologic response patterns in tension headache: effects of tricyclic antidepressants. Cephalalgia 1987;7:55–63.

47. Gannon LR, Haynes SN, Cuevas J, Chaver R. Psychophysiological correlates of induced headaches. J Behav Med 1987;10:411–423.

48. Takeshima T, Takao Y, Takahashi K. Pupillary sympathetic hy-

pofunction and asymmetry in muscle contraction headache and migraine. Cephalalgia 1987;7:257–262.

49. Shimomara T, Takahashi K. Pupillary function asymmetry in patients with muscle contraction headache. Cephalalgia 1986;6:141–145.

50. Carlsson J, Rosenhall U. Occulomotor disturbances in patients with tension headache. Acta Otolaryngol 1988;106:354–360.

51. Schoenen J, Jamart B, Gerard P, Lenarduzzi P, Delwaide PJ. Exteroceptive suppression of temporalis muscle activity in chronic headache. Neurology 1987;37:1834–1836.

52. Firenze C, Del Gatto F, Mazzotta G, Gallai V. Somatosensory evoked potential study in headache patients. Cephalalgia 1988;8:157–162.

53. Covelli V, Ferannini E. Neurophysiological findings in headache patients. Acta Neurol 1987;9:354–358.

54. Holroyd KA, Andrasik F, Westbrook T. Cognitive control of tension headache. Cognit Ther Res 1977;I:121–133.

55. Sternbach RA, Dalessio DJ, Kunzel M, Bowman GE. MMPI patterns in common headache disorders. Headache 1980;20:311–315.

56. Fine BD. Psychoanalytic aspects of head pain. In: The psychotherapy of headache. Res Clin Stud Headache. Basel: Krager, 1969.

57. Friedman AP, VonStorch TJC, Merritt HH. Migraine and tension headaches. A clinical study of two thousand cases. Neurology 1954;4:773–788.

58. Dhopesh VP, Herring CL, Anwar R. Tension headaches in emergency department patients. Psychosomatics 1980;21:631–635.

59. Saper JR. Changing perspectives on chronic headache. Clin J Pain 1986;2:19–28.

60. Tuchman AJ, Daras M. Muscle contraction headache: dexamethasone suppression test and response to amitriptyline. Eur Neurol 1989;29:291–293.

61. Sainsbury P, Gibson JF. Symptoms of anxiety and tension accompanying physiological changes in the musculature system. J Neurol Neurosurg Psychiatry 1954;17:216–224.

62. Chesney MA, Agras S, Benson H, Blumenthal A, Engel BT, et al. Task Force 5: nonpharmacological approaches to the treatment of hypertension. Circulation 1987;76:104–109.

63. Basmajian JV. Research foundations of EMG biofeedback in rehabilitation. Biofeedback Self Regul 1988;4:275–298.

64. Haynes SN, Griffin P, Mooney D, Parise M. Electromyographic biofeedback and relaxation instructions in the treatment of muscle contraction headaches. Behav Ther 1975;5:672–678.

65. Budzynski T. Biofeedback in the training of muscle contraction headache. Biofeedback Self Regul 1978;3:409–434.

66. Philips C. The modification of tension headache pain using EMG biofeedback. Behav Res Ther 1977;15:19–129.

67. Shedivy DI, Kleinman KM. Lack of correlation between frontalis EMG and either neck EMG or verbal ratings of tension. Psychophysiology 1977;14:182–186.

68. Silver BV, Blanchard EB. Biofeedback and relaxation training in the treatment of psychophysiological disorders: or are machines really necessary? J Behav Med 1978;1:217–237.

69. Hart JD, Cickanski KA. A comparison of frontal EMG biofeedback and neck biofeedback in the treatment of muscle contraction headache. Biofeedback Self Regul 1981;6:63–74.

70. Cleary T, Carlson JG. Multisite versus frontalis EMG training: muscular and autonomic generalization. Paper presented at 20th Annual Meeting of the Association for Applied Psychophysiology and Biofeedback, March 17–22, San Diego, 1989.

71. Qualls PJ, Sheehan PW. Electromyograph biofeedback as a relaxation technique: a critical appraisal and reassessment. Psychol Bull 1981;1:21–42.

72. Blanchard EB, Andrasik F, Ahels TA, Teders SJ, O'Keefe DM. Migraine and tension headache: a meta-analytic review. Behav Ther 1980;2:613–631.

73. Holyrod K, Penzien D. Client variables and behavioral treatment of

recurrent tension headache: A meta-analytic review. J Behav Med 1986;9:515–536.

74. Burg HE, Weiss WU. Chronic tension-type headache with and without pericranial muscle disorder: a prospective study of frequency. Paper presented at the 31st Annual Scientific Meeting of The American Association for the Study of Headache, Boston, 1989.

75. Bandura A. Self-efficacy: toward a unifying theory of behavioral change. Psychol Rev 1977;84:191–215.

76. Reich BA. Non-invasive treatment of vascular and muscle contraction headache: a comparative longitudinal clinical study. Headache 1989;29:34–41.

77. Reich BA. Biofeedback treatment of 684 chronic pain patients: a clinical assessment. Paper presented at the Vth World Congress on Pain of the International Association for the Study of Pain. Hamburg, Germany, 1987.

78. Reich BA. Biofeedback and relaxation therapies in the treatment and rehabilitation of cervical trauma. In: CD Tollison, Satterthwaite JR, eds. Painful cervical trauma: diagnosis and rehabilitative treatment of neuromuscular injuries. Baltimore: Williams & Wilkins, 1992.

79. Smith WB. Biofeedback and relaxation training: the effect on headache and associated symptoms. Headache 1987;27:511–514.

80. Marinacci AA, Horande M. Electromyograph in neuromuscular re-education. Bull LA Med Soc 1960;25:57–71.

81. Cataldo MF, Parker LH, Bird BL, Emurian CS, Page JM. Generalization and generality in the behavioral treatment of neuromuscular disorders. In: Gordon WA, Parker MF, Herd JA, eds. Perspective on behavioral medicine (vol 3). San Francisco: Academic Press, 1986.

82. Blanchard EB, Andrasik F, Evans DD, Hillhouse J. Biofeedback and relaxation treatments for headache in the elderly: a caution and a challenge. Biofeedback Self Regul 1985;10:69–73.

83. Speed WG III. Headaches related to muscle contraction. In: Saper JR, ed. Help for headaches: a guide to understanding their cause and finding the best methods of treatment. New York: Warner Books, 1987:99–108.

84. Holroyd KA, Nash JM, Pingel JD, Cordingly GE, Jerome A. A comparison of pharmacological (amitriptyline HCl) and nonpharmacological (cognitive behavioral) therapies for chronic tension headaches. Personal communication, June 1990.

85. Diamond S, Dalessio DJ. The practicing physician's approach to headache. Baltimore: Williams & Wilkins, 1986.

86. Diamond S, Baltes BJ. Chronic tension headache treated with amitriptyline: a double blind study. Headache 1971;11:110–116.

87. Graham JR. Headache: diagnosis and management. Headache 1979;19:133–141.

88. Mathew NT. Photophylaxis of migraine and mixed headache. A randomized controlled study. Headache 1981;21:105–109.

89. Shimomura T, Takahashi K. Alteration of platelet serotonin in patients with chronic tension-type headache during cold pressor test. Headache 1990;30:581–583.

90. Rolf LH, Wiele G, Brune GG. 5-Hydroxytryptamine in platelets of

patients with muscle contraction headache. Headache 1981;21:10–11.

91. Bruhn P, Olesen J, Melgaard B. Controlled trial of EMG feedback in muscle contraction headache. Ann Neurol 1979;6:34–36.

92. Nicholson NL, Blanchard EB, Applebaum KA. Occurrence of psychophysiological symptoms in chronic headache sufferers. Paper presented at 20th Annual Meeting of the Association for Applied Psychophysiology and Biofeedback, March 17–22, San Diego, 1989.

93. Collet L, Cottraux J, Juenet C. Tension headaches: relationship between MMPI score and pain and between MMPI hypochondriasis score and frontalis EMG. Headache 1986;26:365–368.

94. Andrasik F, Blanchard EB, Arena JG, Saunders NL, Barrow DK. Psychophysiology of recurrent headache: methodological issues and new empirical findings. Behav Ther 1982;13:407–429.

95. Ziegler DK, Rhodes RJ, Hassanein RS. Association of psychological measurements of anxiety and depression with headache history in a non-clinic population. Res Clin Stud Headache 1978;6:123–135.

96. Dalessio DJ. Some reflections on the etiologic role of depression in head pain. Headache 1968;8:28.

97. Drummond PD. Predisposing, precipitating and relieving factors in different categories of headaches. Headache 1985;25:16–21.

98. Sheftell FD. Psychophysiological aspects of headache. Headache: changing perspectives and controversies. Proceedings of the American Association for the Study of Headache, Scottsdale, AZ, 1989.

99. Martigoni E, Facchinetti F, Manzoni GC, Petraglia F, Nappi G, Genazzani AR. Abnormal dexamethasone suppression test in daily chronic headache sufferers. Psychiatr Res 1986;19:51–57.

100. Nappi G, Sandrini G, Granella F, Ruiz R, Cerutti G, et al. A new 5-HT2 antagonist (ritanserin) in the treatment of chronic headache with depression. A double blind study versus amitriptyline. Headache 1990;30:439–444.

101. Diamond S. Depression and headache. Headache 1983;23:122–126.

102. Thompson JK, Adams HE. Psychophysiological characteristics of headache patients. Pain 1984;18:41–52.

103. Vaughn R, Pall ML, Haynes SN. Frontalis EMG response to stress in subjects with frequent muscle contraction headaches. Headache 1977;16:313–317.

104. Grazzi L, Frediani F, Zappacosta B, Bioardi A, Bussone G. Psychological assessment in tension headache before and after biofeedback treatment. Headache 1988;28:337–338.

105. Bell NW, Abramowiz SI, Folkins CH, Spensley J, Hutchinson GL. Biofeedback, brief psychotherapy, and tension headache. Headache 1983;23:162–173.

106. Busch E, Wilson PR. Atlanto-occipital and atlanto-axial injections in the treatment of headache [Abstract]. Reg Anesth 1989;11:45.

107. Dwyer A, April C. Bogduk N. Cervical zygapophyseal joint pain patterns. I: A study in normal volunteers. Spine 1990;15:453–457.

108. Aprill C, Dwyer A, Bogduk N. Cervical zygapophyseal joint pain patterns. II: A clinical evaluation. Spine 1990;15:458–461.

Appendix 20.1 Nassau Pain and Stress Center Headache Log

NAME _____ DATE _____ DAY OF WEEK _____

Please rate the degree of _____ you experience during the specified
blocks of time. Use the following numbers:

1 = NONE   2 = SLIGHT   3 = MODERATE   4 = STRONG   5 = INTOLERABLE

TIME	RATING	SETTING	ACTIVITY	ALONE OR WITH WHOM	THOUGHTS	MOOD	HOME EXERCISE OR MEDICATION	COMMENTS
8 - 12 NOON								
12.- 4								
4 - 8								
8 - 12 MIDNIGHT								
MIDNIGHT TO 8								

Appendix 20.2 Medications Associated with High Incidence of Headache[a]

Accutane Capsules (approximately 1 in 20)
Adalat Capsules (10 mg and 20 mg) (23%)
Adrenalin Chloride Solution 1:100 & 1:1,000 (Often)
AeroBid Inhaler System (25%)
Alferon N Injection (15% to 31%)
Anafranil Capsules (28% to 52%)
Anaprox and Anaprox DS Tablets (3–9%)
Ansaid Tablets (3–9%)
Azulfidine Tablets, EN-tabs, Oral Suspension (approximately one-third of patients)
Beconase AQ Nasal Spray (fewer than 5 per 100 patients)
Buprenex Injectable (1% to 5%)
BuSpar (6%)
Cardizem SR Capsules—60 mg, 90 mg, and 120 mg (4.5–12%)
Clinoril Tablets (3–9%)
Clozaril Tablets (more than 5% to 7%)
Cytadren Tablets (1 in 20)
DDAVP Nasal Spray (2% to 5%)
DDAVP Rhinal Tube (2% to 5%)
Deponit NTG Transdermal Delivery System
Dilantin—30 Pediatric/Dilantin—125 Suspension
Dilantin with Phenobarbital Kapseals
Dilatrate—SR (approximately 25%)
Dolobid Tablets (3 to 9%)
Doral Tablets (4–5%)
Eldepryl (2 of 49 patients)
Eminase (less than 10%)
Engerix-B Unit-Dose Vials (1 to 10%)
Enkaid Capsules (5.7%)
Epitrate (frequent)
Epogen for Injection (16.0%)
Ergamisol Tablets (3–4%)
Ethmozine Tablets (8.0%)
Fungizone Intravenous
Gastrocrom Capsules (4 of 87 patients)
Halcion Tablets (9.7%)
Heptavax-B (3.1%)
Hismanal Tablets (6.7%)
Hylorel Tablets (58.1%)
Hytrin Tablets (1.3% to 16.2%)
Indocin Capsules (11.7%)
Indocin Oral Suspension (11.7%)
Indocin SR Capsules (11.7%)
Indocin Suppositories (11.7%)
Indomethacin E.R. Capsules (more than 10%)
Intron A (36% to 47%)
Intropin Injection (among most frequent)
Isordil Sublingual Tablets 2.5 mg, 5 mg, & 10 mg (25%)
Isordil Tembids Capsules (40 mg) (25%)
Isordil Tembids Tablets (40 mg) (25%)
Isordil 5 Titradose Tablets, 5 mg (25%)
Isordil 10 Titradose Tablets, 10 mg (25%)
Isordil 20 Titradose Tablets, 20 mg (25%)
Isordil 30 Titradose Tablets, 30 mg (25%)

Isordil 40 Titradose Tablets, 40 mg (25%)
Isosorbide Dinitrate C.R. Tablets (25%)
Kerlone Tablets (6.5% to 14.8%)
Lariam Tablets
Levatol (7.8%)
Lioresal Tablets (4.8%)
Lopressor HCT Tablets (10 in 100 patients)
Lozol Tablets (greater than or equal to 5%)
Ludiomil Tablets (4%)
Lupron Injection (5% or more)
Marinol (Dronabinol) Capsules (6%)
Marplan Tablets
Meclomen (3–9%)
Mesnex Injection (50%)
Mevacor Tablets (9.3%)
Mexitil Capsules (5.7% to 7.5%)
Midamor Tablets (3% to 8%)
Minipress Capsules (7.8%)
Minitran Transdermal Delivery System (63%)
Minizide Capsules (7.8%)
Moduretic Tablets (3% to 8%)
Mykrox 1/2 mg Tablets (9.3%)
Nalfon Pulvules & Tablets (8.7%)
Naprosyn Suspension (3 to 9%)
Naprosyn Tablets (3–9%)
Nitro-Bid Ointment (50%)
Nitrodisc (63%)
Nitro-Dur (nitroglycerin) Transdermal Infusion System
Nitrogard Tablets
Nitrolingual Spray (50%)
Norpace Capsules (3 to 9%)
Norpace CR Capsules (3 to 9%)
Novantrone (10 to 13%)
Nubain Injection (3%)
Omnipaque (less than 1% to 18%)
Orthoclone OKT3 Sterile Solution (42%)
Orudis Capsules (greater than 3%)
Parlodel Capsules (10–19%)
Parlodel SnapTabs (10–19%)
Pepcid I.V. (4.7%)
Pepcid Oral Suspension (4.7%)
Pepcid Tablets (4.7%)
Permax Tablets (5.3%)
Plague Vaccine (10%)
Prinivil Tablets (5.3%)
Prinzide Tablets (5.2%)
Procardia XL (15.8% to 23%)
Proventil Repetabs Tablets (7%)
Proventil Solutions for Inhalation 0.5% and 0.83% (3%)
Proventil Syrup (4 of 100)
Proventil Tablets (7%)
Prozac Pulvules (20%)
Retrovir Capules (1.6% to 42%)
Retrovir I.V. Infusion (42%)
Retrovir Syrup (1.6% to 42%)
Roferon-A Injection (66% to 71%)
Rowasa Suspension (6.50%)

Rythmol Tablets (1.5% to 4.5%)
Sandimmune Injection (less than 1% to 15%)
Sandimmune Oral Solution (less than 1% to 15%)
Sandimmune Soft Gelatin Capsules (less than 1% to 15%)
Sectral Capsules (6%)
Seldane Tablets (15.8%)
Sorbitrate Chewable Tablets (25%)
Sorbitrate Oral Tablets (25%)
Sorbitrate Sublingual Tablets (25%)
Sorbitrate Sustained Action Tablets (25%)
Stadol (3%)
Synarel Nasal Solution (19% of patients)
Tambocor Tablets (9.6%)
Tegison Capsules (25–50%)
Tenex Tablets (2% to 4%)
Terazol 7 Vaginal Cream (26% of 521 patients)
Terazol 3 Vaginal Suppositories (30.3% of 284 patients)
Tolectin (200, 400, and 600 mg) (3–9%)
Tornalate (4%)
Transderm-Nitro Transdermal Therapeutic System (63%)

Trental (1.2% to 6.2%)
Trexan Tablets (greater than 10%)
Vaseretic Tablets (5.5%)
Vasotec Tablets (1.8% to 5.2%)
Ventolin Rotacaps for Inhalation (6%)
Ventolin Solution for Inhalation (3%)
Ventolin Syrup (4 of 100 patients)
Ventolin Tablets (7 of 100 patients)
Verelan Capsules (5.3%)
Voltaren Tablets (about 7%)
Wytensin Tablets (5%)
Xanax Tablets (12.9%)
Xylocaine Injections (3%)
Yutopar Intravenous Injection (10 to 15% with IV administration)
Yutopar Tablets (10 to 15% with IV administration)
Zestoretic (5.2%)
Zestril Tablets (5.3%)
Zovirax Capsules (0.6% to 5.9%)
Zovirax Suspension (0.6% to 5.9%)

Cluster Headache

21

Clinical Symptomatology and Differential Diagnosis of Cluster Headache

LEE KUDROW

The first descriptive account of cluster headache was provided by Romberg in 1840 (1). According to Heyck (2), clinical characteristics were further refined by Eulenburg, who in 1878, named the disorder angioparalytic hemicrania in his textbook, Lehrbuch der Nervenkrankheiten. Other appellations include migrainous neuralgia (3), ciliary neuralgia (4), and histaminic cephalgia (5). The periodic nature of cluster headache was first described by K. A. Ekbom in 1947 (6). Its "clustering" pattern, described by Kunkle et al.(7) in 1954, provided the origin of the currently accepted term, *cluster headache*.

CLASSIFICATION

Cluster headache was formerly recognized and classified as a primary headache disorder by the Ad Hoc Committee on the Classification of Headache in 1962 (8), and by the Migraine Research Group of the World Federation of Neurology in 1969 (9). In 1988, the Headache Classification Committee of the International Headache Society (10) refined the diagnostic criteria of cluster headache (Table 21.1). Classification of a poorly understood entity remains a dynamic process, subject to change with each new scientific revelation. This discussion is limited to the major types of cluster headache: episodic and chronic cluster headaches, and paroxysmal hemicrania.

Episodic cluster headache is the most common type, affecting 80% of a cluster headache population. It is characterized by attack-susceptible periods (cluster periods) of 1 to 5 months duration, followed by a spontaneous attack-free or remission period of 6 to 24 months (11–14).

Chronic cluster headache, as first described by Ekbom and Olivarious (15), is defined by an absence of remission periods for at least 1-year. Such misfortune is further compounded by an increase in attack-frequency and treatment resistance. Chronicity from the onset of this disorder has been subtyped primary chronic cluster headache; conversion to chronic from episodic states has been termed secondary chronic cluster headache (15).

The third type may be more accurately called a variation of cluster headache. Chronic paroxysmal hemicrania (CPH), first described by Sjaastad and Dale in 1974 (16), resembles cluster headache in pain intensity, distribution, and associated autonomic nervous system signs—but differs most strikingly by its tenfold increase in attack frequency, shorter attack duration, and complete response to indomethacin.

CLINICAL PICTURE
Incidence

Incidence or prevalence rate of cluster headache remains unknown. Only one epidemiologic survey has been reported, limited to 18-year-old Swedish Army recruits—an age of relatively low incidence for cluster headache. In this study, Ekbom et al. (17) reported an incidence rate of 0.09%. Extrapolation from headache clinic populations for migraine and cluster headache patients suggest a possible prevalence rate of 0.4 to 1% among males (18).

Sex, Age, Race, and Ethnicity

Cluster headache is predominantly a male disorder. Male:female ratios range from 4.5:1 to 6.7:1. The mean age of onset is 27 years to 30 years (11–14, 19).

Ethnic representation of cluster headache appears to be equal among groups. In a survey of approximately 500 cluster patients in 1980, little difference was found between ethnic backgrounds (14). Indeed, data from Italian (20) and Scandinavian populations differ little (12). There is, however, an overrepresentation of cluster headache among Afro-Americans, first reported by Lovshin (19) and later corroborated by our own clinic survey (14).

Cluster Headache Attack

Attacks may be preceded by several hours by a sense of euphoria or hypomanic behavior, followed by several minutes of sleepiness and yawning. As often, such prodromal symptoms may either be entirely unnoticed or absent.

The attack often begins with bilateral fullness or pressure in the neck, which may shift to the occipital region, more on one side than the other. Others may experience a

185

Table 21.1.
Classification of Cluster Headache

Cluster headache	3.1
Periodicity undetermined	3.1.1
Episodic	3.1.2
Chronic	3.1.3
Primary chronic	3.1.3.1
Secondary chronic	3.1.3.2
Chronic paroxysmal hemicrania	3.2
Cluster headache-like syndrome	3.3

warmth over the ipsilateral temporal region as the first sign of the impending attack. After 2 to 5 minutes, mild pain may localize about the eye or temple, ipsilaterally. At this point, nasal stuffiness may accompany a sense of panic or anticipatory anxiety. Somewhat agitated, but resigned to the onslaught of agonizing pain for the next 30 to 60 minutes, the patient may withdraw to be alone, select a corner of the room to stand in, pace an area of the floor, or sit in a chair to await the tempest.

Throbbing pain of somewhat greater intensity may stab at the temple, face, or teeth before settling behind an eye. As the focal pain increases, the patient may become restless and begin to hyperventilate, rock forward and backward in the chair, or begin to pace. Nasal stuffiness may now give way to a clear nasal discharge, ipsilaterally.

At peak intensity, the pain has a hot boring quality of such intensity that throbbing is no longer discerned. The patient may cover the affected eye with both hands, alternately pressing and releasing—while rocking or pacing. This agonizing state is celebrated by ipsilaterally profuse lacrimation, conjunctival redness, constrictive pupil, and ptosis. Behavior at this point may be violent, not infrequently associated with striking a wall head-on or with the fists. During mild attacks, one may sit or stand perfectly still in the belief that such meditative posture might actually exert an influence on the attack.

Peak intensities may last from 10 to 60 minutes or longer, at the end of which time, a noticeable decrease of pain appears in waves; crests become less frequent, and intervening nadirs become longer. The pain decreases rapidly. Just minutes from the first decrescendo, patients become aware of being past the peak, allowing themselves to be carried safely to the end of the attack. The only concern is awaiting the next dreaded attack.

Attack Profile

Frequency. The mean frequency of attacks is twice daily, with a range of 1 to 10 per day. Fifty percent of patients experience one attack daily; more than a third, two daily; and 13%, a greater frequency (12, 13).

Duration. The mean duration of attacks is 45 minutes, ranging from 10 minutes to 3 hours. Longer durations may be seen in the occasional patient, which may cause one to question the diagnosis (7, 11, 13, 20, 21).

Rhythmicity and Timing. Attacks more often occur soon after working hours, near dinner time. The second most common time of onset is during sleep, often 90 minutes following sleep onset (14). A temporal relationship between REM-stages of sleep and attack onset has been reported (22, 23).

Location and Intensity. Cluster headache pain is most commonly distributed over oculofrontal or oculotemporal areas, unilaterally. At times, pain may radiate to facial and dental regions. The intensity may be exquisitely severe in most attacks; in some, particularly at the beginning and near the end of the cluster period, the pain may be rather mild. When severe, pain is usually boring, sharp, or burning (11, 13, 24).

Associated Signs and Symptoms. Ipsilateral lacrimation, rhinorrhea, or nasal stuffiness and conjunctival suffusion, are the most common associated features of the cluster headache attack. These signs are reported in 72 to 84% of patients. Ipsilateral ptosis and miosis occur in approximately 60 to 70% of patients (12, 13), becoming permanent in 0.5 to 6.7% of patients (12, 14).

Behavior during attacks is quite similar from patient to patient. The inability to lie still is pathognomonic of this disorder, suggesting a role for position-dependent venous blood flow and possibly involving the cavernous sinus.

Provocation of Attacks. Vasodilators, such as nitroglycerin, alcohol, and histamine may induce cluster headache attacks solely during cluster periods. In the report by Horton (25), attacks were induced in 69% of patients with histamine provocation. In Ekbom's series (26), sublingual nitroglycerin, 1 mg, provoked attacks in 10/10 patients.

Cluster Period

The term *cluster period* applies only to patients with episodic cluster headache. It is the period of attack-susceptibility; and spontaneous and provoked attacks may occur solely during the cluster period.

As with attacks, cluster periods are cyclic. In a recent study (27), approximately 900 cluster period onsets from 400 patients were recorded over a 10-year period. The frequency of cluster periods was found to be related to seasonal photoperiod changes (length of daylight), increasing with shortening or lengthening photoperiods. Peak in cluster period onsets occurred within 2 weeks following the longest and shortest days of the year (July and January) and decreased within 2-weeks following daylight savings and standard time changes (27).

Cluster periods occur 1 to 2 times a year in approximately 70% of patients (21). In an earlier study of 337 episodic cluster headache patients, the mean duration of cluster periods was 2 months, with a range of 2 to 4 months in 84%. The median duration of the cluster period was less than 2 months, confirming other reports (11–14).

Remission Periods

Generally, attacks—either provoked or spontaneous—do not occur during a remission. An occasional patient, however, may experience a single cluster headache attack during a remission period. In our survey of 428 patients, almost 50% experienced remissions of 7 to 12 months duration; almost 20% of 1 to 6 months duration; and the remainder, more than 2 years duration. We had also noted 20-year remission periods in 2 patients (14). Ekbom reported 11 years to 17 years of remission in 5 patients (12).

FAMILY HISTORY

In our earlier survey of 495 patients with cluster headache, a parental and familial history of cluster headache was found in 3.4 and 4.7%, respectively (14). In Ekbom's population of 105 cluster headache patients, 1.9% gave a positive family history (12). Others reported a positive family history ranging between 3.0 and 6.7% (12).

Excluding artifacts and biases as a result of patient reporting, the frequency of positive family histories for cluster headache and cluster headache populations is greater than that expected in a general population. This may suggest a genetic influence. A search for genetic markers within the HL-A histocompatibility antigen system has been somewhat unrewarding (28, 29), with the exception of a report by Martelletti et al. (30). These

investigators reported a decreased frequency for antigen HL-A B14 in their cluster headache population.

DIFFERENTIAL DIAGNOSIS (Table 21.2)

Women patients generally present the greatest diagnostic challenge in assessing cluster headache. In this group, atypical presentations are common and confounded by a high incidence of migraine headache. It sometimes requires long-term follow-up to properly evaluate cluster headache patterns.

Another area of diagnostic difficulty concerns CPH. There appear to be overlapping bell-shaped curves regarding frequency and duration of attacks in these disorders. A dramatic and complete response to prophylactic indomethacin treatment should confirm the diagnosis of CPH.

Other headache conditions that may bear some resemblance to cluster headache include migraine, trigeminal neuralgia, temporal arteritis, pheochromocytoma, and Raeder's syndrome.

Chronic Paroxysmal Hemicrania (CPH)

Sjaastad and Dale (16) first described CPH in 1974. By 1987, Sjaastad (31) reported that he had been informed of

Table 21.2.
Differential Diagnosis

Disorder	Frequency	Duration	Location	Intensity	Quality	Other Findings
Cluster	1–3/day	30–90 min	Unilateral oculofrontal, temporal	Excruciating	Nonthrobbing, boring	Unilateral lacrimation, rhinorrhea, injection, partial Horner's, can't lie down
CPH	4–38/day	3–46 min	Unilateral oculofrontal temporal	Severe	Nonthrobbing, boring	Unilateral lacrimation, rhinorrhea, conjunctival injection, partial Horner's, not restless
Migraine	1–3/month	6–30 hr	Unilateral 60%	Severe	Throbbing 80%	Nausea (85%), vomiting (40%), photophobia (>85%), sonophobia
Trigeminal neuralgia	Several/day	Seconds to minutes	Unilateral, 5th nerve distribution	Severe	Electric, lancinating, nonthrobbing	Trigger zones on face
Temporal arteritis	Persistent		Unilateral, temporal	Severe	Burning, throbbing, nonthrobbing	Chewing, claudication, tender and torturous temporal artery, elevated ESR, polymyalgia
Pheochromocytoma	Daily to monthly	Less than 1 hr	Bilateral, occipital	Severe in supine position	Throbbing	Sweating, pallor, tachycardia within rise in blood pressure
Raeder's syndrome	Persistent	Persistent	Unilateral supraocular	Severe	Burning, throbbing, nonthrobbing	Partial Horner's syndrome

approximately 80 cases throughout the international medical community.

As reported by Russell (32) in 1984, CPH-attack frequency ranges from 4 to 38 per day, with a mean frequency of approximately 14 attacks per day. The duration of attacks may range from 3 to 46 minutes, with a mean of 13 minutes.

Although CPH generally presents as a chronic disorder, a prechronic state has been described (33–35). Recently, an episodic type (EPH) of paroxysmal hemicrania was reported (36). CPH differs from cluster headache in that attacks are more frequent, shorter, associated with less restlessness, completely responsive to indomethacin, and unresponsive to anticluster prophylactic medications (31).

Migraine

The incidence of migraine is approximately 18%; 26% of women and 8 to 10% of men (37). Of the six major types of migraine, common migraine is most frequently encountered, comprising 80% of a migraine population. Migraine differs considerably from cluster headache in that attacks are usually regular at 1–3 times a month with long headache-free intervals between attacks. The migraine attack may last 6 hours to several days and be bilateral in 40% of patients.

Trigeminal Neuralgia

Trigeminal neuralgia differs from cluster headache in the quality of pain, often described as lancinating or electric-like; the duration, usually seconds to minutes; and being frequently triggered by a tactile stimulus of facial areas ipsilaterally. Rarely do attacks waken the patient at night. Trigeminal neuralgia resembles cluster headache in that attacks may occur several times a day, always unilaterally, and with a trigeminal distribution. The pain is severe (38).

Temporal Arteritis

The pain of temporal arteritis, although unilateral, is generally persistent, waxing and waning throughout the day. The pain is generally burning, moderately severe, and located over the temporal artery. The pain of temporal arteritis is exacerbated by chewing claudication. The involved artery may be tender and torturous to palpation and often lacks a pulse. A markedly elevated sedimentation rate supports the diagnosis of temporal arteritis; a biopsy finding of giant cells is confirmatory (39, 40).

Pheochromocytoma

In a review of 100 cases, Thomas et al. (41) describe the headache of pheochromocytoma as severe, throbbing, and often associated with sweating, pallor, tachycardia, and an elevated blood pressure. In contrast to cluster headache, the pain is generally bilateral and occipital.

Raeder's Syndrome

The similarities of Raeder's syndrome to cluster headache include a unilateral supraocular location associated with a partial Horner's syndrome. The pain of Raeder's syndrome (42), however, is generally persistent, and while initially severe, may be followed by decreasing intensity over a period of weeks. In the absence of intracranial disease, Vijayan and Watson (43) have redefined this disorder as a pericarotid syndrome.

In summary, the clinical picture of cluster headache is stereotypic in periodicity, cyclicity, symptomatology, and signs. There is always the exceptional or atypical case that may be confused with other headache disorders, as discussed.

Finally, it should be noted that the pain of cluster headache is severe enough to require immediate attention by the clinician.

REFERENCES

1. Romberg MH. A manual of nervous diseases of man. London: Syndenham Society, 1840 (translated by EH Sieveking).
2. Heyck H. Der cluster-kopfschmerz. Disch Med Wochenschr 1975;100:1292–1293.
3. Harris W. Ciliary (migranous) neuralgia and its treatment. Br Med J 1936;1:457–460.
4. Harris W. Neuritis and Neuralgia. London: Oxford University Press, 1926.
5. Horton BT. Histaminic cephalgia. Lancet 1952;2:92–98.
6. Ekbom KA. Ergotamine tartrate orally by Horton's "histaminic cephalgia" (also called Harris' "ciliary neuralgia"). Acta Psychiatr Scand 1947;46(suppl):106–113.
7. Kunkle EC, Pfeiffer JB Jr, Wilhoit WM, Hamrick LW Jr. Recurrent brief headache in "cluster" pattern. Trans Am Neurol Assoc 1952;77:240–243.
8. Ad Hoc Committee on Classification of Headache. JAMA 1962;179:717–718.
9. World Federation of Neurology's Research Group of Migraine and Headache. J Neurol Sci 1969;9:202.
10. Headache Classification Committee of the International Headache Society. Classification and diagnostic criteria for headache disorders, cranial neuralgias and facial pain. Cephalalgia 1988;8(suppl 7):9–96.
11. Friedman AP, Mikropoulos HE. Cluster headache. Neurology 1958;8:653–663.
12. Ekbom K. A clinical comparison of cluster headache and migraine. Acta Neurol Scand 1970;(suppl 41):46:1–48.
13. Lance JW. Mechanisms and management of headache. 3rd ed. London: Butterworths, 1978.
14. Kudrow L. Cluster headache: mechanisms and management. London: Oxford University Press, 1980:10–150.
15. Ekbom K, Olivarius B de F. Chronic migrainous neuralgia—diagnostic and therapeutic aspects. Headache 1971;11:97–101.
16. Sjaastad O, Dale I. Evidence for a new (?) treatable headache entity. Headache 1974;14:105–108.
17. Ekbom K, Ahlborg B, Schéle R. Prevalence of migraine and cluster headache in Swedish men of 18. Headache 1978;18:9–19.
18. Kudrow L. Cluster headache. In: Blau JN, ed. Migraine. Clinical, therapeutic, conceptual and research aspects. London: Chapman and Hall, 1987:113–132.
19. Lovshin LL. Clinical caprices of histaminic cephalgia. Headache 1961;1:3–6.

20. Manzoni GC, Terzano MG, Bono G, Micieli G, Martucci N, Nappi G. Cluster headache—clinical findings in 180 patients. Cephalalgia 1983;3:21–30.
21. Ekbom K. Pattern of cluster headache with a note on the relation to angina pectoris and peptic ulcer. Acta Neurol Scand 1970;46:225–237.
22. Dexter JD, Riley TL. Studies in nocturnal migraine. Headache 1975;15:51–62.
23. Kudrow L, McGinty DS, Phillips ER, Stevenson M. Sleep apnea in cluster headache. Cephalalgia 1984;4:33–38.
24. Ekbom K, Kugelberg E. Upper and lower cluster headache (Horton's syndrome). In: Brain and mind problems. Rome: Pensiero Sci Publ, 1968:482–489.
25. Horton BT. The use of histamine in the treatment of specific types of headache. JAMA 1941;116:377–383.
26. Ekbom K. Nitroglycerin as a provocative agent in cluster headache. Arch Neurol 1968;19:487–493.
27. Kudrow L. The cyclic relationship or natural illumination to cluster period frequency. [Abstract] Cephalalgia 1987;(suppl 6)7:76–77.
28. Kudrow L. HL-A antigens in cluster headache and in classical migraine. Headache 1978;18:167–168.
29. Cuypers J, Altenkirk H. HLA antigens in cluster headache. Headache 1979;19:228–229.
30. Martelletti MD, Romiti A, Gallo MF, et al. HLA-B14 antigen in cluster headache. Headache 1984;24:152–154.
31. Sjaastad O. Chronic paroxysmal hemicrania: clinical aspects and controversies. In: Blau JN, ed. Migraine: clinical, therapeutic, conceptual and research aspects. London: Chapman and Hall, 1987:135–152.
32. Russell D. Chronic paroxysmal hemicrania: severity, duration and time of occurrences of attacks. Cephalalgia 1984;4:53–56.
33. Sjaastad O, Apfelbaum R, Caskey W, Christofferson B, Diamond S, et al. Chronic paroxysmal hemicrania (CPH). The clinical manifestations. A review. Ups J Med Sci 1980;(suppl):27–33.
34. Sjaastad O. Discussion of chronic paroxysmal hemicrania: two new patients. Presented by Stein H, Rogado A (Headache Rounds). Headache 1980;20:2.
35. Pelz M, Merskey H. A case of pre-chronic paroxysmal hemicrania. Cephalalgia 1982;2:47–50.
36. Kudrow L, Esperanca P, Vijayan N. Episodic paroxysmal hemicrania. Cephalalgia 1987;7:197–201.
37. Waters WE, O'Connor PJ. Prevalence of migraine. J Neurol Neurosurg Psychiatry 1975;30:613–616.
38. Dalessio DJ. A reappraisal of the trigger zones of tic douloureaux. Headache 1969;9:73–76.
39. Horton BT, Magath TB, Brown GE. An undescribed form of arteritis of the temporal vessels. Proc Staff Meet Mayo Clin 1932;7:700–701.
40. Huston KA, Hunder GG, Lie JT, Kennedy BA, Elveback LR. Temporal arteritis. A 25-year epidemiologic, clinical, and pathologic study. Ann Intern Med 1978;88:162–167.
41. Thomas JG, Rooke ED, Kvale WF. The neurologist's experience with pheochromocytoma: a review of 100 cases. JAMA 1966:197–754.
42. Raeder JG. "Paratrigeminal" paralysis of oculo-pupillary sympathetic. Brain 1924;47:149–158.
43. Vijayan N, Watson C. Pericarotid syndrome. Headache 1978;18:244–254.

22

Pathogenesis of Cluster Headache

LEE KUDROW

The etiology of cluster headache is unknown. Various biochemical, hormonal, and vascular changes play a role in the pathogenesis of this disorder. Ordering these data into sequential events is the subject of numerous hypotheses; a difficult undertaking due to many conflicting study results and uncorroborated data. The pathogenesis of cluster headache may be more clearly understood when divided into three major phases: cluster periods, attacks, and induction of attacks.

CLUSTER PERIOD

The cluster period may be defined as a self-limiting attack-susceptible period. With rare exception, provoked or spontaneous attacks occur solely during the cluster period. This altered physiological state appears to be characterized by changes in hypothalamic function. This is evidenced by dyschronic changes in neuroendocrine rhythmicity and impaired autonomic activity.

Chronobiological Changes

Kudrow in 1976 (1) and 1977 (5) found significantly lowered plasma testosterone and LH levels during cluster periods but not during remissions. These results were interpreted to suggest a hypothalamic-pituitary axis involvement in the pathogenesis of cluster headache. These reports were corroborated by others (3–6), although interpretation of findings varied. These included disordered REM-states (4), effects of pain (3, 5), stress (6), and hypothalamic-pituitary axis dysfunction (2, 6). Supportive evidence for hypothalamic-pituitary involvement was reported by Bussone et al. (7) and Leone et al. (8) Thyrotropin response to thyrotropin-releasing hormone was found to be significantly reduced during cluster periods, when compared with response in control subjects or cluster patients in remission.

Further research elucidated mechanisms that might explain these hormonal changes and opened a new window into cluster headache pathogenesis. Alteration or loss of circadian rhythmicity of neuroendocrine substances was subsequently reported. Faccinetti et al. (6) found decreased plasma testosterone levels associated with changes in circadian rhythmicity during cluster periods. Polleri et

al. (9) reported loss of prolactin circadian rhythms in a group of patients during active cluster periods. Additionally, peak values occurred on days in which attacks were experienced. Similarly, Waldenlind et al. (10) found a decrease in 24-hour plasma prolactin secretion and attenuated nocturnal acrophase levels during cluster periods.

Most impressive was the finding of melatonin rhythm changes. Chazot et al. (11) and Waldenlind et al. (12) found decreased nocturnal levels during cluster periods, compared with those in control groups or remission periods, respectively.

Dyschronic changes in plasma cortisol were also noted among patients studied during cluster periods (13–15). Nocturnal peak values were found to be greater and phase-delayed when compared with those in control subjects. Finally, loss of circadian rhythmicity for beta-endorphins (16), blood pressure, and temperature (17) were found during cluster periods.

Circannual Rhythm Changes. Clinically, patients often report that cluster periods are apt to occur at the same time of the year (18, 19). An earlier report suggested a bimodal frequency curve for cluster period onsets (20). The study population, however, was generally too small for accurate analysis, and the study design was retrospective. Recently, in a long-term prospective study, a large cluster headache population was surveyed for cluster period onset frequencies (21, 22). Eight hundred ninety-one cluster period onsets were accurately recorded from approximately 400 male patients over a 10-year period. Mean monthly frequencies of cluster period onset were plotted against length of daylight as mean monthly photoperiods. A bimodal curve revealed peak frequencies in July and January, two weeks following the longest and shortest days of the year, respectively. The bimodal curve was interrupted in May and November, exhibiting decreased period onset frequencies occurring two weeks following resetting of clocks for daylight savings and standard times.

These results demonstrated an association of cluster period onset with photoperiod changes. This suggested possible failure of hypothalamic suprachiasmatic nuclei to synchronize with photoperiods as the magnitude of change increased or decreased. This suggestion is supported by interruption of the increasing period onset frequencies following the resetting of external clocks. The mechanism of this phenomenon may be related to sleep-phase changes produced by resetting of external clocks. An influence of sleep-phase changes on chronobiological pacemakers has been reported elsewhere (23–25).

Impairment of Sympathetic Neuronal Activity

Fanciullacci et al. (26) were first to demonstrate deficient sympathetic responses during cluster periods, between attacks. In their now-classical pupillometric studies, these investigators applied a topical solution of 2% tyramine to the eyes of cluster headache patients during and between attacks. Tyramine causes a release of neuroepinephrine at postsynaptic receptors, to effect a midriatic response. They found that following tyramine instillation the ipsilateral midriatic response was significantly lower than that on the contralateral side. These findings suggested that sympathetic neuronal transmission was impaired on the ipsilateral side (26).

This interpretation gained support from subsequent pupillometric studies by Salvesen et al. (27) and Boccuni et al. (28) Additionally, Boccuni et al. (28) showed that impairment of a sympathetic neuronal activity was not limited to pupillary response. Sympathergic stimulation provoked by hyperventilation produced electrocardiographic changes in cluster patients but not controls. The mechanism, they suspected, was asynchronous repolarization attributed to impaired central sympathetic activity.

Asymptomatic facial sweating patterns have also been demonstrated during cluster periods between attacks. In a study of 18 cluster patients and controls, Saunte et al. (29) demonstrated an ipsilaterally decreased sweating response to thermal stimulation (heat and exercise) and increased sweating response ipsilaterally, following pilocarine administration, compared with controls or contralateral sides among patients. The authors suggested that the pilocarpine response may have reflected a sympathetic denervation supersensitivity phenomenon, but they were cautious in identifying the lesion as preganglionic. As the authors point out, denervation hypersensitivity responses generally result from denervation of postsympathetic ganglia pathways. An exception, described by Lloyd (30), is sweat gland innervation. In this case, denervation of preganglionic sympathetic nerves may cause a hypersensitivity response.

Disturbance of sympathetic activity during cluster periods is further suggested by facial thermographic studies. Friedman and Wood first described ipsilateral forehead cold spots in a significantly high proportion of cluster headache patients between attacks. In subsequent reports, facial thermographic examination of patients between attacks revealed diminished temperature distribution over ipsilateral supraorbital regions in approximately 70% of the study population (31, 32). Similar findings were re-

ported during cluster attacks (33, 34). Changes in supraorbital artery hemodynamics during cluster periods may be associated with impairment of autonomic regulation. Indeed, biopsied specimens of superficial temporal arteries from chronic cluster headache patients and controls, revealed a supersensitive vasodilatory response to in vitro histamine (H_2) administration in the former group (35). However, prophylactic treatment of cluster headache with H_2-blockers has not been successful (36).

INDUCTION OF THE CLUSTER ATTACK

Clinically, spontaneous cluster headache attacks often occur during relaxation, during sleep (often in association with REM-sleep phases) (37, 38), following exertion, and during high-altitude exposure. Attacks may be provoked by vasodilators, such as alcohol (39), histamine (39), and nitroglycerin (40). Ekbom (40) provoked attacks in 10/10 patients following sublingual administration of 1.0 mg nitroglycerin. Attacks were reported to occur 30 to 50 minutes following nitroglycerin administration.

A recent hypothesis (41) speculated that induction of cluster headaches, whether provoked or spontaneous, is due to hypoxemia. An uncompensated hypoxemia would require a blunted chemoreceptor response as a result of impaired autonomic activity. Hypoxemic stimulation above this threshold, it was suggested, may hyperactivate (denervation response) chemoreceptor reflexes and trigger pain-producing pathways. In a polysomnographic study of 10 episodic and chronic cluster patients, Kudrow et al. (38) demonstrated a relationship of cluster attack onset and sleep apnea-induced hypoxemia. A subsequent study showed that the magnitude of hypoxemia may not be as important as the duration of relative hypoxemia. Active cluster patients were compared with remission patients and control subjects for oxygen saturation (SAO_2) changes following nitroglycerin administration (42). SAO_2 values decreased modestly but significantly, following nitroglycerin administration in all patients and in all groups. In remission and control groups, however, SAO_2 values returned to baseline after a mean duration of 26 minutes; significantly decreased SAO_2 values persisted for a mean duration of 40 minutes in the active cluster group. Sustained relative oxygen desaturation culminated in cluster headache attacks in 10/10 active cluster patients. All attacks were aborted by oxygen inhalation associated with a sudden, then sustained increase in SAO_2. Results suggested that once induced, persistent hypoxemia may have been due to impairment of compensatory chemoreceptor autoregulation, a condition inherent to the cluster period (42).

CLUSTER ATTACK

The major focus of investigation in cluster headache has been the cluster headache attack. Involvement of numerous systems has been elucidated. Some (e.g., vasomotor and biochemical changes) appear to be exaggerations of the cluster period; some autonomic nervous system and neurotransmitter changes may be specific to this phase.

Vasomotor Changes

Extracranial Arteries. Horton (43) believed that the pain of cluster headache attacks was due to extracranial vasodilatation. He had observed that a subcutaneous injection of 0.3 to 0.5 mg histamine induced attacks. Headaches were characterized by temporal artery swelling and were relieved by digital compression. Increased facial temperature was noted on the ipsilateral side, which was later corroborated by Lance and Anthony (44).

The role of the external carotid artery and exclusion of internal carotid artery involvement in cluster attacks was suggested in earlier experiments by Kunkle et al. (45). Ekbom (46), however, could not reproduce their results. Involvement of the internal carotid artery and its branches increased in importance in later investigations.

Internal Carotid Artery. Hørvin et al. (47) and Broch et al. (48) studied intraocular changes in cluster headache patients during attacks and demonstrated increased ipsilateral pulse–synchronous indentation pulse waves; and increased ipsilateral pulse–synchronous pressure changes, respectively. Drummond and Anthony (33) obtained plethysmographic records of temporal and supraorbital arteries in cluster headache patients before and after provoked cluster headache attacks. They found increased pulsations ipsilaterally during both phases. These results suggested that attacks may be associated with ophthalmic artery dilation.

The importance of the internal carotid artery (ICA) was further realized in the findings of Ekbom and Greitz (49). Angiograms obtained from several cluster headache patients demonstrated generalized cerebral vessel ectasia. Quite fortuitously, one patient began to experience a cluster attack during angiography. A segmental narrowing of the extradural part of the ICA was noted at the beginning of the attack, which may have been due to the spasm and/or arterial wall edema. This change was associated with a marked dilatation of the ipsilateral ophthalmic artery. Toward the end of the attack, ICA narrowing extended proximally into the upper part of the bony canal. This finding may explain the partial Horner's syndrome associated with attacks, compression of oculosympathetic nerves within the canal. The simultaneous appearance of marked ophthalmic artery dilatation and narrowed ICA was not explained.

An attempt to elucidate the hemodynamics of the ophthalmic artery and supraorbital branches by Doppler flow velocity examinations resulted in conflicting reports. Doppler flow velocity changes between ipsilateral and contralateral supraorbital arteries were reported as slightly lower ipsilaterally (31, 50), significantly higher ipsilaterally (51), and having no significant differences (52).

There is general agreement about facial thermographic changes over supraorbital regions during cluster attacks. During a spontaneous attack in one patient, marked cooling was noted over the ipsilateral supraorbital area. Following the attack, reversal of temperature patterns were noted, demonstrating an increased temperature distribution over the ipsilateral medial canthus and supraorbital region (32). To what extent asymmetrical sweating may have affected this finding is uncertain. Drummond and Lance (34) obtained thermographic images during spontaneous and nitroglycerin-induced attacks. Heat loss was predominant over ipsilateral orbital areas, corroborating the earlier observation.

Cerebral Blood Flow. Sakai and Meyer (53) reported a marked increase in cerebral blood flow (CBF) during attacks in cluster headache patients. This corroborated an earlier finding in one patient by Norris et al. (54). Henry et al. (55), however, could not show CBF changes in three patients with cluster headache. More recently, Aebelholt-Krabbe et al. (56) reported an increased regional CBF in central, basal, and parietotemporal areas during cluster headache attacks.

The attack-related increased cerebral blood flow has been ascribed to impaired autoregulatory responses (53), reactive hyperemia (54), or a pain-related activity (56). Support for impaired regulatory autoregulatory responses was reported later by Sakai and Meyer (57), who demonstrated an impaired autoregulatory response to CO_2 and increased response to O_2.

Biochemical Changes

Histamine. As mentioned earlier, Horton (43) believed that histamine was the major mediator of cluster headache attacks. Urinary excretion of labeled histamine, however, was found to be elevated in only a third of the cluster patients studied (58). In a population of 20 patients with cluster headache, Anthony and Lance (59) obtained blood histamine levels during 22 attacks. They found significantly higher levels than in preheadache samples. Others found plasma histamine levels to be elevated during cluster attacks (60, 61). In view of these findings, cluster headache patients were treated prophylactically in a controlled study with combined H_1- and H_2-receptor blockers (60). No significant improvement was noted when compared with placebo-treated patients.

The role of histamine in the pathogenesis of cluster headache was supported by Appenzeller et al. (62) and Prusinski and Liberski (63). These investigators reported more mast cells from temporal skin biopsies of cluster patients than controls.

Appenzeller et al. (62, 64) further described proximity of mast cells to cutaneous nerves in the cluster group and to perivascular regions in the control groups. Morphological evidence of mast cell degranulation, suggesting extrusion of histamine, was also found. These findings were later corroborated (65–67), but unconfirmed by others (68, 69).

Substance P. Sicuteri et al. (70) presented evidence in support of the role of substance P in the generation of cluster attacks. They suggested that substance P (SP) and allied transmitters, such as vasoactive intestinal peptide (VIP) and CGRP may provoke a rostral spread of neuronal activity in the trigeminal nerve. It was further demonstrated that administration of somatostatin, an inhibitor of SP, alleviated cluster headache attacks (71).

Moskowitz (72) had earlier provided evidence of trigeminal ganglia involvement mediated by neurogenic inflammatory responses in cluster headache attacks. Hardebro (73) suspected a trigeminal nerve–substance P mechanism, with particular respect to the proximity of the sphenopalatine ganglion. These investigators independently suggested that the influence of trigeminal pathways in their respective schemes extended to include a cavernous sinus–carotid syphon region and may account for most of the symptoms and signs of the cluster attack (72, 73).

As noted by Moskowitz (72), the cavernous sinus appears to be an important site in the genesis of cluster headache pain. In almost all cases of symptomatic cluster headache, a condition in which an intracranial lesion is associated with the disorder, the site of involvement is usually in or near the cavernous sinus. Symptomatic cluster headache attacks and autonomic signs are indistinguishable from idiopathic cluster headache (74–78).

Autonomic Nervous System. Involvement of the autonomic nervous system, particularly parasympathetic nerve activity in cluster attacks, may extend beyond its regulation of blood vessels. Stowell (79), in 1970, suggested that the cluster attack may be caused by efferent impulses from greater superficial petrosal nerves, arising from parasympathetic nuclei in the hypothalamus. This may be initiated, he reasoned, by normal impulses arising from cortical areas when cortical control is inhibited by relaxation. Efferent impulses pass from the hypothalamus to the nuclei of the 5th, 7th, and 9th cranial nerves via the dorsal longitudinal fasciculus, but chiefly over the 7th cranial nerve to involve the sphenopalatine ganglion. Sections of the greater superficial petrosal nerve in 32 patients afforded relief in 87.5%. Recurrences, however, were reported to be high at 3-year follow-up. Resection of the first division of the 5th cranial nerve resulted in complete relief of cluster headaches in 5/5 patients (79).

The role of the greater superficial petrosal nerve in cluster headache was first suggested by Gardner et al. (80) as early as 1947. Typical cluster headaches, they reported, could be evinced by stimulation of this nerve, and section of the nerve in 13 patients resulted in partial to excellent success in 75% of cases.

In support of the role of parasympathetic influences in cluster headache, Kunkle et al. (81) found acetylcholine-like substances in the cerebral spinal fluid in 4/14 cluster patients during attacks, but in none of 7 migraine patients.

He hypothesized that parasympathetic storms involving the 7th and 10th cranial nerves may explain all the autonomic features of the cluster attack, including bradycardia.

Recently, de Belleroche et al. (82) reported significantly reduced erythrocyte choline levels during cluster periods, which was reversed by lithium therapy.

According to Dimitriadou et al. (67), the role of parasympathetic hyperactivity may be compatible with mast cell changes and influences of histamine and substance P in the pathogenesis of cluster attacks. They postulated that excessive release of acetylcholine from parasympathetic nerve terminals could stimulate histamine release from mast cells. Histamine and other mediators would stimulate sensitive nerve terminals directly, leading to an antidromic response and release of substance P, resulting in further mast cell degranulation, inflammatory response, and pain.

SUMMARY

It would appear that the cluster period is an altered physiological state, characterized by hypothalamic dysfunction that may result in chronobiological abnormalities and impaired sympathetic and parasympathetic activity, and consequently, autoregulatory deficiencies in vasomotor regulation and chemoreceptor responses to hypoxemia.

This pathophysiological environment is conducive to induction of attacks, either spontaneous or provoked—possibly mediated by sustained hypoxemia due to blunted carotid body activity—and followed by denervation-hyperactive paroxysms of peripheral chemoreceptors (41).

Pathways of the cluster headache attack may involve the 5th, 7th, 9th, and 10th cranial nerves. Hemodynamic changes in arterial and venous channels, particularly in the cavernous sinus, may be mediated via these cranial nerve pathways by histamine, peptide, and cholinergic neurotransmitters, to affect pain and associated signs and symptoms of the cluster headache attack.

REFERENCES

1. Kudrow L. Plasma testosterone levels in cluster headache: preliminary results. Headache 1976;16:28–31.
2. Kudrow L. Plasma testosterone and LH levels in cluster headache. Headache 1977;17:91–92.
3. Nelson RF. Testosterone levels in cluster and non-cluster migraineurs headache patients. Headache 1978;18:265–267.
4. Romiti A, Martelletti P, Gallo MF, Giacovazzo M. Low plasma testosterone levels in cluster headache. Cephalalgia 1982;3:41–44.
5. Klimek A. Plasma testosterone levels in patients with cluster headache. Headache 1982;22:162–164.
6. Facchinetti F, Nappi G, Cicoli C, et al. Reduced testosterone levels in cluster headache: a stress-related phenomenon. Cephalalgia 1986;6:29–34.
7. Bussone G, Frediani F, Leone M, Grazzi L, Lamperti E, Boiardi A. TRH test in cluster headache. Headache 1988;7:43–54.
8. Leone M, Patruno G, Vescovi A, Bussone G. Neuroendocrine dysfunction in cluster headache. Cephalalgia 1990;10:235–239.
9. Polleri A, Nappi G, Murialdo G, Bono G, Martignoni E, Savoldi F. Changes in the 24-hour prolactin pattern in cluster headache. Cephalalgia 1982;2:1–7.
10. Waldenlind E, Gustafsson SA. Prolactin in cluster headache: diurnal

secretion, response to thyrotropin-releasing hormone, and relation to sex steroids and gonadotropins. Cephalalgia 1987;7:43–54.

11. Chazot G, Claustrat B, Brun J, Jordan D, Sassolas G, Schott B. A chronobiological study of melatonin, cortisol, growth hormone and prolactin secretion in cluster headache. Cephalalgia 1984;4:213–220.

12. Waldenlind E, Ekbom K, Friberg Y, Sääf J, Wetterburg L. Decreased nocturnal serum melatonin levels during active cluster headache periods. Opusc Med 1984;29:109–112.

13. Nappi G, Ferrari E, Polleri A, Savoldi F, Vailati A. Chronobiological study of cluster headache. Chronobiologia 1981;2:140.

14. Ferrari E, Canepari C, Bossolo PA, et al. Changes of biological rhythms in primary headache syndromes. Cephalalgia 1983;3(suppl 1):58–68.

15. Waldenlind E, Gustafsson SA, Ekbom K, Wetterbert L. Circadian secretion of cortisol and melatonin in cluster headache during active cluster periods and remission. J Neurol Neurosurg Psychiatry 1987;50:207–213.

16. Nappi G, Facchinetti F, Bono G, et al. Lack of β-endorphin and β-lipotropin circadian rhythmicity in episodic cluster headache: a model for chronopathology. In: Pfaffenrath V, Lundberg P-O, Sjaastad O, eds. Updating in headache. Berlin: Springer-Verlag, 1985.

17. Ferrari E, Martignoni E, Vailati A, Nappi G, Savoldi F, Mandelli B. Chronobiological aspects of cluster headache. Effect of lithium therapy. In: Savoldi F, Nappi G, eds. Headache. Pavia: Palladio Editore, 1979;152–160.

18. Ekbom K. Pattern of cluster headache with a note on the relation of angina pectoris and peptic ulcer. Acta Neurol Scand 1970;46:225–237.

19. Lance JW. Mechanisms and management of headache. 3rd ed. London: Butterworths, 1978.

20. Kudrow L. Cluster headache, mechanism and management. Oxford: Oxford University Press, 1980.

21. Kudrow L: The cyclic relationship of natural illumination to cluster period frequency. [Abstract] Cephalalgia (suppl 6):76–77. 1987.

22. Kudrow L, Cornélissen G, Halberg F. Population study or 3-and 6-monthly changes in cluster headache onsets. Proc. 2nd World Conference on Clinical Chronobiology, Monte Carlo, April, 1990;p.15.

23. Czeisler CA, Richardson GS, Coleman RM, Zimmerman JC, Moore-Ede MC, et al. Chronotherapy: resetting the circadian clock of patients with delayed sleep phase insomnia. Sleep 1981;4:1–21.

24. Lewy AJ, Sacks RL, Miller LS, Hoban TM. Antidepressant and circadian phase-shifting effects of light. Science 1987;235:352–354.

25. Czeisler CA, Kronauer RE, Allan JS, Duffy JF, Jewett ME, et al. Bright light induction of strong (type O) resetting of the human circadian pacemaker. Science 1989;244:1328–1333.

26. Fanciullacci M, Pietrini U, Gatto G, Boccuni M, Sicuteri F. Latent dysautonomic pupillary lateralization in cluster headache. A pupillometric study. Cephalalgia 1982;2:135–144.

27. Salvesen R, Bogucki A, Wysocka-Bakowska MM, Antonaci F, Fredriksen TA, Sjaastad O. Cluster headache pathogenesis: a pupillometric study. Cephalalgia 1987;7:273–284.

28. Boccuni M, Morace G, Pietrini U, Porciani MC, Fanciullacci M, Sicuteri F. Coexistence of pupillary and heart sympathergic asymmetries in cluster headache. Cephalalgia 1984;4:9–15.

29. Saunte C, Russell D, Sjaastad O. Cluster headache: on the mechanism behind attack-related sweating. Cephalalgia 1983;3:175–185.

30. Lloyd DPC. Cholinergy and adrenergy in the neural control of sweat glands. In: Curtis DR, McIntyre AK, eds. Studies in physiology. New York: Springer-Verlag, 1965;169–178.

31. Kudrow L. Thermographic and Doppler flow asymmetry in cluster headache. Headache 1979;19:204–208.

32. Kudrow L. A distinctive facial thermographic pattern in cluster headache—the "Chai" sign. Headache 1985;25:33–36.

33. Drummond PD, Anthony M. Extracranial vascular responses to sublingual nitroglycerin and oxygen inhalation in cluster headache patients. Headache 1985;25:70–74.

34. Drummond PD, Lance JW. Thermographic changes in cluster headache. Neurology 1984;34:1292–1298.

35. Hardebo JE, Aebelholt-Krabbe A, Gjerris F. Enhanced dilatory response to histamine in large extracranial vessels in chronic cluster headache. Headache 1980;20:316–320.

36. Anthony M, Lord GDA, Lance JW. Controlled trials of cimetidine in migraine and cluster headache. Headache 1978;18:261–264.

37. Dexter JD, Riley TL. Studies in nocturnal migraine. Headache 1975;18:261–264.

38. Kudrow L, McGinty DS, Phillips ER, Stevenson M. Sleep apnea in cluster headache. Cephalalgia 1984;4:33–38.

39. Horton BT, MacLean AR, Craig WM. A new syndrome of vascular headache: results of treatment with histamine: preliminary report. Mayo Clin 1939; Proc. 14:257–260.

40. Ekbom K. Nitroglycerin as a provocative agent in cluster headache. Arch Neurol 1968;19:487–493.

41. Kudrow, L. A possible role of the carotid body in the pathogenesis of cluster headache. Cephalalgia 1983; 3:242–247.

42. Kudrow L., Kudrow DB. Association of sustained oxyhemoglobin desaturation and onset of cluster headache attacks. Headache 1990; 30:474–480.

43. Horton BT. Histaminic cephalgia (Horton's headache or syndrome). Maryland State Med J 1961;10:178–203.

44. Lance JW, Anthony M. Thermographic studies in vascular headache. Med J. Aust 1971;1:240–243.

45. Kunkle EC, Pfeifer JP Jr., Wilhoit WM, Hamrick LW Jr. Recurrent brief headache in 'cluster pattern'. Trans Amer Neurol 1952;77:240–243.

46. Ekbom K. Some observations on pain in cluster headache. Headache 1975;14:219–225.

47. Hørven I, Nornes H, Sjaastad O. Different corneal indentation pulse patterns in cluster headache and migraine. Neurology 1972;22:99–98.

48. Broch A, Hørven I, Nornes H. Sjaastad O, Tønsuma A. Studies of cerebral and ocular circulation in a patient with cluster headache. Headache 1970;10:1–13.

49. Ekbom K, Grietz T. Carotid angiography in cluster headache. Acta Radiol (Diagn)1970;10:177–186.

50. Nattero G, Savi L, Pisanti G. Doppler flow velocity in cluster headache. International Congress, Headache '80, Florence, Italy, 1980.

51. Schroth G, Gerber WD, Langohr HD. Ultrasonic Doppler flow in migraine and cluster headache. Headache 1983;23:284–288.

52. Russell D, Lindegaard K- F. Cluster headache: Doppler examination of the extracranial arteries. Cephalalgia 1985;5(suppl 3):276–277.

53. Sakai F, Meyer JS. Regional cerebral hemodynamics during migraine and cluster headaches measured by the ^{133}Xe inhalation method. Headache 1978;18:122–132.

54. Norris JW, Hachinski VC, Cooper PW. Cerebral blood flow changes in cluster headache. Acta Neurol Scand 1976;54:371–374.

55. Henry PY, Vernhiet J, Orgogozo JM, Caille JM. Cerebral blood flow in migraine and cluster headache. Res Clin Stud Headache 1978;6:81–88.

56. Aebelholt-Krabbe A, Henriksen L, Olesen J. Tomographic determination of cerebral blood flow during attacks of cluster headache. Cephalalgia 1984;4:17–23.

57. Sakai, F, Meyer JS. Abnormal cerebrovascular reactivity in patients with migraine and cluster headache. Headache 1979;19:257–266.

58. Sjaastad O, Sjaastad ØV. Urinary histamine excretion in migraine and cluster headache. J Neurol 1977;216:91–104.

59. Anthony M., Lance JW. Histamine and serotonin in cluster headache. Arch Neurol 1971;25:225–231.

60. Anthony M, Lance JW, Lord G. Migrainous neuralgia—blood histamine levels and clinical response to H_1 and H_2 receptor blockade. In: Green R, ed. Current concepts in migraine research. New York: Raven Press, 1978:149–151.

61. Medina JL, Diamond S, Fareed J. The nature of cluster headache. Headache 1979;19:309–322.

62. Appenzeller O, Becker W, Ragas A. Cluster headache. Ultrastructural aspects. Neurology 1978;28:371.

63. Prusinski A, Liberski PP. Is the cluster headache local mastocytic diaethesis? Headache 1979;19:102.

64. Appenzeller O, Becker WJ, Ragaz A. Cluster headache. Ultrastructural aspects and pathogenetic mechanisms. Arch Neurol 1981;38:302–306.

65. Liberski PP, Prusinski A. Further observations on the mast cells over the painful region in cluster headache patients. Headache 1982;22:115–117.

66. Liberski PP, Mirecka B. Mast cells in cluster headache. Ultrastructure, release pattern and possible pathogenetic significance. Cephalalgia 1984;4:101–106.

67. Dimitriadou V, Henry P, Brochet B, Mathiau P, Aubineau P. Cluster headache: ultrastructural evidence for mast cell degranulation and interaction with nerve fibres in the human temporal artery. Cephalalgia 1990;10:221–228.

68. Cuypers J, Westphal K, Bunge ST. Mast cells in cluster headache. Acta Neurol Scand 1980;61:327–329.

69. Aebelholt-Krabbe A, Rank F. Histological examinations of the superficial temporal artery in patients suffering from cluster headache. Cephalalgia 1985;5(suppl 3):282–283.

70. Sicuteri F, Fanciullacci M, Geppetti P, Renzi D, Caleri D, Spillantini MG. Substance P mechanism in cluster headache: evaluation in plasma and cerebrospinal fluid. Cephalalgia 1985;5:143–149.

71. Sicuteri F, Geppetti P, Marabini S, Lembeck F. Pain relief by somatostatin in attacks of cluster headache. Pain 1984;18:359–365.

72. Moskowitz MA. The neurobiology of vascular head pain. Ann Neurol 1984;16:157–168.

73. Hardebro JE. The involvement of trigeminal substance P neurons in cluster headache. An hypothesis. Headache 1984;24:294–304.

74. Herzberg L, Lenman JAR, Victoratos G, Fletcher F. Cluster headache associated with vascular malformations. J Neurol Neurosurg Psychiatry 1975;38:648–649.

75. Thomas AL. Periodic migrainous neuralgia associated with an arteriovenous malformation. Postgrad Med J 1975;51:460–461.

76. Tfelt-Hansen P, Paulsen OB, Krabbe A. Invasive adenoma of the pituitary gland and chronic migrainous neuralgia. A rare coincidence or a causal relationship? Cephalalgia 1982;2:25–28.

77. Mani S, Deeter J. Arteriovenous malformation of the brain presenting as a cluster headache—a case report. Headache 1982;22:184–185.

78. Greve E, Mai J. Cluster headache-like headaches: a symptomatic feature? A report of three patients with intracranial pathologic findings. Cephalalgia 1988;8:79–82.

79. Stowell A. Physiologic mechanisms and treatment of histaminic or petrosal neuralgia. Headache 1970;9:187–194.

80. Gardner WJ, Stowell A, Dutlinger R. Resection of the greater superficial petrosal nerve in the treatment of unilateral headache. J Neurosurg 1947;4:105–114.

81. Kunkle EC. Acetylcholine in the mechanism of headaches of the migraine type. Arch Neurol Psychiatr (Chicago), 1959;84:135.

82. Belleroche deJ, Cook GE, Das I, Joseph R, Tresidder I, et al. Erythrocyte choline concentrations and cluster headache. Br Med J 1984;88:268–270.

23

Medical Management of Cluster Headache

FREDERICK G. FREITAG

The medical management of cluster headache may be divided according to the major approaches to therapy: abortive for acute attacks of cluster headache and the more important, prophylactic treatments for cluster. Prophylactic therapies may be divided (with overlap) into treatments for episodic cluster, chronic cluster, and cluster headache variants. Many well-controlled trials have been conducted on the medical therapies for migraine headache. Cluster headache treatment, by comparison, is represented by comparatively few well-controlled trials of the medical therapies, many of which have been the mainstay of cluster treatment for many years.

ABORTIVE THERAPIES

The use of abortive agents for acute cluster headaches is important, although these medications lack uniform efficacy and convenience for patients. The three primary abortive therapies for cluster headache are oxygen, ergotamine preparations, and local anesthetic agents, applied intranasally.

The use of oxygen in the abortive therapy of cluster headache was originally described by Bayard T. Horton (1), who recommended its use in combination with dihydroergotamine. Kudrow (2) studied the use of oxygen for the acute relief of cluster headache in 52 patients, who each treated 10 acute headaches. The oxygen was administered at 100% concentration rates, via face masks, at a flow rate of 7 liters per minute. Success was defined as relief within 15 minutes, for seven out of 10 cluster attacks. Seventy-five percent of these patients found oxygen inhalation beneficial for treatment of acute cluster. It was more effective in patients with episodic cluster headache than in those with chronic cluster headache, in a small percentage of patients. Oxygen therapy was also found to be more efficacious in patients under age 50, without regard for the chronicity of this disorder. Kudrow (2) compared oxygen to sublingual ergotamine. Using a crossover trail, he showed that oxygen was more likely to be effective in approximately 82% of the patients; sublingual ergotamine was beneficial in only about 70% of treated cases.

A double-blind crossover investigation of oxygen versus air inhalation was conducted by Fogan (3). Of 19 males

with cluster headache participating in this trial, 11 patients completed both phases of the study. The statistical results showed that oxygen was superior to air inhalation in the acute treatment of cluster headache. In patients refractory to standard use of oxygen, its use in a hyperbaric chamber may prove beneficial (4).

For many years, ergotamine preparations have been the "gold standard" in the treatment of migraine and other vascular headaches. Few controlled trials exist of these agents in the acute treatment of cluster headache. Dihydroergotamine, an ergotamine derivative (administered via nasal inhalation) has been compared with placebo in a controlled trial (5). In this trial of 25 patients, 22 completed the study and reported that nasal inhalation of 1 mg of dihydroergotamine was superior to placebo nasal spray. This study was hampered by both technical difficulties and the dose of the inhaled dihydroergotamine that was delivered. These factors played a role in the relatively low numbers of patients who obtained full relief with this treatment.

Ekbom (6) studied the bioavailability of ergotamine tartrate in patients with cluster headache in remission. Inhalation was shown to be the only route of administration likely to produce significant blood levels of this agent. The inhaled form was compared with effervescent tablets, rectal suppositories, and an intravenous administration control.

Clinically, the ergotamine-related medications remain one of the first choices for treatment of acute cluster headache. Routes of administration include inhalation, sublingual, and rectal suppositories. Parenteral administration of dihydroergotamine is the most commonly used and most successful modality. Due to the short duration of most acute cluster attacks, a rapidly acting form of ergotamine must be administered early to achieve efficacy. In patients with migraine headache, ergotamine preparations taken on consecutive days may induce rebound headache. This phenomena is not usually seen in patients with cluster headache. However, adherence to the weekly limits of ergotamine consumption must be followed.

The use of ergotamine preparations as abortive therapy of cluster headache must be avoided in a patient using ergotamine or methysergide for prophylactic therapy. The combined use of these agents could lead to ergotism and its complications.

In 1908, Sluder (7) described a condition which he called sphenopalatine ganglion neuralgia. Vail (8) reported a similar condition which he termed vidian neuralgia. Both conditions appear to be cluster headache. In both of these conditions, the use of cocaine applied by pledget to the sphenopalatine ganglia afforded relief. Barre (9) reported on both the use of applied pledgets as well as self-treatment with cocaine solution in 11 patients with cluster headache. The self-treatment consisted of cocaine applied intranasally through a dropper. Ten of these patients reported at least an 80% reduction in headache severity within several minutes during cluster attacks induced by nitroglycerin. Later, the administration of 10% cocaine solution by dropper for acute attacks, also proved successful. Patients in whom it was not helpful experienced difficulties with application of the solution, had structural abnormalities of the nasal passages, or had marked nasal congestion associated with their cluster attacks. The cocaine solution may relieve cluster attacks because of its local anesthetic abilities. However, its action as a sympathomimetic agent may also contribute to its effectiveness.

A 4% aqueous solution of lidocaine may be applied by a similar method. A study by Kittrele's group (10) found it effective in four of five cluster headache patients. Aqueous lidocaine offers an advantage over cocaine in lacking potential for addiction. However, lidocaine does not possess the sympathomimetic actions found with cocaine. This variation and the difference in concentration between a 4% lidocaine solution and a 10% cocaine solution may contribute to the varying outcomes between the agents.

The local anesthetics, ergots, and oxygen inhalation all provide satisfactory results in the acute treatment of cluster headache. No single therapy is clearly advantageous over the others. Although oxygen therapy is extremely safe, it is ill-suited for the cluster headache patients whose attacks usually occur in public places. The ergots, while more convenient, have poor absorption rates. This delay hampers its use in both abortive and prophylactic therapy of cluster headache. The local anesthetics present difficulties in administration for many patients. The patient must lie down and have proper head positioning for the agent to reach the area of the sphenopalatine ganglia. Cocaine possesses a risk of addiction, although it may be more effective than lidocaine. Both agents are convenient for use in a variety of settings in which cluster may occur.

Several trials of experimental therapies for cluster headache have recently been undertaken. These have involved abortive agents. In a minor clinical investigation, somatostatin appears to relieve the pain of cluster headache through its inhibition of substance P release from trigeminal nerve endings (11). The other therapy currently being investigated for treating acute cluster attacks is sumatrip-

tan. The early results with this serotonergic agonist of the 5-HT$_1$ receptor appears promising (12).

Verapamil, previously used as prophylactic therapy for cluster headache, has been administered intravenously to a small group of patients whose cluster attacks were induced by nitroglycerin. The administration of verapamil at the peak of the acute cluster headache attack significantly decreased pain intensity (13).

Cluster headache may occasionally be considered by patients to be related to sinus disease. The prominence of nasal symptoms and the seasonal preponderance of cluster headache may contribute to their belief. Occasionally patients may have a clinical response of their cluster headaches with over-the-counter sinus remedies (14). Sinutab, one of the over-the-counter remedies, contains acetaminophen, phenyltolamine citrate, and phenylpropanolamine hydrochloride. Three patients with established histories of cluster headache noted a response. A marked shortening of cluster headache attacks was observed with the use of this agent.

Patients with episodic cluster headache are more likely to have a positive response to any of the abortive therapies for cluster headache. Patients with chronic paroxysmal hemicrania may occasionally obtain relief with oxygen inhalation. Difficulty in judging the effectiveness of any of these agents in cluster variants is due to the extremely brief nature of the attacks.

PROPHYLACTIC TREATMENT OF CLUSTER HEADACHE

Prophylactic treatment of cluster headache is preferred for most patients. While the abortive therapies are successful in many patients, they are not uniformly effective. The high frequency of attacks in cluster headache put the patient at risk of increased toxicity from their treatment. For others with cluster headache, especially those with chronic cluster headache, the abortive therapies are less than reliable in relieving the acute attack.

Prophylactic therapies, if started early in cluster headache, are often extremely effective at complete prevention of attacks. Such therapy is more effective in episodic cluster headache and in chronic paroxysmal hemicrania. Patients with chronic cluster headache less often obtain significant remission from their attacks. A decrease in efficacy or breakthrough headaches are far more common with this form of the disease.

There is a good deal of overlap in treating episodic and chronic cluster with the various medical therapies. Many of the therapies have been widely used in clinical practice; others remain in the realm of experimental treatments.

Commonly Used Agents
METHYSERGIDE

The two primary therapies for episodic cluster headache prophylaxis are the ergots and corticosteroids. The ergots that are used primarily are ergotamine tartrate and methysergide.

Methysergide is given in divided doses of 4 to 10 mg per day. The dose is usually titrated to optimize reduction of headache severity as well as the patient's ability to tolerate the therapy. Singular therapy with methysergide tends to be effective in most patients with episodic cluster headache. It has its greatest effect in patients who have never used it previously or have used it only for a few periodic cycles of cluster. The use of singular therapy with methysergide for repeated bouts of cluster headache appears to trigger tachyphylaxis in many patients, making them resistant to this agent. The addition of a corticosteroid in these patients may restore the effectiveness of methysergide. A review of clinical trials with methysergide has been conducted (15). An overall response rate of 73% was demonstrated. The use of methysergide must be restricted to treatment periods lasting no longer than 6 months. The continuous use of methysergide longer than 6 months increases the risk of fibrotic complications involving the retroperitoneal space, lungs, and heart valves. In withdrawing patients from methysergide after 6 months of therapy, the drug should be tapered slowly. These patients should be given a drug-free hiatus of at least one month before methysergide is reintroduced. During this time, appropriate evaluations including chest x-rays, intravenous pyelograms, and laboratory studies should be performed to assess for potential end-organ damage. Monthly evaluation of the patient on methysergide should be conducted to rule out any complications secondary to use of this agent.

ERGOTAMINE TARTRATE

An alternative to methysergide therapy is ergotamine tartrate prescribed in low doses. Typically, a combination preparation containing ergotamine tartrate 0.6 mg, phenobarbital, and belladonna alkaloids (Bellergal-S) can be used, twice daily. As with methysergide, careful evaluations of these patients is necessary monthly, to reduce the risk of complications occurring with the use of this medication.

With both methysergide and ergotamine tartrate, we begin reducing the dose within 2 weeks after the patient's last cluster attack. Decreasing titration of the doses is done at weekly intervals, for most patients. The dose is usually decreased by one tablet of the respective medications, at each weekly interval.

CORTICOSTEROIDS

Corticosteroids may also be used in the prophylactic treatment of cluster headache. Prednisone 10 to 80 mg has been reported to be effective in most patients (16). In this trial, 14 of 19 patients had at least a 50% reduction in attacks. Eleven of the patients became cluster headache–free. These results were comparable to those reported by Kudrow (17) using 40 mg per day of prednisone. Of his 92 patients with cluster headache, 86% showed a significant

benefit from prednisone. Seventy-one percent of the patients in this clinical trial had a greater than 75% reduction in the frequency of their cluster attacks.

With dose reduction, breakthrough of cluster headaches typically occurs as the dose of prednisone is decreased to less than 20 mg per day. In our experience, patients report ing breakthrough cluster headaches during dose reduction may be treated with several techniques to facilitate tapering of the drug. Intramuscular administration of a single dose of ACTH 80 units has proven successful. As an alternative (unless contraindicated), low-dose ergotamine therapy or lithium carbonate given concomitantly with the prednisone may be used. After several days on these agents, the prednisone tapering may be continued. After the patient is completely withdrawn from the prednisone, tapering and discontinuation of the other agents may be achieved.

Alternative corticosteroid therapy have been suggested. Anthony (18) reported successful treatment with methylprednisolone 120-mg injections of the greater occipital nerve. A subsequent trial was undertaken by Bigo's group (19), in which methylprednisolone 160 mg was compared with the dose used by Anthony. Only nine of 16 patients had any type of response. Six of these nine were either at the end of a cluster cycle or the results were partial and transient.

LITHIUM CARBONATE

The two primary therapies for chronic cluster headache are lithium carbonate and verapamil, although other agents may be useful. The use of lithium in cluster headache was advanced by Ekbom in 1974. Subsequently, Kudrow (20) reported its successful use in many patients with chronic cluster headache. Lithium carbonate has also been used successfully in treating episodic cluster headache (17, 21). Ekbom (21) found lithium to have many significant effects in episodic cluster headache. Both Kudrow (17) and Mathew (22) found lithium to be beneficial in most patients treated with the drug.

In chronic cluster headache, Kudrow (20) reported a greater than 90% reduction of attacks in 14 patients. An additional 11 patients had a 60 to 90% reduction in headaches. Mathew (22) found that nine of 11 patients with chronic cluster had a 90% or better response. Of these patients, four had secondary chronic cluster and experienced a complete remission of their headaches. A complete remission in primary chronic cluster headache occurred in five of the 13 patients.

The dose of lithium carbonate required to obtain control of cluster headaches is variable. Although 300 to 900 mg per day is needed in most patients, dose adjustment of lithium carbonate depends on monitoring blood levels of the drug. Optimal levels are between 0.4 and 1.2 mEq/liter, and serum levels should be obtained periodically to avoid toxicity. Lithium carbonate is one of the most widely used agents for long-term treatment of chronic cluster headache. However, no long-term controlled trials with lithium carbonate have been reported. Manzoni and Granella (23) reviewed the published results of its long-term use, noting its safety for long-term use in most patients. Some patients, however, may develop thyroid dysfunction due to chronic use. Some patients fail to maintain remission with this agent, and a small number of patients who initially achieve headache remission will suffer a relapse despite adjustment in the dose of lithium. Most patients continue to maintain their remissions with only rare mild attacks. Approximately one-third of patients report periodic exacerbation of their attacks. Some patients who achieve remission of their cluster headaches remain in remission after drug therapy is discontinued or may convert to episodic cluster headache.

The mechanism by which lithium works in cluster headache is poorly understood. Little correlation is apparent between the action of lithium and the occurrence of depression (22). Genetic markers may play a role in cluster headache and in the response to treatment with lithium as reported by Giacovazzo's group (24). They observed that HLA-b14 is significantly less common in patients with cluster headache than in headache-free controls. The HLA-b18 antigen was also significantly more common in those patients who responded to lithium. The HLA-A1 antigen was present in 35.7% of nonresponders to lithium; only 14.3% of responders tested had this antigen.

Most likely, lithium has its action in cluster headache by altering central mechanisms involved in the headache. Okayasu's group (25) found no change in cerebral hemodynamics in cluster headache patients treated with lithium. Fanciullacci and his colleagues (26) demonstrated a progressive effect in long-term treatment of patients, indicating a correction of the asymmetries in autonomic function and pain sensitivity. Further evidence to suggest the central effects comes from Chazot's group (27). They demonstrated a shift in the secretion of melatonin with a once-daily dose of lithium; a decreased production of cortisol was associated with this time shift in melatonin.

CALCIUM ENTRY BLOCKERS

Verapamil was first reported to be useful in cluster headache by Meyer and Hardenberg (28). Although only four patients were treated with this drug, they all responded to it. Subsequently, Gabai and Spierings (29), in an open trial, found that 33 of 48 patients had at least a 75% reduction in cluster headache. They noted no significant difference in using verapamil in episodic or chronic cluster patients. This study also demonstrated that episodic cluster patients were more likely to have no response, although this same group was more likely to have the most marked reduction in cluster headache. Patients with episodic cluster averaged 6.5 weeks into their cycle of headaches. A response was noted in less than 2 weeks. Chronic cluster headache patients required an average of 5 weeks to respond, and also required a higher average dose. The average dose in chronic cluster headache was 572 mg per day, compared with 354 mg per day for patients with episodic cluster headache.

Bussone's group (30) conducted a placebo-controlled crossover trial of lithium carbonate 900 mg per day versus verapamil 360 mg per day in 25 chronic cluster patients. Both drugs performed comparably. Fifty percent of patients on verapamil achieved a 50% decrease in headache in the first week, compared with 37% on lithium therapy. This difference was equalized by the second week of active treatment. For both agents, equal decrements in analgesic use occurred within the first week. Side effects were slightly more increased during lithium treatment.

Several other calcium entry blockers have also been tried in cluster headache prophylaxis, including nimodopine and nifedipine. Nimodopine proved useful in a small trial of patients with chronic cluster. Meyer and Hardenberg (28) noted, in eight patients, a nearly 50% reduction in the frequency of headaches. Therapy with nimodopine 120 mg per day resulted in all patients obtaining benefit. If the starting dose was 60 mg per day, only 40% of patients responded within the first 2 months. However, if the drug was started at 120 mg per day and then reduced to 60 mg per day after 2 months, the response to nimodopine was maintained. Thirteen patients with episodic cluster headache have also been involved in a trial with nimodopine (31). Using nimodopine 120 mg per day, seven patients obtained relief of their cluster episode within 10 days of starting treatment. All of these patients were in the first 10 days of a headache cycle.

In the previously cited trial by Meyer and Hardenberg (28) nifedipine was also tried. They found uniformly successful results in the 10 patients in whom this agent was used. All 10 experienced a complete remission of their clusters at doses of 30 to 180 mg per day.

SEROTONIN ANTAGONISTS

Pizotifen was tried in 28 patients with cluster headache (32), and compared with ergotamine and placebo. The dose of pizotifen was 1.5 mg per day in divided doses, and the dose of ergotamine was 2 to 3 mg per day in divided doses. Twenty-one percent of the patients became cluster-free during the trial with pizotifen. An additional 36% achieved at least a 50% reduction in their attacks. Ten of the 28 patients did not benefit from pizotifen. Ten patients compared ergotamine with pizotifen, and six found pizotifen to be superior to ergotamine. Comparison with the placebo periods demonstrated that pizotifen was significantly better (p<.001) during the final phase of the study. Pizotifen is not available in the U.S.

Histamine Therapies in Cluster Headache

In 1939, Horton and his colleagues (33) reported on the successful use of histamine injections in the treatment of cluster headache. They recommended that subcutaneous injections of histamine be started at 0.05 mg twice a day for two days, with a gradual titration upward to 0.1 mg twice a day for up to 2 to 3 weeks. These investigators found that 65 of 84 patients obtained relief of their cluster headaches for periods of 2 weeks to 18 months.

Blumenthal (34) recommended using smaller doses of histamine, starting treatment at 0.25 ml of solution containing 0.1 mg of histamine. However, he also found that histamine could be administered as an intravenous solution of histamine phosphate, at doses of 0.55 mg of histamine phosphate in normal saline 100 ml administered over approximately 1 hour. The treatment time was 1 hour regardless of the dose of histamine infused. Gradual titration was accomplished over time. Using a similar technique, Stern (35) found histamine infusion or subcutaneous injections to be uniformly useful in six patients with cluster headache. The patients had been experiencing cluster attacks ranging from 4 to 21 weeks. Remission from cluster attacks persisted for slightly longer than 16 months.

Diamond and his colleagues (36) have also reported the beneficial use of histamine desensitization. Using IV histamine infusion of 5.5 mg of histamine phosphate per 24 hours for 10 days was effective in the treatment of intractable cluster headache. The IV infusions were used in conjunction with H_1 and H_2 antagonists. The histamine desensitization was used as adjunctive therapy to more traditional agents for chronic cluster headache. Significant remission of cluster headache occurred with this protocol. Of interest, patients who had become refractive to more traditional agents, such as lithium carbonate and verapamil, demonstrated a restored response to these agents following completion of the IV histamine desensitization.

Since 1939, when Horton advanced the use of histamine injections for cluster headache, significant disfavor has evolved for its use in cluster headache treatment. Various authors have suggested that there is no place for histamine in the treatment of cluster headache. Several reasons may account for their disdain for this treatment. Histamine desensitization has been inappropriately used by some physicians and has been given for a variety of disorders. This therapy has also been used by some practitioners for treating all of their patients with headaches. Another reason appears to result from several trials using just H_1 and H_2 antagonists as treatment for cluster headache without the use of histamine parenteral administration.

HISTAMINE ANTAGONISTS

A controlled trial of cimetidine was conducted in 20 patients with cluster headache (37). Patients received cimetidine, an H_2 antagonist either alone or in combination with an H_1 antagonist, chlorpheniramine. These two active treatments were compared with placebo. Patients received each treatment for 2 weeks. No significant difference was noted between the three treatments. Russel (38)

also reported on a trial of H_1 and H_2 antagonists in 15 patients with cluster headache, using cimetidine 200 mg per day in divided doses and chlorpheniramine 20 mg per day in a placebo-controlled crossover trial. Twelve patients completed the trial, consisting of 3 weeks on each treatment. Although the results did not reach statistical significance, seven of 12 patients improved while on the regimen. Similar results were reported in a study by Cuyper's group (39). Seven of 9 patients taking the combination of H_1 and H_2 antagonists reported a favorable response. A loss of response was noted within 4 weeks in three of four patients with chronic cluster.

Histamine desensitization and the combined use of H_1 and H_2 antagonists appears to have some efficacy in cluster headache treatment. However, well-controlled trials of this treatment for cluster headache is lacking. This type of therapy is not associated with any of the major complications that may occur in surgical procedures for chronic cluster headache.

Infrequently Used Therapies for Cluster Headache

Lisuride, a derivative of isoergolenyl, has a variety of pharmacological actions. It acts as both a peripheral serotonin antagonist and a central serotonin agonist. Lisuride also possesses dopamine agonist properties. A trial of this agent was conducted in 10 patients (40). Five of the patients had episodic cluster headache, and four of five of these patients improved. A similar result was seen in patients with chronic cluster headache.

Tiospirone was used in a small trial of episodic cluster patients at the Diamond Headache Clinic (41). This drug has serotonergic antagonist action as well as dopaminergic and α-adrenergic agonist action. In the low doses (25 to 125 mg per day) used in this trial, all patients tolerated the medication. Tiospirone demonstrated significant reduction in the frequency and severity of cluster headache. It also reduced the need for abortive medications for acute attacks. Further research with this agent was suspended after adverse effects occurred, at high doses, in patients with a major psychiatric diagnosis.

A mast cell–stabilizing agent, ketotifen, has been tried in 15 patients (42). This agent, which acts similarly to disodium chromoglycate, has a structure similar to pizotifen. It also has H_1-receptor blocking properties. All 15 patients with chronic cluster improved during the trial. Eight patients obtained a complete remission from their attacks. Patients with secondary chronic cluster responded more rapidly than primary chronic cluster patients.

Kudrow (43) and Klimek (44) have reported on decreased levels of testosterone associated with cluster headache. Klimek (45) reported on the use of testosterone porpionicum, administered intramuscularly. A dose of 25 mg per day for up to 10 days was started. Later, a reduced dose of 10 mg per day was given for another period of up to 10 days. A significant improvement was demonstrated in patients with episodic cluster headache. Three patients with chronic cluster did not improve.

The use of antiandrogens was studied by Sicuteri (46). Cyproterone 120 mg per day was given for 2 months to 29 patients with episodic cluster headache. Eleven patients with chronic cluster headache were treated for 4 months. In those with episodic cluster headache, 24% achieved a remission and another 52% improved. The results compared with a 36% remission rate in chronic cluster, and a total improved patient number of 8 of the 11. Significant adverse effects occurred in all patients, including reduced libido. Sicuteri noted that those who had failed with lithium carbonate were most likely to benefit from this treatment.

In 1986, Hardebo reported on a patient who had cluster headache associated with attacks of herpes simplex (47). The patient noted improvement after treatment of the herpes simplex with acyclovir 200 mg five times per day, on two separate occasions.

The use of phenothiazines for the treatment of headache has become increasingly popular in recent years. The mechanism by which these agents exert their influence is not well understood, but it may be related to central effects on dopaminergic and adrenergic transmission or a peripheral adrenergic mechanism. Chlorpromazine, in doses of 75 to 700 mg per day, was studied in an open trial in 13 patients with cluster headache (48). All patients exhibited a favorable response to treatment, and none reported major complications from the use of these agents. Long-term treatment of up to 8 months was carried out in four of the patients. The results are difficult to evaluate, however, since 11 of the 13 patients received concomitant therapy in the first week of treatment. Nine of those patients receiving concomitant medications were treated with ergotamine, methysergide, or prednisone. All of these agents may also induce remissions of cluster headache.

Diamond and his colleagues (49), among others, have reported on alterations in enkephalin and endorphin function associated with cluster headache. Captopril has been shown to have enkephalinase-inhibiting properties (50). An open trial of this agent at doses of 25 to 300 mg per day was undertaken in cluster headache patients. The nine patients with chronic cluster headache had been refractory to conventional therapy. All of the patients had a worsening of their headaches during the first week of treatment, and none preferred the captopril to lithium carbonate.

Budipine, a pharmacological agent with diverse effects, has been tried in various disorders from episodic cluster headache to chronic paroxysmal hemicrania. This agent has an affinity for enkaphalin receptors, monoamine oxidase inhibition, as well as inhibition of the reuptake of biogenic amines (51). The authors did not provide a review of results according to diagnosis. They reported that all but one of 35 patients improved with doses of 15 to 60 mg per day of budipine. Twenty of the patients reported complete remission of their attacks.

An open trial of sodium valproate was conducted in 15 patients (52). Two of the patients had chronic cluster and the remainder were in an acute bout of episodic cluster headache. Both patients with chronic cluster had a marked reduction in their attacks, and 10 of those with episodic cluster had a complete remission.

Indomethacin-responsive Cluster Headache Syndromes

Indomethacin has been used in a variety of cluster headache syndromes, including chronic paroxysmal hemicrania (CPH), atypical cluster headache, multiple jabs, background vascular headache, ice-pick headache, sharp short-lived head pain syndromes, and "jabs and jolts." All of these variants have a common denominator, which is indomethacin as the drug of choice for relief of these headaches.

In chronic paroxysmal hemicrania, a prechronic stage may occur initially. In these patients, low doses of indomethacin provide relief and may be tapered and eventually discontinued without recurrence of the headaches. Once the chronic phase ensues, doses of 25 to 50 mg three times per day afford relief, often within hours of starting treatment (53). As the remission from CPH is maintained, the dose may be tapered to a maintenance dose of 12.5 mg daily to 25 mg four times per day.

In other types of cluster headache variants responsive to indomethacin, Diamond and Medina (54) found that 83% of 54 patients responded to indomethacin. The remainder suffered with what was believed to be a concomitant depression, and they experienced a favorable response to tricyclic antidepressants. Mathew conducted a placebo-controlled trial in five patients with sharp, short-lived head pain syndrome (55). The controlled trial compared aspirin and indomethacin (50 mg, three times per day) with placebo. Aspirin produced a 15% decrease in the average weekly headache index, compared with placebo. Indomethacin therapy resulted in an 89% decrease in the average index. Aspirin also produces a similar degree of benefit in patients with CPH.

PROGNOSIS

The outcome of cluster headache has been examined in two studies. In order to assess outcome, Kudrow (56) contacted patients who had discontinued treatment. He found that approximately half of episodic cluster patients reported no change in the pattern of their headache cycles. About 5% had converted to chronic cluster headache, while 48 of the 124 patients had experienced a prolonged remission from attacks. Twelve of 25 patients with chronic cluster headache continued with their disease unchanged, 20% had converted to episodic cluster headache, and 12% had gone into remission. In a recent unpublished survey, Kunkel and Frame (57) interviewed 68 patients with chronic cluster headache after at least 5 years from their last treatment. Thirty-four percent of their patients continued to have chronic cluster headache that was not well-controlled. An additional 19% of the patients had achieved control of their headaches with treatment. They also found that 23.5% of these patients achieved remission from their headaches, and a similar number had converted to episodic cluster headache. Of those achieving remission, five were relieved by surgery, three each through medications or by discontinuing smoking cigarettes, and one had gone into remission after chiropractic treatment.

REFERENCES

1. Horton BT. Histaminic cephalgia. MD Med J 1961;10:178–203.
2. Kudrow L. Response of cluster headache attacks to oxygen administration. Headache 1981;21:1–4.
3. Fogan L. Treatment of cluster headache, a double blind comparison of oxygen versus air inhalation. Arch Neurol 1985;42:362–363.
4. Weiss LD, Ramasastry SS, Eidelman BH. Treatment of cluster headache patient in a hyperbaric chamber. Headache 1989;29:109–110.
5. Andersson PG, Jespersen LT. Dihydroergotamine nasal spray in the treatment of attacks of cluster headache. Cephalalgia 1986;6:51–54.
6. Ekbom K, Krabbe A, Paalzow G, Tfelt-Hansen P, Waldenlind E. Optimal routes of administration of ergotamine tartrate in cluster headache patients, a pharmokinetic study. Cephalalgia 1983;3:15–20.
7. Sluder S. Etiology, diagnosis, prognosis, and treatment of sphenopalatine ganglion neuralgia. JAMA 1913;61:1201–1205.
8. Vail HH. Vidian neuralgia. Ann Oto Rhin Laryngol 1932;41:837–856.
9. Barre F. Cocaine as an abortive agent in cluster headache. Headache 1982;22:69–73.
10. Kittrele JP, Grouse DS, Seybold ME. Cluster headache local anesthetic abortive agents. Arch Neurol 1985;42:496–498.
11. Caleri D, Marabini S, Panconesi A, Pietrini U. A pharmacological approach to the analgesizing mechanism of somatostatin in cluster headache. La Ricerca in Clinica E in Laboratorio 1987;17:2:155–162.
12. Ekbom K. Presented at the 8th migraine trust. London, September 28, 1990.
13. Boiardi A, Gemma M, Porta E, Peccarisi C, Bussone G. Calcium entry blocker: treatment in acute pain in cluster headache patients. Ital J Neurol Sci 1986;7:5:531–534.
14. Cohen KL. "Sinutabs" for cluster headache. N Engl J Med 1980;303:107–108.
15. Curran DA, Hinterberger H, Lance JW. Methysergide. Res Clin Stud Headache 1967;1:74–122.
16. Couch JR, Ziegler DK. Prednisone therapy for cluster headache. Headache 1978;18:219–221.
17. Kudrow L. Comparative results of prednisone, methysergide and lithium therapy in cluster headache. In: Greene R, ed. Current concepts in migraine research. New York, Raven Press 1978:159–163.
18. Anthony M. Arrest of attacks of cluster headache by local steroid injection of the occipital nerve. In: Rose FC, ed. Migraine. Clinical and research aspects. Karger, Basel, 1985;169–173.
19. Bigo A, Delrieu F, Bousser, MG. Cluster headache: treatment by injection of methylprednisolone into the region of the greater occipital nerve. 16 cases. Rev Neurol 1989; 145:160–162.
20. Kudrow L. Lithium prophylaxis of chronic cluster headache. Headache 1977;17:15–18.
21. Ekbom K. Lithium for cluster headache: review of the literature and preliminary results of long term treatment. Headache 1981;21:132–139.
22. Mathew NT. Clinical subtypes of cluster headache and response to lithium therapy. Headache 1978;18:26–30.
23. Manzoni GC, Granella F. Lithium in chronic cluster headache: side effects and long-term follow-up. In: Mumenthaler M, Van Zweiten PA, Farcot JM, eds. The treatment of chronic pain. New York: Harwood, 1990:8–14.
24. Giacovazzo M, Martelletti P, Romiti A, Gallo MF, Iuvara E. Relationship between HLA system in cluster headache and clinical response to lithium therapy. Headache 1985;25:268–270.
25. Okayasu H, Meyer JS, Mathew NT, Amano T, Hardenberg J. Lithium has no measurable effect on cerebral hemodynamics in cluster headaches. Headache 1984;24:1–4.
26. Fanciullacci M, Pietrini U, Boccuni M, Gatto G, Cangi F. Does lithium balance the neuronal bilateral asymmetries in cluster headache? Cephalalgia 1983;(suppl 1):85–87.
27. Chazot G, Claustrat B, Brun J, Zaidan R. Effects on the patterns of melatonin and cortisol in cluster headache of a single administration of lithium at 7:00 PM daily over one week: a preliminary report. Pharmacopsychiatry 1987;20:222–223.
28. Meyer JS, Hardenberg J. Clinical effectiveness of calcium entry blockers in prophylactic treatment of migraine and cluster headache. Headache 1983;23:266–277.
29. Gabai IJ, Spierings ELH. Prophylactic treatment of cluster headache with verapamil. Headache 1989;29:167–168.
30. Bussone G, Leone M, Peccarisi C, Micieli G, Granella F, et al. Verapamil vs. lithium in prophylactic treatment of chronic cluster headache: a double blind crossover study. In: Rose FC, ed. New advances in headache research. London: Smith-Gordon, 1989:229–234.
31. De Carolis P, Baldrati A, Agati R, De Capoa D, D'Alessandro R, Sacquegna T. Nimodopine in episodic cluster headache: results and methodologic considerations. Headache 1987;27:397–399.
32. Ekbom K. Prophylactic treatment of cluster headache with a new serotonin antagonist, BC 105. Acta Neurol Scand 1969;45:601–610.
33. Horton BT, Maclean AR, Craig W McK. A new syndrome of vascular headache: results of treatment with histamine: preliminary report. Proc Staff Meet MAYO Clin 1939;14:257–261.
34. Blumenthal LS. Current histamine therapy. Mod Med 1950;18:51–54.
35. Stern FH. Histamine cephalalgia—an often overlooked cause of headache. Psychosomatics 1969;10:53–56.
36. Diamond S, Freitag FG, Prager J, Gandhi S. Treatment of intractable cluster headache. Headache 1986; 26:42–46.
37. Anthony M, Lord GDA, Lance JW. Controlled trial of cimetidine in migraine and cluster headache. Headache 1978;18:261–264.
38. Russel D. Cluster headache: trial of combined histamine H1 and H2 antagonist treatment. J Neurol Neurosurg Psychiatry 1979;42:668–669.
39. Cuypers J, Altenkirch H, Bunge S. Therapy of cluster headache with histamine H1 and H2 receptor antagonists. Eur Neurol 1979;18:345–347.
40. Raffaelli E, Martins OJ, Fiho, A.D.S.P.D. Lisuride in cluster headache. Headache 1983;23:117–121.
41. Diamond S, Freitag FG. Unpublished results.
42. Split W, Szmidt M, Prusinski A, Rozniecki J. Ketotifen in the treatment of chronic cluster headache. Headache 1984;24:147–149.
43. Kudrow L. Plasma testosterone levels in cluster headache, preliminary results. Headache 1976;16:28–31.
44. Klimek A. Plasma testosterone levels in patients with cluster headache. Headache 1982;22:162–164.
45. Klimek A. Use of testosterone in the treatment of cluster headache. Eur Neurol 1985;24:53–56.
46. Sicuteri F. Anti-androgenic medication of cluster headache. Int J Clin Pharm Res 1988;8:21–24.
47. Hardebo JE. An association between cluster headache and herpes simplex. N Engl J Med 1986;314:316.
48. Caviness VS, O'Brien P. Cluster headache: response to chlorpromazine. Headache 1980;20:128–131.
49. Diamond S, Mosnaim A, Freitag F, Wolf M, Lee G, Solomon G.

Plasma methionine-enkephalin levels in patients with cluster headache. Longitudinal and acute studies. In: Rose FC, ed. Advances in headache research. London: Smith-Gordon, 1987:209–215.

50. Fanciullacci M, Spillantini MG, Michelacci S, Sicuteri F. Pharmacologic "enkephalinase" inhibition in man. Adv Exp Med Biol 1986;1986:153–160.

51. Kruumlautger H, Kohlhepp W, Reiman G, Przuntek H. Prophylactic treatment of cluster headache with budipine. Headache 1988;28:344–346.

52. Hering R, Kuritzky A. Sodium valproate in the treatment of cluster headache: an open clinical trial. Cephalalgia 1989;9:195–198.

53. Diamond S. Variants of cluster headache. In: Mathew NT ed. Cluster headache. Jamaica, NY: Spectrum 1984: 21–30.

54. Diamond S, Medina L. Cluster headache variant. Arch Neurol 1981;38:705–709.

55. Mathew NT. Indomethacin responsive headache syndromes. Headache 1981;21:147–150.

56. Kudrow L. Natural history of cluster headache—part 1 outcome of drop out patients. Headache 1982;22:203–206.

57. Kunkel R, Frame J. Unpublished results.

24

Surgical Management of Cluster Headache

J. KEITH CAMPBELL and BURTON M. ONOFRIO

Chronic cluster headache can be difficult to treat, often failing to respond to the agents that give relief in the episodic variety. Even in subjects who do respond initially, chronic cluster headache has a tendency to become resistant after a variable period. It is frequently necessary to switch from one treatment regimen to another and to use agents such as methysergide, lithium, and corticosteroids, which are not ideal for long-term administration. Despite these shortcomings, medical management (as described in Chapter 23) provides adequate relief in most persons suffering from chronic cluster headache. In a small minority, however, medical therapy fails either initially or subsequently to prevent the debilitating and agonizing attacks or there is an absolute contraindication to the use of the usually effective agents. For these unfortunate and select few, various surgical procedures have been used for many years.

HISTORY OF SURGICAL MANAGEMENT OF CLUSTER HEADACHE

Since 1926, when Harris (1, 2) recommended interruption of the trigeminal sensory pathways for relief of "ciliary neuralgia," there have been very few reports of successful, long-lasting amelioration of cluster headache by surgical means. Most of the proposed techniques have been directed to the trigeminal sensory system or the parasympathetic fibers in the nervus intermedius and the greater superficial petrosal nerves or the sphenopalatine ganglion and its connections. Cryosurgery of the superficial temporal artery or excision of a portion of the artery and ligation of the middle meningeal artery have been almost uniformly unsuccessful and have been abandoned as surgical options.

Section of the Greater Superficial Petrosal Nerve

Gardner et al. (3) reported their experience with resection of the greater superficial petrosal nerve in 26 patients with intractable unilateral head pain. Half of their subjects suffered "histamine cephalgia" (as described by Horton et al. (4)). Relief was excellent in 25% and fair to good in 50% of cases, and treatment failed in 25%. The authors speculated that surgical division of the greater superficial petrosal nerve interrupted abnormal parasympathetic discharges that might be responsible for dilatation of cerebral, meningeal, and nasal mucosal blood vessels. The pain was thought to result from the vascular changes being felt via the trigeminal nerve. An alternative proposal stated that the operation interrupted painful impulses passing through geniculate somatic afferent fibers (5) from the dura, internal carotid artery, and vidian nerve. Since the original report (3), there have been very few reports of greater superficial petrosal neurectomy in the treatment of cluster headache. Sachs (6) reported pain relief after such neurectomy but noted that the benefit was brief. As recently as 1983, Watson et al. (7) mentioned resection of the greater superficial petrosal nerve in the management of chronic cluster headache. In their series of four patients who were so treated, one had no benefit and three had relief lasting longer than 1 year. Despite reports of isolated successes (8, 9), the tendency for pain to return has led to a search for more effective neurosurgical management.

Section of the Nervus Intermedius

Sachs (6) reported that intraoperative stimulation of the nervus intermedius with the patient under local anesthesia reproduced a painful syndrome resembling cluster headache and that sectioning of the nerve could produce freedom from the attacks of pain. Seven of his nine patients had relief, one for at least 17 years (6, 10). The two failures were attributed to improper selection. More recently, Rowed (11) reported favorably on nervus intermedius section in cluster headache—six of eight patients were pain-free postoperatively during follow-up ranging from 4 to 26 months. Five of the patients successfully treated had delayed but temporary recurrence of pain that was milder than the preoperative pain and was not accompanied by the usual prominent autonomic features such as tearing and rhinorrhea. The benefits of the posterior fossa approach to nervus intermedius section were partially offset by significant ipsilateral hearing loss in two patients and, of lesser importance, moderately severe but temporary vertigo. Not all who have reported on nervus intermedius section have had such success (12).

The theoretical role of the nervus intermedius in cluster headache was exhaustively reviewed by Solomon (13). He postulated that most of the autonomic features and the vasodilatation of the external carotid arterial tree are due to parasympathetic impulses carried by the nervus intermedius and that afferent nociceptive fibers in the mixed nerve might carry the pain from the dilated arterial tree. Vasodilatation is not painful per se, but the intense parasympathetic discharges via the nervus intermedius may result in a perivascular, sterile inflammatory reaction similar to that postulated to occur in migraine.

Sphenopalatine Ganglion Procedures

Cocainization of the sphenopalatine ganglion will abort the pain of cluster headache if performed during an attack. This observation led to attempts to provide long-lasting relief by ganglionectomy or destruction of the ganglion. As with the surgical procedures already described, relief has often been of short duration or incomplete. Meyer et al. (14) discussed surgical removal of the sphenopalatine ganglion in 13 patients with cluster headache, of whom 7 did not have benefit, 4 continued to have pain that could be controlled by analgesics, and only 2 reported complete relief for more than 1 year.

Neurologists familiar with cluster headache generally believe that the syndrome of sphenopalatine ganglion neuralgia is identical with or at least a variant of cluster headache; some otorhinolaryngologists disagree and believe it is a separate condition (15). Whether they are the same or different conditions, destruction or removal of the sphenopalatine ganglion provides such unpredictable or short-lasting relief that the procedure is now rarely performed.

Procedures to Interrupt the Trigeminal Sensory Pathways

The peripheral branches of the trigeminal nerve, the gasserian ganglion, and the main sensory root have each been the site of surgical procedures to obtain relief of pain in cluster headache. Injection of alcohol into the infraorbital nerve or the gasserian ganglion was used by Harris (2, 16) with considerable success. A similar experience with alcohol injections of the ganglion was reported (but not in detail) by McArdle (17). Others have reported failure to relieve pain with alcohol injections into the terminal branches of the trigeminal nerve and no relief after induction of satisfactory anesthesia by gasserian ganglion injection (7).

Favorable experience with radio-frequency thermocoagulation of the gasserian ganglion in the treatment of trigeminal neuralgia led to the application of this percutaneous technique to the treatment of medically resistant cluster headache. Reports by Maxwell (18), Onofrio and Campbell (19), Mathew and Hurt (20), and Watson et al. (7) have shown that if a radio-frequency lesion abolishes the corneal reflex ipsilaterally, it has at least a 66% chance of giving relief from the pain of cluster headache. The

benefit usually persists until the corneal reflex recovers, generally a period of several years or longer. In some of the subjects, painless attacks of ptosis, tearing, and rhinorrhea continue. Maxwell (18) performed a radio-frequency procedure only if a temporary lidocaine block of the gasserian ganglion relieved a spontaneous or induced attack of headache. Sweet (21) stressed the importance of the local anesthetic block before the more permanent procedure.

Retrogasserian injection of glycerol also has been useful in the surgical management of chronic cluster headache (22). The degree of pain relief correlated with the extent of corneal sensory loss.

Trigeminal root section via the posterior fossa has been used as a last resort for completely resistant cluster headache. O'Brien and MacCabe (23), Onofrio and Campbell (19), and others (24–26) have reported that partial or complete retrogasserian sensory root section is the only effective surgical procedure in selected patients. The advantages and disadvantages of such a procedure are discussed below.

Combination Surgical Procedures

Failure to provide relief by a single surgical procedure such as resection of the greater superficial petrosal nerve or nervus intermedius or partial root section of the trigeminal nerve has led to several combination operations. Kunkel and Dohn (27) reported their experience in 12 male patients who underwent section of the greater superficial petrosal nerve and neurolysis of the sensory root of the trigeminal nerve. Three subjects were not helped by the procedure, although the postoperative attacks of pain were no longer accompanied by autonomic features. Three patients were temporarily relieved of the painful attacks, and the remaining six patients remained pain-free during follow-up (duration not stated). Morgenlander and Wilkins (28) severed the nervus intermedius and performed a partial section of the sensory root of the trigeminal nerve in nine patients. All subjects had a recurrence of cluster headaches postoperatively. One of the patients who underwent a repeat of the procedures was pain-free 2 years postoperatively. Neurovascular decompression of the trigeminal nerve and section of the nervus intermedius have been used in combination (28) with a limited duration of freedom from pain.

INDICATIONS FOR SURGICAL MANAGEMENT

On the basis of our experience (19) and that of others (18, 20), operation is considered only when all medical options have been exhausted and when the clinical course indicates that a spontaneous remission is unlikely. By definition, chronic cluster headache is present when the patient has had attacks of pain for 1 year without remission or when remission lasts for fewer than 14 days (29). In practice, operation should be considered only when attacks have been present for at least 1 year and they cannot be prevented by any reasonable medical means, when the attacks cannot be aborted by oxygen inhalation or appropriate use of ergotamine preparations, and when they are causing major suffering. The reasons for withholding operation until all medical means are exhausted are that no single procedure will guarantee pain relief and all of the procedures have some risk and some adverse effects.

Avoidance of operation is essential in persons with psychologically unstable personalities and in those with atypical pain features. A history of bilateral attacks of cluster headache, even if one side predominates, should lead to a careful review of the possible effects of a surgical attempt to control the pain. Experience has shown that surgical relief on one side sometimes leads to an apparent reactivation of cluster headache contralaterally. No procedure resulting in any significant degree of trigeminal sensory or motor loss should be performed bilaterally. Bilateral corneal insensitivity on both sides significantly increases the risk of keratitis and other corneal damage, and bilateral weakness of the masseter muscles seriously compromises chewing.

CURRENT RECOMMENDATIONS

When it has been determined that a patient has medically intractable chronic cluster headaches and when computed tomography or magnetic resonance imaging has been done to exclude a structural cause for the headaches, the implications of a trigeminal nerve procedure should be fully discussed.

During the past 10 years, we have used a percutaneous radio-frequency trigeminal gangliorhizolysis or, less commonly, a posterior fossa trigeminal sensory rhizotomy in an attempt to provide relief from chronic cluster headache. Our results (19) with the initial 26 patients indicated that relief of pain was excellent in 54%, fair to good in 15%, and poor in 31%. Subsequent procedures in a similar number of patients have confirmed this earlier experience and confirmed the observation that corneal sensory loss is essential if pain relief is to occur. Others have validated this finding (20, 22).

The advantages of the radio-frequency procedure, including the low morbidity and mortality in experienced hands (30, 31), the brief stay in the hospital, and the ability to repeat the procedure if pain returns, make it our procedure of choice. A posterior fossa sensory rhizotomy of the trigeminal nerve is performed only if, for technical reasons, it is not possible to obtain complete sensory loss in the first division of the trigeminal nerve by the percutaneous radio-frequency procedure. In a small percentage of subjects, the shape of the face precludes satisfactory placement of the radio-frequency electrode through the foramen ovale into the appropriate portion of the gasserian ganglion. For these patients, a failed radio-frequency procedure is followed by a complete trigeminal sensory root section through the posterior fossa. The motor branch is

spared if possible. A partial sensory root section has not proved effective because it rarely results in complete corneal sensory loss. Reoperation to complete a root section is rendered difficult and hazardous by the development of postoperative scarring, which makes correct identification of the trigeminal nerve uncertain.

Risks of a Radio-Frequency Lesion of the Gasserian Ganglion

Preoperatively, the patient must be fully informed of the specific risks of the radio-frequency procedure and the anticipated effects of the trigeminal nerve ablative procedure. The discussion must include a full disclosure of the risks attendant with corneal anesthesia and the possible development of anesthesia dolorosa of the face. Table 24.1 lists most of the risks of a radio-frequency lesion of the trigeminal nerve. The frequency of anesthesia dolorosa is usually stated to be between 2% and 4% after a destructive trigeminal nerve procedure, and it can occur after a radio-frequency lesion or root section. The development of this painful dysesthetic sensation cannot be predicted by a temporary lidocaine block of the nerve, and therefore we have not used this procedure, as Maxwell advocated (18). Provided the patient understands the risks and is willing to accept facial numbness in exchange for the pain of cluster headache, an ablative procedure is offered.

Percutaneous Radio-Frequency Gangliorhizolysis

With the patient awake, an 18-gauge needle is introduced into the forehead as a ground electrode. A small amount of lidocaine is then infiltrated just lateral to the corner of the mouth on the affected side (2 cm lateral for third division analgesia and 3 cm lateral for first and second division analgesia) (Fig 24.1). With the head hyperextended and rotated 15° to the opposite side, an anteroposterior skull roentgenogram is obtained to delineate the foramen ovale. The electrode is inserted with this trajectory under fluoroscopic imaging. The depth of the electrode through the foramen ovale will then determine the divisional analgesia. The average depth from the inner aspect of the foramen ovale to the opening of Meckel's cave into the posterior fossa is 2.1 cm. A lateral skull roentgenogram will ensure

Table 24.1.
Risks of a Radio-Frequency Lesion of the Gasserian Ganglion

Infection, including meningitis
Intracranial hemorrhage
Damage to structures adjacent to the ganglion
Trigeminal motor weakness
Temporal lobe seizures
Complication of anesthesia
Postoperative herpes simplex eruption in denervated area
Failure to relieve the target pain
Anesthesia dolorosa
Neuroparalytic keratitis
Death

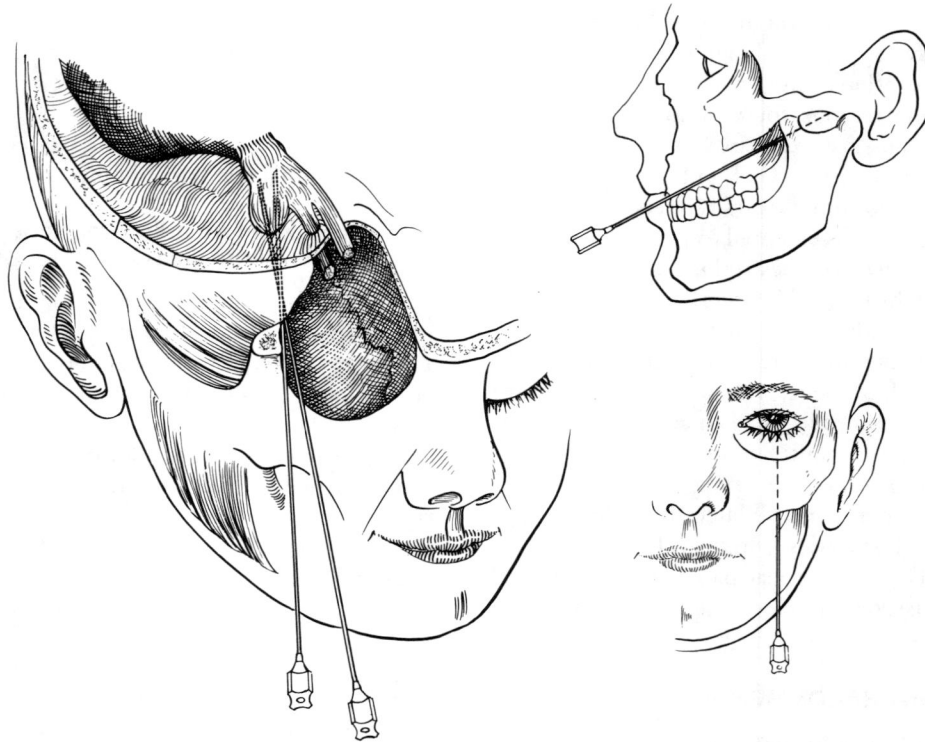

Figure 24.1. Placement of electrode for various divisions is shown with relationship to angle of mouth, external auditory meatus, and pupil. (From Onofrio BM. Stereotaxic gasserian ganglion ablation using a new stereotaxic probe. Mayo Clin Proc 1972;47:196–198.)

accurate placement—shallow for third division, midposterior for second division, and 1 mm short of the opening of Meckel's cave for first division. Cerebrospinal fluid should be seen flowing from the needle when final positioning has been achieved.

Once Meckel's cave is entered, the thermistor stylet is then inserted (Fig 24.2). The active electrode side-arm lead and the ground forehead electrode are attached to the R_2G frequency generator. Then, under methohexital sodium drip, the lesion is made at 90°C until the desired level of hypalgesia is achieved. Once the desired result is achieved, the needle is removed and the patient is sent to the post-anesthesia room. The parameters for producing the lesion are detailed elsewhere (30, 32). A successful lesion for relief of cluster headache must result in analgesia and anesthesia of V^1 and at least the upper portion of the V^2-innervated facial structures. As indicated previously, corneal sensory loss with abolition of the corneal reflex appears to be essential if pain relief is to result.

RESULTS

When a successful radio-frequency lesion results in the desired sensory loss, most patients are immediately free from painful attacks, and a small percentage have attacks that continue for a few days and then cease. Failure to prevent the pain has almost always been associated with less than complete V^1 and corneal sensory loss. Several authors have reported an occasional subject in whom the pains persisted despite adequate sensory loss (7, 19, 20). The explanation for these failures is unknown, although pain transmission through the nervus intermedius or facial nerves is suggested.

Recurrence of attacks is to be expected as the effects of the radio-frequency lesion are repaired, just as may occur when the procedure is used for the management of trigeminal neuralgia. Our impression is that the benefits of the radio-frequency lesion are less long-lasting than in trigeminal neuralgia. In our patients treated for cluster headache, recovery of corneal sensation usually has been followed by a return of the painful attacks in 1 to 3 years or occasionally much longer. Repeating the radio-frequency procedure is possible and appropriate if the recurrent attacks fail to respond to medical management.

POSTOPERATIVE CARE

Corneal sensory loss demands careful preoperative and postoperative education of patients. They are instructed to use artificial tears every 4 hours while awake for the first few weeks and then less often if the eye remains normal. They must be instructed to examine the eye every day in a mirror and to see a physician immediately if the conjunctival sac is injected or if the cornea is cloudy. They should enlist the aid of their friends and relatives to report any redness or unusual appearance of the eye. Those who work in a dirty or hazardous place should either wear goggles or have a clear side shield added to their prescription or safety

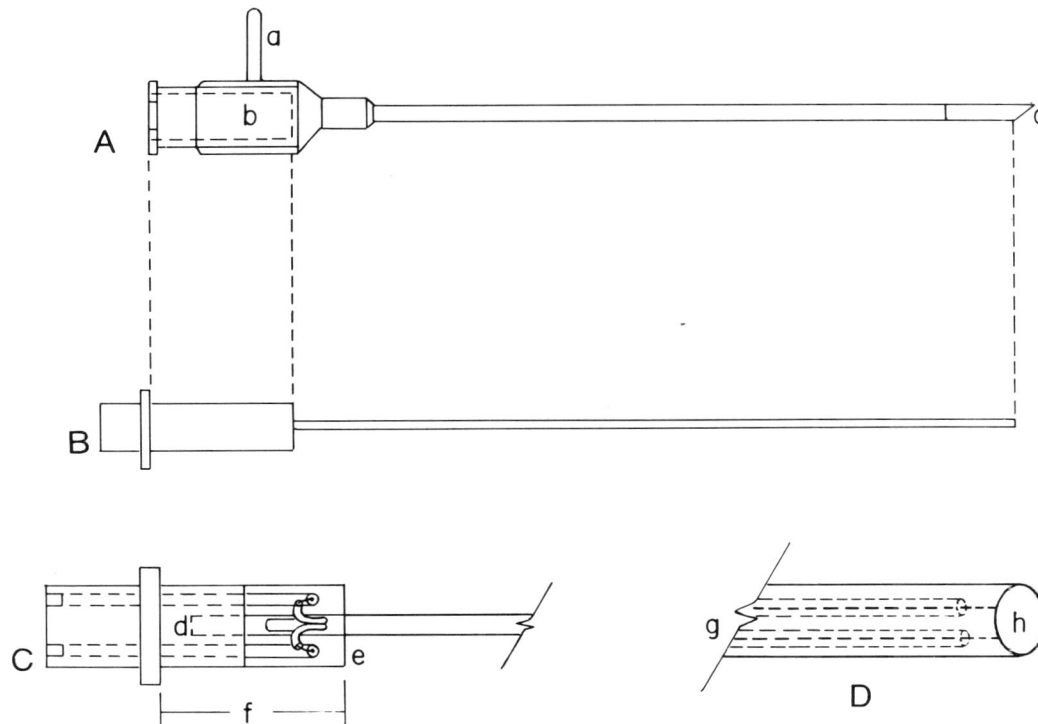

Figure 24.2. *A,* Stereotaxic needle is a 20-gauge, thin-walled spinal needle; hub and needle are entirely coated with three coats of Epoxylite 6001-M except for stud (*a*) and 5- to 8-mm exposed soft-beveled tip (*c*); (*b*) is a 4.5-mm diameter × 9-mm hole. *B,* Stylet. *C,* Enlarged view of thermistor connector assembly: (*d*) hole bored into receptacle to accept a 23-gauge stylet; (*e*) slot in stylet for thermistor leads; (*f*) pins and stylet are epoxied in place to form a barrel with a total length of 9 mm and a diameter of 4.4 mm. *D,* Enlarged view of the tip assembly: (*g*) wire insulated with no. 33 micro ML nylar tubing; (*h*) 0.13-mm diameter thermistor (resistance at 25°C = 2000 ohms). Thermistor is embedded in needle with epoxy. (From Onofrio BM. Stereotaxic gasserian ganglion ablation using a new stereotaxic probe. Mayo Clin Proc 1972;47:196–198.)

eyeglasses. A tarsorrhaphy should be performed if corneal ulceration occurs.

Temporary weakness of the motor branch of the trigeminal nerve occurs with radio-frequency procedures; in some series weakness has occurred in up to 40% of patients (33), but in the majority it resolves within a few months. The patients quickly learn to chew on the unaffected side of the mouth and to avoid foods requiring hard biting. If sensory loss extends to the upper lip, they should be warned of the possibility of biting or burning the lip.

Posterior Fossa Trigeminal Sensory Root Section

This procedure is performed only as a last resort in the treatment of chronic cluster headaches and only when a radio-frequency lesion has been unsuccessful in producing long-lasting, dense sensory loss in V^1 and V^2. It is not an appropriate operation when a radio-frequency lesion has produced the required numbness and the pain has persisted. The risks are similar to those of the percutaneous procedure with the additional risks of a posterior fossa procedure: intraoperative complications such as an air embolism, hemorrhage, and damage to other posterior fossa structures, including the adjacent cranial nerves. Postoperative leakage of cerebrospinal fluid through the craniec-

tomy or via the mastoid air cells can occur and requires further surgical intervention.

Our current practice is to recommend a complete sensory root section if a posterior fossa operation is to be performed. A partial root section can, surprisingly, be followed by significant recovery of facial sensation. Such a phenomenon is usually associated with return of cluster headache.

Postoperative care of the eye is the same as after a radio-frequency lesion. The greater degree of sensory loss after a root section is more difficult to accept because it includes the teeth and tongue as well as all other structures receiving trigeminal sensory innervation. Damage to the motor root is no more frequent than with the radio-frequency procedure. The incidence of anesthesia dolorosa is about the same as with other ablative procedures. Failure to relieve the painful attacks of cluster headache can occur even after complete root section (9, 19).

SUMMARY OF SURGICAL MANAGEMENT

It is well to remember that, as stated by Watson et al. (7), "no [surgical] procedure is consistently associated with long-standing relief" from chronic cluster headache. Our experience confirms this view and emphasizes the significant differences in the results of surgical procedures in this condition compared with the surgical management of trigeminal neuralgia, in which failure to provide relief is relatively uncommon.

Although there has recently been renewed interest in nervus intermedius section, our bias is to use the less-invasive radio-frequency lesion of the trigeminal ganglion in that we (19) and others (7, 18, 20) have shown satisfactory relief of pain in approximately two-thirds of subjects. Subsequent recurrence of pain can be dealt with by a repeat procedure if medical management is again ineffective. Production of complete corneal anesthesia by the radio-frequency lesion is associated with pain relief in such a high percentage of cases that we advise an open root section if, for technical reasons, the radio-frequency procedure cannot be performed. The risks of corneal sensory loss and the small but unpredictable risk of anesthesia dolorosa are considered acceptable for hapless sufferers of medically intractable cluster headache, many of whom have reached a point of desperation and who not infrequently consider suicide. Development of an effective medical treatment for this group would immediately put an end to neuroablative procedures, but until that time, a trigeminal nerve destructive operation should be considered when all medical management has failed.

REFERENCES

1. Harris W. Neuritis and neuralgia. London: Oxford University Press, 1926: 301–313.
2. Harris W. Ciliary (migrainous) neuralgia and its treatment. Br Med J 1936;1:457–460.
3. Gardner WJ, Stowell A, Dutlinger R. Resection of the greater superficial petrosal nerve in the treatment of unilateral headache. J Neurosurg 1947;4:105–114.
4. Horton BT, MacLean AR, Craig WM. A new syndrome of vascular headache: results of treatment with histamine: preliminary report. Proc Staff Meet Mayo Clin 1939;14:257–260.
5. Chorobski J, Penfield W. Cerebral vasodilator nerves and their pathway from the medulla oblongata: with observations on the pial and intracerebral vascular plexus. Arch Neurol Psychiatry 1932;28: 1257– 1289.
6. Sachs E Jr. The role of the nervus intermedius in facial neuralgia: report of four cases with observations on the pathways for taste, lacrimation, and pain in the face. J Neurosurg 1968;28:54–60.
7. Watson CP, Morley TP, Richardson JC, Schutz H, Tasker RR. The surgical treatment of chronic cluster headache. Headache 1983;23:289–295.
8. Stowell A. Physiologic mechanisms and treatment of histaminic or petrosal neuralgia. Headache 1970;9:187–194.
9. Wake M, Hitchcock E. A review of treatment modalities for periodic migrainous neuralgia. Pain 1987;31:345–352.
10. Sachs E Jr. Further observations on surgery of the nervus intermedius. Headache 1969;9:159–161.
11. Rowed DW. Chronic cluster headache managed by nervus intermedius section. Headache 1990;30:401–406.
12. Wilkins RH, Morgenlander JC. Results of surgical treatment of cluster headache: initial relief followed by recurrence. Neurosurgery 1989;24:948.
13. Solomon S. Cluster headache and the nervus intermedius. Headache 1986;26:3–8.
14. Meyer JS, Binns PM, Ericsson AD, Vulpe M. Sphenopalatine ganglionectomy for cluster headache. Arch Otolaryngol 1970; 92:475–484.
15. Ryan RE Jr, Facer GW. Sphenopalatine ganglion neuralgia and cluster headache: comparisons, contrasts, and treatment. Headache 1977;17:7–8.
16. Harris W. Alcohol injection of the gasserian ganglion for migrainous neuralgia. Lancet 1940;2:481–482.
17. McArdle MJ. Variants of migraine. In: Smith R, ed. Background to migraine. New York: Springer-Verlag, 1969.
18. Maxwell RE. Surgical control of chronic migrainous neuralgia by trigeminal ganglio-rhizolysis. J Neurosurg 1982;57:459–466.
19. Onofrio BM, Campbell JK. Surgical treatment of chronic cluster headache. Mayo Clin Proc 1986;61:537–544.
20. Mathew NT, Hurt W. Percutaneous radio-frequency trigeminal gangliorhizolysis in intractable cluster headache. Headache 1988;28: 328–331.
21. Sweet WH. Controlled thermocoagulation of trigeminal ganglion and rootlets for differential destruction of pain fibers: facial pain other than trigeminal neuralgia. Clin Neurosurg 1976;23:96–102.
22. Ekbom K, Lindgren L, Nilsson BY, Hardebo JE, Waldenlind E. Retro-gasserian glycerol injection in the treatment of chronic cluster headache. Cephalalgia 1987;7:21–27.
23. O'Brien MD, MacCabe JJ. Trigeminal nerve section for unremitting migrainous neuralgia. In: Rose FC, Zilkha KJ, eds. Progress in migraine research. London: Pitman Books, 1981: 185–187.
24. White JC, Sweet WH. Pain and the neurosurgeon: a forty-year experience. Springfield, IL: Charles C Thomas, 1969: 345–434.
25. Dott NM. Discussion. Proc R Soc Med 1951;44:1034–1037.
26. Earl CJ, McArdle MJ. Chronic migrainous neuralgia. In: Locke S, ed. Modern neurology. Boston: Little, Brown and Co, 1969: 583–588.
27. Kunkel RS, Dohn DF. Surgical treatment of chronic migrainous neuralgia. Cleve Clin Q 1974;41:189–192.
28. Morgenlander JC, Wilkins RH. Surgical treatment of cluster headache. J Neurosurg 1990;72:866–871.
29. Headache Classification Committee of the International Headache Society. Classification and diagnostic criteria for headache disorders, cranial neuralgias and facial pain. Cephalalgia 1988;8(suppl 7):12–92.
30. Onofrio BM. Radio-frequency percutaneous gasserian ganglion lesions: results in 140 patients with trigeminal pain. J Neurosurg 1975;42:132–139.
31. Sweet WH, Wepsic JG. Controlled thermocoagulation of trigeminal ganglion and rootlets for differential destruction of pain fibers. Part 1: Trigeminal neuralgia. J Neurosurg 1974;40:143- 156.
32. Rovit RL. Percutaneous radio-frequency thermal coagulation of the gasserian ganglion. In: Rovit RL, Murali R, Jannetta PJ, eds. Trigeminal neuralgia. Baltimore: Williams & Wilkins, 1990:109–136.
33. Sweet WH. The treatment of trigeminal neuralgia (tic douloureux). N Engl J Med 1986;315:174–177.

Selected Topics

25

Migraine Headache Variants

ROBERT S. KUNKEL

This chapter discusses some of the complications of migraine as well as several syndromes that are felt to be related to an underlying migraine mechanism. Uncommon varieties of migraine such as ophthalmoplegic migraine, basilar migraine, and migraine aura without headache (migraine equivalents) are discussed in Chapter 10.

The overwhelming majority of patients suffering from migraine have migraine without aura (common migraine) or migraine with aura (classic migraine). A fair number of migraineurs have some episodes of migraine aura without headache (see Chapter 10). Migrainous infarction (complicated migraine) may be more frequent than is realized. Total global amnesia is felt by many to be basically a migrainous phenomenon. The relationship of recurrent vertigo to migraine in both children and adults has become more evident in recent years. Recurrent abdominal pain in childhood (abdominal migraine) is most likely to be a manifestation of migraine when other organic causes have been excluded.

A few other headache syndromes are felt often to be related to migraine or at least have a vascular etiology. These include exertional headache, cold stimulus headache, cough headache, coital headache, and "ice-pick headache." These are discussed in Chapter 37.

MIGRAINOUS INFARCTION (COMPLICATED MIGRAINE)

In the new IHS classification, migrainous infarction and complicated migraine are separated. Migrainous infarction is defined as one or more migrainous aura symptoms not fully reversible within 7 days and/or neuroimaging demonstration of an ischemic infarction in a relevant area. In addition, other causes of infarction must have been ruled out (1).

Complicated migraine is now known as migraine with prolonged aura. The aura symptoms last longer than 60 minutes but less than 7 days with neuroimaging studies being normal (1). The neurological or visual symptoms usually start as an aura prior to the pain, but at times they may commence after the actual headache has been present for a while.

It is important to recognize that any migraineur can have an infarction or complicated migraine attack at any time. It would be quite unusual with the first attack, and most who develop this complication have had migraine attacks for years. Visual symptoms are more common than other neurological symptoms in complicated migraine or migrainous infarction, just as they are in migraine with aura. Visual defects occur about twice as often as other neurological defects (2).

The incidence of cerebral infarction associated with migraine is unknown. Whether or not migraine sufferers are more prone to strokes has been debated for years. In reviewing records of over 4800 migraine patients under age 50, 20 were found to have had brain infarction associated with a migraine attack (3). The same investigators found that 25% of cerebral infarctions occurring in persons under age 50 were associated with migraine. Similar figures were found in persons under age 40 suffering a cerebral infarction (4). Other studies of strokes in young people have found an incidence of 5% and 10% occurring in migraine sufferers (5, 6).

Thus strokes occurring in persons with migraine are not very common, whereas migraineurs make up a fairly significant number of those patients under age 40 suffering from a stroke. Because of the increased incidence of migraine in women, migraine-related strokes occur more often in women under the age of 50, whereas strokes in nonmigrainous persons under the age of 50 occur more frequently in men.

Since most permanent neurological defects occurring as a consequence of a migraine attack are visual, most infarctions involve the posterior cerebral artery distribution (7). The middle cerebral artery is the second most common area involved. Infarction of the brainstem, which might occur during an attack of basilar artery migraine, is quite rare (8).

It is essential to investigate persons under 50 years of age who have evidence of cerebral infarction for other causes than migraine. Vasculitis, coagulopathy, infection, occlusive cerebral vascular disease, mass lesions, aneurysms, embolism, and arterial venous malformations have all been reported to cause strokes in young persons. Since migraine is such a common disorder, if another condition coexists it is very difficult to know which is the underlying cause. In one study, if a stroke occurred during a migraine attack, only about 9% had another underlying disease; whereas 91% of patients with migraine who had a stroke not associated with a migraine attack were found to have other possible causes (9). Therefore, a stroke occurring during an attack of migraine is most likely secondary to migraine.

Persons with migraine that is associated with visual or neurological symptoms should avoid other risk factors of stroke such as smoking, hypertension, hyperlipidemia, and estrogens. These known risk factors in a patient with migraine who has neurological or visual symptoms undoubtedly increase the likelihood of a migraine-related cerebral infarction occurring. The prognosis is generally good, and the Mayo Clinic group found significant residual abnormalities in only two of their 20 patients with migraine-associated stroke (3).

RETINAL MIGRAINE

Retinal migraine is felt to be quite rare. It is attributed to retinal ischemia from prolonged central retinal artery constriction occurring as an aura preceding a migraine attack. Monocular scotoma or blindness due to migraine should last less than 60 minutes, and according to the IHS classification, headache follows within 60 minutes or precedes the visual symptoms (1). Headache is almost always present, and monocular symptoms occurring in the absence of a headache are most likely due to thromboembolic disease of the carotid artery, but they could represent migraine aura without headache.

Corbett prefers the term *ocular migraine*, since optic nerve ischemia has been reported to occur as a migrainous phenomenon, and it would cause monocular visual symptoms as well (10). Retinal or ocular migraine usually occurs in young persons, whereas the monocular symptoms due to vascular disease occur in older persons. Like most transient neurological or visual symptoms occurring with migraine, the duration is usually longer (30 to 60 minutes) than that of the more typical transient ischemic attack of amaurosis fugax due to carotid artery disease (11). Therefore, persons with unilateral eye symptoms, especially if they are of a few minutes duration and are not accompanied by a headache, should be thoroughly worked up, for the cause is most likely thromboembolic or vascular disease rather than migraine.

HEMIPLEGIC MIGRAINE

Migraine accompanied by unilateral motor deficits is termed hemiplegic migraine. In the past, this term has been applied to migraine with unilateral sensory or motor deficits, but to strictly adhere to the definition of this term, there should be weakness. Sensory changes are usually associated with weakness. The hemiparesis lasts more than 60 minutes (if less it is called migraine with aura) and less than 7 days (if longer it is a migrainous infarction) (1).

Hemiplegic migraine has typically been separated into familial hemiplegic migraine and hemiplegic migraine. Prolonged hemiparesis may occur sporadically in persons who have migraine with aura, but it is quite rare. Most persons with weakness preceding the migraine attack have restoration of function within 60 minutes, which fulfills the criteria for migraine with aura.

Familial hemiplegic migraine is a well-recognized entity (12–14). To fit this definition, a first-degree relative must have identical attacks (1). The neurological symptoms usually commence as an aura but may come on during the attack of migraine. Usually the pattern is the same with each attack. Other migrainous symptoms such as nausea, vomiting, photophobia, and phonophobia usually occur in addition to the hemiparesis. Glista and his co-workers have described a family in which the attacks of hemiplegic migraine were triggered by minor head trauma (13).

Usually the hemiplegia lasts several days but resolves completely without any residual deficit. This is probably because the deficits are due to cerebral edema rather than a true infarction (12, 15). Like other neurological or visual symptoms of migraine, weakness will not hit abruptly but will develop gradually and move or spread from proximal to distal or distal to proximal muscles.

If a person is seen during the first attack of hemiplegic migraine, a thorough workup is needed to exclude any underlying lesion in the cardiovascular or central nervous system. Sources of emboli and causes of vasculitis need to be excluded. Usually there is a history of similar attacks in family members, but such a history may be difficult to obtain.

DYSPHRENIC MIGRAINE

Many migraineurs have disturbances of cognitive function during the attack of migraine. It is not unusual for some confusion and impairment of concentration to occur, either as an aura or during the attack. When mental symptoms such as confusion or agitation occur without any significant headache (migraine aura without headache), the diagnosis can be quite difficult, especially when such symptoms have not occurred in the past.

Transient global amnesia (TGA) is characterized by retrograde amnesia for events prior to the attack: repetitive questioning, inability to form new memories, and the absence of any focal neurological signs or symptoms (16). A typical migraine attack may be accompanied by transient global amnesia or the symptoms may occur in the absence of a headache.

It is likely that total global amnesia is often a manifestation of a migrainous event involving the posterior cerebral circulation without accompanying headache. Electroencephalographic abnormalities consisting of slow waves have been reported during attacks of TGA (17, 18). These findings are similar to what has been seen in migraine and ischemia. In the past, TGA has been felt by some to be a manifestation of epilepsy and classified as a seizure disorder.

Acute confusional migraine is a condition usually seen in adolescence (19, 20). Confusion, agitation, and disorientation occur with or without a headache. Often the headache is mild and occurs after the confusion clears; occasionally a headache precedes the confusion, which makes the diagnosis of migraine more likely. The confusion may last a few minutes to several hours. Although a familial history of migraine is usually present, if the first attack is one of confusion with very little headache, the symptoms can be quite alarming.

Drug use, encephalitis, postictal state, and other metabolic abnormalities must be excluded. It is felt that the confusional state is due to cortical or subcortical dysfunction secondary to ischemia and/or edema. Electroencephalographic recordings are normal or show slow waves during the attack, with an absence of epileptiform discharges (19). Acute confusional episodes and transient global amnesia usually occur as a single episode in persons with migraine and rarely reoccur. When they occur as the initial manifestation of migraine without any previous migraine attacks, the diagnosis of migraine usually is not made until more typical attacks of migraine occur.

VERTIGO AND MIGRAINE

Growing evidence indicates a relationship between migraine and vertigo. Vertigo is a common symptom occurring in basilar artery migraine. It is often an aura prior to the attack. Vestibular symptoms (vertigo, ataxia) are more prevalent than auditory symptoms in patients with migraine (21). Vertigo may precede a migraine attack, occur during an attack, or occur as an aura symptom without a headache following. It has been estimated that about one-third of persons with migraine will suffer from vertigo at one time or another (22, 23).

If vertigo occurs in close proximity to a migraine attack, either as an aura or during the attack, it is probably a manifestation of migraine. Diagnosing recurrent vertigo as a migrainous aura without headache may be difficult. Episodic vertigo occurring for years without causing any demonstrable vestibular abnormalities on testing should suggest a migrainous origin. Vestibular abnormalities are usually present in reoccurring peripheral disorders such as Ménière's disease or vestibular neuronitis (24). Many patients with recurrent vertigo respond to antimigrainous prophylactic therapy.

Benign paroxysmal vertigo of childhood, first described by Basser in 1964, is considered to be a precursor to migraine (15). These attacks occur in children, usually beginning before age two. The child looks fearful and may fall or grab something to keep from falling. The attack lasts a few minutes and is usually associated with nausea, vomiting, and pallor. Nystagmus may be present during the attack. A significant number of children suffering from benign paroxysmal vertigo go on to develop migraine (26, 27).

Ménière's disease seems to be more prevalent in migraineurs than in the general population (28). It, like migraine, is a paroxysmal disorder and perhaps shares a similar pathophysiology, with episodic focal vascular spasm being prevalent in both conditions.

ABDOMINAL MIGRAINE

Abdominal migraine occurs mostly in children but can occur in adults (29). Children usually have recurring attacks of abdominal pain with nausea and vomiting (30). A family history of migraine is usually present in children with this symptom. Some children have migraine headache as well, but they can have the abdominal symptoms without migraine attacks. Most adults with abdominal migraine attacks have had migraine headaches. Abdominal pain, along with nausea and vomiting, can occur with a headache, but the term *abdominal migraine* should be used when persons have recurring abdominal symptoms that are not associated temporally with the headache attacks.

The terms *periodic syndrome, abdominal epilepsy,* and *abdominal migraine* have all been used for recurring attacks of abdominal pain with nausea and vomiting. Most feel that such spells are not epileptogenic (31). Further evidence that such recurrent symptoms are migrainous is found in a study showing that 27 of 28 children with the diagnosis of abdominal migraine and a group of migraine children had similar differences in fast wave activity, as measured by visually evoked responses, compared with controls (32).

In children, the attacks last 1 to 6 hours and are usually eased with sleep. Abdominal migraine is diagnosed only after an extensive workup excludes gastrointestinal, biliary, or pelvic disease. As with any of the syndromes that might occur as an aura without headache (migraine-equivalent), this diagnosis should be considered in anyone with recurring abdominal symptoms for which no cause is evident. Children may also have recurring cyclic vomiting without any pain as a manifestation of abdominal migraine.

Other migrainous symptoms may accompany the abdominal pains. Photophobia, irritability, dizziness, chilling, and sweats, all of which are common with the more usual migraine attacks, may occur along with the abdominal symptoms.

THERAPY OF MIGRAINE VARIANTS

Any of these syndromes that are felt to be migrainous in etiology are treated just as one would treat the more typical migraine attacks. If the nonheadache symptoms occur quite frequently, then prophylaxis should be used in the form of a β-blocker or calcium channel antagonist. In children who have some of these nonheadache phenomena, sleep may be all that is necessary to end the attack. For the most part, the conditions discussed do not occur very frequently in any one person and necessitate no specific treatment. There is very little in the literature regarding pharmacological management of any of the discussed syndromes with acute abortive therapy. Ergotamine tartrate, which has been used for years very effectively in the more typical migraine headache attack, is usually avoided because most of the symptoms have been felt to be due to vascular constriction and spasm. With growing evidence that migraine actually begins as a central nervous system dysfunction, ergotamine might very well be useful in aborting these attacks, and most people who have used ergotamine have not noted any worsening of the symptoms following its use. Rapid-acting antiinflammatory agents or even corticosteroids might also be useful in those rare situations where the symptoms are prolonged.

REFERENCES

1. Headache Classification Committee of the International Headache Society. Classification and diagnostic criteria for headache disorders, neuralgias and facial pain. Cephalalgia 1988;8(7):19–28.
2. Bartelson JD. Transient and persistent neurological manifestations of migraine. Stroke 1983;18:21–25.
3. Broderick JP, Swanson JW. Migraine related strokes. Arch Neurol 1987;44:868–871.
4. Spaccavento LJ, Solomon GD. Migraine as an etiology of strokes in young adults. Headache 1984;24:19–22.
5. Hart RG, Miller VT. Cerebral infarction in young adults: a practical approach. Stroke 1983;14:110–114.
6. Sacquegna T, Andreoli A, Baldrati A, et al. Ischemic strokes in young adults: the relevance of migrainous infarction. Cephalalgia 1989;9:255–258.
7. Connor R. Complicated migraine: a study of permanent neurological and visual defects caused by migraine. Lancet 1962;2:1072–1075.
8. Bernsen H, Van de Vlasakker C, Verhagen W, Prick M. Basilar artery migraine stroke. Headache 1990;30:142–144.
9. Bogousslavsky J, Regli F, Van Melle G, et al. Migraine stroke. Neurology 1988;38:223–227.
10. Corbett J. Ocular aspects of migraine. In: Blau JN, ed. Migraine, clinical and research aspects. Baltimore: Johns Hopkins University Press, 1987:625–633.
11. Fugino T, Akiya S, Takagi S, et al. Amaurosis fugax for a long duration. J Clin Neuro Ophthalmol 1983;3:9–12.
12. Bradshaw P, Parsons M. Hemiplegic migraine, a clinical study. Q J Med 1965;34:65–85.
13. Glista GG, Mellinger JF, Rooke ED. Familial hemiplegic migraine. Mayo Clin Proc 1975;50:307–311.
14. Whitty CWM. Familial hemiplegic migraine. J Neurol Neurosurg Psychiatry 1953;16:172–177.
15. Rosenbaum HE. Familial hemiplegic migraine. Neurology 1960;10:164–170.
16. Caplan L, Chedra F, Lhermitte F, Mayman C. Transient global amnesia and migraine. Neurology 1981;31:1167–1170.
17. Mathew NT, Meyer JS. Pathogenesis and natural history of transient global amnesia. Stroke 1974;5:303–311.
18. Steinmetz EF, Vroom FQ. Transient global amnesia. Neurology 1972;22:1193–1200.
19. Emery ES. Acute confusional state in children with migraine. Pediatrics 1977;60:110–114.
20. Gascom G, Barlow C. Juvenile migraine presenting as an acute confusional state. Pediatrics 1970;45:628–635.
21. Kayan A, Hood JD. Neuro-otological manifestations of migraine. Brain 1984;107:1123–1142.
22. Shelby G, Lance JW. Observations on 500 cases of migraine and allied vascular headaches. J Neurol Neurosurg Psychiatry 1960;23:23–32.
23. Kuritzy A, Ziegler DK, Hassanein R. Vertigo, motion sickness, and migraine. Headache 1981;21:227–231.
24. Harker LA, Rasekh CH. Episodic vertigo and basilar artery migraine. Otolaryngol Head Neck Surg 1987;96:239–250.
25. Basser LS. Benign paroxysmal vertigo of childhood. Brain 1964;87:141–152.
26. Koenigsberger MR, Chutorian AM, Gold AP, Schivey MS. Benign paroxysmal vertigo of childhood. Neurology 1970;20:1108–1113.
27. Parker W. Migraine and the vestibular system in children and adolescence. Am J Otol 1989;10:364–371.
28. Hood JD, Kayan A. Neuro-otology and migraine. In: Blau JN, ed. Migraine, clinical and research aspects. Baltimore: Johns Hopkins University Press, 1987:613.
29. Kunkel RS. Migraine aura without headache. Pain Manage 1990;3:176–182.
30. Lundberg PO. Abdominal migraine—diagnosis and therapy. Headache 1975;15:122–125.
31. Lanzi G, Balottin A, Ottolini F, et al. Cyclic vomiting and recurrent abdominal pain as migraine or epileptic equivalents. Cephalalgia 1983;3:115–118.
32. Mortimer MJ, Good PA. The VER as a diagnostic marker for childhood abdominal migraine. Headache 1990;30:642–645.

26

Headache Associated with Head Trauma

WILLIAM G. SPEED III

Ninety percent of nervous system head trauma is caused by injury to the head, which produces one of the most devastating health problems in the United States (1). About 3 million head injuries occur per year in the United States (2, 3), and the annual national financial burden resulting from this is estimated to be more than 3 billion dollars. The loss of income from the disabilities associated with head injuries is undoubtedly huge, and the impact on the quality of life including marriage, family, career, financial independence, and social life can be disastrous.

Most head injuries result from falls or automobile accidents in which alcohol may play a significant role. The remainder are caused by recreational activities (e.g., football, wrestling, boxing), industrial accidents, self-inflicted injuries, injuries inflicted by others, military activities, and blows by objects (1). It is estimated that 30 to 50% of such head injuries result in headaches persisting for more than 2 months (4, 5). These are termed chronic posttraumatic headaches.

There is no correlation between the severity of the head injury and the severity of the headache as evidenced by such parameters as (a) coma or its duration, (b) amnesia, (c) increased intracranial pressure, and (d) EEG abnormalities (2, 6). In fact, headache may be less frequent after major cerebral injury than after minor concussion. Some of the most intractable cases of posttraumatic headache occur after trivial injury (7).

POSTTRAUMATIC SYNDROME

In addition to headache, there are frequently other symptoms that develop in association with head injury. They are so closely allied to the injury that produces the headache that it would be inappropriate to discuss one to the exclusion of the other. These symptoms are strikingly consistent from patient to patient, although they may vary in the degree to which they are experienced. These are as follows (8–15):

Lightheadedness or true vertigo
Hyperacusis
Tinnitus
Impaired memory
Reduced attention span

Easy distractibility
Impaired ability to comprehend
Forgetfulness
Deterioration of logical thinking
Inability to grasp new or abstract concepts
Insomnia
Apathy
Easy fatiguability
Reduced motivation
Decreased libido
Alcohol intolerance
Irritability
Anger outbursts
Mood swings
Anxiety, depression, and frustration
Syncope

The posttraumatic syndrome may be characterized by all of these symptoms or by only a few. Lightheadedness, memory impairment, reduced attention span, impaired ability to concentrate, anxiety, anger outbursts, depression, and frustration are the most common. They usually develop within 24 to 48 hours following trauma, although rarely there may be a more delayed onset. These complaints may persist for months, years, or decades.

PATHOGENESIS

The number of neurons that make up the 3 pounds or so of a human brain is on the order of 100 billion. A typical neuron may have from 1000 to 10,000 synapses and may be fed by hundreds or thousands of other neurons (16). The extensive combinations and permutations that this structuring permits truly boggles the mind.

The pathogenesis of posttraumatic headache and posttraumatic syndrome has not yet been proven with certainty. However, as investigative techniques become more sophisticated, increasing evidence indicates that even minor trauma to the head may result in prolonged malfunction of the brain (17–21), strongly supporting an organic basis for this disorder.

Head injury results from mechanical forces transmitted directly to the underlying brain tissue. In closed head injury, (which is much the most common type except in war conditions), the skull itself remains intact, and the amount of

215

energy delivered to the cerebrum, brainstem, and cerebellum determines the extent of brain injury. The strength of the force reaching the intracranial structures is greater when the skull remains intact than when it is fractured or penetrated. When the skull is fractured or penetrated, significant energy is absorbed, thereby reducing the amount that reaches the intracranial structures. This is probably why some "minor" head injuries produce more posttraumatic symptoms than some more extensive injuries.

Nerve fiber degeneration occurs in the cerebral hemispheres and brainstem as a result of trauma, and it occurs often in mild as well as severe head injury. Strich suggests that this degeneration is the consequence of the tearing or stretching of nerve fibers due to mechanical forces acting at the time of injury (19).

In 1943 Holbourn (22), a physicist, using gelatin models of the brain, established that in some cases of trauma to the head the force responsible for producing neurological dysfunction was not impact itself but rather acceleration/deceleration of the brain. He also advanced the concept that head injury occurring with the head free (i.e., allowed to accelerate) is potentially more harmful than head injury with the head fixed. Denny-Brown and Russell in 1941 (23) demonstrated in cats that it required less force to produce concussion when the head is free to move than when it is fixed.

If the accepted popular concept is true, that head injury occurring in sports such as football, boxing, or wrestling is associated with a lesser incidence of posttraumatic headache than that following industrial or automobile injury, then this phenomenon offers a possible explanation for that difference. Sports participants are trained and conditioned and are in a constant anticipatory state of protection, lessening the probability of unexpected free movement of the head as the result of a blow. Industrial and automobile accidents occur without warning, and there is no chance to set up protective forces. In other words, the head is in a free state and therefore vulnerable to an acceleration/deceleration injury.

Oppenheimer (20) described widely scattered lesions composed of microglial clusters in more than 75% of 59 cases with survival times of more than 12 hours. After 24 to 48 hours of survival, axonal retraction balls could be seen in the neighborhood of these microglial clusters, indicating that the clusters were associated with axonal rupture. It is of particular interest that microglial clusters have been found in the brains of patients who have had a history of concussional head injury but who died from other causes (24).

Experiments on guinea pigs from 1945–1950 by Windle and Groat (25–27) show that after single or multiple concussive blows to the head, insufficient to produce death, nerve cell damage in the brainstem is produced. In addition, Becker et al. (28) have shown that similar guinea pigs performed poorly in maze-running tests when compared with controls, although they appeared otherwise normal.

Striking, swirling movements of the brain, following even subconcussive blows to the heads of rhesus monkeys whose skulls have been replaced with transparent material, have been demonstrated cinematographically (21). Brain movement during and immediately after impact has been confirmed with more refined methods, including arteriography, by Ommaya (29). These findings suggest a means by which minor head injury may produce significant alteration of brain function.

In 1983, further evidence that demonstrable injury to the brain occurs with minor head injury was presented by Povlishock et al. (17) in a unique experiment. These authors implanted pellets of horseradish peroxidase (HRP) gel into the brains of cats. After 24 hours very minor head injury was produced using a hydraulic pressure transient device producing a fluid percussion injury force of no more than 1.8 to 1.9 atmospheres for a duration of 18 to 22 milliseconds. Because the injury was produced under general anesthesia, there were no clinical correlates, but all of the cats recovered and seemed to be perfectly normal. The cats were then sacrificed at varying intervals and an orderly sequence of pathological events, demonstrated only by the sophisticated methods of HRP technology and electron microscopy, became evident.

Briefly, within an hour of injury, distinct intraaxonal pooling of HRP was noted in a limited number of efferent axons coursing through the brain. Within 2 hours there were more marked changes in axons and occasional instances of cut-off of HRP transport along the distant axon, suggesting a block, either functional or from anatomical discontinuity. Within 12 to 24 hours there were enlarged ball-like swellings in direct continuity with a proximal portion of labeled axons but not in continuity with the distal portion. These were counterstained with silver and were shown to be typical "retraction balls," as demonstrated years previously by Strich (19). Electronmicroscopy showed that HRP pooling areas contained focal aggregation of organelles within 1 hour of injury, and at longer intervals, these changes were more pronounced. Standard light microscopy and hematoxylin and eosin (H & E) staining showed no abnormalities.

It is clear therefore that damage to nerve fibers is produced in head injury, and there is little doubt that it occurs frequently in both mild and severe injury (19). Other studies (18, 30) have demonstrated a slowing of cerebral circulation for months or years after head injury, indicating that at least one measurable phenomenon remained in an abnormal state for long periods of time even after "nonserious" deceleration injury.

Other reported disturbances following trauma include (a) altered vasomotor regulation (18), (b) vestibular dysfunction, (c) asymmetrical hearing loss, (d) abnormal brainstem evoked potential (31–33), (e) impaired visual evoked responses (34), (f) altered neurotransmitter function (35), and (g) an indication of continued metabolic abnormality connected with carbohydrated oxidation and acid-base regulation (24). Although the significance of these findings in the chronic symptomatology of the posttraumatic syndrome is not yet conclusively understood, they clearly implicate organic factors in this disorder.

CLINICAL FEATURES

Posttraumatic headache may mimic almost any of the chronic headache disorders. The headache may be constant or intermittent (less likely) and may involve any areas of the head (e.g., frontal, ocular, retroocular, temporal, parietal, vertex, occipital) in various combinations or include the entire head. There may be more than one type of headache in the same patient. Some headaches are described as a broad band around the head or an ache located deep inside the head, but more often they are described as aching, pressing, squeezing, expanding, burning, stabbing, and/or throbbing and pounding. Depending on the specific mechanism(s) involved, the headache may be aggravated by bending over, coughing, sneezing, straining, jarring the head, exposure to bright lights or loud noises, touching the head, ingestion of alcohol, physical exertion, stress, or anxiety.

HEADACHE MECHANISMS

A variety of mechanisms are responsible for posttraumatic headaches, and these may occur singly or in various combinations.

Tension-type

This headache is clinically indistinguishable from the chronic tension-type headache that occurs unrelated to trauma. It is a constant, nonthrobbing, dull pressure pain that may be posterior cervical, occipital, vertex, temporofrontal, or almost any combination of these. These headaches are probably associated with neuronal or neurotransmitter disturbances in the pain modulation areas of the brain. Why this disorder develops as the result of trauma is not known with certainty, but the pathogenesis described above, leading to interference with the normal function of neurotransmitters, offers an attractive hypothesis.

Vasodilatation

Pulsating, pounding, throbbing headaches are common in posttraumatic headaches and are produced by vasodilatation. Although some of these headaches are nonmigrainous vascular headaches, it is clear that the migraine disorder can be triggered by head injury (36, 37). Both classical and common migraine have been precipitated by head injury (38, 39). Trauma may precipitate the first attack of migraine in a susceptible individual or increase the frequency and/or severity of preexisting migraine and sometimes produce the features of chronic migraine. It is believed that migraine has a genetic basis, probably biochemical, and presumably, a blow to the head, even though trivial, is capable of activating this genetic abnormality. It is not clear why the migraine disorder may be disturbed for many months or longer following head injury, but most probably this is related to neuronal and axonal abnormalities secondary to trauma.

Combined Muscle Contraction and Vasodilatation

These mechanisms may be disturbed simultaneously, and the term mixed type headache is used to describe this entity.

Scar Formation

If the soft tissue of the head is injured, a localized area of tenderness results. This occurs from entrapment of sensory nerve endings at the site of scarring or the stimulation of nerve endings involved in the locally damaged tissue even if scarring did not develop (40). Headache is felt for the most part around the site of the injury, and the pain may be intermittent or continuous. The involved site is always strikingly tender to external pressure.

Tension-Type, Vasodilatation, and Scar Formation

These may occur simultaneously in the same patient.

Injuries to the Cervical Region

Injuries to the superficial and deep structures of the neck, involving muscle, ligaments, discs, bone, or nerve roots, produce cervical pain that may be referred to the head. "Whiplash injury" results from sudden hyperextension of the neck followed by hyperflexion. It is most commonly caused by rear-end automobile accidents. The pain occurs immediately or shortly after the injury. The headache may be limited to the occipital area or spread to include the vertex, temple, frontal, and retrobulbar areas as well. Pain is described as dull, aching, and squeezing with, at times, pounding and throbbing components. The cervical pain is aggravated by movements of the neck. The head and neck pains persist for days or weeks and in some cases become chronic and last for months or much longer. Exacerbation of preexisting arthritis or discogenic disease may occur. In some cases, the occipital neurovascular bundle (consisting of the occipital nerve, artery, and vein) at the level of the occipital ridge may be traumatized secondary to prolonged muscle contraction or excessive vascular dilatation impinging on the occipital nerve itself. "Occipital neuralgia" is the term used to describe this condition.

Psychological Factors

Psychological factors must be assessed in the posttraumatic syndrome. Although the etiological relevance of psychological factors has been extensively compared to the relevance of organic ones, the relative role of each in the production of emotional symptomatology and chronic headache remains somewhat controversial. The weight of evidence at present is swinging the pendulum almost entirely to the organic point of view. It may not be possible in all cases to clearly differentiate psychological symptoms produced by the patient's reaction to the injury from those produced by an organic disorder caused by the injury itself. This is probably a fruitless exercise, since both of these factors, in all likelihood, are operating to varying degrees. However, the stereotyped nature of the symptomatology seen over and over again points strongly in the direction of organicity.

DIAGNOSES

The diagnosis depends on a detailed history, since usually there are few objective abnormalities. In a headache history one must look for the time of onset of the headache in relation to the injury; frequency, duration, and location of the pain; intensity variations of the pain; associated neurological symptomatology (and whether it is occurring before, during, or after the headache), nausea, vomiting, or a positive family history for headaches. In assessing the patient with posttraumatic syndrome, a CT or MRI scan of the head is usually indicated but is most often normal.

MANAGEMENT

Tension-type headaches respond best to tricyclic compounds such as amitriptyline, imipramine, or doxepin. The average dose is 50 to 100 mg per day but may vary from 25 to 150 mg depending on the patient's response and tolerance. Occasionally cyclobenzaprine, a tricyclic compound with muscle-relaxant properties, may prove useful. The dose is 10 mg t.i.d.

When tension-type and vascular headaches occur together, they should be treated in the same manner but with the addition of a β-adrenergic blocking agent. Several β-blockers have been used successfully: propranolol, metoprolol, atenolol, nadolol, and timolol. The usual doses are for propranolol 10 to 80 mg q.i.d., for metoprolol 100 to 200 mg b.i.d., for atenolol 50 mg once or twice daily, for nadolol 20 to 80 mg b.i.d., and for timolol 10 to 20 mg b.i.d. In highly resistant and selected cases the addition of an MAO inhibitor to the above combination (not given with imipramine) may prove beneficial. Phenelzine sulfate 15 mg t.i.d. is the one most often used. This is a relatively safe combination provided the prescribing physician knows the properties of an MAO inhibitor and properly instructs the patient in the necessary precautions when using this agent. Biofeedback is frequently useful as an additional modality.

Posttraumatic migraine should be managed exactly as one manages migraine unrelated to trauma. A combination of a β-blocker and a tricyclic compound is frequently helpful, but other agents such as periactin, sansert, ergotamine, ergonovine, clonidine, verapamil, diltiazem, or midrin used appropriately may be beneficial. Side effects or even absence of response to one β-blocker does not mean that the same response will be found to all of those just listed. The combination of β-blockers and various tricyclic compounds shows

a better response than either of these compounds used alone. If it is tolerated, amitriptyline is the best of the tricyclic compounds. The dose is that described above.

The pain from local tissue damage or scar formation may improve following infiltration of the involved area with 8 ml of 1% Xylocaine containing 4 mg of dexamethasone. The site is easy to find since it is pinpoint tender to finger pressure. The occipital neurovascular bundle can be more specifically localized if one uses a Doppler device to identify the occipital artery that is adjacent to the occipital nerve.

The treatment of cervical strain or "whiplash" should be conservative, a cervical collar, heat, and massage to start. Occasionally, Xylocaine and dexamethasone infiltrated into specifically localized tender areas of the neck may be useful. Biofeedback may be quite helpful.

It may be appropriate to address the psychological factors in a few of these patients. When such factors appear to be playing a paramount role in the continuation of posttraumatic symptoms, consultation with psychologists, behavioral medicine specialists, or psychiatrists may be indicated. Are mood changes an understandable psychological reaction of the individual to the new cognitive or physical impairment or are they the direct consequence of the site of brain injury? Considerable evidence supports the concept that they are directly related to the site of brain injury (41–44).

Posttraumatic headache and related symptomatology have an impact not only on the patient but on the patient's family, friends, employer, and work colleagues. The symptoms generated by brain injury—chronic head pain, impaired memory, impaired concentration, diminished attention span, insomnia, easy fatiguability, and decreased libido, etc.—produce an enforced and distinctly unpleasant change in one's life routine. It is difficult to imagine a more perfect situation for a self-perpetuating cycle (i.e., an organically induced malfunction of physiological processes which results in devastating symptomatology that leads to anxiety, fear, depression, and frustration, which in turn enhances the physiological malfunction, completing the vicious circle).

The most appropriate management of the posttraumatic syndrome involves consideration of all of the above. In addition, the physician should address the impact these symptoms have on the patient's immediate family. The controlling issue here is education. Both the patient and family must understand the consequences of the injury and the resulting forces that produce the devastating situation for the patient. When feasible, the employer, lawyer, and insurance and other disability agencies should be included in this educational process, but this is a difficult, impractical, unrealistic, and probably impossible task.

PROGNOSIS

Recovery from posttraumatic headaches depends in part on the mechanism of the headache. Patients who have vascular headaches seem to be more prone to prolonged headaches than others, but this is certainly not absolute. Jacobson (45), in a follow-up evaluation of 46 minor head-injured patients, concluded that most of those who were going to lose their headaches had lost them within 2 months, and all of those who were going to lose their headaches have done so in 4 years. Fourteen of these patients had headaches beyond 4 years, a few from 8 to 20 years following the injury. It appears to be rather well established that the symptomatology of the posttraumatic syndrome may be prolonged for years and that about 15 to 20% of such patients will be in this category (46–49). In other reports (50) many patients who did return to work had to work in down-graded jobs, mainly because the persistence of their symptoms prevented them from carrying out heavy physical or mental work.

Unfortunately, there are no solid, reliable prognostic guidelines for physicians to follow. Whether the headache is totally related to an organic disturbance or in part to a conversion reaction, the patient is often considerably disabled for very long periods. Experience teaches (and the literature supports the concept) that patients who continue to have posttraumatic symptomatology for more than 4 years following their injury have a poor prognosis regardless of the pathogenesis.

DISCUSSION

The medicolegal disability aspect of the posttraumatic syndrome is of great importance to the patient and the physician. There seems to be almost no difficulty in obtaining a reasonable legal settlement for one who has suffered from posttraumatic syndrome, provided there has been a demonstrable lesion such as a laceration, skull fracture, or a significant loss of consciousness. Many of these cases never come to trial and are settled promptly, particularly if there are objective signs on testing or examination. Unfortunately, most cases that come to trial because of the posttraumatic syndrome involve persons with no residual objective injury to tissue, no history of loss of consciousness or significant amnesia, and no other acceptable evidence of substantial injury. No matter how incapacitating the symptoms might be, these patients usually face a tough and medically unjustifiable legal battle to receive warranted compensation.

Recognition that minor head trauma can lead to devastating effects for individuals, to the point of totally disrupting their lives for long periods of time, has been slow in developing. Only very recently have Social Security regulations recognized that headache may be a legitimate reason for disability. Whether prior statements have or have not been changed is not certain, but in the recent past they stated "abnormalities which manifest themselves only as symptoms are not medically determinable." Another portion of the regulations state (or used to state) that "the Secretary only will decide whether one is disabled and the weight given to the physician's statement depends upon the extent to which it is supported by specific and complete physical findings." Since there usually are no objective clinical or laboratory findings in patients with long-standing symptoms of the posttraumatic syndrome, patients applying for disability under these circumstances have a most difficult road to travel.

The concept that settlement of litigation is all that is needed to stop the symptoms of the posttraumatic syndrome is no longer tenable. Legal settlement has nothing to do with the termination of symptoms, nor does it play any role in whether or not a patient can or cannot return to work (47, 49, 51). Patients with relatively normal preexisting personalities appear to be just as vulnerable to posttraumatic symptomatology as others (52).

The posttraumatic syndrome is so stereotyped and seen with such repetition by those who specialize in headache problems that it becomes unreasonable to believe that these patients are faking this disorder, prolonging it for the sake of litigation, or have developed psychological symptomatology because the injury "was the straw that broke the camel's back" in their ability to cope with life. The dilemma faced by the physician is one of distinguishing the legitimately impaired patient, whose symptoms are produced or aggravated by trauma, from those in whom the continuation of symptoms is instigated by compensation motives, revenge, greed, or the avoidance of responsibility. Malingering is defined as the conscious simulation of symptoms of illness with intent to deceive. It implies willful deceit, and I submit that the symptomatology of the posttraumatic syndrome is so complex and yet so stereotyped that no one but the most knowledgeable and devious individual with an exceptional memory for detail could succeed in simulating it. Malingering in the posttraumatic situation is rare, and we must guard ourselves as physicians against projecting a cynical attitude toward trauma patients for fear that we may be duped by a clever malingerer. Although there is no stereotype for a malingerer, there are certain things in the patient's background that may make the physician suspicious, such as (a) emotional instability, (b) vocational instability, (c) job dissatisfaction, (d) lack of work motivation, and (e) sociopathic character disorder.

SUMMARY

Chronic headache and other associated constellations of symptoms are a common sequel to head injury. The consistency of symptoms from one patient to the next, observed with monotonous repetition and supported by findings of malfunctions within the brain, are strong indications that this syndrome is an organic process induced by injury. Most patients with this syndrome will improve with appropriate management over time, but one can expect prolonged disability in about 15 to 20% of such patients. A supportive and well-structured therapeutic program that includes pharmacotherapy, behavioral and psychological management, and rehabilitation counseling is important.

REFERENCES

1. Report of the Panel on Strokes, Trauma, Regeneration, and Neoplasms to the National Advisory Neurological and Communicative Disorders and Stroke Council. National Institutes of Health. 1979.
2. Caveness WF. Incidence of cranial cerebral trauma in the United States. Ann Neurol 1977;1:507.
3. Cartlidge NEF, Shaw DA. Head injury. Philadelphia: WB Saunders, 1981:2.
4. Brenner CT, Friedman AP, Merrit HH, Denny-Brown D. Posttraumatic headache. Ann Neurosurg 1944;1:379.
5. Merritt HH, Friedman AP, Brenner CT. Headache and posttraumatic syndrome. Trans Am Neurol Assoc 1944;70:57.
6. Friedman AP, Merritt HH. Relationship of intracranial pressure in the presence of blood in the cerebrospinal fluid to the occurrence of headache in patients with injuries to the head. J Nerv Ment Dis 1945;102:1–7.
7. Miller H. Accident neurosis. Br Med J 1961;1:919–925, 992–993.
8. Silfverskiold BP. The postconcussion syndrome and its treatment. In: Walker AE, Caveness WF, Critchley M, eds. Late effects of head injury. Springfield, IL: Charles C Thomas, 1969:33–45.
9. Lusk MD, Knott JA. Effect of head injury on libido. Med Aspects Hum Sex 1982;16:22–39.
10. Weinstein EA. Sexual disturbance after brain injury. Med Aspects Hum Sex 1974;8:10.
11. Zulch KD. Medical causation. In: Walker AE, Caveness WF, Critchley M, eds. Late effects of head injury. Springfield IL: Charles C Thomas, 1969:467.
12. Rutherford WH, Merritt JD, McDonald JR. Sequelae of concussion caused by minor head injury. Lancet 1974;1:1–4.
13. Gronwall D, Wrightson P. Delayed recovery of intellectual function after minor head injury. Lancet 1974;2:605–609.
14. Jacobson SA. Mechanism of the sequelae of minor craniocervical. trauma. In: Walker AE, Caveness WF, Critchley M, eds. Late effects of head injury. Springfield, IL: Charles C Thomas, 1969:33–45.
15. Osler, LD, Fusillo MG. A peculiar type of post concussive "blackout." J Neurol Neurosurg Psychiatry 1965;28:344–349.
16. Flanagan D, ed. The brain. Scientific American. New York: WH Freeman, 1979.
17. Povlishock JT, Becker DP, Cheng CLY, Vaughn GW. Axonal change in minor head injury. J Neuropath Exp Neurol 1983;42:225–242.
18. Taylor AR, Bell RR. Slowing of the cerebral circulation after concussional head injury. A controlled trial. Lancet 1966;2:178–180.
19. Strich SJ. The pathology of brain damage due to blunt head injuries. In: Walker AE, Caveness WF, Critchley M, eds. Late effects of head injury. Springfield, IL: Charles C Thomas, 1969:501–526.
20. Oppenheimer DR. Microscopic lesions in the brain following head injury. J Neurol Neurosurg Psychiatry 1968;31:299.
21. Pudenz RH, Sheldon CH. The lucite calvarium. A method for direct observation of the brain. J Neurosurg 1946;3:487.
22. Holbourn AHS. Mechanics of head injury. Lancet 1943;2:438–441.
23. Denny-Brown D, Russell WR. Experimental cerebral concussion. Brain 1941;64:93.
24. Taylor AR. The cerebral circulatory disturbance associated with the late effects of head injury. In: Walker AE, Caveness WF, Critchley M, eds. Late effects of head injury. Springfield, IL: Charles C Thomas, 1969:501–526.
25. Windle WF, Groat RA. Disappearance of nerve cells after concussion. Anat Rec 1945;93:201.
26. Windle WF, Groat RA, Fox CA. Experimental structural alteration in the brain during the after concussion. Surg Gynecol Obstet 1944;79:561.
27. Groat RA, Simmonds JQ. Loss of nerve cells in experimental cerebral concussion. J Neuropath Exp Neurol 1950;9:150.
28. Becker RF, Groat RA, Windle WF. Effects of concussion upon the retention of learning in the guinea pig. Fed Proc 1945;4:6.
29. Ommaya AK. In: Caveness WF, Walker AE, eds. Head Injury Conference Proceedings. Philadelphia: JB Lippincott, 1966:268.
30. Skinhoj E. Determination of regional cerebral blood flow in man. In: Walker AE, Caveness WF, Critchley M, eds. Head Injury Conference Proceedings. Philadelphia: JB Lippincott, 1966:431.
31. Noseworthy JH, Miller J, Murray TJ, et al. Auditory brain stem evoked responses in postconcussion syndrome. Arch Neurol 1981;38:275–278.
32. Rowe MJ. The brain stem evoked response in postconcussion vertigo [Abstract]. Electroencephalog Clin Neurophysiol 1977;43:454.
33. Toglia JU, Rosenberg RE, Ronis ML. Posttraumatic dizziness. Arch Otolaryngol 1970;92:485–492.
34. Ommaya AK, Gennarelli TA. Cerebral concussion and traumatic unconsciousness. Brain 1970;97:633–654.
35. Van Woerkom TCAM, Teelken AW, Minderhond JM. Difference in neurotransmitter metabolism in frontotemporal lobe contusion and diffuse cerebral contusion. Lancet 1977;1:812–813.
36. Haas DC, Pineda GS, Lourie H, et al. Juvenile head trauma syndromes and their relationship to migraine. Arch Neurol 1975;32:727–730.
37. Kalenak ER, Petro DJ, Brennar RW. Migraine secondary to head trauma in wrestling. Am J Sports Med 1978;6:112–113.
38. Bennet ER, et al. Migraine precipitated by head trauma in wrestling. Am J Sports Med 1974;8:202–205.
39. Behrman, S. Migraine as a sequela of blunt head injury. Injury 1977;9:74–76.
40. Jones OW, Brown HA. The measurement of posttraumatic pain. J Nerv Ment Dis 1944;99:668.
41. Gainotti G. Emotional behavior and the hemispheric side of the brain. Cortex 1972;8:41–55.
42. Follstein MF, Maiberger R, McHugh PR. Mood disorders as a specific complication of stroke. J Neurol Neurosurg Psychiatry 1977;40:1018–1020.
43. Robinson RG, Szetela B. Mood changes following left hemispheric brain injury. Ann Neurol 1981;9:447–453.
44. Milner B. Residual intellectual and memory deficits after head injury. In: Walker AE, Caveness WF, Critchley M, eds. The late effects of head injury. Springfield, IL: Charles C Thomas, 1969.
45. Jacobson SA. Mechanism of the sequelae of minor craniocervical trauma. In: Walker AE, Caveness WF, Critchley M, eds. The late effects of head injury. Springfield, IL: Charles C Thomas, 1969:501–526.
46. Denker PG. The post-concussion syndrome: prognosis and evaluation of organic factors. N Y State J Med 1943;271:379–384.
47. Kelly R, Smith BN. Post-traumatic syndrome: another myth discredited. J Roy Soc Med 1981;74:275–277.
48. Caveness WF. Head Injury Conference Proceedings. Caveness WF, Walker AE, eds. Lippincott, Philadelphia 1966:209.
49. Glaser MA, Shafer FP. Skull and brain traumas: their sequelae. JAMA 1932;98:271–276.
50. Balla J, Moraitis S. Knights in armour. A follow-up study of injuries after legal settlement. Med J Aust 1970;2:355–361.
51. Mersky H, Woodford JM. Psychiatric sequelae after minor head injury. Brain 1972;95:521–528.
52. Kozol H. Pre-traumatic personality and psychiatric sequelae of head injury. Arch Neurol Psychiatry 1945;53:358–364.

27

Headache Associated with Intracranial Abnormalities

THOMAS E. GRETTER

This chapter discusses intracranial abnormalities, some with specific identifiable causes, such as tumors, high and low spinal fluid pressure syndromes, iatrogenic disorders and some without identifiable causes, such as benign intracranial hypertension, that cause severe headache. Intracranial abnormalities such as arachnoid cysts may exist that are incidental to headaches, and aggressive treatment will not alter the typical course. Aggressive treatment is needed in other headache causes to preserve neurological function and life.

Headache as a common illness has been discussed earlier in this book. The prevalence of headache had been estimated at 97% in the general population. It may be higher, but patients seek medical care at a lesser rate. The vast majority of individuals with headache do not have a specific structural lesion or intracranial abnormality that can be identified as the agent responsible. Headaches are classified into three general groups: tension-type; migraine and its subtypes; and those referring to a specific organic lesion or associated medical condition (increased intracranial pressure, cranial arteritis, subarachnoid hemorrhage, medical illness, toxic condition, etc.). This chapter focuses on intracranial abnormalities that are conditions in the latter category.

There are intracranial lesions and conditions that cause headache which in some instances produce symptoms and signs that mimic specifically described headache symptom complexes including cluster, migraine, and tension-type headaches. Trauma, medical illness, sinus disease, cerebral vascular diseases and other causes of headache are discussed elsewhere in this book. The challenges to the physician are to determine when underlying intracranial pathology may be causing the headache symptoms and signs the patient manifests and when to investigate further into the headache cause. In today's cost-conscious atmosphere, there is resistance to using high technology studies such as computerized tomography (CT) and magnetic resonance imaging (MRI) to determine the presence or absence of a structural abnormality. Certainly, an abnormal neurological examination without adequate explanation or a recent change in the headache character are indicators for additional studies. An index of suspicion is based on the temporal profile of the headache. Recent onset of a sudden severe headache or a change in the

pattern of a subacute headache or a chronic headache warrants further study. Focal neurological symptoms during a headache attack (complex or complicated migraine) have been associated with a high incidence of structure abnormalities (1). There is no specific headache pattern that can be allocated to a type of headache such as migraine with 100% assurance that there is not a structural abnormality. This author feels that an investigation using high technology studies is not warranted if a benign headache type is established. However, if the benign nature of the headache cannot be established using historical and physical facts, then further study is warranted.

The severity and location of the head pain are probably of least value in determining a benign or life-threatening cause and the headache course. It is useful to look at the headache profile and the factors relating to the pain. A several-year history of unchanging pain or pain precipitated by factors such as specific foods, alcohol, stress, menses, or illness indicates a non-life-threatening headache. A new or changing headache pattern should arouse suspicion for an intracranial abnormality or other cause for the headache.

The intracranial source of the pain has long been discussed, as the exact mechanism is not known. The brain itself has been felt insensitive to pain. Pain can originate from other intracranial structures by traction, inflammation, or pressure on cranial nerves, arteries, veins, sinuses, and the meninges.

PRESSURE HEADACHE

Benign Intracranial Hypertension

Benign intracranial hypertension (pseudotumor cerebri) presents with a headache, visual loss or changes in vision, and papilledema. The nature of the pain varies with each patient. Migraine-like symptoms, including pounding pain, hallucinations, vomiting, are reported (2). The diagnosis is made by exclusion and established by ruling out brain tumors and other mass lesions, intracranial infections, hemorrhage, aqueductal stenosis, obstructive hydrocephalus and encephalopathy secondary to multiple other factors including hypertension. The term "benign" may not be appropriate, as sight is threatened and prompt treatment is needed to save vision. However, "benign" is appropriate in the absence of the noted life-threatening causes and the spontaneous remissions that occur.

The pathogenesis of the condition is not understood. This condition is commonly seen in young, healthy women who may have a history of menstrual irregularity and are slightly to severely overweight. Endocrine studies have not demonstrated an abnormality. Several mechanisms have been suggested but there are no supporting data for any hypothesis. These mechanisms include CSF absorption rate slowing, increased CSF production, and increased brain volume suggestive of brain edema.

The physical findings include papilledema, sometimes with hemorrhages and enlargement of the blind spot on formal visual fields. A sixth cranial nerve palsy presenting as diplopia has been reported, but other neurological signs are absent.

Brain imaging using CT or MRI fails to show a mass lesion or structural abnormality. The ventricles are not dilated and are usually small.

Treatment of this condition is individualized. When the signs are acute and rapidly progressive with progressive visual loss then treatment must be prompt to save sight. Medical therapy is initiated before surgical intervention and sometimes resolves the problem. Acetazolamide (Diamox), a carbonic anhydrase inhibitor that reduces CSF production, is given orally, and is more effective with a drug holiday 1 day a week. Furosemide (Lasix) also reduces pressure. If the signs progress, lumbar puncture, performed daily, reducing the CSF pressure to normal has been advocated. A shunt is the indicated procedure with intractable high pressure after a medical regimen or progressive visual loss. Temporal decompression is probably not effective (3).

A variety of conditions with similar symptoms of the condition including headache, papilledema and visual change have been reported but from a purely logical point do not represent benign intracranial hypertension. These causes though uncommon, have found their way into the literature and are found in academic discussions on the differential diagnosis. The list includes medication, medical illness, and other conditions. These should stand alone, as the pathogenesis is not understood, and in the case of association with specific medications, the signs resolve with discontinuing the medication. The medications commonly referred to include vitamin A, lithium carbonate, tetracycline, aminodrome, and nalidixic acid. Medical diseases referred to include endocrine diseases, anemia (iron deficient), collagen vascular disease, and several other illnesses and conditions.

High Intracranial Pressure

Increased intracranial pressure as a cause for headache is the source for discussion. Cerebral spinal fluid pressure was elevated to over 680 mm H_2O and did not result in headache in human subjects in 1943 (4). Headache is a part of acute obstructive hydrocephalus and certainly a symptom of shunt malfunction in patients treated with that system. Whether structure shift is necessary for pain is unclear.

Increased intracranial pressure secondary to a lesion obstructive to cerebral spinal fluid outflow from the ventricles may develop symptoms of migraine with aura. Colloid cysts of the third ventricle and brainstem tumors are noted to cause CSF outflow obstruction with hydrocephalus which is the common mechanism for the headache symptoms (5).

The pain description usually consists of pain on awakening, increasing with position change and straining (cough, bowel movement), and accompanied by nausea and vomiting, visual blurring, dizziness, and vertigo. There is usually neck stiffness and later papilledema. Visual loss is a serious but late manifestation. Acute obstruction is more likely to cause pain than slow obstruction. Neurological examination does not show focal findings. A CT or MR scan will establish the diagnosis and should be done before consideration of a lumbar puncture. The treatment is a shunt or surgical relief of the obstruction.

Obstruction of the aqueduct of Sylvius by an infection involving the meninges, including fungal, tubercular, bacterial, and viral, may be gradual or acute and presents diagnostic challenges. Hydrocephalus developing slowly may not have a history of headache in spite of hugely dilated ventricles.

Acute hydrocephalus from the ball-valve action of a colloid cyst of the third ventricle or from a rapidly expanding posterior fossa lesion can produce severe headache. The headache is not localized and can fit any description, including that of a specific migraine pattern. Nausea, vomiting, and altered level of consciousness, from lethargy to coma, may ensue. Prompt diagnosis with CT or MRI and shunting are necessary to sustain life.

CONGENITAL CONDITIONS

Congenital conditions can manifest in adult life with headache as the presenting complaint. Arnold Chiari malformation (cerebellar tonsil herniation through the foramen magnum) may obstruct cerebral spinal fluid flow. The headache is nonspecific, and the neurological signs may include cranial neuropathies, (especially extraocular movement abnormalities), cerebellar signs (nystagmus, dysmetria, ataxia) and long tract signs (increased tone, increased deep tendon reflexes, extensor plantar responses, etc.). The MRI is diagnostic, and the treatment is surgical in the face of progressive neurological deficits.

COMMUNICATING HYDROCEPHALUS

Communicating hydrocephalus with failure of absorption of cerebral spinal fluid secondary to trauma, subarachnoid hemorrhage, infection, etc. may present with a headache, which is usually generalized and sometimes more posterior in location. Normal pressure hydrocephalus (NPH), occurring in older individuals, presents with gait disturbance, incontinence, and decreasing mental status. Headache is very unusual in NPH. The diagnosis is established by ruling out a mass lesion through CT or MRI and a cystometrogram (radionuclide CSF flow study). There is an improvement in neurological signs following removal of 30 to 50 ml of CSF. A shunt procedure is the definitive treatment.

Arachnoid Cysts

The advent of CT scan and later MRI has led to finding arachnoid cysts during headache investigation. Rarely are arachnoid cysts the cause of headache, and surgical drainage or excision does not alter the headache pattern. Sometimes arachnoid cysts may communicate with the normal CSF system by a valve-like structure that does not allow drainage, only expansion. CSF pulsations will cause the cysts to expand and lead to pressure symptoms. Serial studies (CT or MRI) will show cyst enlargement that indicates the need for surgical intervention. The headache, if present, may be secondary to distortion and be either generalized or localized.

Subarachnoid spaces on CT or MRI may be enlarged as an anatomical variant, such as the cisterna magna or cisterna ambiens, and not be pathological as a cause for headache. Surgery is not indicated.

LOW-PRESSURE SYNDROME

Post Lumbar Puncture Headache

Quincke introduced the lumbar puncture as a diagnostic tool in 1891. Since then, the incidence of postspinal headache has fluctuated, depending upon the author and the technique used. The headache can occur immediately or develop several days after the procedure. The pain is generalized, sometimes with neck stiffness, and is position-dependant. The pain is relieved by lying down and made worse by standing. Dizziness, nausea, and vomiting may accompany the headache. There are no focal neurological signs, although a sixth nerve palsy, either unilateral or bilateral, may (rarely) accompany the headache. The patient is usually afebrile and responds to bed rest for a few days. Sometimes it is necessary with persistent pain to use a blood patch, an injection of autologous blood in the epidural space to seal the dural leak. Epidural fibrin preparations have been reported to be helpful (6). The recognized technique of lumbar puncture is to use a small (20 gauge) needle with the bevel aligned to split, not cut, the longitudinally running dural fibers and leave the patient lying down for 30 minutes afterward.

Cerebrospinal Fluid Fistula Headache

Lumbar puncture is the commonest cause for low cerebral spinal pressure syndrome, but there are other considera-

tions. CSF rhinorrhea secondary to trauma (fracture of the cribriform plate) may produce a low-pressure syndrome and may be associated with repeated bacterial meningitis. The cause may be trauma, spontaneous or associated with tumors. Spontaneous idiopathic CSF hypotension as a rare, unexplained entity has been described (7). The diagnosis is established by demonstrating the CSF leak, using albumin isotopes and scanning or Metrizamide using CT.

Neurological Sarcoidosis

Headache may be an early rare sign of sarcoidosis, which affects the leptomeninges and the brain. This generalized disease is characterized by developing noncaseating epithelioid granulomatous nodules that can be distributed anywhere. The lungs, skin, lymph nodes, eyes, parotid gland, and central nervous system are most commonly affected. The first signs and symptoms may be neurological with headache, bilateral facial weakness, and other central nervous signs. Seizures can occur. The etiology is not known. The more common signs are mediastinal adenopathy, diffuse pulmonary infiltrates, skin lesions, and hepatic nodules. There is a mild fever and anemia with elevated serum calcium and globulin levels in some cases. The diagnosis is established by biopsy after clinical suspicion. The treatment includes corticosteroids and chlorambucil as an alternative.

Toxic Headache

Headache that results from exposure to toxins is described as generalized, pulsating, moderate, and constant. There are few localizing symptoms and signs. The toxic state may be secondary to infection, alcoholism, uremia, heavy metals, carbon monoxide poisoning, etc. The exact mechanism of this type of headache is not known and has been subject to debate. The toxic cause is suspected by a history of exposure, and appropriate studies based on the toxin are initiated. Treatment is symptomatic, usually involving mild analgesics.

BRAIN TUMORS

Headaches secondary to brain tumors can take on any description. The headache caused by an intracranial neoplasm can take on any clinical symptom complex and cannot be differentiated from nontumor headaches by clinical description alone.

For discussion, headache associated with brain tumors can be divided into two distinct categories based on pathophysiology: (a) increased intracranial pressure produced by tumor volume or impingement on cerebral spinal fluid outflow channels and (b) no change in intracranial pressure or the effect of the tumor itself.

The mechanism for pain production by the tumor alone in the second category is unclear unless specific pain-sensitive structures are evolved. The patient may be free of neurological signs. The pain description may be the text-book description of a headache pattern (migraine) or have other characteristics to arouse suspicion such as new onset, pain that varies with changing position, and pain that occurs at unusual intervals without an associated event. This second category can have a wide variety of neurological signs and symptoms that are based on localized destruction of brain tissue, compression of tissue, edema, and other unknown factors. Other neurological signs and symptoms may be present such as a changing mental status, convulsions, or focal neurological deficit. The triad of headache, vomiting, and papilledema is usually a late manifestation of increasing pressure, although it can appear early (8).

Tumor pathological type has little correlation with head pain, but location may. Posterior fossa tumors are more apt to cause increased pressure than supratentorial tumors.

To differentiate headache caused by intracranial tumors from other causes is difficult, based on clinical grounds. The frequency of reported headaches with tumors is high but so is the overall incidence of headache. No special characteristics are attributable to tumor-caused headache. The clinician is sometimes left with an index of suspicion as the indicator to request MRI or CT. Probably the best indicator is the onset of headache in a person who has been previously headache-free. The pain can be intermittent, nonlocalized, and increased with change in position, and can last for varying periods of time. Although the pain characteristics may vary and the neurological examination is normal at first, headache seldom remains the only manifestation of a brain tumor.

Primary Brain Tumor

No specific headache symptoms or types differentiate the pathological tumor type. Both benign and malignant tumors by the methodology described above may present as headaches. The headache description may take on any or several descriptive features (Table 27.1). The frequency of headache in tumor patients related to that cause is about 20% (9). Paroxysmal headache symptoms with nausea, vomiting, and vertigo mimicking basilar migraine were the initial symptoms of a brainstem glioma (10). Donaldson reported two patients with headache with aura (classical migraine), who had a several-year-history, who developed hydrocephalus secondary to colloid cysts of the third ventricle and a tumor of the ventral midpons.

Cluster headache symptoms may be associated with intracranial neoplasms, and several pathological types and locations have been reported (11). Parasagittal meningiomas with Tolosa Hunt syndrome, adenoma of the pituitary gland, and an upper cervical meningioma have been reported. Lymphoma of the leptomeninges involving the trigeminal nerve has mimicked cluster migraine (12). The pain is probably a manifestation of trigeminal dysfunction

Table 27.1.
Headache Description with Tumor[a]

Intermittent	85%
Nonthrobbing	75%
Awake from sleep	15%
Morning headache	15%
Change of position	20%
Exertion	25%
Nausea and vomiting	50%
Ipsilateral	8%

[a]Data from Rushton JG, Rook ED. Brain tumor headache. Headache 1962;2:147–152.

secondary to involvement by the tumor and will more often present as face pain rather than migraine symptoms.

Metastatic Tumor

Metastases to the brain can have headaches as part of the symptom complex. The headache characteristics are equal to primary brain tumors in that the cause of the pain is similar. Cerebral metastases even have been reported as presenting as migraine with aura (13).

Cranial nerves are susceptible to metastases during their course within the skull and may be primarily involved or trapped secondary to bone evolvement. Pain or loss of function of the involved nerve or adjacent nervous tissue tends to be progressive. Greenberg et al. reviewed the more typical clinical syndromes that carry eponyms that sound like a "Who's Who in Neurology" (14).

The pain is usually focal with tenderness. The diagnosis is established using CT and MRI. Plain x-rays are infrequently used because of the ability to do serial sections on CT and attain fine resolution. In spite of modern technology, not all the cases are verified radiographically. Radiation is the treatment of choice and is sometimes done on a clinical basis alone. Cerebral spinal fluid should be studied to determine the presence of meningeal carcinomatosis. The treatment is radiation for palliation.

REFERENCES

1. Drexler ED. Severe headaches. When to worry, what to do. Postgrad Med 1990;87 (4):164–170,173–180.
2. Murali R. Neurosurgical considerations in headaches. Otolaryngol Clin North Am 1989;22 (6):1229–1250.
3. Johnston I, Paterson A, Besser M. The treatment of benign intracranial hypertension: a review of 134 cases. Surg Neurol 1981;16(3): 218–224.
4. Kunkle E, Ray BS, Wolff HG. Experimental studies in headache: analysis of the headache associated with changes in intracranial pressure. Arch Neurol Psychiatry 1943;49:323–358.
5. Donaldson IM. Migraine due to hydrocephalus. Headache 1984;24(5):272–273.
6. Schlenker M, Ringelstein EB. Epidural fibrin clot for the prevention of post-lumbar puncture headache: a new method with risks (letter). J Neurol Neurosurg Psychiatry 1987;50(12):1715.
7. Bell WE, Joynt RJ, Sahs AL. Low spinal fluid pressure syndrome. Neurology 1960;10:512–521.
8. Joseph R, Cook GE, Steiner TJ, Clifford-Rose F. Intracranial space-

occupying lesions in patients attending a migraine clinic. Practitioner 1985;229(1403):477–481.

9. Rushton JG, Rooke ED. Brain tumor headache. Headache 1962;2:147–152.

10. Novak GP, Moshe SL. Brainstem glioma presenting as paroxysmal headache. Dev Med Child Neurol 1985;27(3):379–382.

11. Hannerz J. A case of parasellar meningioma mimicking cluster headache. Cephalalgia 1989;9(4):265–269.

12. DeAngelis LM, Payne R. Lymphomatous meningitis presenting as atypical cluster headache. Pain 1987;30(2):211–216.

13. Pepin EP. Cerebral metastasis presenting as migraine with aura (letter). Lancet 1990;336(8707):127–128.

14. Greenberg H, Deck MDF, Vikram B, Chu F, Posner JB. Metastases to the base of the skull: clinical findings in 43 cases. Neurology 1981;31:530–537.

28

Headache Associated with Medication and Substance Withdrawal

ALAN M. RAPOPORT and FRED D. SHEFTELL

Headaches can be caused by medications in non-headache-prone individuals, and certain existing headache syndromes can be worsened by the abuse of medications or the withdrawal of medications or substances such as caffeine, analgesics, and ergots. Understanding this relationship between medication and headache can help physicians to better diagnose and treat their patients.

DRUGS INDUCING HEADACHE

Vasodilator drugs such as nitroglycerin can cause headaches even in the non-headache-prone individual. Cardiac patients using nitroglycerin will frequently develop throbbing headaches. Long-acting nitroglycerin, nitropaste, and the sublingual form can cause throbbing headaches. Workers in plants manufacturing explosives may also develop a nitroglycerin headache, but they sometimes become tolerant to nitroglycerin and stop having their headaches over a period of time. The headaches are throbbing, appear within 1 hour, and are usually described as being worse with any type of physical exertion. Patients with migraine are more sensitive to the effects of nitroglycerin than patients who do not usually have headaches (1). Nitrites are used in cured meats to produce a more uniformly colored product. Nitrites are contained in hot dogs, salami, bologna, ham, bacon, and other cured meats. Patients who are sensitive to nitrites may develop a bilateral throbbing headache and facial flushing within 20 minutes after ingestion. As little as 1 mg of sodium nitrite can cause a headache (2).

Alcohol is a complex substance that can produce headaches in many ways. It is a vasodilator and may contribute to causing headaches even in non-headache-prone individuals. The hangover syndrome is more complex and lasts 5 to 10 hours, long after the alcohol has been metabolized (3).

Histamine is a natural substance that, when injected under the skin or intravenously, can cause headaches. Although controversial, the use of intravenous histamine desensitization for chronic and severe cluster headache has been beneficial to certain patients. Patients are given small doses of intravenous histamine phosphate slowly throughout most of the day and over the course of several days. The purpose is to desensitize the body to histamine and decrease the cluster headache. If the rate of intravenous administration is too rapid for the individual, a typical cluster headache can be induced. The treatment is to slow the rate of administration or stop it temporarily and treat the patient with 7 liters/minute of pure oxygen by mask in a seated position or give dihydroergotamine (D.H.E. 45) intravenously.

Dipyridamole (Persantine) has been used in patients with transient ischemic attacks. It has a slight vasodilating effect and theoretically can cause headache in susceptible individuals.

Certain vasoconstrictor drugs and substances can cause withdrawal headaches. Caffeine is a vasoconstrictor and actually can be helpful in treating an acute headache. If an individual has too high an intake of caffeine on a daily basis, caffeine withdrawal headaches can occur. These occur in individuals consuming a higher than normal amount of caffeine who wake up later than usual on the weekend and develop weekend headaches. There is 100 to 150 mg of caffeine in a cup of coffee. Patients may be susceptible to these headaches if their caffeine intake is over 350 mg per day and much more susceptible at an intake of 500 to 800 mg per day. If they wake up 2 hours later than they ordinarily do, they may develop headaches. Or they could go longer than normal to have their next cup of coffee and develop one. Ergotamine tartrate works in a somewhat similar way to produce ergotamine-withdrawal headaches (described later in this chapter).

Certain drugs can cause hypertension, either when they are given or when they are withdrawn, and this can induce headache. Monoamine oxidase inhibitor drugs such as phenelzine sulphate (Nardil) as well as many others are excellent drugs for treatment of depression and certain types of headaches. They have as potential side effect the ability to cause either hypotension or hypertension. Patients taking these drugs must avoid dietary ingestion of tyramine. Patients who consume tyramine may develop the "cheese-effect," which is acute hypertension due to the inability of the body to detoxify the tyramine via monoamine oxidase pathways. This can also be caused by taking over-the-counter drugs that contain sympathomimetic amines, such as drugs used for the common cold and sinus problems. The hypertensive crisis that ensues is usually associated with a severe throbbing headache.

A similar problem can be seen in patients taking too high a dose of sympathomimetic drugs such as amphetamines, methamphetamine, and phenylpropanolamine, which is frequently found in over-the-counter sinus medication. The same problem can be seen in patients on certain antihypertensive medication when they are withdrawn rapidly. This is seen with clonidine hydrochloride (Catapres) and can be seen with the β-blockers (e.g., propranolol).

Patients on certain medications can have intracranial bleeding as a side effect that causes sudden severe headache with decreased level of consciousness. Anticoagulant drugs such as intravenous heparin or oral dicumarol (Coumadin), used to prevent emboli and treat clots, can cause this serious side effect. Also, any drug acutely elevating blood pressure can cause intracranial bleeding, which would cause headache.

Drugs can cause benign intracranial hypertension (pseudotumor cerebri). In this condition, patients taking these drugs develop severe headaches, associated with papilledema and sometimes bilateral sixth nerve palsies with diplopia. CT scans are usually normal, but their spinal fluid pressures are markedly elevated. Medications that can do this are certain antibiotics such as tetracycline and nalidixic acid (NegGram), vitamin A, corticosteroids, thyroxine, lithium, and phenytoin (Dilantin). Patients with acne are frequently taking a combination of tetracycline and vitamin A, and if they do so in too high a dose, they may develop this syndrome. The treatment is to stop the offending drug and sometimes to use acetazolamide (Diamox) and/or steroids.

Finally, certain drugs can worsen preexisting headaches. Women placed on estrogen cyclically will often develop headaches as the estrogen is withdrawn. Progesterone sometimes causes headaches and sometimes relieves them. Danazol (Danocrine) has been known to cause headaches. Alcohol has been mentioned and analgesics and ergotamines are mentioned below.

ANALGESIC-REBOUND HEADACHE

A significant cause of refractory headache in patients with chronic daily headache is the abuse of analgesics, ergots, and other abortive headache medication. It is no wonder that a patient who has 3 to 5 days a week of headache, or certainly a patient with daily headache, will begin to overmedicate with abortive headache medications. The patient is in constant or frequent pain, medication is readily available off-the-shelf (i.e., nonprescription) or by a

doctor's prescription, and guidelines are usually not carefully set by the physician because they are unknown or not thought about. This potential abuse of abortive headache medication does not exist in patients who have only occasional headaches. They develop this syndrome only if the headaches become so frequent that they begin to medicate with abortive agents frequently and prophylactically to prevent the next headache from starting or the current headache from worsening. Nonheadache patients who take large amounts of analgesics for other reasons such as arthritis do not develop analgesic-rebound headache (4).

It is important to emphasize that many abortive headache agents are extremely helpful to the occasional headache sufferer when used properly. The following medications are all helpful in certain headache syndromes:

Aspirin and aspirin-containing combination medications
Acetaminophen and acetaminophen-containing combination medications
Nonsteroidal antiinflammatory compounds
Vasoactive substances such as isometheptene mucate (Midrin)
Ergotamine tartrate (Cafergot and Wigraine)
Dihydroergotamine (D.H.E. 45)
Butalbital-containing compounds (Fiorinal, Fiorinal with codeine, Fioricet and Esgic)
Narcotics
Steroids
Antiemetics (Phenergan and Reglan)
Sedative-hypnotics

All these medications can be effective in the treatment of the occasional headache sufferer when the guidelines are adhered to. However, the abuse of these medications may lead to dependency and/or analgesic-rebound headache or ergotamine-rebound headache. Other medications such as nasal sprays, antihistamines, sinus medications, and tranquilizers are often abused by the headache sufferer.

Analgesic-rebound headache (ARH) is an often unrecognized clinical syndrome in which the frequent and excessive use of analgesics (e.g., aspirin, acetaminophen, narcotics) by chronic headache sufferers perpetuates and worsens head pain rather than relieves it. Such consumption also interferes with the therapeutic efficacy of standard, usually effective pharmacological and nonpharmacological treatment regimens, thus preventing expected improvement.

Patients who use small amounts of analgesics may note some relief from tension-type headache early in the course of that syndrome. But patients with frequent or daily headache seem to habituate to the therapeutic action of such agents. This begins a cycle of increased consumption that not only fails to provide pain reduction, but seems to perpetuate and intensify the headache. This paradoxical effect of analgesics is called analgesic-rebound headache. Patients continue to take the medication long after it stops relieving pain, because they feel they have to do something. At the beginning, the medicine seems to work for 3 to 4 hours to decrease the headache.

The term *rebound* refers both to the worsening of the headache as the analgesic effect wears off, 3 to 4 hours after taking the previous pills, and to the apparent withdrawal phenomenon, whereby the patient experiences an escalation of pain after totally discontinuing the medication. This may go on for several days. The analgesic wash-out period is the time required for reregulation of the nociceptive system and the renewed potential for pain relief following the cessation of analgesic intake.

Our group at The New England Center for Headache in Stamford, CT (including Dr. Randall Weeks and Dr. Steve Baskin) has studied 2500 patients with ARH. Certain clinical trends have emerged. Most patients with ARH are in their thirties or forties and have had mild, subacute, or chronic tension-type headache for many years. Prior to that, they had intermittent migraine. They usually experience pain 2 to 4 times per week prior to abusing analgesics, but they may have daily pain that waxes and wanes throughout the day.

The headaches last from 6 to 24 hours and are described as mild, dull, nonthrobbing, steady, bilateral, frontooccipital, or diffuse discomfort. Early in the syndrome, these headaches are not associated with visual complaints or autonomic symptoms such as nausea, vomiting, diarrhea, sweating, pupillary changes, or stuffed nostrils. There are no focal symptoms such as weakness, paresthesias, or speech problems. Frequency of pain and/or pain duration slowly increases, and patients gradually begin to use over-the-counter or prescription analgesics in larger amounts. With time, the headaches develop the characteristics of migraine, and the syndrome becomes a mix of several types of headaches. Patients also have sleep disturbances such as difficulty falling asleep and early morning awakening, depression, irritability, trouble concentrating, restlessness, and tremor. There is frequently a family history of depression, substance abuse, and headache.

Some patients use only one type of analgesic tablet, but a significant number of patients will use two and sometimes three. Each tablet usually contains one to three substances, so that a patient may be taking six or eight different medications on a daily basis. The most common preparation used is a combination of either aspirin or acetaminophen with a short-acting barbiturate and sometimes caffeine. But it is very common for patients to use off-the-shelf medication in large quantities, and they can cause the "rebound" effect. It is not yet clear whether nonsteroidals such as ibuprofen cause rebound as much as aspirin and acetaminophen do. Narcotics will also cause rebound headaches and are frequently more difficult to deal with because of more significant withdrawal problems and dependency.

Patients note only temporary, partial relief and begin to medicate 3 to 4 times per day often as soon as relief wears off. Some will start to take medication in anticipation of a severe headache, to ensure that their level of activity will not be compromised by pain. They will frequently jump the gun and medicate for a very mild headache, because they are concerned about it becoming more severe.

Patients may often awaken in the morning either without a headache or with a very mild headache and medicate before getting out of bed. They continue to medicate every day, their intake ranging from 5 to 20 tablets per day, but averaging 5 to 6 tablets per day. Some patients take up to 5 tablets at one time for a bad headache, even if they know that it will not be effective. There is little relief, and the headache appears to worsen in spite of increased amounts of medication. They are at high risk to develop toxicity from medication, especially hepatic and renal toxicity, and ulcers.

RELEVANT RESEARCH

Kudrow studied the paradoxical effect of frequent analgesic use in 200 daily headache sufferers (5). One hundred patients were given amitriptyline HCI (Elavil, Endep) and 100 were not. The two groups were further subdivided into two equal subgroups of 50 each; one discontinued analgesics, the other did not. At the end of 4 weeks, the amitriptyline-treated group had a mean improvement of 30% in the subgroup using analgesics compared with 72% improvement in the analgesic-free subgroup. In the nonamitriptyline group the corresponding figures were 18 and 43%, respectively. These data support and underscore the need to have patients discontinue analgesics to maximize the likelihood of therapeutic benefit from usually effective preventive medications. Even in the absence of treatment, a significant number of patients improved by discontinuing analgesics.

Mathew studied 200 patients who were consuming excess symptomatic medications, yet suffering almost daily headaches (6). He included patients taking pain medication, sleeping medication, ergotamines, nasal spray, and antihistamines. All groups studied showed initial withdrawal reactions and improvement over a period of several weeks. The group that did the best was the one placed on appropriate prophylaxis after discontinuation of symptomatic medication. He concluded that the daily use of symptomatic or immediate relief medications results in chronic daily headache. Discontinuing the daily symptomatic medication itself resulted in improvement in the headache and enhanced the beneficial effect of prophylactic medications.

Isler studied 235 migraine patients who were consuming analgesics at a rate of 30 or more tablets per month (many of whom were also taking ergotamine (7)). He found that they had twice as many headache days per month as those who took fewer than 30 tablets per month. It was found that the slow withdrawal of analgesics and ergotamine while maintaining appropriate prophylactic treatment (mostly β-blocking agents combined with tricyclic antidepressants) improved chronic headache and decreased the frequency of headache days. He concluded that the chronicity of headache was a direct consequence of abuse of medication designed for immediate effect. Restriction of the use of such drugs to once a week or less was recommended. A limitation of the study was that it combined analgesic abusers with ergotamine abusers and studied only migraine patients without addressing tension-type headache.

Dichgan and colleagues studied the effects of the abrupt withdrawal of mixed analgesics in 52 patients with chronic headache (8). Patients developed withdrawal symptoms but improved markedly for long periods.

Wilkinson studied nonheadache patients who took large amounts of analgesics for other conditions (i.e., arthritis) and found that they do not develop analgesic-rebound headache (4).

CLINICAL STUDIES AT THE NEW ENGLAND CENTER FOR HEADACHE

Our first two studies on ARH at The New England Center for Headache showed that most patients improved when taken off their analgesics, some doing better with the addition of cyproheptadine (Periactin) or amitriptyline HCI (Elavil). Our most recent study on ARH was an attempt to ascertain the length of time that the analgesic detoxification process (wash-out period) may take (9). Ninety patients took part in this study, and all took a minimum of 14 analgesic tablets per week. Significant improvement was defined as greater than 67% reduction in the frequency of headache. Physiological data showed no significant changes, but there was a trend for patients treated with amitriptyline to have lower levels of frontalis EMG. Those on no medication had the highest finger temperature readings. Thirty percent of the patients were significantly improved during the first month; 37% more during the second month; 13% more during the third month; and 2% during the fourth month for a total of 82% of patients improving over the 4 months. All patients were asked to discontinue analgesics, and some were treated with small doses of cyproheptadine and vitamin B_6 and others with small doses of amitriptyline.

The data suggest that the analgesic wash-out period may be as long as 12 weeks for some patients, but is often at least 8 weeks. To fully evaluate any headache treatment modality, a period of 8 to 12 weeks off analgesic medication is necessary when treating patients who have ARH as part of their clinical picture.

DISCUSSION

The pain from chronic tension-type headache was thought at one time to be peripheral, possibly secondary to contracted muscles and painful nerves in the head and neck. An emerging body of data suggests that it may be a central nervous system disorder and that analgesics may be more centrally active than the peripheral role they play in inhibiting prostaglandins. If the pain of chronic daily headache is central in origin and associated with tolerance, habituation, and rebound pain, then it may be secondary to suppression of a central antinociceptive system such as the ascending and descending serotonergic system controlling sleep, dull pain, migraine, and feeling of well-being. It is known that aspirin works centrally to increase serotonin levels, but there is a paradoxical effect with increased pain.

It used to be thought that the rate-limiting step in the availability of cerebral serotonin was the concentration of the enzyme 5-tryptophan hydroxylase in the brain. It is now known that the level of cerebral tryptophan is the limiting factor.

Tryptophan is the only amino acid bound to serum protein. Salicylates (aspirin) break that bond and increase the availability of free tryptophan and hence serotonin in the brain. Studies show that 1 to 2 hours after administration of tryptophan, there is an increase in brain serotonin. Thus, large amounts of aspirin may greatly increase brain serotonin concentration.

In spite of high serotonin levels, there is a paradoxical increase in the amount of headache. Probably there is a down-regulation of serotonin receptors with a reduction in the number of serotonin receptor sites in the brain or some other receptor dysfunction or blockade. This reduces the effectiveness of the increased amount of serotonin and the result is increased pain.

ERGOTAMINE-REBOUND HEADACHE

Ergotamine tartrate is an effective drug to arrest a migraine attack in progress. But its misuse can cause tolerance, dependence, and an increase in frequency of migraine-type headache as well as ergotism. A patient using ergotamine 2 to 3 times weekly notes its effectiveness but also a possible increase in the frequency of headaches. Before long, the headaches may become daily and respond rapidly to a small dose of ergot. According to Saper, as little as 0.5 mg of ergotamine three times per week is enough to produce dependence (10). The problem is perpetuated because stopping the ergotamine for just 24 hours produces a severe withdrawal headache, which is quickly relieved by taking another dose; hence the patient does not want to stop the medication. In addition, the patient becomes refractory to the usually effective modes of treatment, be they behavioral or pharmacological. Treatment begins with ergot withdrawal, usually in a hospital setting.

TREATMENT OF ANALGESIC AND ERGOTAMINE-REBOUND HEADACHE

Our strong belief is that the patient must be withdrawn from all analgesics and ergotamines. In our experience, this is best done over 3 to 5 days, but it could be done abruptly, as long as no barbiturates, narcotics, or ergots are involved. This can sometimes be done on an outpatient basis, but it may be necessary to hospitalize the patient. It is certainly safer, more comfortable, and ultimately more beneficial to the long-term improvement of the chronic headache sufferer to hospitalize these patients in a specialized, multidisciplinary headache treatment unit. Attention to cognitive/psychological factors is important, as patients may feel more helpless without their usual ritual of medication consumption. Cognitive/behavioral work and relaxation therapy (e.g., biofeedback training) are important during withdrawal.

The widespread usage of analgesics for headache and the lack of understanding of the concept of analgesic rebound by both patients and treating physicians, leads to the ubiquitous problem of analgesic-rebound headache today. Physicians who are unaware of this concept will have much more difficulty treating their patients effectively. As Dr. Kudrow has shown, even treating the patient with the proper prophylactic medication is not very effective when analgesics continue to be taken in large quantities. So purely from the treatment point of view, understanding analgesic-rebound headache is vital. From the diagnostic point of view, the lack of understanding of analgesic rebound by neurologists and headache specialists adds to the problem of the lack of reliability in headache diagnosis.

CONCLUSION

Certain medications can cause headache, and other medications used to treat headache can actually worsen the headache syndrome when they are abused. Understanding these concepts and treating patients appropriately leads to much more effective headache treatment in the chronic headache sufferer.

REFERENCES

1. Schnitker MT, Schnitker MA. A clinical test for migraine. JAMA 1947;135:89.
2. Henderson WR, Raskin NH. "Hot dog" headache; individual susceptibility to nitrite. Lancet 1972;2:1162–1163.
3. Goldberg L. Alcohol, tranquilizers and hangover. Q J Stud Alcohol 1961;1(suppl):32–58.
4. Lance F, Parkes C, Wilkinson M. Does analgesic abuse cause headaches de novo? Headache 1988;28(1):61–62.
5. Kudrow L. Paradoxical effects of frequent analgesic use. Adv Neurol 1982;33:335–341.
6. Mathew N, Kurman R, Perez F. Drug induced refractory headache—clinical features and management. Headache 1990;30(10):634–638.
7. Isler H. Migraine treatment as a cause of chronic migraine. In: Rose FC, ed: Advances in migraine research and therapy. New York: Raven Press, 1982;159–164.
8. Dichgans J, Diener HC, Gerber WD, et al. Analgetica-induzierter Dauerkopfschmerz. Dtsch Med Wochenschr 1984;109:369–373.
9. Rapoport AM, Weeks RE, Sheftell FD, et al. The "analgesic washout period": a critical variable in the evaluation of headache treatment efficacy. Neurology 1986;36(suppl 2):100–101.
10. Saper JR, Jones JM. Ergotamine tartrate dependency: features and possible mechanisms. Clin Neuropharmacol 1986;9:244–256.

29

Headaches Associated with Medical Diseases

MICHAEL R. JAFF and GLEN D. SOLOMON

The most common causes of headache in clinical practice are the so-called benign headache disorders—migraine, tension-type, and cluster headache. Headache is a symptom rather than a diagnosis, and the diagnosis of a benign headache disorder requires that other diseases that may cause headache be excluded. This chapter seeks to familiarize the reader with systemic illnesses that have headache as a common symptom.

When approaching the patient who complains of the symptom "headache," the practitioner must consider the medical diseases that may cause headache. A thorough medical history and physical examination usually allows the physician to exclude medical disease, or conversely, raise the possibility of underlying disease as etiology of headache. Without consideration of the many disorders that include headache as a symptom, the headache treatment may be unsuccessful, and the patient may suffer needlessly.

The structures that cause intracranial pain include cerebral blood vessels, cerebral veins and venous sinuses, and the dura mater (1). In addition, prolonged contraction of skeletal muscles of the scalp and neck can cause headache. Any lesion, infection, or inflammatory process that affects these structures, from whatever cause, may provoke headache. Unfortunately, none of the pain patterns are pathognomonic for specific systemic illnesses. Therefore, the historical clues concerning the nature of the head pain must be combined with other medical history and physical examination to elicit a diagnosis.

New case reports appear quite often, making a complete list of every medical condition associated with headache impractical. This chapter lists major groups and classes of disease.

INFECTIOUS CAUSES

Sinusitis has long been recognized as a cause of headache, especially if the ethmoid and maxillary sinuses are involved (see Chapter 22). Sphenoid sinusitis is a cause of headache, which may often be difficult to diagnose (2). The headache is generally transient, and often retroorbital. These headaches are exacerbated by activities that increase facial pressure, such as straining or bending (3). Dental

infections have been well described, and dentists often see patients initially with complaints of headache. Other entities can be confused with dental pain, including cluster headache (particularly lower half syndrome) (4). The physician must discern between upper respiratory infections and nasal allergies. This may be a difficult distinction, requiring shrewd diagnostic acumen (5). A CT scan of the sinuses or nasal endoscopy may be needed to differentiate these disorders.

Meningitis is a life-threatening central nervous system infection that requires prompt diagnosis and therapy. The most common bacterial pathogens include *Haemophilus influenzae*, *Neisseria meningitidis*, and *Streptococcus pneumoniae* in the adult population (6). Headache is common in this disorder, along with the classic signs and symptoms of fever, nuchal rigidity, photophobia, and altered consciousness. Definitive diagnosis requires cerebrospinal fluid examination documenting a polymorphonuclear pleiocytosis, elevated protein and depressed glucose content, and microbiologic confirmation of a pathogen. Prompt initiation of antimicrobial therapy is warranted before results of microbiologic data are available. Other types of meningitis occur as a result of infection by viruses, parasites, fungi, and mycobacteria. The latter two classes may produce a less "typical" and more indolent course, more likely to present as chronic headache.

Scalp infections and skull infections including osteomyelitis and epidural and subdural abscesses are unusual infectious causes of headache.

Recurrent episodes of "aseptic meningitis," often referred to as Mollaret's meningitis, may be associated with headache. Other transient neurological manifestations may be seen including coma, seizures, delirium, hallucination, dysequilibrium, and altered speech patterns (7). This entity is distinctly uncommon.

Brain abscess is often a chronic, serious medical condition. Headache often does not manifest itself early in the course of the illness. If chronic, the headache of a brain abscess is dull and unrelenting. Diagnosis is best made with CT scanning or magnetic resonance imaging (MRI). Antibiotic therapy must be accompanied by surgical drainage of the abscess.

Viral encephalitis is another serious infectious illness associated with headache. The two endemic causes of encephalitis in the United States are herpes simplex virus (HSV) and rabies virus. Arboviruses and postinfluenza encephalitis have been reported (8). Cerebrospinal fluid analysis reveals a mononuclear cell pleiocytosis and an elevated protein content. The CSF may occasionally be normal. MRI and electroencephalography may be helpful in securing a diagnosis. Brain biopsy should be reserved for desperate clinical settings. Acyclovir has proved useful for treatment of HSV encephalitis (9) but not the other viral encephalitides.

Although lumbar puncture (LP) is needed in the diagnosis of many infectious causes of headache, it is not without risk. Lumbar puncture headache can occur within 48 hours of the procedure and is worsened by upright posture. The pain is generally throbbing and can persist for weeks to months. Techniques suggested to decrease the incidence of the LP headache include lying supine after the procedure, use of small-diameter needles, and adequate hydration before the procedure (10).

In the correct clinical setting, headache may be a symptom of underlying infection with the human immunodeficiency virus, HIV. AIDS patients develop a multitude of neurological manifestations including aseptic meningitis, subacute encephalitis, and painful peripheral neuropathy (11). The HIV virus is both lymphotropic and neurotropic, allowing the virus to invade the central nervous system early in the course of the infection (12). In a patient with documented HIV infection, new onset of headache must prompt a diagnostic search for central nervous system disease, including cryptococcal meningitis, lymphoma, or sinusitis.

COLLAGEN VASCULAR DISEASES

The collagen vascular diseases are often difficult to diagnose because of protean manifestations, many of which are nonspecific. The classic connective tissue disease associated with headache is temporal (giant cell) arteritis. This is a disease caused by giant cell infiltration into the walls of arteries, commonly the temporal artery. This giant cell infiltration may also affect other arteries, thereby producing a different pain syndrome. The headache of temporal arteritis is nonspecific and may occur in any location in the head (13). The major risk of temporal arteritis is involvement of retinal arteries with subsequent blindness. Diagnosis is supported by an elevated sedimentation rate and confirmed by pathological demonstration of giant cell infiltration into arterial walls on temporal artery biopsy. Therapy with rapid initiation of corticosteroids at a dose of prednisone 60 mg per day is needed to prevent blindness. Corticosteroids are tapered at a rate determined by the clinical course.

The headache in collagen vascular disease is usually throbbing and relentless. Other evidence of vasculitis

should be sought, including multiorgan system involvement, focal neurological deficits, skin lesions (such as palpable purpura), fever, and weight loss.

Other collagen vascular diseases associated with headache include polyarteritis nodosa, scleroderma, Wegener's granulomatosis, and systemic lupus erythematosus. Some investigators believe that headache is the most frequent neurological complication among patients with SLE (14). Patients may manifest serious neurological consequences associated with headache, such as subdural hematoma (15). Treatment of the underlying connective tissue disorder may relieve the headache. Corticosteroids and other immunosuppressive agents may be necessary.

The chronic fatigue syndrome must be included in this discussion. Although the etiology and pathogenesis of this illness remain elusive, we are gaining tremendous clinical experience in diagnosing this pervasive illness. A recent study assessing the efficacy of intravenous immunoglobulin therapy in chronic fatigue syndrome reported headache in 93% of the patients enrolled (16). In addition, headache is listed as one of 11 minor criteria in the working case definition of the chronic fatigue syndrome (17). Therapy of chronic fatigue syndrome remains unsatisfactory, and the headaches are managed symptomatically.

NEUROLOGICAL DISEASE

The most prevalent neurological disease with associated headache is ischemic and hemorrhagic cerebrovascular disease. The classic scenario is the "warning" headache preceding a subarachnoid hemorrhage (SAH). The headache is usually of sudden onset, unilateral or occipital, and can occur at varying intervals preceding the actual hemorrhage. One study of 30 patients with proven aneurysmal subarachnoid hemorrhage revealed that 43% of these patients recalled a warning headache, and the interval between the headache and hemorrhage ranged from 1 to 80 days (18). Mechanisms of headache in subarachnoid hemorrhage include the irritant effect of blood, the rise in intracranial pressure, and stimulation of vascular nerve endings in ruptured vessels (19). Due to the potentially catastrophic nature of SAH, angiography is indicated if one suspects a "warning" headache.

Headache in ischemic stroke is not as well understood. The headache is usually mild and brief and may occur before the event or at the onset of the vascular event. Carotid circulation events generally cause frontal headache; vertebrobasilar strokes cause posterior headache (19). The incidence of headache in ischemic cerebrovascular disease has been noted to be 27 to 30% (20). One reported case noted an unusual type of exertion headache, cough headache, as a marker for ischemic cerebrovascular disease in a patient with other neurological signs (21).

The incidence of headache in the antiphospholipid antibody syndrome is being clarified. The lupus anticoagulant and anticardiolipin are acquired antiphospholipid antibodies that are found in SLE, other autoimmune disorders, and occasionally in normal subjects. The presence of these "autoantibodies" in association with recurrent arterial and venous thrombosis, thrombocytopenia, recurrent fetal loss, and neuropsychiatric disorders comprise the antiphospholipid antibody syndrome (22). In a recent study of 51 patients with stroke and transient ischemic attacks, only three had clinical and laboratory criteria sufficient to diagnosis this syndrome (23). Clearly, the headaches in patients with this disorder should suggest arterial or venous thrombosis. This disorder may be particularly common in patients with "migrainous stroke."

Increased intracranial pressure is a feared underlying cause for headache, especially if a mass lesion is present. A mass lesion in the brain displaces cerebrospinal fluid, blood, or brain mass. The headache is often referred to as a traction headache (1), described as a dull aching pain, located in proximity to the tumor. Exertion worsens the headache pain. Approximately 60% of patients with brain tumors have headache (24). Many authors feel that a normal neurological examination, along with a lack of other signs suggesting increased intracranial pressure rule against a mass lesion as the cause for headache (25).

Disorders of the cervical spine and headache are reviewed in detail elsewhere. The pain-sensitive structures of the cervical spine include the vertebral column, cervical muscles, cervical nerve roots, and vertebral arteries. Diseases involving the cervical spine include rheumatoid arthritis, ankylosing spondylitis, and congenital bony abnormalities (26). However, the most common cervical spine abnormality associated with headache is cervical spondylosis. Although there are reports that as many as 80% of patients with cervical spondylosis have headaches, other authors report headache rates as low as 13% (27). It is generally accepted that patients with radiculopathy have a more severe headache.

Other neurological illnesses associated with headache include benign intracranial hypertension (pseudotumor cerebri), multiple sclerosis (28), epilepsy (29), brain herniation (30), posttraumatic headache (31), and postendarterectomy hemicrania (32).

ENDOCRINE DISORDERS

Vasodilation and vascular causes are the accepted mechanisms for headache resulting from endocrine diseases. The most common "endocrine disorder" associated with headache is "relative" hypoglycemia. When a patient with a prior diagnosis of migraine headache misses a meal, it often stimulates the onset of headache. Investigators have documented disorganized electroencephalographic activity as blood glucose concentrations fall (33). However, in Service's landmark review of 60 cases of insulinoma, headache was not noted in these patients during hypoglycemic events (34). Other endocrine disorders associated with headache and hypoglycemia include hypothyroidism and

adrenal insufficiency. The headache of hyperthyroidism is felt to be related to anxiety and tension, along with increased metabolic demands.

Hyperparathyroidism may have associated headache that is felt to be related to hypercalcemia and, perhaps, magnesium deficiency. One interesting case report of hyperparathyroidism documented a patient with intractable headache and fever of unknown origin (35).

Headache has been associated with various pituitary tumors. The mechanisms are either direct pressure on surrounding cerebral structures by the tumor or the result of end-organ dysfunction by glands under the influence of pituitary tumors. A recent report revealed improvement in headache pain in two patients with acromegaly with the use of somatostatin analogue (36).

A study of 212 women with prolactinomas revealed that hyperprolactinemia was associated with headache only if a prolactinoma was present (37). It is important to note that headache can occur, even in patients with the empty sella turcica syndrome (1, 38).

Two cases of migraine that resolved after treatment for hyperlipoproteinemia have been reported. Although many variables remain unexplained, our improved ability to diagnose and treat lipid disorders may uncover similar therapeutic effects (39).

HYPERTENSION

Although many believe that headache is a common symptom of patients with hypertension, studies have demonstrated no difference in the frequency of headache between normals and hypertensives with diastolic blood pressures below 130 mm Hg (40). Hypertensive headaches have been described as morning headaches, mild to moderate in intensity, and occipital in location. These headaches tend to resolve with ambulation (41). The association of deteriorating mental status, headache, and severe hypertension suggests hypertensive encephalopathy. Treatment of this entity requires intensive care with close monitoring, along with the use of parenteral antihypertensive agents such as sodium nitroprusside, labetalol, or diazoxide (42).

Pheochromocytoma is a secondary cause for hypertension. Headache is often associated with this and is paroxysmal, coincident with the sudden rise in blood pressure. In a study of 27 patients with documented pheochromocytoma, 74% had headache. These headaches correlated with excess catecholamine production (43).

Various medications may cause hypertension and headache, including the tyramine/monoamine oxidase inhibitor reaction, abrupt withdrawal from numerous antihypertensive drugs, and treatment with agents with sympathomimetic activity, such as pseudoephedrine and dextroamphetamine. Cocaine has been reported to cause migraine headache and may also cause headache with associated paroxysmal hypertension (44).

The syndrome of exertional headache (cough, exercise,

benign coital) is though to result from transient elevations in blood pressure. Some investigators believe that benign coital headache is a vascular headache or a headache due to low cerebrospinal fluid pressure, as in post–lumbar puncture headache (45).

CARDIOVASCULAR DISEASES

Ischemic coronary artery disease has been associated with headache. Classic angina pectoris is substernal chest heaviness, occasionally radiating to the neck, jaw, and arm. It is usually associated with exertion or stress. Occasionally, headache can also occur during anginal episodes (46). However, isolated patients have been reported with exertional headache as the only manifestation of coronary artery disease (47).

Severe aortic insufficiency may be associated with headache, presumably due to the increased volume of blood being forcibly ejected into the carotid arteries (48). Apparently, symptoms may persist even after corrective valvular surgery.

PULMONARY DISEASE

Sarcoidosis is a chronic granulomatous disease that classically involves multiple organ systems, predominantly lung, ocular, and skin. Neurological involvement occurs in 5% of cases and generally causes granulomatous meningitis. The most common neurological symptoms include cranial nerve palsies (1, 49). Cranial nerves 2, 5, 7, or 8 are most classically involved. CNS sarcoidosis usually results in spontaneous remission. If remission does not occur, corticosteroids may be useful (50).

Hypoxia and hypercarbia, regardless of the cause, are potent stimuli for headache. Hypoxemia causes cerebral vasodilation, as does elevated carbon dioxide concentration. The headache related to hypoxia and hypercarbia is generally nocturnal and in the early morning. Classic pulmonary diseases associated with headache include chronic obstructive pulmonary disease, chronic congestive heart failure, polycythemia (51), and obstructive sleep apnea (52). Some authors feel that headache is not a consistent or reliable finding in sleep apnea; however, high-altitude headache has been associated with hypoxia. The headaches are usually intense and throbbing, associated with facial flushing, photophobia, and a sensation of head fullness. The symptoms generally resolve when patients return to sea level (53).

RENAL DISEASE

Patients with end-stage renal disease requiring dialysis often complain of headache with characteristics of migraine. These headaches seem to occur near the termination of a dialysis period. Renal transplantation seems to improve or abolish the headaches. Some researchers suggest that these headaches are related to hypertension, decrease in blood pressure during dialysis, and to osmolality and electrolyte changes. Other postulated mechanisms include changes in circulating renin and aldosterone levels (32).

CHEMICAL AGENTS, TOXINS, AND HEADACHE

A myriad of substances can cause headache. Some of these are noted in other sections of this text. One of the most common syndromes is the "Chinese restaurant syndrome" or Kwok's disease. Symptoms include headache, tightness and numbness of the face and throat, paresthesias of mouth, nausea, flushing and sweating of the face, palpitations, and weakness. The causative agent is monosodium glutamate, a flavor enhancer widely used in oriental cooking. Other substances proven to provoke headache include licorice; nitrites; food, drug, and cosmetic dyes; alcohol; chocolate; various vitamins and minerals including nicotinic acid; caffeine; and various pesticides (54, 55).

Chronic carbon monoxide inhalation may also cause headache, generally via hypoxia. Poor ventilation and automobile exhaust or furnace fumes lead to carbon monoxide inhalation.

GASTROINTESTINAL DISEASE

Scattered anecdotal reports suggest headache as an associated symptom in inflammatory bowel disease, gallbladder disease, and constipation. One report even suggests an increased prevalence of headache in patients with the irritable bowel syndrome (56).

GYNECOLOGIC HEADACHE

Headache is a well-known complication of menstruation and the premenstrual syndrome. Menstrual migraine is quoted to be 10 to 70% of all migraine headaches, and up to 60% of all women have menstrual migraine (57). Some authors even suggest that the use of oral contraceptives in patients with menstrual migraine can worsen the headaches (57).

Headaches can be associated with menopause in a number of women. Migraineurs may note an exacerbation in migraine around the time of menopause. The headaches are felt to be related to vasomotor instability and may be improved by supplemental estrogens.

SUMMARY

No single list can include all the diseases that may present with headache. Since fever may be the most common medical cause of headache, any illness that manifests fever can present with headache. Because headache is such a common symptom, many headache sufferers will be found to have underlying medical diseases. Whether headache is associated with the underlying disease or merely a symptom of an additional benign headache disorder is not always clear.

In this chapter, we sought to review diseases that commonly include headache as either a presenting symptom or as a frequent manifestation. Hopefully, readers will be more cognizant of the medical disorders associated with headache and remain vigilant in conducting complete medical histories and physical examinations.

REFERENCES

1. Murali R. Neurosurgical consideration in headaches. Otol Clin North Am 1989;22(6):1229–1250.
2. Friedman WH, Rosenblum BN. Paranasal sinus etiology of headaches and facial pain. Otol Clin North Am 1989;22(6):1217–1228.
3. Lee K, Yanagisawa K. An obscure etiology for headache: sphenoid sinus disease. Yonsei Med J 1988;29(3):209–218.
4. Faermark W. Dental pain and histaminic cephalgia. J Am Soc Psychosom Dent Med 1972;19(2):57–61.
5. Moore GF, Massey JD, Emanuel JM, et al. Head pain secondary to nasal allergies. Ear Nose & Throat J 1987;66:41–53.
6. Tunkel AR, Wispelwey B, Scheld WM. Bacterial meningitis: recent advances in pathophysiology and treatment. Ann Intern Med 1990;112:610–613.
7. Hermans PE, Goldstein NP, Wellman WE. Mollaret's meningitis and differential diagnosis of recurrent meningitis. Am J Med 1972;52:129–140.
8. Whitley RJ. Viral encephalitis. N Engl J Med 1990;323(4):242–248.
9. Whitley RJ. Herpes simplex virus infections of the central nervous system; a review. Am J Med 1988;85(suppl 2):61–67.
10. Raskin NH. Lumbar puncture headache: a review. Headache 1990;(Mar):197–200.
11. Gabuzda DH, Hirsch MS. Neurologic manifestations of infection with human immunodeficiency virus. Ann Intern Med 1987;107:383–391.
12. Dalakas M, Wichman A, Sever J. AIDS and the nervous system. JAMA 1989;261(16):2396–2399.
13. Blaiss MS, Waxman J, Lange RK. Occipital headache as a manifestation of giant cell arteritis. South Med J 1982;75(7):887–888.
14. Anzola GP, Dalla Volta G, Balestrieri G. Headache in patients with systemic lupus erythematosus: clinical and telethermographic findings. Arch Neurol 1988;45:1061–1062.
15. Bovim G, Jorstad S, Schrader H. Subdural hematoma presenting as headache in systemic lupus erythematosus. Cephalgia 1990;10:25–29.
16. Peterson PK, Shepard J, Macres M, et al. A controlled trial of intravenous immunoglobulin G in chronic fatigue syndrome. Am J Med 1990;89:554–560.
17. Holmes GP, Kaplan JE, Gantz NM, et al. Chronic fatigue syndrome: a working case definition. Ann Intern Med 1988;108:387–389.
18. Verweij RD, Wijdicks EFM, van Gijn J. Warning headache in aneurysmal subarachnoid hemorrhage. Arch Neurol 1988;45:1019–1020.
19. Edmeads J. Headaches in cerebrovascular disease. Postgrad Med 1987;81(8):191–198.
20. Loeb C, Gandolfo C. Headache in ischemic cerebrovascular disease. Neurology 1987;37:1266.
21. Britton TC, Guiloff RJ. Carotid artery disease presenting as cough headache. Lancet 1988;(June):1406–1407.
22. Love PE, Santoro SA. Antiphospholipid antibodies: anticardiolipin and the lupus anticoagulant in systemic lupus erythematosus (SLE) and in non-SLE disorders. Ann Intern Med 1990;112:682–698.
23. Trimble M, Bell DA, Brien W, et al. The antiphospholipid antibody syndrome: prevalence among patients with stroke and transient ischemic attacks. Am J Med 1990;88:593–597.
24. Raskin N. Headaches associated with organic diseases of the nervous system. Med Clin North Am 1978;62(3):459–466.
25. Barlow CF. Headaches and brain tumors. Am J Dis Child 1982;136:99–100.
26. Edmeads J. Headaches and head pains associated with diseases of the cervical spine. Med Clin North Am 1978;62(3):533–544.
27. Iansek R. Cervical spondylosis and headaches. Clin Exp Neurol 1982;May:175–178.
28. Headache in multiple sclerosis. Br Med J 1969;(Jun)713–714.
29. Laplante P, Saint-Hilaire JM, Bouvier G. Headache as an epileptic manifestation. Neurology 1983;33:1493–1495.
30. Nightingale S, Williams B. Hindbrain hernia headache. Lancet 1987;(Mar):731–734.
31. Khurana RK. Post traumatic headache with ptosis, miosis and chronic forehead hyperhidrosis. Headache 1990;30:64–68.
32. Appenzeller O. Cerebrovascular aspects of headache. Med Clin North Am 1978;62(3):467–480.
33. Kudrow L. Systemic causes of headache. Postgrad Med 1974;56(3):105–111.
34. Service FJ, Dak AJ, Elveback LR, et al. Insulinoma: clinical and diagnostic features of 60 consecutive cases. Mayo Clin Proc 1976;51:417–429.
35. Blair DC, Fekety FR. Primary hyperparathyroidism presenting as fever of unknown origin with unremitting headache. Ann Intern Med 1979;91(4):575–576.
36. Musolino NR, Marins JR, Bronstein MD. Headache in acromegaly: dramatic improvement with the somatastatin analogue SNS 201-995. Clin J Pain 1990;6:243–245.
37. Strebel PM, Zacur HA, Gold EB. Headache, hyperprolactinemia, and prolactinoma. Obstet Gynecol 1986;68(2):195–199.
38. Browne JD, Kohut RI. Headache and the primary empty sella syndrome. Arch Otol Head Neck Surg 1986;112:883–885.
39. Leviton A, Camenga D. Migraine associated with hyper-pre-beta lipoproteinemia. Neurology 1969;19:963–966.
40. Hatfield WB. Headache associated with metabolic and systemic disorders. Med Clin North Am 1978;62(3):451–458.
41. Edmeads J. The worst headache ever: ominous causes. Postgrad Med 1987;86(1):93–104.
42. Calhoun DA, Oparil S. Treatment of hypertensive crisis. N Engl J Med 1990;323(17):1177–1183.
43. Lance JW, Hinterberger H. Symptoms of pheochromocytoma, with particular reference to headache, correlated with catecholamine production. Arch Neurol 1976;33:281–288.
44. Jaff MR. Recognition and treatment of cocaine abuse. Cleve Clin J Med 1990;57(7):595–596.
45. Porter M, Jankovic J. Benign coital cephalgia: differential diagnosis and treatment. Arch Neurol 1981;38:710–712.
46. Lefkowitz D, Biller J. Bregmatic headache as a manifestation of myocardial ischemia. Arch Neurol 1982;39:130.
47. Caskey WH, Spierings ELH. Headache and heartache. Headache 1978;18:240–243.
48. Harvey WP, Segal JP, Hufnagel CA. Unusual clinical features associated with severe aortic insufficiency. Ann Intern Med 1957;47:27–31.
49. LeWitt PA. Neurosarcoidosis and headache. South Med J 1984;77(2):272–273.
50. Reik L Jr. Disorders that mimic CNS infections. Neurol Clin 1986;4(1):223–248.
51. Hatfield WB. Headache associated with metabolic and systemic disorders. Med Clin North Am 1978;62(3):451–458.
52. Kaplan J, Staats BA. Obstructive sleep apnea syndrome. Mayo Clin Proc 1990;65:1087–1095.
53. Kassirer MR, Von Pelejosuch R. Persistent high-altitude headache and ageusia without anosmia. Arch Neurol 1989;46:340–341.
54. Seltzer S. Food, and food and drug combinations, responsible for head and neck pain. Cephalalgia 1982;2:111–124.
55. Friedman AP. Recurring headache: diagnosis and differential diagnosis. Prim Care 1974;1(2):275–292.
56. Watson WC, Sullivan SN, Corke M, et al. Globus and headache common symptoms of the irritable bowel syndrome. Can Med Assoc J 1978;118:387–388.
57. Digre K, Damasio H. Menstrual migraine, differential diagnosis, evaluation and treatment. Clin Obstet Gynecol 1987;30(2):417–430.

30

Cranial Neuralgias and Atypical Facial Pain

RONALD BRISMAN

The cranial neuralgias—trigeminal neuralgia is the most common type—respond extraordinarily well to carbamazepine and neurosurgical intervention and must be clearly distinguished from atypical facial pain, which may be helped with antidepressants but not carbamazepine or surgery. When only some of the features of trigeminal neuralgia are present, the condition may be called atypical trigeminal neuralgia, or trigeminal neuralgia with atypical features—a condition that often responds to the same medications and surgical procedures as pure trigeminal neuralgia.

TRIGEMINAL NEURALGIA

Clinical Features

Trigeminal neuralgia is characterized by paroxysmal, triggered, episodic pain in the trigeminal distribution. It is unilateral at any one time, is usually associated with normal neurological examination, and responds well to carbamazepine and denervation (1, 2).

The pain is *paroxysmal* and is characterized by sudden bursts of extremely intense pain lasting from a few seconds to a few minutes (3) or 20 to 30 seconds (4). The pain is like an "electric shock" and is followed by relative freedom from pain for a few seconds to a minute (4), to be followed again by another jab of severe pain. During bouts of pain, the patient may say that the pain is constant, but when encouraged to be immobile and silent, the patient will note that the pain temporarily subsides. Attacks of this recurring pain may occur for hours. Sometimes milder forms of the pain are present.

The pain is *triggered* by light touch about the face, especially in the perioral area. Talking, eating, brushing the teeth, washing the face, a light wind, and in severe cases, any movement of the body may precipitate the pain. The pain is followed by a refractory period of up to 2 to 3 minutes during which it is difficult to elicit pain (5).

The condition is *episodic*, and there may be weeks or months of remission interspersed with varying intervals of pain. In a study of 155 cases, 78 (50%) had one or more spontaneous remissions lasting 6 months or longer and 38 (24.5%) had similar remissions of 12 or more months (6).

Spontaneous remission may explain the apparently good responses from treatments that are probably ineffective. Such remissions lasted up to 4 years in 17 out of 39 patients after the extraction of apparently sound teeth (6).

According to Harris (7), trigeminal neuralgia becomes more chronic with time, and the intervals decrease between the episodes of pain, although some patients have periodic bouts of pain for several weeks or months every year. He describes one case where the pain disappeared with advancing age, but says that is a very rare occurrence (7).

At any one time, the pain of trigeminal neuralgia is *unilateral*. The right side is more likely to be affected (61% of the time, Table 30.1) than the left. Contralateral pain may develop sometime in the course of the illness (8) in 8.6% of patients who do not have multiple sclerosis (Table 30.1) and in 31% of 26 patients with multiple sclerosis. Bilateral simultaneous trigeminal neuralgia is rare but has occurred in 0.5% of 409 patients.

Trigeminal neuralgia is in the *distribution of the trigeminal nerve*, usually the second or third divisions, either alone or in combination. First-division pain occurred in 17.7% of patients and was frequently accompanied by second-division pain (Table 30.2).

In patients who have not had previous denervation, the *neurological examination is usually normal*. Definite hypoalgesia in the absence of previous surgical denervation should raise the suspicion of a structural lesion involving the trigeminal nerve, such as a brain tumor or multiple sclerosis. Under these circumstances, there often are other neurological abnormalities. Approximately 20% of patients with typical trigeminal neuralgia and normal computerized tomography may have abnormal areas of decreased sensation in the face, as detected by a careful sensory examination and the aesthesiometer (9).

Carbamazepine (Tegretol) is so effective in treating trigeminal neuralgia (10, 11), that the diagnosis should be doubted if there is no response to this medication (1).

Trigeminal neuralgia responds to *denervation*. Peripheral nerve blocks of the trigeminal nerve with local anesthetics such as Xylocaine or Marcaine characteristically relieve the pain, although the effect is temporary.

Table 30.1.
Characteristics of 383 Patients with Trigeminal Neuralgia: 1976–1990[a]

Female	63.4%
Right-sided pain	60.9%
Bilateral face pain, by history	8.6%
Average age at onset of symptoms	56.6 years

[a]None of these patients had multiple sclerosis or brain tumor.

Table 30.2.
Division of Pain in 383 Patients with Trigeminal Neuralgia: 1976–1990

Division	2 & 3	3	2	1 & 2	1–3	1	1 & 3
No. pts	136	101	82	46	10	7	1
Percentage	35.5	26.4	21.4	12.0	2.6	1.8	0.3

Incidence, Age, Sex

Approximately 11,750 new cases of trigeminal neuralgia develop each year in the United States. This is based on an overall age- and sex-adjusted incidence rate of 4.7 per 100,000 (12) and the 1990 census projection of 250,000,000 people. Older patients are more likely to be affected than younger ones, although the age at onset of the first symptom in patients without multiple sclerosis or brain tumor has varied from 12 to 89 years, with an average of 56.6 years (Fig. 30.1, Table 30.1).

Patients with multiple sclerosis are more likely to develop trigeminal neuralgia than others (13). Approximately 1% of patients with multiple sclerosis have trigeminal neuralgia (14). They develop trigeminal neuralgia at a younger age than those without multiple sclerosis, and in the 26 patients with multiple sclerosis in our series, the average age of onset of trigeminal neuralgia was 47 years.

Most patients (63.4%) with trigeminal neuralgia are female, but an important reason for this is that there are more females among older people. The age-adjusted sex ratio has been estimated at either 1.17 females to 1.00 males (13) or 1.74:1 (12).

Related Conditions

Twenty-six (6.4%) of 409 patients with trigeminal neuralgia also had *multiple sclerosis*. *Multiple sclerosis* should be suspected in younger patients whose symptoms of trigeminal neuralgia begin before the age of 45 and in those with bilateral trigeminal neuralgia (14, 15). Most of these patients will have evidence by history or physical examination of malfunction in other parts of the nervous system. Internuclear ophthalmoplegia or nystagmus was present in 12 of 16 patients with multiple sclerosis and trigeminal neuralgia (15).

Only a few patients with trigeminal neuralgia will have a *brain tumor*. This occurred in 9 (2%) of 418 patients in the present series, and in 1 to 5% in other series (16). Many of these patients will have other neurological abnormalities caused by the brain tumor (17). Hearing loss from an acoustic neurinoma is one of the more common cranial neuropathies in brain-tumor-associated trigeminal neuralgia (18). It is easy for this to go undetected because many patients, especially the elderly, may have hearing impairment due to causes other than a brain tumor (16).

Rarely, a patient with trigeminal neuralgia and no other signs or symptoms will have a brain tumor causing the trigeminal neuralgia. In those whose face pain symptoms are intractable enough to require a neurosurgical procedure, computerized tomography (with and without contrast) or magnetic resonance imaging (19) should be done to exclude the possibility of a brain tumor, even though most patients will not have one.

It has recently been suggested that patients with hypertension may be more likely to develop trigeminal neuralgia (12).

Medical Treatment

Carbamazepine (Tegretol) is an anticonvulsant that is also highly effective in relieving the pain of trigeminal neuralgia (10, 11). Almost all patients will respond to this medication. It is not unusual to find that patients who initially were helped by small nontoxic doses of carbamazepine later require higher doses that may no longer relieve the pain or may be associated with toxic side effects. Those few patients with trigeminal neuralgia that is otherwise typical, who report that carbamazepine never relieved their pain, usually took too low a dose, often because they had or feared unpleasant side effects.

Patients who are symptomatic from trigeminal neuralgia should be treated with carbamazepine. The medication is available in 200-mg tablets, 100-mg chewable tablets, and a suspension of 100 mg/5ml. Treatment is usually begun at a dose of 100 mg twice a day. The daily dose is increased by 100 or 200 mg until the patient gets relief. The usual maintenance dose is a total of 400 to 800 mg daily, which is given in divided doses from two to four times a day. Most patients can be managed with less than 1200 mg daily, but infrequently, it is necessary to give more. After the patient is free of pain for several weeks, attempts should be made to reduce the dose gradually to the minimum necessary for continued pain relief.

Patients are advised to take the carbamazepine right after a meal or with some milk to minimize the likelihood or severity of gastrointestinal disturbances such as nausea or vomiting.

Many unpleasant side effects may occur from carbamazepine. The most common are dizziness, drowsiness, unsteadiness, nausea, and vomiting, and they are most likely to develop when carbamazepine is initiated or the dose is too high. They usually subside when the dose is lowered. Central nervous system toxicity is more likely to develop in the elderly (a common group afflicted with trigeminal neuralgia) and in those with multiple sclerosis. Carbamazepine is contraindicated in those with a known sensitivity

Age at 1st symptom, Trigeminal Neuralgia

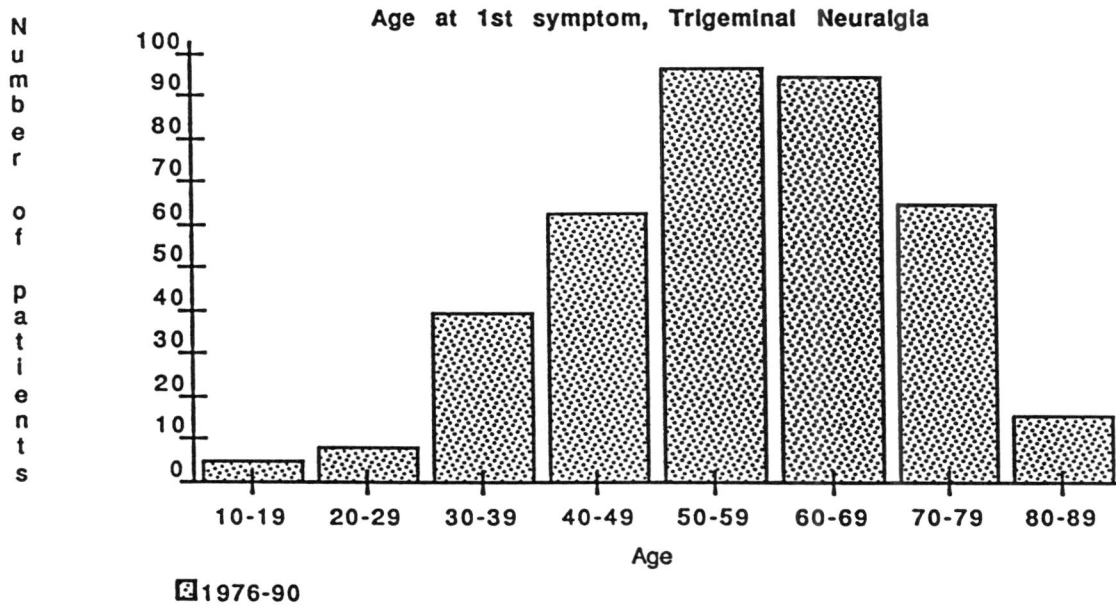

Figure 30.1. Trigeminal neuralgia without multiple sclerosis or brain tumor. MS, 26 patients, bilateral in 8 (30.77%); average age onset of symptoms 47.06 years; MS, 26 of 409 patients (6.36%); 9 (2.15%) of 418 had brain tumor.

to tricyclic compounds. Its use with monamine oxidase inhibitors is not recommended. The possibility exists that carbamazepine may activate a latent psychosis and confusion or agitation in the elderly.

Because of the possibility of dizziness and drowsiness occurring from the use of carbamazepine, patients should be cautioned about the hazards of operating machinery or automobiles or engaging in other potentially dangerous tasks.

Other toxic effects that may appear from the use of carbamazepine include rashes, bone marrow suppression, and liver or renal impairment. A complete blood and platelet count and liver and renal chemistries should be done before beginning treatment, after 2 weeks, and at approximately 8- to 12-week intervals, more frequently if there are abnormalities in the blood test results or clinical suspicion of bone marrow suppression. Complete blood counts every 2 weeks during the first 2 months of treatment have been recommended (20). Substantial changes require that the medication be stopped.

Aplastic anemia is a rare but sometimes fatal complication of carbamazepine therapy; 20 cases (13 fatal) were reported between 1964 and 1982 (20). Patients with abnormalities on the baseline blood and platelet counts and those taking other myelotoxic drugs should be considered at special risk for hematologic toxicity from carbamazepine therapy (20). In these patients, carbamazepine therapy should be monitored closely or avoided (20). Patients should be advised of signs and symptoms of early hematologic toxicity, such as fever, sore throat, ulcers in the mouth, pallor, easy bruising, and petechial or purpuric

hemorrhage, and should be advised to report to the physician immediately if any of the above develop.

Carbamazepine has mildly anticholinergic effects and may worsen eye problems associated with elevated intraocular pressure. Patients with glaucoma who are also being treated with carbamazepine for trigeminal neuralgia should have their extraocular pressure carefully monitored.

Elevated levels of carbamazepine, sometimes with toxicity, may occur when it is used with erythromycin, cimetidine, propoxyphene, isoniazid, or calcium channel blockers.

Blood levels for carbamazepine can be easily obtained. Usual adult therapeutic levels are between 4 and 12 μg/ml.

Baclofen (Lioresal) is a muscle relaxant and antispastic medication that may relieve the pain of trigeminal neuralgia in some patients (21). Baclofen may be effective alone or in combination with doses of carbamazepine or phenytoin that were ineffective when used without baclofen. The dose of baclofen is gradually titrated for each individual; an initial dose of 5 mg three times a day is given for 3 days, then increased every 3 days by a total daily dose of 15 mg until the optimal dose (usually 40 to 80 mg) is achieved. The most common adverse reactions are drowsiness, dizziness, and fatigue.

Although it is not effective in many patients, the anticonvulsant *phenytoin (Dilantin)* may be tried if treatment is not successful with carbamazepine or baclofen. The usual dose of phenytoin is 100 mg three or four times a day. In only 5 of 70 patients was a medical regimen including phenytoin successful without surgical treatment, although another 8 patients were taking it as an effective supplement to surgical denervation (3). Others have reported that phenytoin-induced pain relief was complete in 8 of 20 patients and partial in six (22).

Clonazepam (Klonopin) is a benzodiazepine anticonvulsant that was effective in 65% of cases with trigeminal neuralgia (23). The initial dose was 0.5 mg three times a day, and it was increased every 3 days by a total daily increment of 0.5 to 1 mg until pain was relieved. Somnolence developed in 80% and unsteadiness of gait in 88%; these were severe and incapacitating in nine of 25 patients.

Mephenesin carbamate and chlorphenesin carbamate (Maolate) are muscle relaxants that are now used infrequently but have relieved pain in some patients with trigeminal neuralgia (4, 24). Mephenesin carbamate provided sufficient comfort in 60% of 52 patients to make a surgical procedure unnecessary (24). One to 3 gm were given orally every 3 hours. Patients who were unable to take oral medication were treated with intravenous mephenesin; 4 gm were added to 5% glucose in water, and this was given by slow intravenous drip over a 12-hour period. Some unpleasant side effects were light-headedness and unsteady gait. The dose of chlorphenesin carbamate was from 800 to 2400 mg per day (4), and drowsiness sometimes developed.

The anticonvulsant *sodium valproate* (600 to 1200 mg per day) lessened the symptoms of trigeminal neuralgia in 13 (65%) of 20 patients (25). Four of the 13 responders also required other medications as well as the sodium valproate. One patient was unable to tolerate sodium valproate because of persistent nausea.

A recent report from the Institute of Experimental Medicine of the Central University of Venezuela School of Medicine indicates that *pimozide*—an antipsychotic drug that blocks dopaminergic receptors—may reduce symptoms of trigeminal neuralgia in patients who were refractory to other medical therapy (26). Oral doses of from 4 to 12 mg per day were used. All 48 patients responded to pimozide, and the total trigeminal neuralgia score was reduced by 78%. Adverse effects including physical and mental retardation, hand tremors, memory impairment, involuntary movements during sleep (jerkings), and slight Parkinson's disease manifestations were frequently observed during pimozide treatment and occurred in 40 (83.3%) patients. These symptoms diminished when patients received small doses of biperiden or when the dose of pimozide was reduced.

Although many medications have been used in the treatment of trigeminal neuralgia, medical treatment is primarily treatment with carbamazepine because it is so effective. For those who cannot be managed with carbamazepine, either because it is no longer effective or because of adverse side effects, and still want to try further medical treatment, it is reasonable to offer baclofen. Most of the other medicines are either ineffective or associated with so many adverse effects that patients who continue to have severe and incapacitating pain in spite of carbamazepine and/or baclofen are best managed with neurosurgical procedures, especially the percutaneous ones.

Surgical Treatment

When properly done, the *percutaneous, controlled, partial denervation of the gasserian ganglion and retrogasserian rootlets with radiofrequency (RFE)* (27) *and/or glycerol* (28, 29) is an extremely safe and effective procedure. Patients are discharged home from the hospital several hours after it is completed.

The procedure is done in the radiology suite, where submentovertex and lateral skull x-rays are taken to help localize the needle. The needle is insulated except for the distal several millimeters. It is inserted in the cheek and directed toward the foramen ovale. When x-rays indicate that the position is proper, the foramen ovale is penetrated. Final position is confirmed not only by x-ray localization but also by the response of the patient to low-voltage electrical stimulation. Controlled thermocoagulation of the trigeminal nerve is then performed.

During the procedure, hemodynamic changes such as hypertension, tachycardia, or bradycardia are often seen, especially when the foramen ovale is penetrated or the nerve is heated. Noninvasive monitoring of pulse, blood pressure, and electrocardiogram, and treatment of hypertension with small doses of hydralazine, and bradycardia with atropine, can minimize the hemodynamic changes. Respiratory insufficiency may occur from medications given during the procedure for analgesia and sedation. By using pulse oximetry to monitor oxygen saturation, encouraging the patient to breathe deeply, administering nasal oxygen, and supporting the oral airway, the surgeon can prevent hypoxia. All the above noninvasive monitoring techniques have been done on the last 97 of 588 consecutive percutaneous trigeminal procedures; in the entire group (588), there have been no hemodynamic or ventilatory complications (30).

It is desirable to make most of the denervation in the trigeminal division where light touch triggers pain. As the cannula is advanced deeper into the retrogasserian cistern, it often will pass from third to second, then first divisions. A more anteromedial placement through the foramen ovale will facilitate a second- or first-division lesion. Sometimes it is not possible to position the electrode in the exact division that is desired. The use of glycerol at this point is particularly helpful (29). Glycerol is a mildly denervating agent that is most effective when there is free flow of cerebrospinal fluid from the cannula, something that occurs approximately 60% of the time. Small volumes of glycerol, such as 0.25 ml, are rarely associated with profound denervation. When the RFE electrode is not in the exact trigeminal division that is sought, it is better to add a small dose of glycerol, especially if there is a free flow of CSF, rather than denervate profoundly an inappropriate division. This is especially the case when one is trying to make a second- or first-division lesion. The surgeon who is prepared to use RFE or glycerol, either alone or together, has additional flexibility that enhances the precision of the denervation.

The degree of denervation is an important factor that will influence recurrence and unpleasant sequelae of trigeminal denervation such as dysesthesias and keratitis. The more denervation that is achieved, the less likely is recurrence, but the chance of dysesthesias and keratitis developing is increased. Partial denervation is preferable to total or profound denervation. Although a partial lesion will increase the possibility of recurrence, recurrence is easily managed, either with medication such as carbamazepine or a repeat procedure. The RFE/glycerol procedure can be repeated without additional difficulty and with an excellent chance that it will relieve pain. In my experience with 444 patients treated between 1976 and 1990 with percutaneous RFE/glycerol procedures, I have found that 25.5% of the patients have required more than one procedure. Those who are younger at the time of the first procedure and those who are followed for a longer period are more likely to require another procedure. Of the first 158 patients (between 1976 and 1983), when a more denervating lesion was made, major dysesthesias occurred in 9% and keratitis in 2.5% (31). Between 1983 and 1990, a milder denervation has been accomplished; major dysesthesias occurred in only 2.8% of 287 patients, and none developed keratitis.

It is important to make the patient comfortable during the RFE/glycerol procedure. This will make patients more willing to undergo this procedure initially and subsequently if recurrence develops. It also provides better working conditions for the surgeon. Originally I used intravenous fentanyl, droperidol, and methohexital to give the patient sedation and analgesia during the procedure. This was the standard that had been described in the literature (27). More recently I have found that patient comfort during the procedure is significantly improved when I use premedication with oral diazepam and give high doses of midazolam (average of 5.5 mg) as well as fentanyl and methohexital (32).

Percutaneous microcompression (PM) of the trigeminal ganglion with a Fogarty balloon is a newer percutaneous method for denervating the trigeminal nerve and has been used to treat trigeminal neuralgia (33, 34). Although pain relief may be obtained from this procedure, there are probably more complications than are associated with a moderate RFE/glycerol procedure (35). When percutaneous microcompression is done, a larger needle is used and facial hematomas are more likely to occur than with RFE. The percutaneous microcompression is probably less selective than RFE, and trigeminal motor loss, though it usually eventually resolves, is much more frequently seen with PM. The use of general anesthesia with PM also increases the complexity of the procedure and potential morbidity.

Suboccipital craniectomy and microvascular decompression is a more major intracranial procedure for treatment of trigeminal neuralgia. It is based on the idea that blood vessels may compress the trigeminal nerve at its root entry zone and may therefore cause trigeminal neuralgia. Blood vessels are frequently seen near the trigeminal nerve and sometimes mechanically deform the nerve, but their etiologic relationship to trigeminal neuralgia has been disputed (36).

An intracranial operation to decompress the trigeminal nerve is done under general anesthesia (37). The patient is placed in the lateral position, and the head is secured with a three-pointed Mayfield headrest. A small retromastoid craniectomy is done and the operating microscope is used. If a blood vessel is found compressing the nerve—usually a tortuous superior cerebellar artery—the nerve may be decompressed by placing a small prosthesis of either Ivalon foam sponge (Unipoint Industries, High Point, NC) or Teflon felt between the nerve and blood vessel. Sometimes, when compression is not found, the caudal 30 to 50% of the sensory part of the trigeminal nerve is divided. If a vein is found to be compressing the nerve, the vein is cauterized and divided.

There is no doubt that this operation can often relieve the pain of trigeminal neuralgia. As in all operative procedures for trigeminal neuralgia, recurrence sometimes occurs. Unfortunately death may result from the operation in approximately 1% of cases, and another 2% may have a permanently disabling stroke or hemorrhage (35). A number of other complications also may occur, such as ipsilateral hearing loss in 4 to 19.5% of the patients, permanent facial palsy in 1 to 6%, and aseptic meningitis in as many as 30% when Teflon felt is used (35, 37).

Because of the much lower risks associated with the percutaneous RFE/glycerol procedure, it is preferable for initial treatment of patients with intractable pain that is not well managed with medication. Repeat RFE/glycerol can be done for recurrent pain. For those few patients who cannot be managed well with RFE/glycerol, the suboccipital microvascular operation is appropriate (38).

ATYPICAL TRIGEMINAL NEURALGIA

Some patients with paroxysmal, triggered pain in the trigeminal distribution have one or more features that are not typical of trigeminal neuralgia. Usually these patients have constant pain between the paroxysms, and the pain is not always triggered. Atypical trigeminal neuralgia sometimes occurs in patients with multiple sclerosis or brain tumor. Patients with atypical trigeminal neuralgia are often helped by carbamazepine. If this is not satisfactory, then neurosurgical procedures such as the percutaneous radiofrequency/glycerol denervation may help, although the results are not so reliable as for those patients with pure trigeminal neuralgia (2).

VAGOGLOSSOPHARYNGEAL NEURALGIA

Vagoglossopharyngeal neuralgia is a paroxysmal, triggered pain in the distribution of the ninth and tenth nerves

(2, 39). The pain is located in the ear, tonsil, larynx, and/or posterior aspect of the tongue, with occasional spread to other parts of the face (39).

Vagoglossopharyngeal neuralgia is often triggered by swallowing (especially cold drinks), chewing, coughing, talking, or eating certain highly spiced, sweetened, or acidic foods (39); but the pain of vagoglossopharyngeal neuralgia is triggered less often than is the pain of trigeminal neuralgia. Although patients with vagoglossopharyngeal neuralgia may have paroxysmal pain, they often have a more constant, dull aching, burning, or pressure sensation (39). Infrequently, vagoglossopharyngeal neuralgia may be associated with syncope (39, 40).

The incidence of vagoglossopharyngeal neuralgia is approximately 0.04% per 100,000 people per year; that is one hundredth as often as trigeminal neuralgia. The average age of onset of vagoglossopharyngeal neuralgia is a little less than trigeminal neuralgia, although the age of onset has been anywhere from the 20s to the 80s (39). The left side of the face is affected with vagoglossopharyngeal neuralgia in 83% of cases (39), and that is much more frequent than in trigeminal neuralgia, where the left side is affected in 42% of patients (41). Multiple sclerosis is extremely rare with vagoglossopharyngeal neuralgia and occurred in fewer than 0.3% of cases. Brain tumor is much more common with vagoglossopharyngeal neuralgia and was present in from 15 to 25% of patients (42). Approximately 25% of patients with vagoglossopharyngeal neuralgia will also have trigeminal neuralgia (39).

Vagoglossopharyngeal neuralgia often responds to carbamazepine. Surgery is reserved for patients with intractable pain that does not respond to carbamazepine. Section of the ninth and upper 15 to 20% of the rootlets of the tenth cranial nerve provides excellent relief of pain with minimal morbidity (41–43). Elderly patients or those who have severe medical illness that precludes suboccipital craniectomy should have percutaneous radiofrequency electrocoagulation of the ninth and tenth cranial nerves. Complications such as bradycardia with hypotension, and impaired phonation and deglution can result from excessive vagal denervation (44, 45). These can be minimized by proper x-ray localization in the anteromedial part of the jugular foramen, continuous monitoring of electrocardiogram and blood pressure (46), and small incremental lesions (47).

GENICULATE NEURALGIA

Otalgic geniculate neuralgia is a rare condition that is caused by impairment of the sensory part of the seventh cranial nerve. Patients with geniculate neuralgia have pain primarily in the ear, although it may radiate toward other parts of the face. It may be constant or intermittent and is sometimes associated with herpes zoster infection (41, 48). It is sometimes triggered by light touch in or near the ear.

Diagnosis and treatment of neuralgic ear pain is difficult because of the multiple sensory innervations of the ear, which may be supplied by the upper cervical, fifth, seventh, ninth, and tenth cranial nerves. Local anesthetics applied to the back of the throat may temporarily relieve the pain of glossopharyngeal (ninth nerve), but not geniculate neuralgia (39).

Intractable pain from geniculate neuralgia that does not respond to carbamazepine may be relieved by cutting the sensory part of the seventh nerve. This may be accomplished by cutting the nervus intermedius (49, 50), but sometimes the vestibular nerve (51), geniculate ganglion, and anterior 20% of the diameter of the motor portion of the facial nerve (52) may have to be excised.

Prosopalgic geniculate neuralgia is a very different condition from the otalgic form. In prosopalgic geniculate neuralgia, the pain is in the deeper structures of the face, including the posterior orbit and posterior nasal, malar, and palatal areas (48). This condition is probably a cluster headache. It has also been named nervus intermedius neuralgia (51), and surgical section of the nervus intermedius has been done (51, 53). The surgical results have been unpredictable, and neurosurgical denervation for this condition is not recommended (41).

ATYPICAL FACIAL PAIN

Atypical facial pain is not paroxysmal or triggered. It is not in the distribution of any cranial nerve. It is often continuous and sometimes bilateral. Many symptoms of depression and anxiety are seen in these patients (54–56). Atypical facial pain does not respond to carbamazepine but may be helped by tricyclic or other kinds of antidepressants. Surgery is contraindicated because it does not help and often makes the patient worse (1).

REFERENCES

1. Brisman R. Trigeminal neuralgia and other facial pains: diagnosis, natural history, and nonsurgical treatment. In: Brisman R, ed. Neurosurgical and medical management of pain: trigeminal neuralgia, chronic pain, and cancer pain. Boston: Kluwer, 1989:25–33.
2. Brisman R. Medical treatment of orafacial pain. In: Tollison CD, ed. Handbook of chronic pain management. Baltimore: Williams & Wilkins, 1987.
3. White JC, Sweet WH. "Trigeminal neuralgia, tic douloureux" pain and the neurosurgeon. Springfield, IL: Charles C Thomas, 1969: 123–178.
4. Dalessio DJ. The major neuralgias, postinfectious neuritis, intractable pain, and atypical facial pain. In: Dalessio DJ, ed. Wolff's headache and other head pain. 4th ed. New York: Oxford University Press, 1980:233–255.
5. Kugelberg E, Lindblom U. The mechanism of pain in trigeminal neuralgia. J Neurol Neurosurg Psychiatry 1959;22:36.
6. Rushton JG, MacDonald HNA. Trigeminal neuralgia: special considerations of nonsurgical treatment. JAMA 1957;165:437.
7. Harris W. Neuritis and neuralgia. London: Oxford University Press, 1926:418.
8. Brisman R. Bilateral trigeminal neuralgia. J Neurosurg 1987;67:44–48.
9. Terrence CF. Differential diagnosis of trigeminal neuralgia. In: Fromm GH, ed. The medical and surgical management of trigeminal neuralgia. New York: Futura Publishing, 1987:43–60.
10. Blom S. Trigeminal neuralgia: its treatment with a new anticonvulsant drug (G-32883). Lancet 1962;1:839–840.

11. Rockliff BW, Davies EH. Controlled sequential trials of carbamazepine in trigeminal neuralgia. Arch Neurol 1966;15:129–136.

12. Katusic S, Beard CM, Bergstralh E, Kurland LT. Incidence and clinical features of trigeminal neuralgia, Rochester, Minnesota, 1945–1984. Ann Neurol 1990;27:89–95.

13. Rothman KJ, Monson RR. Epidemiology of trigeminal neuralgia. J Chron Dis 1973;26:3–12.

14. Rushton JG, Olafson RA. Trigeminal neuralgia associated with multiple sclerosis: report of 35 cases. Arch Neurol 1965;13:383–386.

15. Brisman R. Trigeminal neuralgia and multiple sclerosis. Arch Neurol 1987;44:379–381.

16. Brisman R. Trigeminal neuralgia and brain tumors. In: Brisman R, ed. Neurosurgical and medical management of pain: trigeminal neuralgia, chronic pain, and cancer pain. Boston: Kluwer, 1989:65–70.

17. Bullitt E, Tew JM, Boyd J. Intracranial tumors in patients with facial pain. J Neurosurg 1986;64:865–871.

18. Revilla AG. Tic douloureux and its relationship to tumors of the posterior fossa. Analysis of twenty-four cases. J Neurosurg 1947;4:233–239.

19. Tanaka A, Takaki T, Maruta Y. Neurinoma of the trigeminal root presenting as atypical trigeminal neuralgia: diagnostic values of orbicularis oculi reflex and magnetic resonance imaging. A case report. Neurosurgery 1987;21:733–736.

20. Hart RG, Easton JD. Carbamazepine and hematological monitoring. Ann Neurol 1982;11:309–312.

21. Fromm GH, Terrence CF, Chattha AS. Baclofen in the treatment of trigeminal neuralgia: double-blind study and long-term follow-up. Ann Neurol 1984;15:240–244.

22. Braham J, Saiz A. Phenytoin in the treatment of trigeminal and other neuralgias. Lancet 1960;2:892–893.

23. Court JE, Kase CS. Treatment of tic douloureux with a new anticonvulsant (clonazepam). J Neurol Neurosurg Psychiatry 1976;39:297.

24. King RB. The value of mephenesin carbamate in the control of pain in patients with tic douloureux. J Neurosurg 1966;25:153–158.

25. Peiris JB, Perera GLS, Devendra SV, Lionel NDW. Sodium valproate in trigeminal neuralgia. Med J Aust 1980;2:278.

26. Lechin F, van der Difs B, Lechin ME, Amat J, Lechin AE, et al. Pimozide therapy for trigeminal neuralgia. Arch Neurol 1989;46:960–963.

27. Sweet WH, Wepsic JG. Controlled thermocoagulation of trigeminal ganglion and rootlets for differential destruction of pain fibers: Part 1 trigeminal neuralgia. J Neurosurg 1974;39:143–156.

28. Hakanson S. Trigeminal neuralgia treated by the injection of glycerol into the trigeminal cistern. Neurosurgery 1981;9:638–646.

29. Brisman R. Retrogasserian glycerol injection with or without radiofrequency electrocoagulation for trigeminal neuralgia. In Brisman R, ed. Neurosurgical and medical management of pain: trigeminal neuralgia, chronic pain, and cancer pain. Boston: Kluwer, 1989:51–56.

30. Brisman R. Hemodynamic and respiratory monitoring during percutaneous radiofrequency electrocoagulation for trigeminal neuralgia. 59th Annual Meeting of American Association of Neurological Surgeons. New Orleans, 1991:550.

31. Brisman R. Treatment of trigeminal neuralgia by radiofrequency electrocoagulation. In: Brisman R, ed. Neurosurgical and medical management of pain: trigeminal neuralgia, chronic pain, and cancer pain. Boston: Kluwer, 1989:41–49.

32. Brisman R. Analgesia and sedation during percutaneous radiofrequency electrocoagulation for trigeminal neuralgia. Neurosurgery 1993;Mar:

33. Mullan S, Lichtor T. Percutaneous microcompression of the trigeminal ganglion for trigeminal neuralgia. J Neurosurg 1983;59:1007–1012.

34. Brown JA, Preul MC. Percutaneous trigeminal ganglion compression for trigeminal neuralgia. J Neurosurg 1989;70:900–904.

35. Brisman R. Cranial pain surgery. In: Post KD, Friedman E, McCormick P, eds. Postoperative complications in intracranial neurosurgery. New York: Thieme, 1993:181–206.

36. Adams CBT. Microvascular compression: an alternative view and hypothesis. J Neurosurg 1989;57:1–12.

37. Jannetta PJ. Trigeminal neuralgia: treatment by microvascular decompression. In: Wilkins RH, Rengachary SS, eds. Neurosurgery. New York: McGraw-Hill, 1985:2357–2362.

38. Brisman R. Suboccipital craniectomy and treatment of trigeminal neuralgia. In: Brisman R, ed. Neurosurgical and medical management of pain: trigeminal neuralgia, chronic pain, and cancer pain. Boston: Kluwer, 1989:57–63.

39. Rushton J, Stevens JC, Miller RH. Glossopharyngeal. (Vagoglossopharyngeal) neuralgia. A study of 217 cases. Arch Neurol 1981;38:201–205.

40. Bohm E, Strang RR. Glossopharyngeal neuralgia. Brain 1962;85:371–388.

41. Brisman R. Neuralgia of the seventh, ninth, and tenth nerves. In Brisman R, ed. Neurosurgical and medical management of pain: trigeminal neuralgia, chronic pain, and cancer pain. Boston: Kluwer, 1989:83–90.

42. Dandy WE. Glossopharyngeal neuralgia (tic douloureux). Its diagnosis and treatment. Arch Surg 1927;15:198–214.

43. Robson JT, Bonica J. The vagus nerve in surgical consideration of glossopharyngeal neuralgia. J Neurosurg 1950;7:482–484.

44. Tew JM, Tobler WD. Percutaneous rhizotomy in the treatment of intractable facial pain (trigeminal, glossopharyngeal, and vagal nerves). In: Schmidek HH, Sweet WH, eds. Operative neurosurgical techniques, vol 2. New York: Grune & Stratton, 1982:1083–1106.

45. Ori C, Salar G, Giron G. Percutaneous glossopharyngeal thermocoagulation complicated by syncope and seizures. Neurosurgery 1983;13:427–429.

46. Isamat F, Ferran E, Acebes JJ. Selective percutaneous thermocoagulation rhizotomy in essential glossopharyngeal neuralgia. J Neurosurg 1981;23:575–580.

47. Arias MJ. Percutaneous radio-frequency thermocoagulation with low temperature in the treatment of essential glossopharyngeal neuralgia. Surg Neurol 1986;25:94–96.

48. Hunt JR. Geniculate neuralgia (neuralgia of the nervus facialis); a further contribution to the sensory system of the facial nerve and its neuralgic conditions. AMA Arch Neuro Psychiatry 1937;37:253–285.

49. Furlow LT. Tic douloureux of the nervus intermedius (so-called idiopathic geniculate neuralgia). JAMA 1942;119:255–259.

50. Wilson AA. Geniculate neuralgia; report of a case relieved by intracranial section of the nerve of Wrisberg. J Neurosurg 1950;7:473–481.

51. Sachs E Jr. The role of the nervus intermedius in facial neuralgia. Report of four cases with observations on the pathways for taste, lacrimation, and pain in the face. J Neurosurg 1968;28:54–60.

52. Pulec JL. Geniculate neuralgia: diagnosis and surgical management. Laryngoscope 1976;86:955–964.

53. Solomon S, Apfelbaum RI. Surgical decompression of the facial nerve in the treatment of chronic cluster headache. Arch Neurol 1986;43:479–481.

54. Weddington WW, Blazer D. Atypical facial pain and trigeminal neuralgia: a comparison study. Psychosomatics 1979;20:348.

55. Lesse SE. Atypical facial pain syndrome. Arch Neurol 1960;3:122–123.

56. Engle GL. "Psychogenic" pain and the pain prone patient. Am J Med 1958;26:899–918.

31

Headache Associated with Sinus Disease

HOWARD L. LEVINE

Sinusitis has become the most common chronic disorder in the United States, surpassing diseases like arthritis. There are over 30 million Americans, approximately one out of eight individuals, who suffer from chronic sinusitis (1). It is a rare individual who has neither suffered from nor known someone with sinusitis. In 1989, there were nearly 16 million visits to physicians for sinusitis (2). Nearly all of these sinus sufferers have facial and head pain.

Recently, great progress has been made in the diagnosis and management of sinusitis through the use of nasal endoscopy for office diagnosis (3, 4), computed tomographic (CT) imaging of the sinuses (5), and more efficient medical and surgical management (6–10). Each of these has contributed to better understanding of the pathophysiology of sinusitis.

ANATOMY OF THE LATERAL NASAL WALL

Diagnosis and management of sinusitis has become dependent upon an understanding of the anatomy of the lateral nasal wall and mucociliary clearance from the sinuses.

Upon the lateral nasal wall are three turbinates (occasionally a fourth is present), which are bone covered with mucosa (Fig. 31.1). The turbinates change in size cyclically over several hours, creating periods of nasal congestion and nasal patency. Turbinate congestion is also gravity-dependent and alternates between the two sides of the nose. Inferior to each of the turbinates is a meatus with the same name as the turbinate superior to it. In the middle meatus, between the middle and inferior turbinate lies a slit-like opening, the hiatus semilunaris. The hiatus semilunaris is the opening into the infundibulum, the funnel-like space posterior and inferior to it (Fig. 31.2). It is into this narrow infundibular space that the maxillary and anterior ethmoid, and occasionally frontal sinuses drain. The medial wall of the infundibulum is the thin "boomerang-shaped" bony uncinate process. At the posterior end of the infundibulum and hiatus semilunaris is the bulla ethmoidalis, which is the largest of the anterior ethmoid air cells. This entire region is frequently referred to as the ostiomeatal complex (OMC). Many slight anatomical and

pathological abnormalities in the OMC may cause recurrent sinusitis.

The superior meatus is the space into which the posterior ethmoid air cells drain. Abnormalities in this region may cause posterior ethmoid sinusitis.

The sphenoid sinus drains into the sphenoid-ethmoid recess, which is the narrow space between the sphenoid ostium and the posterior aspect of the superior turbinate. Like the other sinuses, anatomical and pathological abnormalities in the region may cause recurrent sinusitis.

CLASSIFICATION OF SINUSITIS

Many patients come to the physician believing that their headache and facial pain is sinus in origin, when in fact it has some other etiology. For this reason, accurate history and diagnostic evaluation is crucial in making the correct diagnosis. Many of these individuals will have taken over-the-counter sinus medications, felt better, and therefore assumed incorrectly that their headache was truly sinus in origin. Most of these individuals will feel symptomatically better from the sedative effect of the antihistamine or the pain relief from the analgesic contained in combination "sinus-cold" remedies.

A biochemical theory for the origin of sinus pain has been proposed (Fig. 31.3) (11). Chemical, infectious, or thermal irritants may cause the release of substance P, which causes an orthodromic impulse and referred pain. Mechanical pressure within the nasal and sinus cavities may occur from mucosal contact and anatomical abnormalities that also cause the release of substance P. This may produce an antidromic impulse at the level of the nasal mucosa and subsequent vasodilatation and hypersecretion. This in turn produces more mechanical pressure and release of substance P. A vicious cycle is initiated.

Acute Purulent

Acute purulent sinusitis often is part of or follows an acute upper respiratory tract infection. For this reason, it is frequently viral in origin, but it may become secondarily infected by bacteria. Most patients with acute purulent sinusitis present with pain over the infected sinus. The

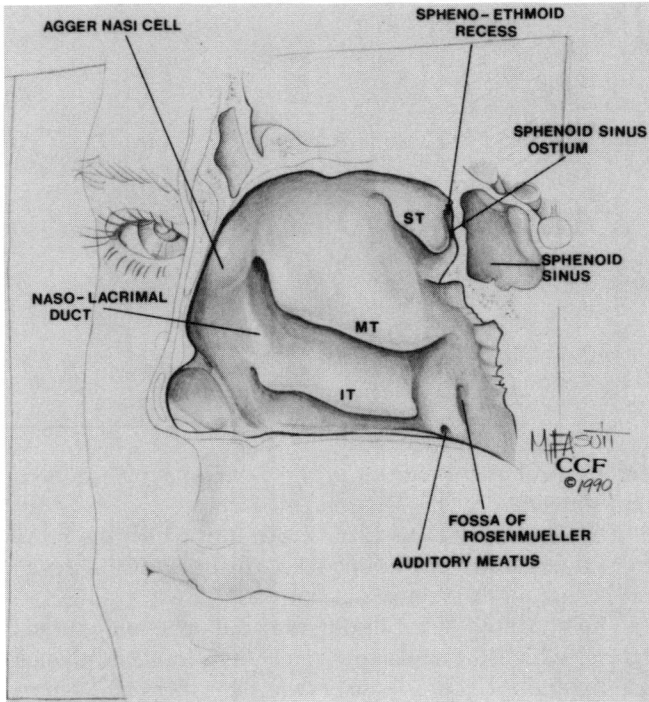

Figure 31.1. Oblique view of the right side of the lateral nasal wall with the turbinates and their respective meati.

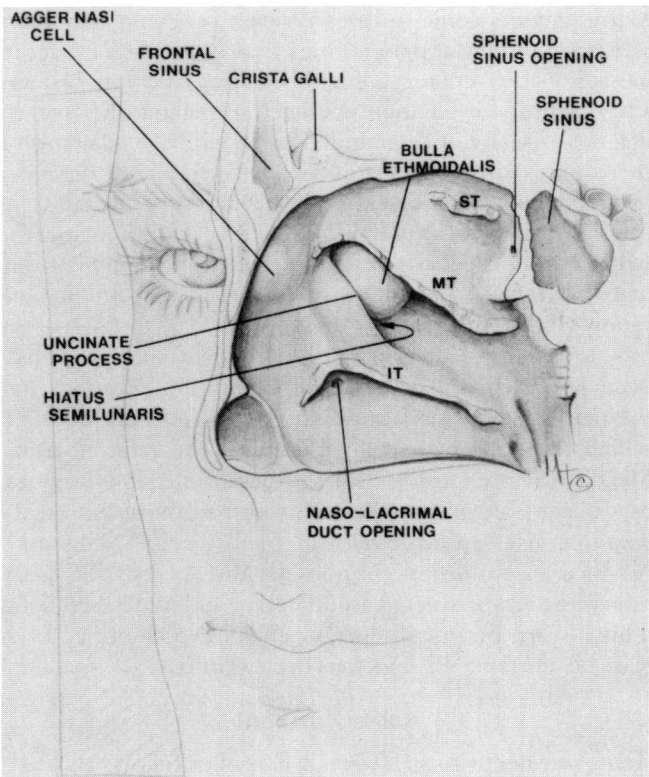

Figure 31.2. Oblique view of the lateral nasal wall with a portion of the middle turbinate removed exposing the *hiatus semilunaris, uncinate process,* and *ethmoid bulla.*

BIOCHEMICAL CAUSE OF SINUS PAIN

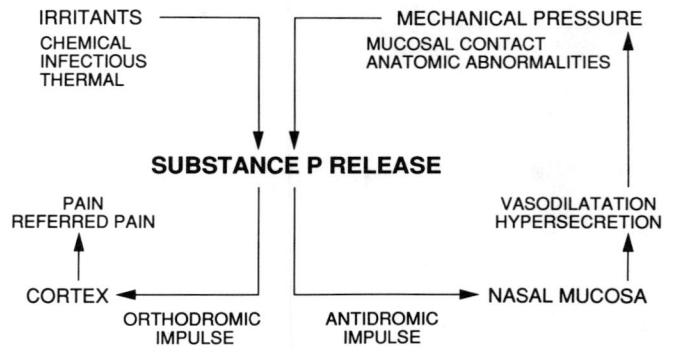

Figure 31.3. A proposed theory of the creation of a vicious cycle through mechanical and chemical irritants causing the release of substance P and pain.

pain is usually sharp, but it may be a throbbing dull ache. It may radiate some distance from the infected sinus. The pain of frontal sinusitis is most often felt immediately over that sinus. Maxillary sinusitis is sensed not only over the maxillary sinus but also into the upper teeth, mimicking a dental infection. Ethmoid sinusitis is manifest by pain in the lacrimal fossa, medial canthal, and temporal regions. Sphenoid sinusitis produces pain that is deep-seated, retro-orbital, vertex, and/or occipital. Sinus pain is often worse when moving the head or when bending over. Because the sinus is usually filled with infected fluid during acute sinusitis, there may be the sensation of fluid movement when bending over. Percussing the involved sinus will elicit the pain. Often, there is an accompanying fever. Patients experience purulent nasal or postnasal secretions, especially upon awakening. Imaging studies demonstrate either an opacified sinus (Fig. 31.4) or an air-fluid level within the sinus (Fig. 31.5). A simple, screening CT scan has recently been used to view each of the sinuses. It gives far more detailed information about each of the sinuses than the traditional plain sinus roentgenograms (Fig. 31.6). The radiation exposure to the patient is less than that with plain sinus roentgenographs.

Examination of the nose reveals an erythematous, inflamed mucosa (Fig. 31.7). If the natural outflow pathway from the sinus is completely obstructed, there are no purulent secretions seen. Most often, however, there is pus seen within the nasal cavity and especially within the region of the middle turbinate and middle meatus. Posterior rhinoscopic examination usually demonstrates pus running over the posterior end of the inferior turbinate into the nasopharynx.

The most common pathogens in acute purulent sinusitis are *Streptococcus pneumoniae, Haemophilus influenzae,* and *Moraxella catarrhalis* (12, 13). There is little correlation between nasal cultures and sinus pathogenic organisms. Therefore, unless gross purulent secretions are seen coming from the region of sinus outflow (i.e., OMC), treat-

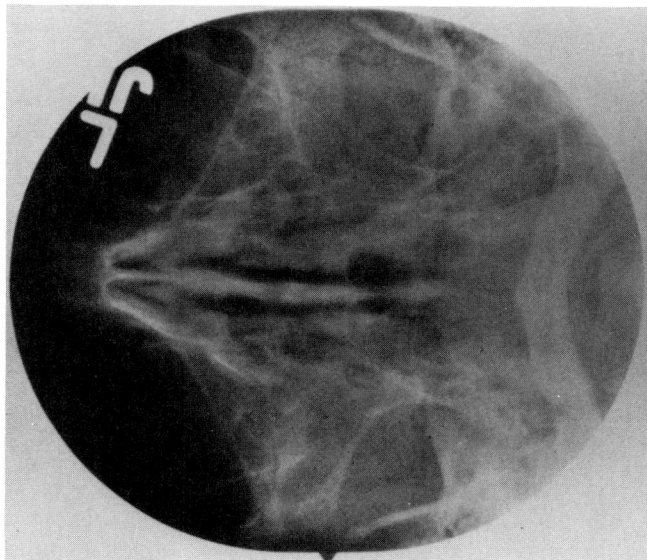

Figure 31.4. Plain sinus roentgenography demonstrating an opacified maxillary sinus.

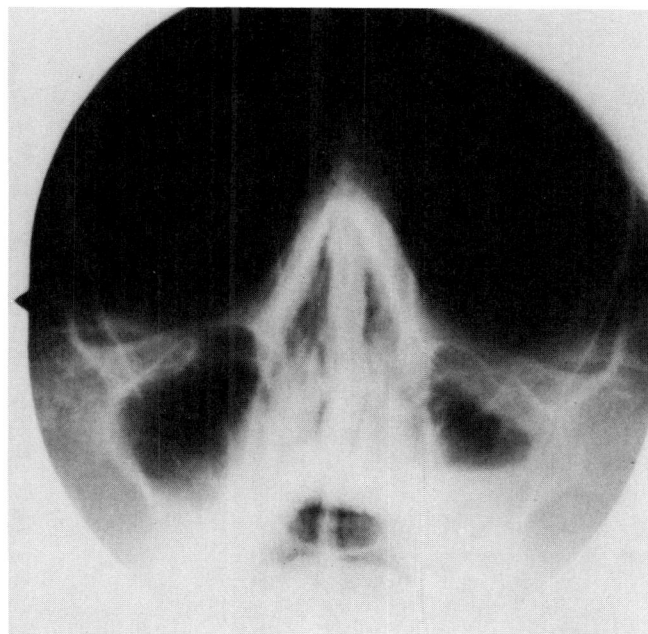

Figure 31.5. Plain sinus roentgenography demonstrating an air-fluid level during acute sinusitis.

ment is empiric. An antibiotic that is appropriate to the most common offending organisms is chosen. Topical and systemic decongestants are used to reduce nasal congestion and improve sinus drainage. Mucolytics help by thinning secretions and promoting drainage. Treatment with antibiotics is maintained for 2 weeks. Systemic decongestants and mucolytics are continued for an additional week after the completion of the antibiotics. Topical decongestants are used for a maximum of 5 days, to avoid rebound nasal congestion when the decongestant ceases to be active. Antihistamines should be avoided, since they cause drying and thickening of secretions.

Irrigation of the infected sinus has been commonly used in the past in attempts to decrease the bacterial load and remove purulent secretions. Many otolaryngologists today do not irrigate the sinuses, but medically decompress them with topical and systemic decongestants.

Acute Barosinusitis

Acute barosinusitis occurs with changes in weather (i.e., barometric pressure) or altitude. It very well may be one of the most common causes of "sinus headaches". The sinus ostium becomes obstructed, air is absorbed from within the sinus, and a vacuum is formed. The pain that is produced is initially severe and sharp but most often becomes a dull aching pressure several minutes or hours later. There is no fever, purulent drainage, or nasal congestion unless the sinus remains obstructed and becomes secondarily infected. Barosinusitis is treated symptomatically with systemic or topical decongestants. If mucosal edema is present, a topical corticosteroid spray (e.g., beclomethasone) is used.

While nasal endoscopy and sinus imaging may be abnor-

mal, several anatomical abnormalities may predispose to recurrent barosinusitis. Each should be looked for and treated, especially when medical management has failed.

A concha bullosa of the middle turbinate is an ethmoid air cell within the turbinate (Figs. 31.8, 31.9). While often not pathological, it may narrow the middle meatus, especially with minor mucosal swelling of the turbinate or OMC mucosa. This in turn causes obstruction of the OMC. The lateral wall of the concha bullosa can easily be removed surgically, leaving the mucosally lined medial portion to form a new middle turbinate and open the OMC.

The middle turbinate is normally curved, with its concavity lateral toward the OMC. Sometimes the turbinate has a paradoxical bend with the convexity lateral toward the OMC, obstructing the middle meatal outflow (Fig. 31.10). If the paradoxical middle turbinate is causing barosinusitis, the anterior inferior portion of the middle turbinate can be resected or a submucous resection of the middle turbinate can be performed. This opens the OMC and relieves the symptoms.

The uncinate process can be elongated (Fig. 31.11), shortened and widened (Fig. 31.12), or have an air cell (bullosa of the uncinate) within it. The uncinate may be rotated medially up against an enlarged bulla ethmoidalis. With minor amounts of nasal congestion and mucosal edema, these different configurations of the uncinate can obstruct the infundibulum and cause barosinusitis. This can be corrected surgically by removing the uncinate process, thereby opening the infundibulum.

Figure 31.6. Screening axial computed tomographic scan demonstrating acute sinusitis
with an air-fluid level.

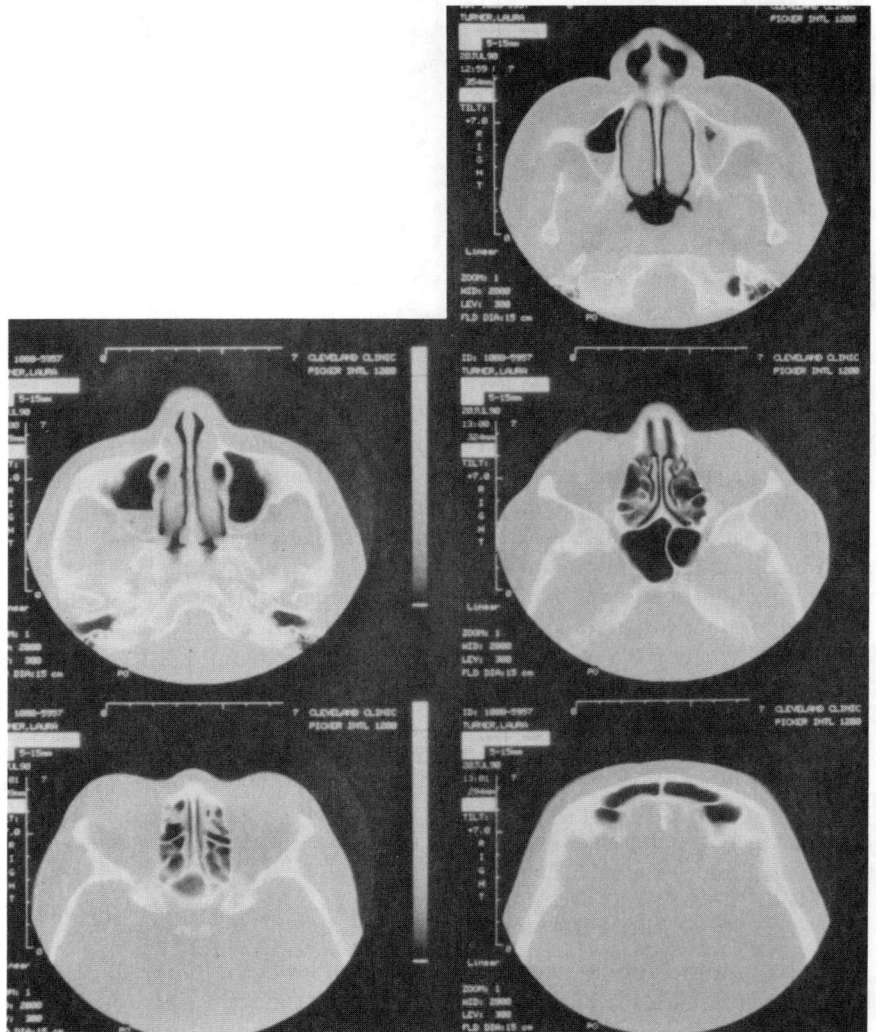

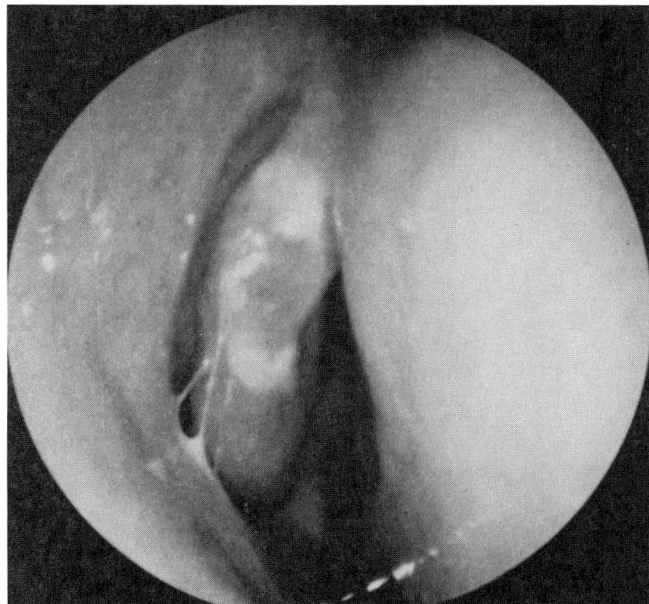

Figure 31.7. Marked erythema, engorgement, and purulent secretions in the middle meatus with acute sinusitis.

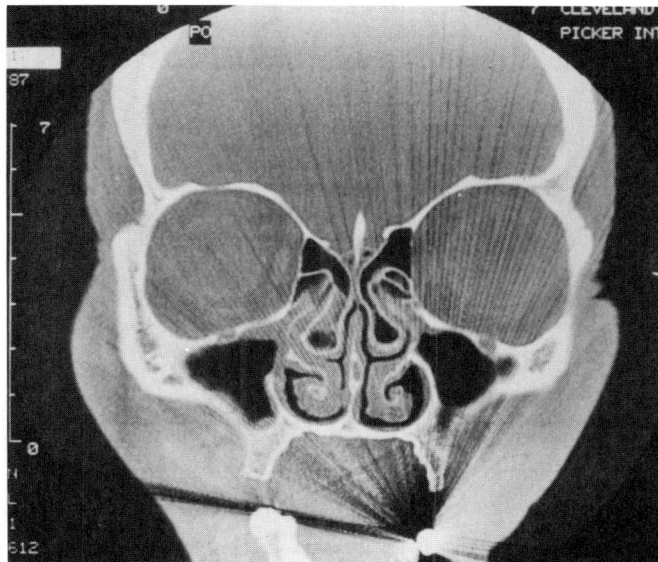

Figure 31.9. Concha bullosa obstructing the infundibulum.

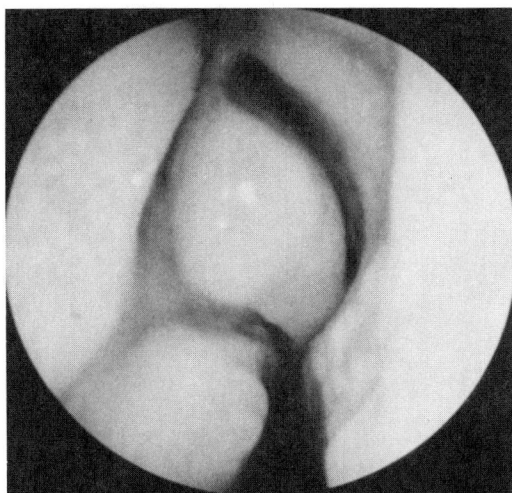

Figure 31.8. Enlarged and rounded head of the middle turbinate seen with an air cell within the turbinate known as a concha bullosa.

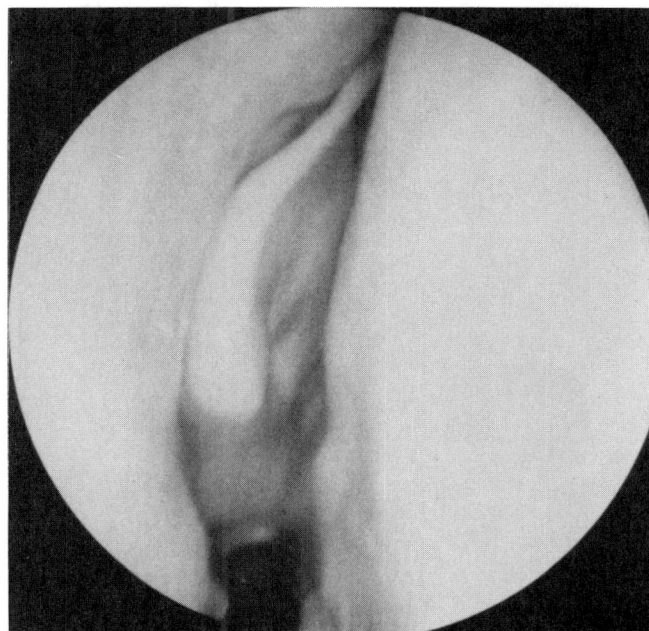

Figure 31.10. A paradoxically bent middle turbinate with the concavity medial, producing obstruction of the ostiomeatal complex and sinusitis.

Acute Recurrent Sinusitis

Patients with acute recurrent sinusitis will have all the symptoms of acute sinusitis. Even though they are treated appropriately with antibiotics and decongestants, within a few weeks after completing treatment, the symptoms recur. Most often the physician prescribes another course of treatment with the same or another antibiotic appropriate to the suspected organisms. The same events take place. Many of these patients describe getting a common upper respiratory tract infection, often at the same time as someone else in their home. The other individual is over the

infection in a matter of days, while the patient has it linger for weeks. During that time there is persistent drainage, nasal obstruction and congestion, facial pain, and pressure.

Most of these patients, when examined endoscopically in the ambulatory clinic and imaged with coronal CT scan will have some anatomical or pathological source for their recurrent disease (Figs. 31.13–31.15). Any of the anatomical abnormalities that cause acute barosinusitis may cause acute

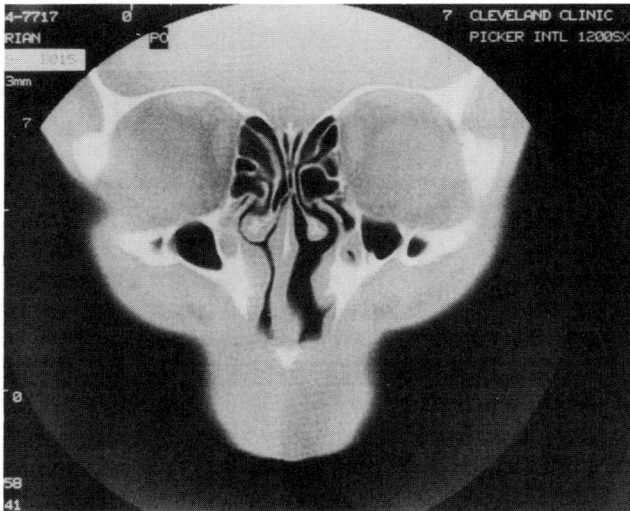

Figure 31.11. An elongated uncinate process impacting into the ethmoid bulla and producing sinusitis.

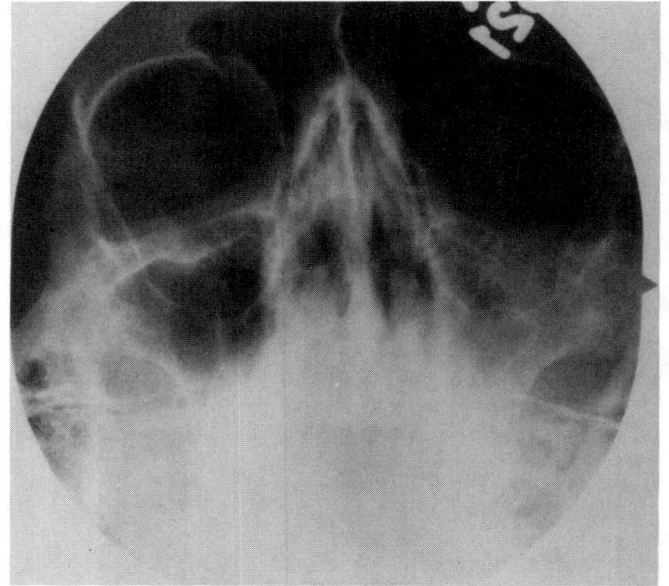

Figure 31.13. Plain sinus roentgenograph in a patient with recurrent acute sinusitis, demonstrating an opacified maxillary sinus.

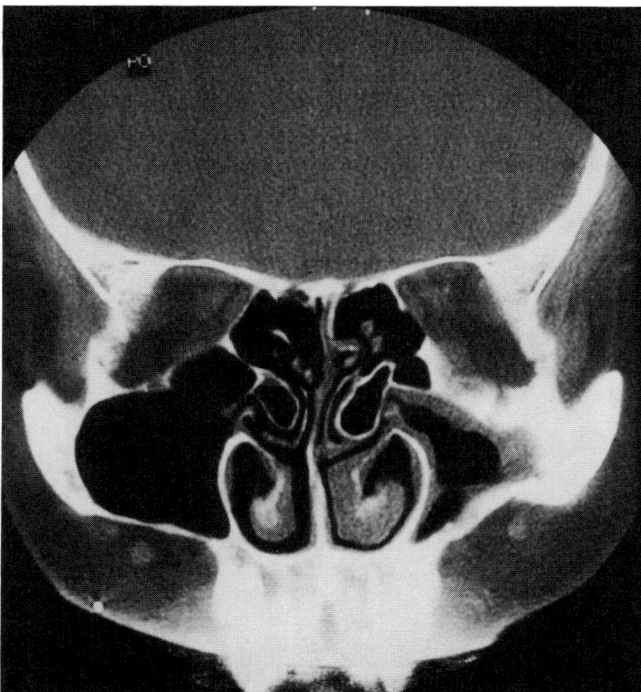

Figure 31.12. A shortened and widened uncinate process obstructing the ostiomeatal complex and producing sinusitis.

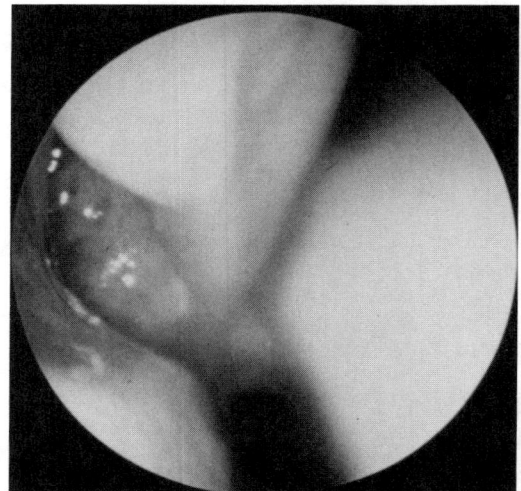

Figure 31.14. Nasal endoscopic view of the middle meatus of patient (Fig. 31.13), revealing a polypoid mass obstructing the ostiomeatal complex.

recurrent sinusitis. Plain, traditional sinus roentgenographs will only show the result of the disease, such as maxillary, ethmoid, or frontal sinus mucosal thickening or opacification. Obtaining a coronal CT scan when the patient is least symptomatic often visualizes the offending pathology without the associated surrounding mucosal edema and fluid within the sinuses. Most of the time an anatomical or pathological abnormality is seen in the OMC.

Haller cells are another anatomical cause for recurrent sinusitis. These are ethmoid sinus air cells that are present within the superior and medial walls of the maxillary sinus (Fig. 31.16). While often present and not pathological, they may obstruct the outflow from the maxillary sinus and cause sinusitis. This occurs especially during times of an upper respiratory tract infection when mucosal edema and the presence of Haller cells together compromise the OMC.

Polyps in and around the OMC can obstruct the outflow from the maxillary, ethmoid, and frontal sinuses (Fig.

31.17). Likewise, polyps in the sphenoid-ethmoid recess may cause sphenoid sinusitis.

Treatment for acute recurrent sinusitis is removal of the anatomical or pathological cause. If mucosal edema or polyposis is visualized endoscopically, topical (beclometh-asone) and/or systemic steroids are used. If purulent secretions are present, antibiotics and a decongestant are used. If there is persistent repetition of infection in spite of medical management, an appropriate surgical procedure should be considered. For many, this is a relatively minor procedure in which the uncinate process is removed and the natural ostium of the maxillary sinus opened. This provides drainage through the natural ostium of the maxillary sinus and the infundibulum. Others need a more extensive ethmoidectomy.

Chronic Sinusitis

While acute sinusitis is usually diagnosed by the presence of pain, purulent drainage, mucosal edema, and air-fluid level on sinus imaging, chronic sinusitis is not as clearly defined and therefore is often misdiagnosed. At some times, it is underdiagnosed, with physicians not recognizing many of its subtle symptoms, and at other times, it may be overdiagnosed, with patient and/or physician believing that every upper respiratory infection, episode of rhinitis, and headache is an episode of sinusitis. Adequate history and the use of nasal endoscopy coupled with coronal CT imaging of the sinuses has greatly facilitated the accuracy of the diagnosis of chronic sinusitis.

While patients with acute sinusitis most often complain of severe pain over the infected sinus, those with chronic sinusitis generally complain of a dull aching either over the sinus or (more often) over the midface. While initially saying that they have a headache, with further inquiry, patients say that the discomfort is facial. With questioning about the nature of the discomfort, patients do not typi-

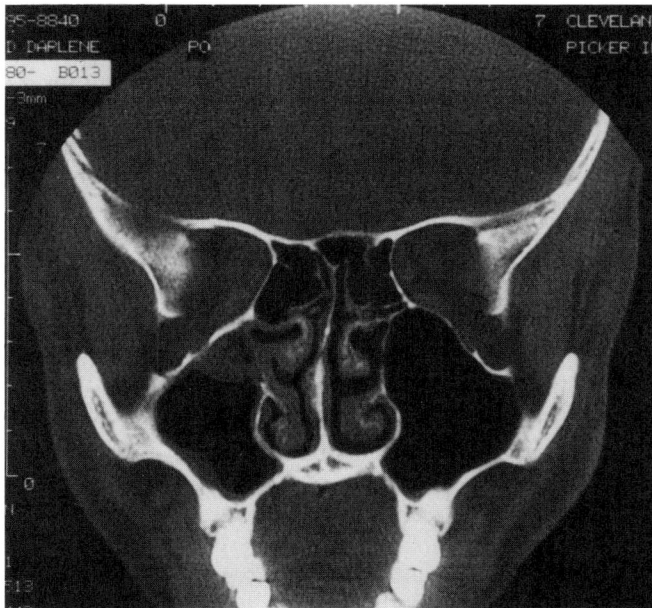

Figure 31.15. Computed tomographic scan of patient (Figs. 31.13, 31.14) taken after treatment at a time of well-being, revealing the obstruction within the ostiomeatal complex.

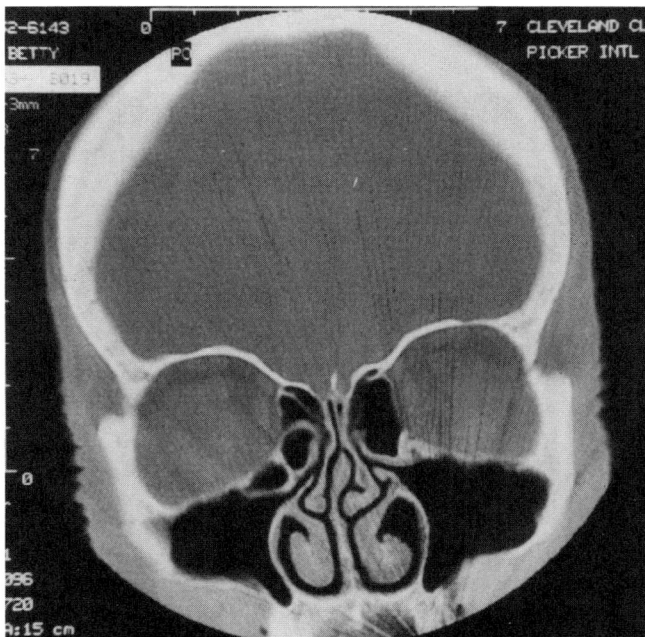

Figure 31.16. Haller cells produced by pneumatization of the ethmoid sinus along the orbital floor and into the maxillary sinus, producing narrowing of the infundibulum.

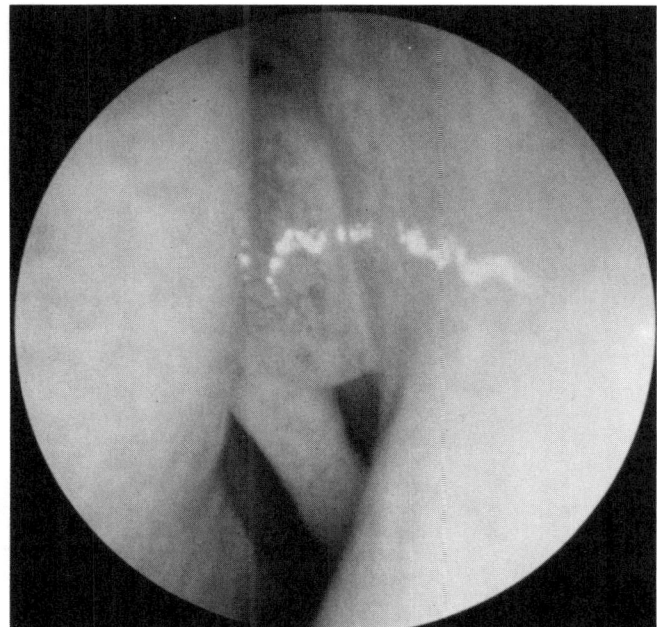

Figure 31.17. Polyps in the middle meatus, producing obstruction of the ostiomeatal complex, recurrent sinusitis, and pain.

cally call this pain, but rather a constant pressure or fullness. It is unusual for the pain to be constant for days or weeks as with some headaches, but rather, it fluctuates as the mucosal edema and congestion alter. There is rarely any throbbing, pulsating, photophobia, nausea, vomiting, or sleepiness. However, some patients with migraine and/or vascular headaches have these episodes exacerbated by an episode of sinusitis.

In addition to the dull aching and pressure over the face, there is intermittent nasal congestion and obstruction. These symptoms may erroneously be attributed to turbinate dysfunction (i.e., allergic or vasomotor rhinitis) or to nasal septal deformity. Thick purulent postnasal secretions are nearly always present. At times the secretions may be milky white, with periods of thicker, more colored secretions. These are worse upon awakening and during times of the year or environments with low humidity. Like patients with acute recurrent sinusitis, most of these patients are treated with antibiotics appropriately and then have periods of well-being, only to have an exacerbation of their symptoms. These postnasal secretions often cause sore throat, halitosis, and even gastrointestinal upset.

Patients with chronic sinusitis may have had an episode of acute sinusitis that caused enough edema and inflammation in the OMC to produce persistent obstruction. This obstruction causes stasis of secretions within the sinus, which becomes secondarily infected. Because of the changes in the oxygen tension within the sinus, the normal aerobic flora become anaerobic. These infected secretions cause more inflammation in the sinus outflow tract and more edema and inflammation. The anaerobic bacteria are usually anaerobic *Streptococcus*, *Corynebacterium*, *Veillonella*,

and *Bacteroides*. *Staphylococcus* is also seen to much greater extent than in acute sinusitis. For this reason, an antistaphylococcal or augmented penicillin is a first antibiotic of choice. A second choice would be clindomycin or cephalosporin.

On examination endoscopically, there may be any of the anatomical abnormalities seen with acute, acute recurrent, or barosinusitis. Polyposis may be seen minimally within the OMC or massively filling the nasal and sinus cavity (Figs. 31.18, 31.19). Scarring may be present within the nose and sinus cavity secondary to surgical attempts that have failed (Fig. 31.20). The scarring makes for a poorer subsequent surgical result, since there is less chance that functioning cilia will return in these scarred regions. This loss of cilia causes stasis of secretions and recurrent infections.

The vicious cycle of obstruction, inflammation, and infection must be broken by either medical or surgical management. Medical management includes the appropriate antibiotics to cover pathogenic flora that exist in chronic sinusitis along with a decongestant and mucolytic agent. Treatment is usually for 3 weeks. When nasal polyposis is part of the etiology of chronic sinusitis, a short burst of systemic steroids accompanied by topical nasal steroids (beclomethasone) for at least 6 weeks is used. The antibiotic/decongestant/mucolytic regimen is combined with steroids when both infection and polyposis are seen together.

Septal Contact and Impaction

Abnormalities of the nasal septum may cause and contribute to facial pain and "sinus-like" symptoms. The nasal septum may have a spur of bone that arises from the

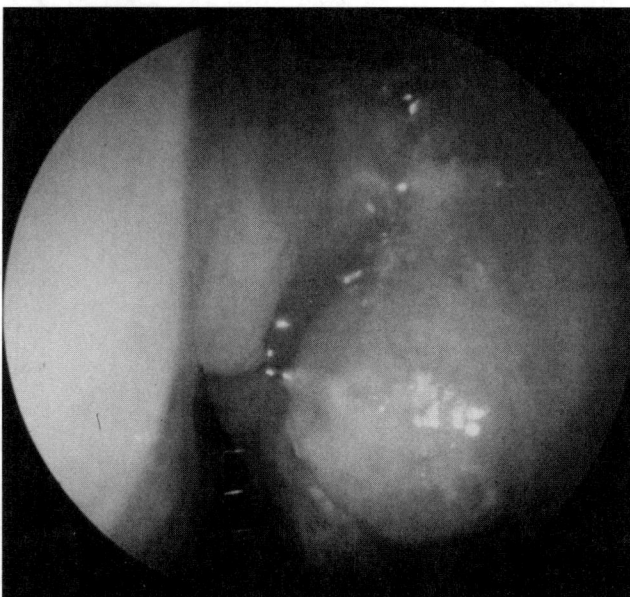

Figure 31.18. Massive polyposis within the ostiomeatal complex, producing pain, pressure, and sinusitis.

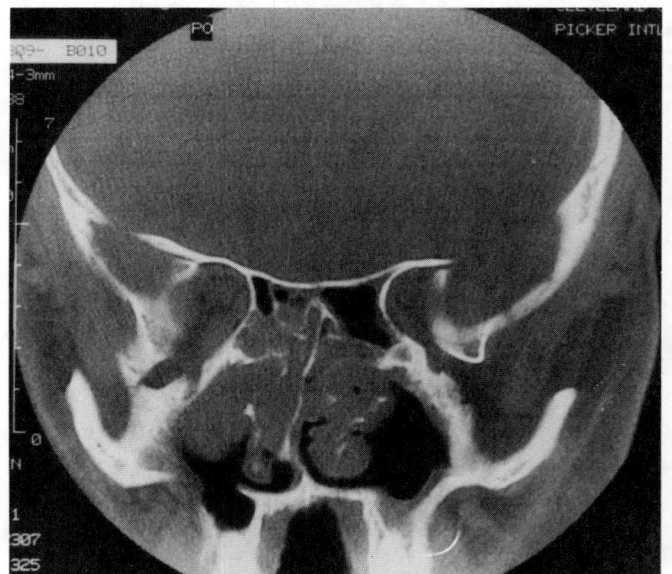

Figure 31.19. Massive polyposis filling and obstructing the ostiomeatal complex and producing recurrent sinusitis and pain.

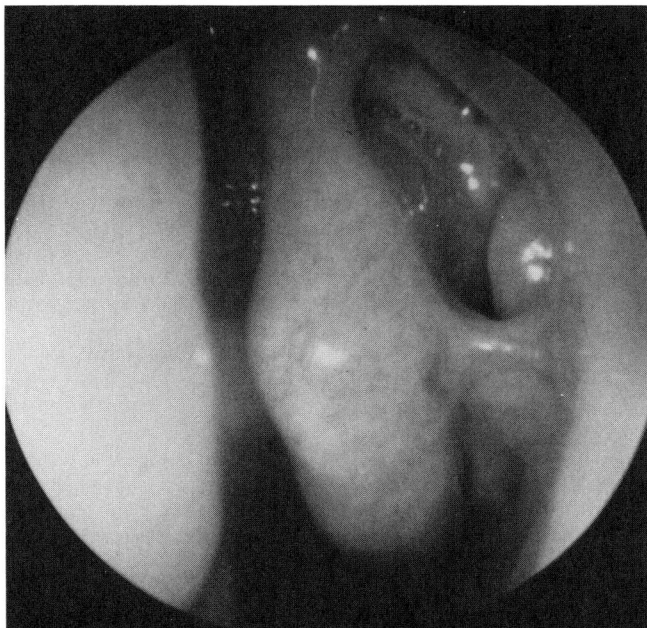

Figure 31.20. Scar tissue within the middle meatus from previous surgery causing repeated episodes of sinusitis.

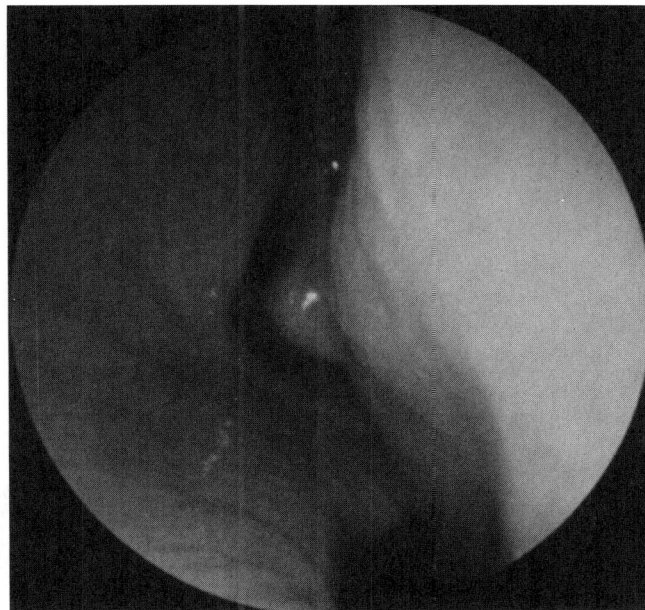

Figure 31.21. Nasal septal spur impacting upon the lateral nasal wall and producing pain.

maxillary crest to contact the lateral nasal wall. At times when the nasal turbinates are congested, there is contact between the spur and the lateral wall (Fig. 31.21). In other instances, the nasal septal spur impacts into the lateral nasal wall, regardless of any nasal congestion. In either of these instances, there may be pain. It is not clear whether this pain is related to an irritative phenomenon by the spur to the sensory fibers of the lateral nasal wall, or to obstruction of the sinus ostia, specifically the OMC.

These patients have a spectrum of pain, which may be severe, lancinating, and intermittent or constant, dull, and aching. The pain is nearly always in the medial canthal and lacrimal fossa region. Unilateral nasal congestion and eye tearing may be associated with this.

If a patient is seen at a time of pain, decongesting the nose and applying topical anesthesia to the area of the spur most often relieves the discomfort. If a secondary sinusitis has occurred, pain may remain. If there is no pain at the time of the examination, yet the clinician is suspicious of septal contact or impaction as the etiology, the patient can be given a spray for 4% Xylocaine with 1% Neo-Synephrine mixed in equal amounts. This can be used at the time of the pain in attempt to get pain relief. The patient should keep track of how often and how quickly pain relief is achieved. If there appears to be a correlation between the use of the spray and pain relief, consideration is given to removal of the septal spur.

Allergic and Vasomotor Rhinitis

Facial pain and pressure may occur due to engorgement of the nasal turbinates. While the turbinates swell and con-

tract alternately from side to side as part of the normal nasal cycle, there are phenomena that will exaggerate this response. Typically, the patient describes pressure and pain over the nasal dorsum, medical canthal area, and midface.

Patients with allergic rhinitis usually present with itchy nose and itchy and watery eyes. There is clear, watery rhinorrhea and often fits of sneezing. Symptoms may be perennial or seasonal, depending upon the etiology. The nasal examination reveals the watery nasal secretions and the turbinates that appear pale, boggy, and edematous.

Patients with mild-to-moderate allergic rhinitis may be treated symptomatically with an antihistamine to control the watery secretions and a decongestant for the nasal turbinate engorgement. Topical beclomethasone or nasal cromolyn is also helpful. Patients with severe and uncontrolled symptoms should be evaluated by an allergist and desensitization considered.

Vasomotor rhinitis is a nonallergic, usually perennial rhinitis manifest by profuse watery nasal drainage. There is rarely any itching of the eyes or nose. Sneezing fits do occur. Many of these patients do get turbinate engorgement and subsequent midfacial pain and pressure. Many of these patients mistake these symptoms for being sinus in origin.

Vasomotor rhinitis is due to an imbalance of the autonomic innervation of the nose. There is a hyperactivity of the parasympathetic or hypoactivity of the sympathetic innervation. This results in a net hypersecretion and vascular leakage within the nose. On examination, the turbinates appear watery and spongy.

Vasomotor rhinitis may be caused by irritants such as

smoke, pollutants, perfumes, and cold dry air. During times of stress, there is increased nasal congestion. Vasomotor rhinitis may also be caused by various pharmacological agents such as sympathetic blocking agents (e.g., propranolol, reserpine, methyldopa), antidepressants (e.g., thioridazine), anticholinesterase inhibitors (e.g., estrogen), and systemic disorders such as hypothyroidism. However, most individuals do not have an identifiable cause.

Treatment should include removal or avoidance of the cause if possible. Symptomatic treatment includes an antihistamine for the watery nasal drainage and a decongestant for the turbinate engorgement. If there are persistent symptoms, a beclomethasone spray is used. Ipratropium spray is often effective for the rhinorrhea.

When conservative management with environmental control and medication is ineffective, laser photocoagulation of the turbinates is effective (14). This creates a layer of scar tissue in the submucosa, prevents rapid extremes of congestion and decongestion, and decreases the watery nasal drainage that comes from the turbinates.

Neoplasms

Some neoplasms of the nose and paranasal sinuses produce "sinus-like" symptoms. A benign or malignant neoplasm may cause sinusitis as the tumor obstructs any or all of the sinus ostia. Facial pain or pressure may be present.

While most patients who have sinusitis and/or nasal polyposis have bilateral disease, nearly every neoplasm is unilateral. Therefore, it is imperative to be suspicious of a neoplasm when there is unilateral or single-sinus disease. Initially, it is appropriate to treat the patient medically when there is uncertainty whether the disease is inflammatory or neoplastic. However, there must be follow-up and repeat examination and imaging performed to be sure that the opacified sinus has cleared.

REFERENCES

1. Moss AJ, Parsons VL. Current estimates from the National Health Interview Survey, United States—1985. Hyattsville, MD: National Center for Health Statistics, 1986:66–67; DHHS Publication no. (phs)86–1588. Vital Health Stat; series 110; no. 160.
2. National Disease and Therapeutic Index. Plymouth Meeting, PA: IMS, Inc., 1988–1989:487–488.
3. Kennedy DW, Zinreich SJ, Rosenbaum A, Johns ME. Functional endoscopic sinus surgery: theory and diagnostic evaluation, Arch Otolaryngol 1985;111:576–582.
4. Levine HL. The office diagnosis of nasal and sinus disorders using rigid nasal endoscopy. Otolaryngol Head Neck Surg 1990;102:370–373.
5. Zinreich SJ, Kennedy DW, Rosenbaum AE, Gayler BW, Kumar AJ, Stammberger H. CT of the paranasal sinuses: imaging requirements for endoscopic surgery. Radiology 1987;163:769–775.
6. Kennedy DW, Zinreich SJ, Kuhn F, Shaalan H, Naclerio R, Loch E. Endoscopic middle meatal antrostomy: theory, technique, and patency. Laryngoscope 1987;97:8(part 3, suppl 43).
7. Levine HL. Functional endoscopic sinus surgery: evaluation, surgery and follow-up of 250 patients. Laryngoscope 1990;100:79–84.
8. Rice DH, Schaeffer SD. Endoscopic paranasal sinus surgery. New York: Raven Press, 1988.
9. Schaeffer SD, Manning S, Close LG. Endoscopic paranasal sinus surgery: indications and considerations. Laryngoscope 1989;99:1–5.
10. Stammberger H. Endoscopic sinus surgery: concepts in the treatment of recurring rhinosinusitis. Part I. Anatomic and pathophysiologic considerations. Part II. Surgical technique. Otolaryngol Head Neck Surg 1986;94:143–156.
11. Stammberger H, Wolf G. Headaches and sinus disease: the endoscopic approach. Ann Otol Rhinol Laryngol 1988;(suppl 134):3–23.
12. Frederick J, Braude A. Anaerobic infection of the paranasal sinuses. N Engl J Med 1974;290:135–137.
13. Wald ER, Milmoe GJ, Bowen A, Ledsma-Median J, Salamon N, Bluestone CD. Acute maxillary sinusitis in children. N Engl J Med 1981;304:749–754.
14. Levine HL. The KTP/532 laser for the treatment of turbinate dysfunction. Otolaryngol Head Neck Surg 1991;104:247–251.

32

Headache Associated with Temporomandibular Dysfunction

JEROME D. BUXBAUM and NORBERT R. MYSLINSKI

The conceptualization of headache is almost as broad as the entire sphere of pain and nociception. This chapter discusses the relationship between headache and temporomandibular joint dysfunction (hence referred to as TMD). A significant number of headaches have had at least a part of their etiology and pathology in the stomatognathic system. Therefore, no discussion of headache would be complete without a discourse of its relationship with the stomatognathic system.

For the purposes of this textbook, the term headache is used to describe head pain, as opposed to facial pain. However, a number of patients refer to pain in the preauricular area as well as some other facial areas as headache. The above statement notwithstanding, any discussion of the interrelationship between headache and TMD necessitates a brief description of the TMD syndrome.

Historically, discussions of pain and nociception in the orofacial area have been rather fragmented, narrow, and confusing to some degree. This statement is exemplified by the perturbations that have existed for many years in the area of TMD. TMD per se is not a pathological entity. Just as the term coronary disease may indicate any one of a number of specific pathologies, TMD simply denotes a family of symptoms indicative of a number of specific pathologies. To date, these number approximately 110 to 120 pathological entities. Some are dental in origin, some systemic, some psychological, some arthrogenous, and some myogenous (1).

The symptom set common to all of these pathologies includes one or more of the following: perturbations of the range and/or gait of mandibular movement, joint sounds, muscle spasm, otic symptoms, pain in the orofacial area (usually preauricular), headache, and cervical discomfort. This symptom set indicates the inherent anatomical and physiological interrelationships in the stomatognathic system. The system is a closed five-part system consisting of the dentition, periodontium, temporomandibular joint, associated neuromusculature, and the cervical area from C1 to C3. Therefore, it encompasses an area from the skull superiorly to the sternoclavicular area inferiorly and the entire ventrodorsal extent of this area except for portions of the brain (See Fig. 32.1). As this is a closed system, an abnormality in any single component will result in functional changes in one or more of the other components. This effect may or may not be large enough to produce clinically apparent alterations.

The discomfort of most patients with TMD is multifactorial. As such, the most important factor in the management of these individuals is an accurate diagnosis. As simplistic as this statement may appear, it is often violated. The complexity of the system frequently requires the expertise of a team of health care specialists to determine an accurate diagnosis and an appropriate treatment plan. As a result, many patients have a tortuous prior history consisting of numerous clinicians from a number of health disciplines, but no coordinated or comprehensive diagnostic workup. Due to the length of the patient's nociceptive experience, most must be classified as one of the three types of chronic pain patients (2). Although a discussion of chronic pain ramifications is beyond the scope of this text, the reader should refer to an appropriate source for information in this area (3). This chapter focuses on areas of TMD that most frequently involve headache as a significant symptom. It also defines the role of the dentist as part of the clinical team.

EPIDEMIOLOGY

The percentage of patients with TMD symptoms has been extensively studied over many years and in numerous countries. The results of these studies have not been consistent, due mainly to deficiencies in research design. Fortunately, there has been publication of several excellent studies using random samples drawn from the general population. These reports have been more consistent in their conclusions. They conclude that between 50 and 60% of the general population have one or more symptoms of some form of TMD (4, 5). The variability noted above notwithstanding, the inescapable conclusion is that a significant percentage of the general population displays some symptomatology associated with temporomandibular dysfunction in its broadest context.

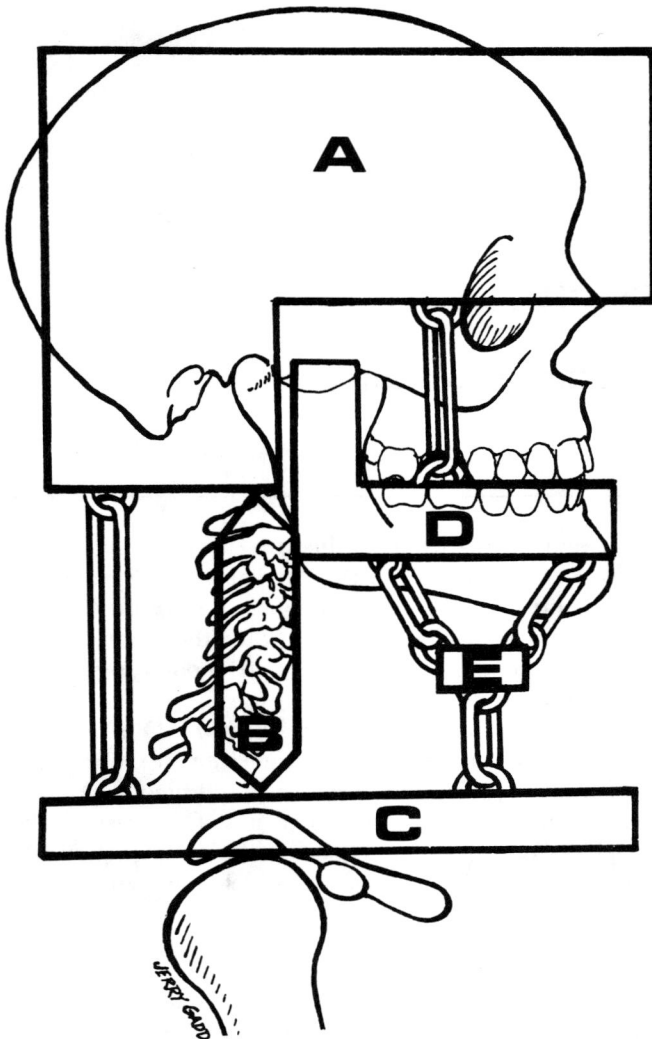

Figure 32.1. *A,* Skull; *B,* cervical area of the vertebral column; *C,* shoulder, clavicular, and sternal areas; *D,* mandible; *E,* hyoid bone.

The studies also indicate that more females are involved than males (6). In addition, there appears to be significant evidence that TMD symptoms become more pronounced and more numerous with increasing age (7). This fact assumes greater significance considering our society's ever-increasing numbers of elderly individuals, which may, in part, account for the increasing numbers of patients seeking remediation from this syndrome.

Most epidemiologic studies of TMD symptoms reveal that headache is a frequent and significant symptom. For example, in a sampling of 739 students, the most frequently mentioned TMD symptom was headache (8). A study of 120 consecutive patients in a TMD clinic revealed that 42% listed headache as a major symptom (9). A recent study reported 55 out of 100 patients with chronic headache who were referred consecutively to a neurologist, displayed symptoms indicating pathology in the stomatognathic system. Patients were randomly assigned to ei-

ther a dentist or a neurologist for further treatment. The results of this study showed that more patients treated by the dentist reported a greater decrease in the intensity and frequency of their headaches than those treated by the neurologist (10). A number of studies of common migraine, now termed migraine without aura, have shown the probability of a relationship between headache and parafunctional oral habits. The conclusion is that a significant percentage of common migraine patients display evidence of some stomatognathic system dysfunction (11). This relationship does not appear to apply to classic migraine (migraine with aura) patients.

The interrelationship between pathology in the orofacial area and headache has been most dramatically illustrated by the most recent diagnostic classification of the International Headache Society. Emphasis was placed on the expansion of three categories in the Society's Classification and Diagnostic Criteria for Headache Disorders, Cranial Neuralgias, and Facial Pain. These expanded areas are 11.1 cranial bones, 11.7 disorders of the temporomandibular joint, and 11.8 masticatory muscle disorders (12). The classification reinforces the complexities of a highly integrated and closed stomatognathic system. Consider the example of the effects of an internal disc derangement affecting one side of the TMJ. Obviously, the intracapsular structures on the affected side are dysfunctional. However, this dysfunction affects the contralateral side of the joint, the interocclusal relationship, the masticatory, cervical and associated neuromusculature, and otic structures.

Several conclusions can be drawn from these various studies. The first is that a significant percentage of the general population manifests one or more symptoms of dysfunction in the stomatognathic system. Secondly, one of the more predominant of these symptoms is headache. Lastly, there is ample evidence that for some patients, treatment of their TMD pathology results in a diminution of headache in frequency and/or intensity. However, not all TMD patients report headache as a major symptom. Also, the headache pain of many patients remains intractable even after appropriate diagnosis and treatment of the stomatognathic system.

PATHOPHYSIOLOGY OF TMD PAIN

Obviously, an inherent relationship exists between some TMD pathologies and some forms of headache. The basis for this coexistent set of symptoms is found in both the neural and muscular anatomy, and physiology of the region in question. Although nerve and muscle are interdependent and mutually functional, discussion shall be separate for clarity and understanding.

Nerves

The peripheral areas innervated by the trigeminal nerve are extensive (Fig. 32.2). As you can observe from the

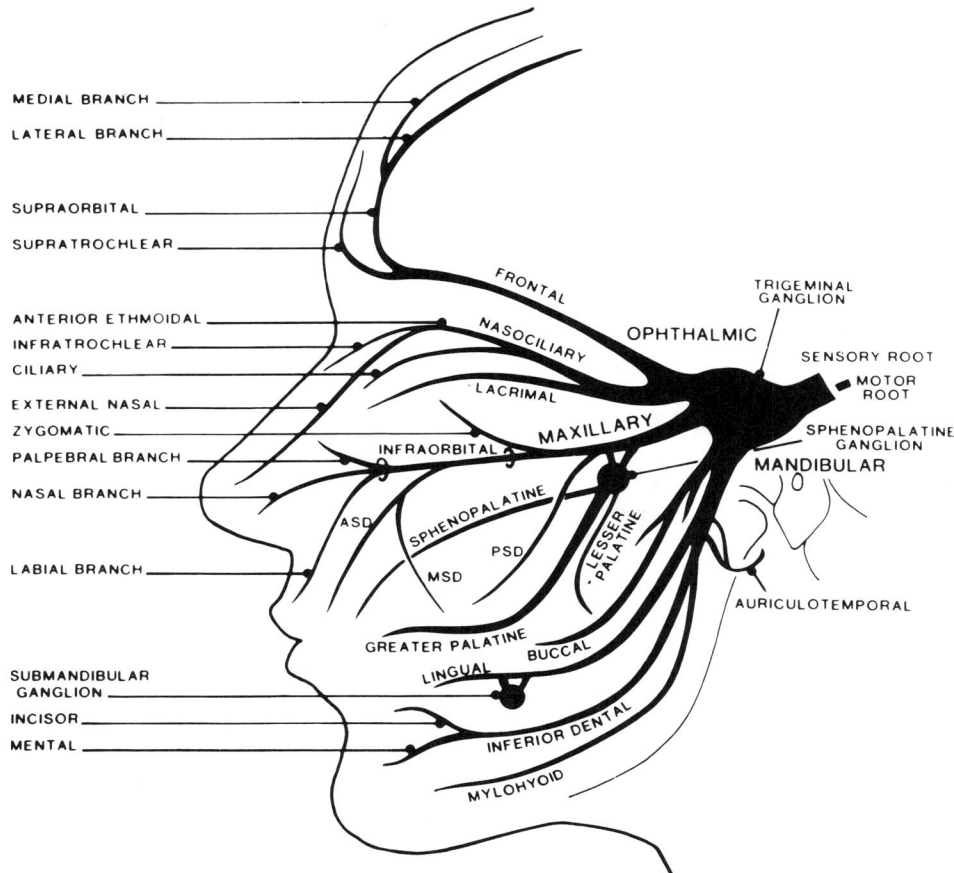

Figure 32.2. Areas innervated by the trigeminal nerve.

MEDIAL BRANCH

LATERAL BRANCH

SUPRAORBITAL

SUPRATROCHLEAR

ANTERIOR ETHMOIDAL

INFRATROCHLEAR

CILIARY

EXTERNAL NASAL

ZYGOMATIC

PALPEBRAL BRANCH

NASAL BRANCH

LABIAL BRANCH

SUBMANDIBULAR GANGLION

INCISOR

MENTAL

FRONTAL

NASOCILIARY

OPHTHALMIC

LACRIMAL

MAXILLARY

INFRAORBITAL

ASD

SPHENOPALATINE

PSD

MSD

LESSER PALATINE

GREATER PALATINE

BUCCAL

LINGUAL

INFERIOR DENTAL

MYLOHYOID

TRIGEMINAL GANGLION

SENSORY ROOT

MOTOR ROOT

SPHENOPALATINE GANGLION

MANDIBULAR

AURICULOTEMPORAL

diagram, it alone may account for muscular, optic, and sinus type headaches. Composing the primary nociceptive afferents of the trigeminal (N.V) are both nonmyelinated C fibers and thinly myelinated A delta fibers. The peripheral extensions of these fibers function as dendrites. Physiologically, the C fibers terminate as polymodal nociceptive receptors and the A delta fibers as either high-threshold mechanoreceptors or heat nociceptors. Compared with a typical spinal nerve, the trigeminal has a greater ratio of myelinated to unmyelinated nerve fibers, a greater number of nociceptive receptor-fiber units, and a shorter conduction distance. The cell bodies of these first-order nociceptor receptor-fiber units are located in the trigeminal ganglion (also known as gasserian, semilunar). The cell bodies are small- and medium-sized pseudounipolar cells. The central projections from these cells enter the brainstem and only descend. The descending fiber group is called the spinal tract of the trigeminal nerve, and the tract descends through the pons and medulla ipsilaterally. It terminates about the level of the third cervical vertebra. As it descends, the tract gives off fibers that pass into the spinal nucleus of the trigeminal. The spinal nucleus lies medial to the trigeminal tract. The spinal nucleus is divided into three component portions. Moving rostrocaudally, these sections are the subnucleus oralis, subnucleus interpolaris,

and subnucleus caudalis. Subnucleus caudalis merges caudally with the dorsal horn of the spinal cord. Although some nociceptive units, primarily from tooth pulp, may be found in oralis and interpolaris, most nociceptive units have their initial synapse in subnucleus caudalis. Two general types of secondary nociceptive neurons have been identified in caudalis: (*a*) nociceptive-specific neurons that respond only to noxious thermal and mechanical stimuli and (*b*) wide-dynamic-range neurons that respond to both nonnoxious and noxious stimuli (13). Similar to the dorsal horn of the spinal cord, the spinal nucleus is layered cytoarchitecturally. The primary nociceptive fibers terminate superficially in layers I, II, and III, and more deeply in layer V. After synapsing, the fibers decussate and ascend. Some fibers project to other areas of the spinal nucleus. Most however, ascend to the thalamus.

It is important to note that the spinal nucleus receives sensory input from more than just the trigeminal nerve. In addition to the trigeminal, the spinal nucleus is the first-order termination of afferents from the facial, glossopharyngeal, vagus, and cervical nerves 1 through 3. This convergence is of profound importance in considering the interaction between TMD pathology and headache, especially in relation to referred pain.

Muscles

The musculature of the stomatognathic system may be grossly divided into four groups: the masticatory muscles, infrahyoid group, suprahyoid group, and the associated muscular group (Fig. 32.3). Of these, the muscles most involved in TMD head and neck pain, either directly or referred, are the masseter, temporalis, lateral (external) pterygoid, medial (internal) pterygoid, and digastric (Fig. 32.3). These move the mandible and are innervated by branches of the mandibular division of the trigeminal nerve. The sternocleidomastoid and trapezius muscles help move the head and are innervated by the accessory nerve.

The masseter muscle is innervated by the masseteric nerve, and its main action is to elevate the mandible and close the jaw. Trigger points located in the deep portions of this muscle refer pain to the ear and TMJ. Tinnitus described as a "low roaring noise" is a common complaint. Trigger points located in the superficial layers refer pain to the face, jaw, and posterior mandibular and maxillary teeth. Toothache in the patient is a frequent complaint. The masseter was found to be the second most commonly involved muscle in TMD (14), and it has the second highest number of active trigger points (15). However, these re- sults differ from those of others (16).

The temporalis muscle is innervated by the mandibular nerve, and it functions primarily to close the mandible.

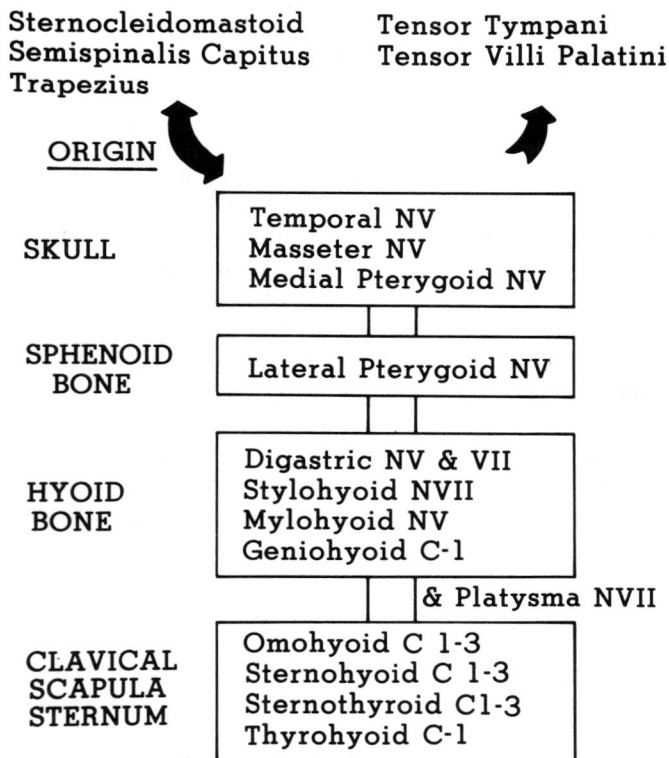

Figure 32.3. Stomatognathic muscles.

Some fibers are also used for retrusion and lateral deviation of the jaw to the same side. Trigger points in this muscle refer pain to the upper portion of the face and the maxillary teeth. Patients complain of head pain but usually not of restricted jaw opening.

The lateral pterygoid muscle is innervated by the lateral pterygoid nerve and is anatomically and functionally divided into inferior and superior divisions. Electromyographically the two divisions are antagonists. The functions of the inferior division include mandibular depression, pro- trusion, and lateral deviation to the opposite side. It refers pain to the TMJ. Although the superior division does not insert directly on the articular disc, it is anatomically positioned to stabilize it. Physiologically it performs stabi- lization of the disc during jaw closing. The lateral pte- rygoid refers pain to the zygomatic area. Diffuse pain in the malar region occurs after anterior displacement of the disc. The superior lateral pterygoid is probably the most commonly involved muscle in TMD (14, 15).

The medial pterygoid, innervated by the medial pterygoid nerve, primarily functions to elevate the mandible. Acting alone it deviates the jaw to the opposite side. It conveys pain to the TMJ, the infraauricular areas, and the posterior part of the mouth.

Innervation of the anterior belly of the digastric muscle is by the mylohyoid nerve, and the posterior belly of this muscle is innervated by the facial nerve. The digastric assists in depressing and retruding the mandible. The anterior belly refers pain to the mandibular incisor area.

The sternocleidomastoid muscle helps to stabilize and fix the position of the head while chewing or talking. It helps to tip the head back and raise the chin. Working unilaterally it approximates the ipsilateral ear to the shoulder. It refers pain through the entire face and head, especially the ear, postauricular region, and the frontal area. It is a frequent cause of tension headaches.

Most of the action of the trapezius is on the shoulder, suspending, squaring, shrugging, and pulling it in. It is also a rotator of the scapula. Fixing the shoulder, it assists in pulling the head posteriorly and laterally. The trapezius refers pain to the temple area, the postauricular area, the mandibular angle, and the posterolateral part of the neck. This muscle is also a source of tension headaches.

Muscle Pain

Most patients with TMD suffer primarily from a muscle disorder. In studies by Forsell (17), headache patients demonstrated a high prevalence of TMD signs and symptoms. In these studies, the frequency of headache correlated with the occurrence of clinical TMD signs. Studies by Magnusson and Carlsson (18, 19) of TMD and other dental patients found that the frequency and severity of headache varied with the severity of TMD. The only variable of TMD, however, that showed a distinct relationship to headache in their study was masticatory muscles that were painful to palpation.

Headaches of a dull, steady nature may be the result of inappropriate pericranial muscle activity. Literature has often described the tenderness of these muscles in various types of headaches. Headache patients often have difficulty relaxing their muscles in general. However, the relationship between headache and measurable muscle activity is complex and controversial, as indicated by Chapman (20) and Pikoff (21). Therefore, more complicated mechanisms have replaced the earlier theory of headache pain being caused simply by an increase in muscle tension.

Mechanisms of Muscle Pain

Theoretical mechanisms of muscle pain that may be pertinent to headache include (a) long-lasting ischemia, (b) low-grade inflammation, (c) trigger points, (d) muscle strain, and (e) altered skeletal muscle length. Any combination of these mechanisms may exist in any particular clinical situation.

Ischemia

The cause of ischemic pain is an accumulation of slowly diffusible, pain-producing metabolites that are produced in the muscle and stimulate or sensitize nociceptors. Muscles adapted for tonic activity (type I fibers) are less likely to become ischemic during contractions than those adapted for fast activity (type II fibers). The lateral pterygoid in normal adults is dominated by type I fibers; however, the temporalis frontalis and most other muscles of the head and neck do not have a predominance of type I fibers.

The grinding and clenching of teeth causes an increase in blood flow (22); however, if contractions are strong enough, they may produce an ischemia (23). These contractions increase intramuscular pressure, but it does not, on the average, rise above the arterial blood pressure, and therefore it cannot be the total cause of the ischemia. Another possibility is that the arteries are cut off at their point of entry through the muscle fascia by the displacement of tissue during contraction (24). Lower-grade contractions may cause smaller areas of muscle ischemia through a similar mechanism.

Inflammation

Some headaches are associated with inflammatory diseases, such as temporal arteritis and dermatomyositis. Most headache patients do not show classic signs of acute inflammation; however, a low-grade inflammation with the release of pain-producing metabolites is possible.

Trigger Points

Trigger points are knots of hyperactive and hypersensitive muscle that give rise to tenderness and referred pain. They are palpable and produce a local twitch when adequately stimulated. Trigger points in the muscles of the head and neck give rise to referred pain in the head. Evocation of the same anatomical pattern of referred pain can occur, if one injects hypertonic saline into the muscle (25).

Different movements or conditions are responsible for the activation of trigger points in different muscles. Trigger points can be activated by such things as occlusal imbalance, bruxism, cracking nuts or ice between the teeth, clenching on a pipe, thumb sucking late in childhood, "whiplash" due to auto accidents or other extension-flexion trauma, direct trauma such as the impact of a baseball, long periods of jaw immobilization, or sustained contractions such as playing the violin. The etiology of trigger points is still unknown; however, ischemia has been suggested as a cause (26).

Histological studies of trigger points have shown any number of abnormalities, including edema and different levels of degeneration from swelling of mitochondria to loss of the contractile substance (27, 28). The muscle fibers appear to be connected by a network of reticular fibers that are absent in normal muscle (29). There is a deficiency of ATP and ADP, which may be partly explained by hypoxia (30).

Muscle Strain

Severe exercise produces two types of muscle pain: (a) immediate pain produced by an accumulation of metabolites, and (b) delayed-onset pain probably due to microtrauma to the myofascial tissue.

The cause of the delayed-onset pain is controversial, but plausibly it is due to torn or damaged tissue. Asmussen (31) reported that delayed-onset pain is more likely after work that lengthens muscle than after work that shortens muscle. Newham et al. (32) argue that this is because more mechanical damage is likely after work that lengthens muscle. Christensen (33) has demonstrated that pain is more likely to persist after tooth grinding than after tooth clenching. Jensen et al. (34) showed that 30 minutes of sustained forceful tooth clenching in a group of migraine suffers did not cause more headache than did a similar but weak, just-noticeable tooth clenching.

Alterations in Skeletal Muscle Length

One of the unique aspects of the stomatognathic system is the latitude that exists in alterations of length of its muscular component. The dimension between the mandible and the maxilla is determined by the dentition. The extent of tooth eruption is a factor of the neurosensory input from mechanoreceptors located in the periodontal ligaments, and masticatory musculature. Alterations in the dentition resulting from orthodontia, prosthodontia, loss of posterior dentition, and other causes will affect the skeletal muscle length of the system. Although the musculature is capable of some adaptation, the adaptive capability is finite. All skeletal muscles have an optimal length. When a muscle is at or near this ideal length it can perform "work" with the least amount of expended energy. If significantly above or below this length, the muscle must expend markedly more energy to perform the same amount of "work." The musculature of the stomatognathic system as stated, frequently undergoes alterations in its length. As such, it often does not function at or near its optimal length and, in this state, is under constant but varying degrees of stress. These factors have been well established in the literature for many years (35).

Electromyography Studies

Numerous studies of headache have included EMG recordings from muscles of the head and neck. Bakke et al. (36) and Clifford et al. (37) discovered that EMG levels rose during migraine attacks.

However, the relationship between baseline EMG levels in headache versus nonheadache subjects is still undetermined. Using surface electrodes, Sturgis et al. (38) discovered that patients with muscle-contraction headaches had higher baseline EMG levels; on the other hand, Sutton and Belar (39) did not find any significant difference. Bakal and Kaganov (40) found that migraine patients exhibited higher baseline levels, but Anderson and Franks (41) did not. Using needle electrodes, Posniak-Patewicz (42) showed that patients with muscle-contraction or migraine headaches produced muscle potentials at rest, but controls without headache did not.

EMG biofeedback produces a decrease in baseline EMG values. Muscle-contraction headache and migraine patients show similar amounts of improvement after EMG biofeedback (20).

Referred Pain

Muscle injury discussed in the last section is sometimes felt in areas of the body other than the injured tissue itself. This is called referred pain. The pain is usually referred from the muscle to a more superficial area of the body, and it usually does not stray beyond the embryonic segment to which the originating muscle belongs. However, there are exceptions. There is no general rule for guessing the referred pain pattern of a muscle. The pain pattern of each muscle must be learned individually. In addition, the muscle's referred pain pattern enlarges as the activity of the trigger point increases (43).

Referred pain is felt in an area innervated by a different nerve than that which innervates the source of the pain. This differentiates it from projected pain, which is felt in the peripheral receptive field of the same nerve as the source of the pain. In many cases the patient is only aware of the referred pain and not of the source.

The muscles of mastication have specific patterns of referred pain that are predictable and reproducible (44). The temporalis muscle refers pain to the side of the head and upper teeth. The deep layers of the masseter muscle refer to the TMJ and ear. The superficial layers refer to the gingiva, molar teeth, and jaws. The internal pterygoid

refers to the TMJ and the mouth. The external ptyergoid is the main source of referred pain to the TMJ.

Convergence of the neuronal input is the most likely explanation for referred pain. There is convergence of input from both the referring and the referred sites into secondary neurons (transmission cells of the spinal nucleus of the trigeminal) or elsewhere in the central nervous system. Activity in the cells of this pathway is eventually interpreted by the cerebral cortex as pain at the referred site. Since pain is more common at the referred site, the brain has "learned" that activity arriving in that particular pathway is caused by pain in the referred site. When the same pathway is stimulated by activity in the referring site, the signal reaching the brain is no different, and the pain is mistakenly attributed to the referred site. This is called the convergence theory, where input from the referring site suffices to produce pain in the referred site. Sessle and Greenwood (45) have demonstrated convergence of somatic input onto the trigeminal brainstem neurons.

The facilitation theory (a variation of the convergence theory) holds that activity from the referring site lowers the threshold of the secondary neurons so that minor activity from the referred site (that would normally die out) is passed on to the higher centers. Therefore, activity from both sites is necessary to feel the pain at the referred site.

If the convergence theory were correct, then anesthetizing the referred site would have no effect on the pain; if the facilitation theory were correct, then the pain would disappear. In actuality, the effects of local anesthesia at the referred site vary. When the pain is mild, it may be completely abolished; when the pain is severe, it is usually unaffected. Both convergence and facilitation probably play a role in the pathogenesis of referred pain.

CLINICAL EVALUATION

It is now obvious that not all headaches have an orofacial component. It is also true that not all TMD pathology results in headache as a reported symptom. However, if a thorough clinical evaluation has eliminated any neurological, vascular, or other systemic cause for the patient's head pain, then current research and clinical data indicate the necessity for a TMD evaluation. The same indication exists if treatment for any of the above pathologies does not result in a marked reduction in the patient's symptomatology. The reverse of this is equally applicable. It has been reported (46) that approximately 80% of all reported headaches are associated with some form of aberrant muscular activity. Therefore, TMD should be clinically considered as an etiologic source without neurological or vascular findings. If a patient is treated initially for TMD and the therapy does not result in diminution of headache, then other systemic causes should be taken into consideration.

A number of procedures are involved in a complete TMD workup. Some are simple and can, and indeed should, be performed by any clinician. Execution of the more complex procedures requires an appropriate specialist. The complete TMD evaluation entails the following: (a) a very thorough history and systems review, (b) an examination of the oral and perioral hard and soft tissues, (c) a study of the occlusal relationships, (d) measurements of the mandibular range of motion, (e) assessment of pain on mandibular distraction, (f) perturbations in the pattern of mandibular gait, (g) auscultation of the TMJ, (h) palpation of the TMJ and all of its adnexal musculature, (i) radiographs, (j) cine' MRI studies, (k) deprogrammed occlusal analysis, (l) electromyographic studies, and (m) indicated laboratory tests. It is beyond the scope of this work to discuss each of these entities in detail. (For additional information the reader may consult any of the numerous and excellent texts available devoted to the diagnosis and treatment of TMD.) However, it is appropriate to elaborate on several of the basic diagnostic entities.

Enough emphasis cannot be placed upon the importance of the history and systems review. It is vital to attempt to discover if there is any known cause for the patient's discomfort. Establishment of the headache's location, frequency, intensity, quality, and duration is important. Note that there are two components to "duration." The first involves the length of time that the complaint has been present, the second concerns how long the pain is present in each episode. The clinician should ask patients about any differences in the type of headache they experience. Frequently, the clinician discovers that the patient is suffering from more than one type of headache.

Any clinician can simply assess the mandibular range of motion. The determination of the measurement of the vertical opening is accomplished by first measuring the number of millimeters an upper incisor vertically overlaps its lower counterpart. Then the patient is asked to open as far as possible, and the space between the previously mentioned teeth is measured. The vertical range of mandibular movement is the sum of these two parameters. The normal value for mandibular opening is 50.3 ± 6.9 mm. A very gross determination of the ability to open normally is that any subject should be able to insert three fingers, held vertically between the upper and lower anterior dentition.

Lateral excursion is the distance the lower incisors can move either left or right from their normal, centered position. The normal value for this maneuver is 9.1 mm. The lateral excursions should be approximately equal. A reduced excursion indicates pathology in the contralateral joint. For example, if left lateral is normal and right lateral below normal, it would indicate pathology in the left TMJ.

Protrusion refers to the forward movement of the mandible. The normal value for this excursion is at least 6.1 mm. The movement should be made without deviation to either side. If the mandible demonstrates deviation during protrusion, it indicates pathology in the contralateral joint.

The mandibular opening maneuver in normal subjects generates no deviations or deflections. Mandibular opening with repeated deviations or deflections indicates pa-

thology in the TMJ. Joint auscultation is performed by placement of a stethoscope over the preauricular area bilaterally. The patient is then instructed to open the mandible, move it left and right and protrude. Notes should be made of the presence of any "clicks" (a readily discernible snapping sound) or crepitus (a sound similar to that of a vehicle riding over gravel). Joint sounds without any other symptom do warrant treatment. Joint "clicking" may indicate an anterior disc displacement. If "clicking" is present, have the patient protrude the mandible. Then repeat the opening and closing movements from this protruded position. If the "click" disappears after the first opening and closing cycle in the protruded position, it indicates that the disc displacement is probably reversible.

The TMJ should be palpated both directly and intrameatally. In addition all of the following muscles should be palpated and the presence of pain and/or myospastic areas noted. The muscles are the deep and superficial masseter, anterior middle and posterior temporalis, semispinalis capitis, trapezius, levator scapulae, sternocleidomastoid, splenius capitis, medial pterygoid, hyoid-digastric area, and the lateral pterygoid area. These techniques are easily mastered by observation.

The patient should be referred to an appropriate specialist if TMD is suspected of contributing to the headache problem. During the referral process, the patient can be supported in several ways. Most TMD patients have some myospastic activity. The myospastic cycle can most easily be broken by use of trigger point injections of lidocaine without vasoconstrictor, or refrigerant sprays such as Ethylchloride-fine (Gebauer) coupled with gentle exercise. Muscle relaxants, tranquilizers, and narcotics are of little value in alleviating the patient's discomfort. TMD symptoms can best temporarily be handled medically by the judicious use of nonsteroidal antiinflammatory drugs and tricyclic antidepressants.

Classic migraine headaches do not appear to respond to TMD therapy. However, the reduction of common migraine intensity and frequency can occur if TMD pathology is a complicating factor and if it is treated appropriately. The reader is cautioned that this may be the result of inaccurate initial diagnosis of the common migraine. It would be erroneous to assume that all common migraine, when coupled with TMD pathology, is responsive to TMD therapy alone.

SUMMARY

The number of patients presenting to a physician with a primary symptom headache is nearly 2%. The number of TMD patients with a primary symptom of headache is approximately 50%. The authors have presented the physiological, anatomical, and pathophysiological factors that account for this interrelationship. In the absence of neurological findings, the stomatognathic system should be considered as a possible etiologic site for headache.

REFERENCES

1. Buxbaum JD, Myslinski N. The physiology, pathology, pathophysiology, diagnosis and treatment of the stomatognathic system and related facial pain. 2nd ed. Baltimore: University of Maryland, 1990:7–10.
2. Casey KL, Dubner R. Animal models of chronic pain: scientific and ethical issues. Pain 1989;38(3):249–252.
3. Tollison CD. Handbook of chronic pain management. Baltimore: Williams & Wilkins, 1989.
4. Locker D, Slade G. Prevalence of symptoms associated with temporomandibular disorders in a Canadian population. J Community Dent Oral Epidemiol 1988;16(5):310–313.
5. Functional disorders of the masticatory system in southwest Finland. Community Dent Oral Epidemiol 1979;7(3):177–182.
6. Schubert R, Frank S. Epidemiology of myoarthropathy. A longitudinal study over 5 years. Dtsch Zahnaerztl Z 1988;35(2):303–305.
7. Makila E. Frequency of mandibular dysfunction symptoms in institutionalized elderly people. Gerontology 1979;25(4)283–243.
8. Solberg, WK, Woo MW, Houston JB. Prevalence of mandibular dysfunction in young adults. J Am Dent Assoc 1979;98(1):25–34.
9. Chua EK, Tay DK, Tan BY, Yuen KW. A profile of patients with temporomandibular disorders in Singapore—a descriptive study. Ann Acad Med Singapore 1989;18(6):675–680.
10. Schokker RP, Hansson TL, Anskin BJ. The result of treatment of the masticatory system of chronic headache patients. J Cranio Disord Facial Oral Pain 1990;4(2):126–130.
11. Moss RA, Lombardo J, Hodgson JM, O'Carroll K. Oral habits in common between tension headache and non-headache populations. J Oral Rehab 1989;16(1):71–74.
12. McNeil C, ed. Craniomandibular disorders—guidelines for evaluation, diagnosis and management. Chicago: Quintessence Publishing, 1990:13–19.
13. Roth GI, Calmes R. Oral Biology. St. Louis: CV Mosby, 1981:9–13.
14. Greene CS, Lerman MD, Sutcher HD, Ladkin DM. The TMJ pain-dysfunction syndrome: heterogeneity of the patient population. J Am Dent Assoc 1969;79:1168–1172.
15. Sharav EP, Tzukert A, Refaeli B. Muscle pain index in relation to pain, dysfunction and dizziness associated with the myofascial pain-dysfunction syndrome. Oral Surg 1978;46:742–747.
16. Hansson T, Wilner M. A study of the occurrence of symptoms of diseases of the temporomandibular joint, masticatory musculature and related structures. J Oral Rehabil 1975;2:313–324.
17. Forsell H. Mandibular dysfunction and headache. Proc Finn Dent Soc 1985;81 (suppl II):591.
18. Magnusson T, Carlsson GE. Comparison between two groups of patients in respect to headache and mandibular dysfunction. Swed Dent J 1978;2:85–92.
19. Magnusson T, Carlsson GE. Recurrent headaches in relation to temporomandibular joint pain-dysfunction. Acta Odontol Scand 1978;36:333–338.
20. Chapman SL. A review and clinical perspective on the use of EMG and thermal biofeedback for chronic headaches. Pain 1986;27:1–43.
21. Pikoff H. Is the muscular model for headache still viable? A review of conflicting data. Headache 1984;24:186–198.
22. Petersen FB, Christiansen LV. Blood flow in human temporalis muscle during tooth grinding and clenching as measured by 133-xenon clearance. Scand J Dent Res 1973;81:272–275.
23. Rasmussen OC, Bonde-Petersen F, Christensen LV, Moller E. Blood flow in human mandibular elevators at rest and during controlled biting. Arch Oral Biol 1977;22:539–543.
24. Moller E, Rasmussen OC, Bonde-Petersen F. Mechanism of ischemic pain in human muscles of mastication: intramuscular pressure, EMG, force and blood flood of the temporal and masseter muscles during biting. In: Bonica JJ ed. Advances in pain research and therapy. Vol 3. New York: Raven Press, 1979:271–281.
25. Kellgren JH. On distribution of pain arising from deep somatic structures, with charts of segmented pain areas. Clin Sci 1939;4:35–46.
26. Good MG. The role of skeletal muscles in the pathogenesis of diseases. Acta Med Scand 1950;138,285–292.
27. Christenssen LV, Moesmann G. On the etiology, pathophysiology and pathology of muscular fibrositis due to hyperfunction: a discussion based on recent investigations. Tandlaegebladet 1967;71:30–237.
28. Yunus MB, Kalyan-Raman UP, Kalyan-Raman K, Masi AT. Pathologic changes in muscle in primary fibromyalgia syndrome. Am J Med 1986;81(suppl 3A):38–42.
29. Bartels EM, Danneskiold-Samsoe. Histological abnormalities in muscle from patients with certain types of fibrositis. Lancet 1986;1:755–757.
30. Bengtsson A, Henriksson KG, Larson J. Reduced high-energy phosphate levels in the painful muscles of patients with primary fibromyalgia. Arthritis Rheum 1986;29:817–821.
31. Asmussen E. Observations of experimental muscle soreness. Acta Rheum Scand 1956;2:109–116.
32. Newham DJ, Mills KR, Quigley BM, Edwards RH. Pain and fatigue after concentric and eccentric muscle contractions. Clin Sci 1983;64:55–62.
33. Christensen LV. Facial pain from experimental tooth clenching. Tandlaegebladet 1970;74:175–182.
34. Jensen K, Bulow P, Hansen H. Experimental tooth clenching in common migraine. Cephalalgia 1985;5:245–251.
35. Storey AT. Physiology of a changing vertical dimension, J Prosth Dent 1962;12(6):912–921.
36. Bakke M, Tfelt-Hansen P, Olesen J, Moller E. Action of some pericranial muscles during provoked attacks of common migraine. Pain 1982;14:121–135.
37. Clifford T, Lauritzen M, Bakke M, Olesen J, Moller E. Electromyography of pericranial muscles during treatments of common migraine headache attacks. Pain 1982;14:137–147.
38. Sturgis ET, Schaefer CA, Ahles TA, Sikora TL. Effect of movement and position in the evaluation of tension headache and nonheadache control subjects. Headache 1984;24:88–93.
39. Sutton EP, Belar CD. Tension headache patients versus controls: a study of EMG parameters. Headache 1982;22:133–136.
40. Bakal DA, Kaganov JA. Muscle contraction and migraine headache: psychophysiological comparison. Headache 1977;17:208–215.
41. Anderson CD, Franks RD. Migraine and tension headache: Is there a physiologic difference? Headache 1981;21:63–71.
42. Pozniak-Patewicz E. "Cephalic" spasm of head and neck muscles. Headache 1976;15:261–266.
43. Travell JG, Simons DG. Myofascial pain and dysfunction: the trigger point manual. Baltimore: Williams & Wilkins, 1983:46–50.
44. Travell J. Temporomandibular joint pain referred from muscles of the head and neck. J Prosthet Dent 1960;10:745–763.
45. Sessle BJ, Greenwood LF. Inputs to trigeminal brain stem neurones from facial, oral, tooth pulp and pharyngolaryngeal tissues: I. Responses to innocuous and noxious stimuli. Brain Res 1976;117:211–226.
46. Diamond S. Muscle contraction headaches. In: Dalessio DJ. Wolff's headache and other head pain. 5th ed. New York: Oxford University Press, 1987:172.

33

Chronic Daily Headache: Combined Migraine/Muscle-Type Headache

NINAN T. MATHEW

Many patients present with headaches that recur almost daily. Careful analysis of their symptoms and history reveals that these patients suffer from more than one type of headache. The headaches may vary in location, severity, quality, and accompanying symptoms. Most patients describe two types of headache. One is a bilateral, low-grade, diffuse, nagging head pain that is felt as "pressure" around the head or in the posterior regions of the head, including the neck. This type of headache is present most of the time, but it may vary in intensity from time to time. In addition, patients complain of episodes of a much more severe, usually unilateral, usually throbbing headache, associated with nausea, vomiting, and certain migraine accompaniments. These severe headaches may last for 2 or 3 days, subsiding only to give way to the chronic nagging, achy sensation of the first type. Severe attacks can be triggered by any of the factors listed in Table 33.1, the most common trigger in women being menstruation. A combination of these two types of headache in the same patient can be called a "mixed headache" of migraine and chronic tension-type headache. The other synonyms used in the literature are combined headache (1), migraine with interparoxysmal headache (MIH), and chronic daily headache. The new international headache classification (2) does not recognize mixed headache as a separate entity, and these patients are supposed to be classified as migraine, usually common migraine (1.1) and chronic tension-type headache (2.2).

These patients exhibit features of vascular head pain, such as aggravation by movements and activity, throbbing character, associated nausea and vomiting, plus features of pericranial muscle spasm and tenderness. Many patients will have both migraine and tension-type headache occurring independently of one another at different times. Many patients with migraine also have tension-type occurring as a continuation of migraine attacks. At least three different clinical patterns of mixed headaches are recognized.

CLINICAL SUBTYPES

Predominantly Migrainous Type

The first subtype is characterized by headache attacks with predominantly migrainous features occurring periodically over many years until the clinical expression subsides. Although most attacks are clearly migrainous (pulsatile, throbbing, unilateral with photophobia, sonophobia, and nausea and vomiting), minor less distinct "tension-type" may accompany the attack. The tension-type consists of dull, constant aching or perhaps pressure or "tightness" around the head and neck, with nonlocalizing discomfort for many days. This sometimes precedes the migrainous attack, or it may follow it. Tenderness of the scalp and neck may be present. Combing the hair may become painful, and often patients cannot rest their heads on pillows because of tenderness of the scalp.

Predominantly Tension-Type

The second clinical pattern is a dull, constant discomfort onto which is superimposed throbbing pain, nausea, photophobia, and sometimes unilateral exaggeration of pain occurring at irregular intervals, lasting for a number of hours.

Transformed Migraine: Chronic Daily Headache

The third and probably the most common pattern is that of a **transformation of episodic migraine into a daily headache** syndrome (3, 4). Most of these patients start out having typical common migraine attacks, usually related to menstrual cycle. Then, after a number of years, especially after 15 years or so, they start having a daily headache syndrome. Most of these patients wake up in the morning with daily or almost daily head pain that might fit the description of tension-type headache. They also continue to have vascular or migrainous attacks, but less frequently, and perhaps with somewhat less intensity as years go by.

Table 33.1.
Triggers of Migraine

Common factors	Less common factors
Menstruation	High humidity
Anxiety, stress, worry	Excessive sleep
Oral contraceptives	High altitude
Glare, dazzle	Drugs (nitroglycerin, reserpine,
Physical exertion, fatigue	indomethacin, hydralazine)
Lack of sleep	Cold foods
Hunger	Reading, refractive errors
Head trauma	Pungent odors
Certain foodstuffs and alcoholic	Fluorescent lighting
beverages	Allergic reactions
Weather or ambient tempera-	
ture change	

In a retrospective study of daily headache syndrome at the Houston Headache Clinic we found that 75% of patients with daily headaches had a history of episodic migraine, and that more than half of them were hormone-dependent headaches such as menstrual migraine. We identified various factors that might have influenced the transformation of the episodic migraine into daily headache. These included an abnormal personality profile (especially neuroticism including depression), excessive stress, excessive use of caffeine and medication containing analgesics and ergotamine, and development of hypertension. We suggested that most of these types of daily headaches are a continuum of episodic migraine influenced and perpetuated by these same factors, i.e., neuroticism, excessive medication, stress, and development of hypertension. A diagnosis of tension headache under such circumstances is not justified.

CONCEPT OF CONTINUUM IN PRIMARY HEADACHE DISORDER

Distinguishing the various clinical manifestations of headache in these patients may become very difficult. In a given case, at times it is impossible to distinguish between a common migraine attack and a tension-type headache. A review of the current concepts of headache is revealing (5).

Electromyographic activity of the frontalis muscle at one time was thought to be a characteristic of tension-type headache, but recent studies have shown that most migraine patients also show increased frontalis muscle electromyographic activity. There are patients who are diagnosed as having tension-type headache who show very little spontaneous electromyographic activity in the frontalis muscle. In fact, the international classification has recognized two types of tension-type headache: one with pericranial muscle tenderness and one without. Amyl nitrate, a vasodilator, intensified headache severity in 43% of patients in trials involving tension-type patients. Intravenous administration of histamine produced throbbing head pain in 24 of 25 migraine patients and up to half of the tension-type patients, while none of the 13 controls experienced similar symptoms.

Platelet serotonin, considered important in migraine pathogenesis, has been shown to be lower in patients with tension-type headache than in normal controls and headache-free migraine patients.

Biofeedback training using electromyographic feedback, temperature training, and simple relaxation leads not only to similar reductions in headache within groups of migraine and tension-type headache patients, but also to a similar reduction of headache across diagnostic groups. Propranolol, an effective migraine prophylactic, and amitriptyline, an antidepressant, can be combined effectively for treatment of the patient with mixed headache. It is pointed out in the population studies that considerable overlap in the clinical features exists between migraine and tension-type headache, and there is a lack of concrete evidence of two discrete types of pain. Most patients with migrainous attacks continue to have low-grade, dull headaches following the migraine. Many patients report migrainous attacks preceding a constant head pain of the tension-type headache or vice versa.

Ziegler (6), using a factor analysis form of statistical method on various symptoms in 1198 headache patients, came to the conclusion that none of the traditional nosologic criteria of migraine occur with frequency high enough to be a sensitive diagnostic index capable of distinguishing migraine from tension-type headache. It is an error to equate all frequent generalized headaches with tension-type. Migraine headaches are often generalized. Frequency or duration of headache cannot be used to define tension-type headache. It is well known that common migraine can last for a number of days in some patients.

Given such data, the common headache disorder may be thought of as one entity with a wide spectrum of clinical manifestations. The mixed headache syndrome and the daily headache can be considered as falling in the middle of a wide spectrum of clinical manifestations (Fig. 33.1). At one end of the spectrum is the migraine with aura, which can be easily distinguished, and at the other end of the spectrum is the pure tension-type headache.

A number of other observations point to the possibility of a central mechanism for chronic recurrent headaches. Changes in platelet serotonin have been demonstrated in both migraine and muscle contraction headaches, and changes in the endogenous opioids have been noted in cerebrospinal fluid during migraine attacks and chronic recurrent headaches. Such data, combined with the fact that most medications now used in the prophylaxis of migraine and tension-type headache are centrally acting, support the idea that benign recurrent headaches are probably of central nervous system origin involving the neurotransmitter systems of the brainstem and other related areas (7).

BEHAVIORAL COMPLICATIONS OF MIXED HEADACHES

Chronic recurrent headaches can be associated with a number of behavioral factors that might have a bearing on

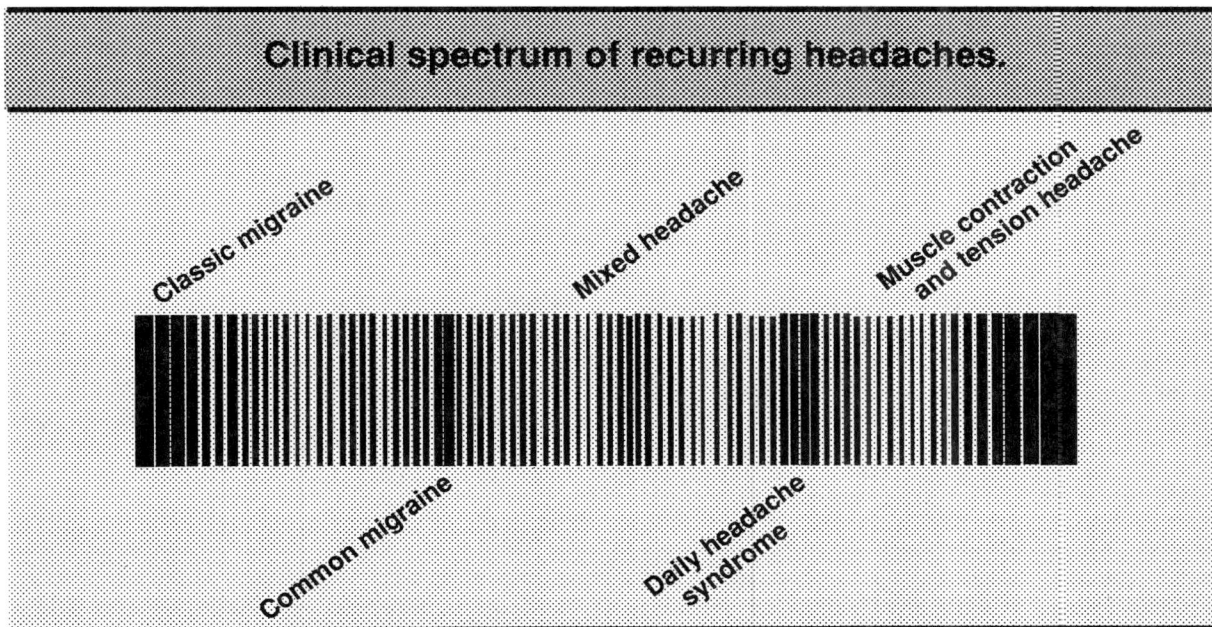

Figure 33.1. Clinical spectrum of recurring headaches.

Table 33.2.
Average Self-Rating Depression Scales among Headache Patients[a]

Category of Headache	Number of Patients	Depression Scale Score	Average Age	Percentage of Women
Migraine	1219	37	36	81
Cluster	222	35	37	12
Mixed vascular and tension-type	1113	52	44	79
Tension-type	379	55	47	54

[a]Scores above 50 are considered to indicate clinical depression.

the management and prognosis of chronic mixed headache syndrome (5). **Depression** has been identified as an associated feature of mixed headache syndrome. The causal relationship between headache and depression has been controversial. Some authors consider depression to be a cause of headache, while others consider depression to be secondary to headache. Tricyclic antidepressants have been shown to reduce the frequency and severity of migraine, and more so in mixed headache (8). A self-rating depression scale done at the Houston Headache Clinic (Table 33.2) shows that groups of patients with mixed headache and tension-type headache show elevated scales compared with episodic migraine or cluster headache patients. This may indicate the relationship of depression with the chronicity and duration of the headache and lack of substantial headache-free intervals in the first two groups.

Neuroticism as evidenced by elevated scores on scales 1, 2, and 3 (hypochondriasis, depression, and hysteria) of the Minnesota multiphasic personality inventory has been documented in patients with chronic recurrent headaches. Pure migraine and cluster headache patients obtain lower scores than do tension-type and mixed headache groups.

This may be due to more frequent and longer headache-free intervals. There is some indication that neuroticism is an integral part of the headache etiology.

The third and probably most difficult complication of the chronic mixed headache syndrome is the **chronic pain behavior** that may ensue in these patients. This may interfere with successful management and prognosis. Learned pain behavior is chronic and is based on conditioning; it can be influenced by contingent reinforcement. Common reinforcers of chronic headache behavior include medications taken "as needed," attention from people around the patient, and frequent emergency room visits. Headache behaviors are reinforced by leading to "time out" and by enabling the patient to avoid adverse consequences. Examples are absence from work, avoidance of household duties, or avoidance of sexual relations because of headache. Chronic headache behavior might also be perpetuated if positive activity and behavior is punished or is not reinforced.

Apart from the development of chronic headache behavior in patients, the behavior and attitude toward the patient by others, such as physicians, nurses, family, and spouse, change. Excessive sympathy and overprotection, or neglect, rejection, or abuse may occur. After the physician has dealt with one of these patients for a while without success, the next step is usually rejection of the patient, often by means of psychological labels such as "hysteric," "suggestible," "conversion reaction," "secondary gain," "psychogenic headache," and "difficult." Sometimes patients are told that it is all in their heads, or this message is indirectly communicated by referring them to psychologists or psychiatrists for evaluation.

Traditional psychiatric interventions do not work well with patients like this, and often the patient is advised to live with the headache. This advice typically produces anger on the part of the patient and leads to further medical assessment and evaluation. Since the patient knows there is pain, being told the headache is imaginary seems absurd, and the health-care professionals involved lose credibility. From such interactions an iatrogenic illness may develop that includes chemical dependency, increased headache associated with long-term use of ergotamine analgesics and caffeine (drug-induced headache) (9), and drug-induced psychological symptoms such as depression, anxiety, sleeplessness, and social withdrawal. The mixed headache group is especially vulnerable to iatrogenic complications of headache (Table 33.3).

DRUG-INDUCED HEADACHE

Analgesic and ergotamine overuse can result in headache resembling mixed headaches. The characteristic features of drug-induced headache are a self-sustaining, rhythmic headache, medication cycle characterized by daily or almost daily headache, and an irresistible and predictable use of symptomatic medication as the only means of relieving headache attacks. The drug-induced headache has many characteristics, including varying severity, location, and type and the tendency to be precipitated by the slightest physical or intellectual effort. Most of the time it is difficult to distinguish it from primary headache disorders, such as tension-type headache and migraine. Most of those

Table 33.3.
Iatrogenic Complications of Mixed Headache

Ergot compounds: Toxicity; dependency (withdrawal and rebound headache); peripheral vascular spasm (gangrene); coronary artery symptoms; seizures, amaurosis, hemiparesis and cerebral effects; peripheral neuropathy

Caffeine: Headache due to excessive use of caffeine-containing products; caffeine-induced nervousness, restlessness, insomnia

Methysergide: Retroperitoneal fibrosis; pleuropulmonary fibrosis; endocardial fibrosis

Phenacetin: Nephropathy and tumors

Paradoxical effects of analgesics: Interfere with endorphin system

Benzodiazepine dependency: Withdrawal seizures, delirium

Propranolol: Fatigue, bradycardia

with a history of migraine exhibit some features of migraine during some of the daily headache attacks, although they rarely show the typical and distinct pattern of migraine attacks. A drug-induced headache can be throbbing. Accompanying symptoms are very striking in drug-induced headache and include asthenia, nausea, restlessness, irritability, memory problems, difficulty in intellectual concentration, and behavioral abnormalities such as depression and neurotic behavioral patterns.

Sleep Abnormalities. Difficulty in initiating and maintaining sleep and early-morning awakening with severe headache are very common in patients with drug-induced headaches. This was observed in 71% of our patients (9). Predictable early morning (between 2 AM and 6 AM) headache occurred in 46%. There is usually a correlation between predictable early morning headache and a high intake of butalbital, caffeine, or ergotamine. Most patients take their analgesic or ergotamine tablets in the early morning hours when they wake up with a headache.

Tolerance. Tolerance develops to symptomatic medications including analgesics, analgesic sedatives, caffeine preparations, narcotics, nasal decongestants, and vasoconstrictor analgesic combinations like isometheptene mucate (Midrin, Carnrick Laboratories, Cedar Knolls, NJ), resulting in gradually increasing frequency of consumption and total quantity of medication. As with ergotamine, medication may be consumed in anticipation of headache or long before the actual headache attack occurs. Fear of an impending severe headache leads to consumption of symptomatic medications unnecessarily. This phenomenon is not entirely the fault of the patient, because there is no reliable way for a patient to predict which of the minor headaches will lead to a severe episode.

Withdrawal Headache and Related Symptoms. Abrupt cessation of daily excessive symptomatic medications may result in increased intensity of headache, accompanied by nausea, abdominal cramps, diarrhea, restlessness, sleeplessness, and mental anguish. These symptoms are especially common in patients who consume butalbital and caffeine analgesic combinations. Seizures have been reported in certain instances. The increased headache intensity may start within 24 to 48 hours, and in most cases it subsides in 5 to 7 days.

Headache Improvement after Withdrawal of Symptomatic Medications. The most striking feature of drug-induced headache is the continued improvement in headache frequency and severity, general well-being, sleep patterns, and a reduction in irritability, depression, and lethargy after the initial withdrawal is over. In our series of 200 patients, mere discontinuation of symptomatic medication resulted in a 52% improvement in the headache index (9). Addition of prophylactic medication, after discontinuation of daily symptomatic medications, resulted in 78% improvement in a 12-week period.

Concomitant Prophylactic Agents. From our study (9), it is clear that daily excessive use of symptomatic medications nullifies the beneficial effects of concomitant prophylactic agents. Of our 200 patients, 116 (58%) were on prophylactic antimigraine medications, yet they continued to have daily headache. Withdrawal of daily symptomatic medication enhanced the effect of prophylactic agents.

TREATMENT OF MIXED HEADACHE

Because of the complications described above, prophylactic therapy designed to reduce the frequency and severity of headaches is often preferred to repeated use of analgesic or narcotic medications. There are three main modalities of prophylactic pharmacotherapy, biofeedback therapy, and behavioral management. Prophylactic pharmacotherapy offers substantial long-term benefits and has now come to be accepted as the most important modality of treatment for chronic recurrent headache (7, 8).

While prophylactic therapy appears to be promising, a number of problems may be encountered. These include individual differences among patients in responsiveness to different medications and an inability to sustain good therapeutic response as time progresses. Under these circumstances it may be logical to use combinations of medication and other modalities of treatment concomitantly to achieve better long-term results (8).

The key to successful management of chronic recurrent headache is correct diagnosis. Organic conditions that may mimic benign recurrent headache have to be ruled out with proper history, physical examination, neurological examination, and whenever indicated, ancillary neurological workup. Emotional history, family history, and behavioral history are extremely important in the overall management of the patient. Physicians should take an interest in the patient's complaints, explore the headache in its entirety, make the diagnosis and explain it to the patient, foster a positive attitude toward prognosis, and provide continuity of care.

Continuity of care and a close patient-physician relationship are extremely important for effective handling of chronic headache patients. Over the past few years, a few well-organized headache clinics have been established in various parts of the world where the approach to the treatment of chronic headache differs from that of a busy physician whose interests are not particularly directed to headache. Headache clinics emphasize complete evaluation of the patients, and their emotional environment, making an adequate diagnosis, initiating prophylactic treatment (often involving several modalities), and ensuring continuity of care.

Since the biochemistry and mechanism of pain in migraine and related headaches differ from those of other chronic pains, it is imperative that chronic recurrent headache be addressed separately from other chronic pain. There are numerous abortive and prophylactic pharmaceutical agents, other than analgesics, that can be successfully used in the treatment of headache. Headache clinics differ from pain clinics in their pharmacological approach and in their less extensive physical and behavioral approach, even though the behavioral approach is used to a significant degree in headache clinics as well.

The simple mixed headache in which muscular and vascular features coexist during a well-circumscribed attack is best treated with medication for the symptomatic relief of the predominant headache element. For a simple muscular pain, simple analgesics and nonsteroidal antiinflammatory agents may be useful. For an acute migrainous attack, ergotamine tartrate or Midrin, often in conjunction with antinausea medications, is appropriate. At times medications useful for both elements are required.

The long-term prophylactic management of chronic mixed headache syndrome involves a number of other factors. Elimination of daily analgesics is extremely important. Many patients who become habituated may require hospitalization to end chronic analgesic or narcotic use.

Medications most appropriate to the prophylaxis of common migraine headache include combinations of propranolol and tricyclic antidepressants (8). A randomized controlled study was undertaken at the Houston Headache Clinic (8). The three most commonly used modalities in the prophylactic treatment of headache—propranolol, amitriptyline, and biofeedback training—were compared individually and in combination. Three hundred forty patients with mixed headache were randomly allotted to eight therapeutic categories. The total duration of the study was 3½ years, and the therapeutic groups were evaluated for a period of 7 months, including 1 month of pretreatment observation. Improvement was assessed by percentage of change in the average headache index during the last 3 months of evaluation from the pretreatment headache index.

In the migraine group, 273 patients completed the study. Improvement was significantly higher in patients receiving prophylactic treatment than in control patients who were on abortive ergotamine treatment. Propranolol plus biofeedback yielded the best results in the migraine group, and addition of amitriptyline did not significantly change the percentage of improvement. Propranolol alone (62%) was significantly superior to amitriptyline (42%) (P<.01) The difference between propranolol alone and propranolol plus amitriptyline was not statistically significant.

In the mixed headache group, 281 patients completed the study. The most effective treatment was a combination of amitriptyline, propranolol, and biofeedback training. Amitriptyline alone was superior to propranolol alone in the treatment of mixed headache (P<.01). A combination of propranolol and amitriptyline was superior to either alone. Biofeedback alone did not appear to be the treatment of choice, but it significantly contributed to better results as an adjunct when it was combined with pharmacological agents. Concomitant use of propranolol and amitriptyline did not result in any adverse reaction or clinical incompatibility.

Nonsteroidal antiinflammatory agents also have a definite place in prophylactic management. In some patients who do not tolerate tricyclic compounds, monoamine oxidase inhibitors are beneficial; however, they should be used with extreme caution because of the inherent side effects of that particular group of medications. Methysergide is a useful prophylactic agent in chronic recurrent migraine syndrome. However, it is the author's belief that it should be prescribed only under close supervision and monitoring, with full knowledge of the possible long-term side effects, especially retroperitoneal fibrosis.

REFERENCES

1. Ad Hoc Committee. Classification of headache. JAMA 1962;6:717.
2. Headache Classification Committee of the International Headache Society. Headache classification. Cephalalgia 1988;8(suppl 7):9–96.
3. Mathew NT, Stubits E, Nigam MP. Transformation of episodic migraine into daily headache: analysis of factors. Headache 1982;22:66–68.
4. Mathew NT, Reuveni U, Perez F. Transformed or evolutive migraine. Headache 1987;27:102–106.
5. Mathew NT. New horizons in the management of headache: the headache clinic. Neurol Clin 1983;1(2):533–549.
6. Zeigler DK, Hassanein RS, Couch JR. Headache syndrome suggested by statistical analysis of headache symptoms. Cephalalgia 1982;2:125–134.
7. Saper JR. The mixed headache syndrome: a new perspective. Headache 1982;22:284–286.
8. Mathew NT. Prophylaxis of migraine and mixed headache. A randomized controlled study. Headache 1981;21:105–109.
9. Mathew NT, Kurman R, Perez F. Drug induced refractory headache—clinical features and management. Headache 1990;30:634–638.

34

Headache in the Pediatric and Adolescent Population

A. DAVID ROTHNER

Headache is a frequent symptom in children and adolescents. Acutely it may be an incidental symptom accompanying fever, respiratory infections, systemic infections, or a "serious" symptom in an acute central nervous system disorder. Chronically, it may be seen in children and adolescents with migraine, stress, and increased intracranial pressure. Headache affects the lifestyle of both children and their parents and may result in significant time lost from school. Differentiating non-life-threatening acute illness from life-threatening acute illness and recognizing psychological distress requires that all physical and psychological causes be investigated in order to make the correct diagnosis and begin appropriate treatment. The evaluative process may be difficult for even the most experienced clinician. Although the vast majority of headaches in children and adolescents are not associated with organic disease, parents frequently seek a physician's aid, fearing that their child has a brain tumor. These fears must be dealt with in a realistic and sympathetic fashion when evaluating the child with headache.

HISTORICAL ASPECTS

Although Hippocrates described migraine more than 25 centuries ago, very few references were made concerning the subject of headaches in children until 1873, when William Henry Day, a British pediatrician, devoted a chapter in his book *Essays On Diseases In Children* to the subject of headaches (1). He recognized that nonorganic, nonvascular headaches were the most common type in children and stated, "Headaches in the young are for the most part due to bad arrangements in their lives." Lewis Carroll brought his migrainous hallucinations to life when he created Alice in *Through the Looking Glass*. The fact that the images of Alice's changes in size appear in a children's story is particularly appropriate, since headaches are so common in children. Bille reported on the incidence and nature of headaches in 9000 school children in 1962 (2). He noted that by age seven, 1.4% of children had true migraine headaches, 2.5% had frequent nonmigrainous headaches, and 35% had infrequent headaches of other varieties. By age 15, 5.3% had migraine headaches, 15.7% had frequent nonmigrainous (muscle-contraction headaches),

and 54% had experienced infrequent nonmigrainous headaches. Since that time, three books on the subject of headaches in children have appeared: by Friedman and Harms in 1967 and more recently by Barlow and Hockaday (3–5). A recent study by Stewart et al. once again established the concept that headaches appearing under the age of 20 are quite common (6).

PATHOPHYSIOLOGY

Both extracranial and intracranial structures are sensitive to pain. The extracranial structures sensitive to pain include the larger vessels. Intracranial tissue sensitive to pain include the sinuses, larger veins, dural arteries, and the arteries at the base of the brain. Pain in and about the face and the front half of the skull is mediated via the fifth cranial nerve; smaller areas are innervated by branches of cranial nerves 7, 9 and 10. Pain in the occipital portion of the skull is mediated via the upper cervical nerves. Certain areas such as the brain itself, the cranium, and portions of the dura, ependyma, and choroid plexus are insensitive to pain. Any condition causing inflammation, displacement, or invasion of these innervated structures causes pain (7). There is no reason to suspect that the mechanism for transmitting pain to the cortex and/or the biochemical and neural mechanisms of initiating a migraine attack are any different in a child than in an adult (8).

CLASSIFICATION

The classification of headaches is based on the presumed location of the abnormality, its origin, its pathophysiology, or the symptom complex. The International Headache Society has recently updated its classification (9). This classification is useful for those doing research in the field of headache. A simpler classification divides the headaches into those that are vascular in etiology such as migraine and cluster headache, those that are due to intracranial abnormalities such as brain tumors, and those that are secondary to stress. Such a classification is outlined in Diamond and Dalessio in their recent text (10). Clinically, I find it useful to classify headaches by incorporating their temporal pattern. By plotting the severity of the headache over time, four sequences result: acute, acute and recurrent, chronic and progressive, chronic and nonprogressive (Fig. 34.1) (11). The fifth sequence, the mixed headache syndrome, combines symptoms of acute recurrent headache, superimposed upon chronic nonprogressive headaches. This is most frequently seen in adolescents.

An acute headache is a single event with no history of a previous similar event. If this event is associated with a fever and a flu-like syndrome, symptomatic treatment is indicated. However, if this event is associated with neurological symptoms or signs, a quick and accurate diagnosis is critical since intervention can be lifesaving. The differential diagnosis of this type of headache involves a wide variety of potential disorders including systemic illness, central nervous system infection, subarachnoid hemorrhage, trauma, and toxins such as lead and carbon monoxide. The history and physical examination are critical in differentiating these etiologies.

Acute recurrent headaches are events that *recur* periodically in a similar fashion. Most often they are migrainous, with severe throbbing head pain associated with nausea and vomiting.

Chronic progressive headaches worsen in severity and frequency over time. When these headaches are accompanied by symptoms of increased intracranial pressure such as lethargy, personality change, vomiting, or abnormal neurological signs, an organic process should be suspected.

Chronic nonprogressive headaches may be constant, occur daily, or several times weekly without significant change in severity. These headaches are not usually associated with symptoms of increased intracranial pressure or an abnormal neurological examination. They are usually related to stress and are psychological.

The fifth category, the mixed headache syndrome, is acute recurrent headache, superimposed upon chronic nonprogressive headaches. The episodic headache is migrainous. The nonprogressive headache is similar to that seen in chronic stress syndromes. The patient is able to differentiate between the two types of headache when

questioned. Symptoms of increased intracranial pressure are not present and the neurological examination is normal. The practitioner is aided by this dimension of time to determine the need and the urgency of intervention.

MEDICAL EVALUATION

The medical model for the evaluation of the child or adolescent with headaches includes a thorough history, general physical examination, and detailed neurological examination (12). The history is the key to the correct diagnosis and allows the examiner to differentiate between "benign" headache types and headaches that are symptomatic of central nervous system pathology. The clinician should suspect the etiology of the headache syndrome at the conclusion of the history. Questions should be directed to both the child and the parent. Even a young child can provide useful information, although somewhat less reliable and less specific. In adolescents a private interview is useful. Answers to the questions listed in Figure 34.2 provide a data base upon which to formulate a diagnosis. Additional questions concerning symptoms of increased intracranial pressure such as ataxia, lethargy, seizures, weakness, personality change, and visual disturbance should also be obtained. The standard pediatric history regarding pregnancy, labor, delivery, growth, development, behavior, previous encephalopathic events, academic function, and systems review provide additional information pertinent to the headache problem. When one obtains further information concerning hypertension, chronic sinus disease, recurrent abdominal pain or limb pain, previous emotional disorders, significant head trauma, and the use of medications for other conditions, a better understanding of the headache problem results. Pay attention to the affect of the child and the parents during the interview, as useful clues concerning depression, anxiety, conflict, and hostility can be obtained.

The general physical examination must include the measurement of blood pressure, even in the young child, as

Figure 34.1. Headache types.

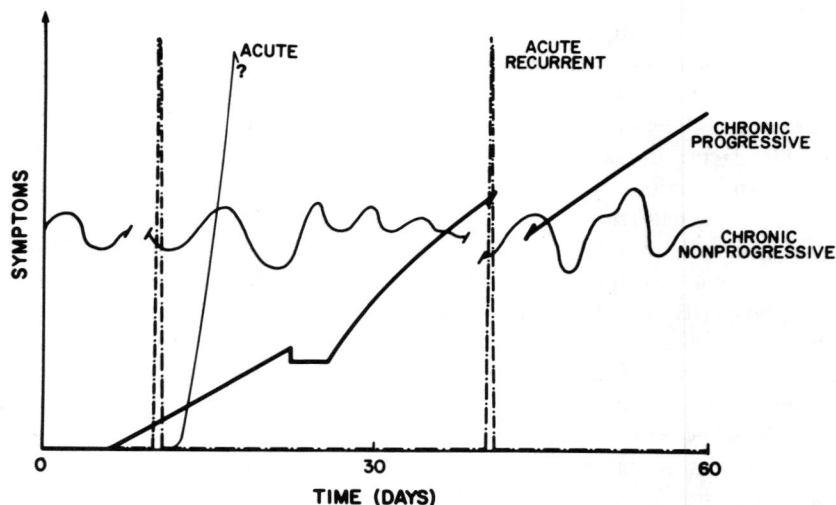

1. Do you have single or multiple types of headache?
2. How did the headache(s) begin?
3. How long have they been present?
4. Are your headaches worsening or staying the same?
5. How frequently do they occur?
6. How long do they last?
7. Do they occur under any special circumstances or at any special time?
8. Are they preceded by warning symptoms?
9. Where are they located?
10. What are the characteristics of the pain?
11. Do you have associated symptoms during the headache?
12. Do you stop what you are doing during the headache?
13. Are symptoms of increased intracranial pressure present between headaches?
14. Do you have any chronic medical problem?
15. Does any particular medication make the headache better?
16. Does any particular activity make the headache worse?
17. Do you take any medication on a regular basis?
18. Does anyone else in your family have headaches?

Figure 34.2. Questions for use in evaluating patients complaining of headache.

this may be the only clue to hypertension. Each organ system should be examined, since it may participate in the genesis of a headache problem. The skin should be examined closely, looking for petechiae, striae, café au lait spots, or hypopigmented macules that may indicate a central nervous system etiology for the headache.

The thorough neurological examination begins with the measurement of the cranial circumference compared with normal values. If the head is significantly enlarged and this is not a familial trait, one should seek hydrocephalus or an occult tumor as a possible cause. An underlying vascular malformation may be suspected if auscultation of the cranium reveals a machinery-like bruit. Tenderness of the scalp may indicate trauma in a battered child. The fundoscopic examination, which may be difficult in a small child, is frequently left until the end of the examination, to avoid losing the child's cooperation. Findings such as optic atrophy, papilledema, or hemorrhages require further diagnostic testing. A sixth nerve palsy or the inability to move the eye laterally may indicate nonlocalized increased intracranial pressure. Any combination of lower cranial nerve abnormalities, cerebellar dysfunction, or long track signs may indicate a brainstem or posterior fossa lesion. If the neurological examination is abnormal, neuroimaging is necessary.

Throughout the history and examination, the mental status of the patient should be monitored, since behavioral

problems, a thought disorder, or encephalitis may be pertinent to the diagnosis.

CHOOSING APPROPRIATE TESTS

At the conclusion of the history and physical examination and before selecting laboratory tests, the clinician should classify the headache type. If the patient is acutely ill, a rapid evaluation is in order. If the patient has episodic headaches that appear to be migrainous, no laboratory testing is usually required. Patients with progressive headache and neurological symptoms and signs require further evaluation and a neuroimaging procedure. Patients with nonprogressive daily headaches may need a neuroimaging study to include their sinuses as well as a more in-depth investigation of psychological issues.

LABORATORY STUDIES

The choice of laboratory tests rests upon the differential diagnosis (13). Roentgenograms of the skull are no longer used routinely. The electroencephalogram is of limited value in the routine evaluation of children with headaches. Nonspecific abnormalities are frequently found not only in children with a wide variety of central nervous system disorders but in many normal children. In acute disorders, persistent slowing must be evaluated with neuroimaging. Epileptiform abnormalities occur to a slightly greater degree in migrainous patients, but their clinical significance and relevance to therapy is unclear (14).

Computerized tomography (CT) and magnetic resonance imaging (MRI) are safe, rapid, accurate methods of evaluating the intracranial contents (15). They are useful in a wide variety of conditions including malformations, CNS infections, trauma, neoplasms, degenerative disorders, and vascular disorders. Their accuracy exceeds that of roentgenograms of the skull, EEG, angiography, and pneumoencephalography combined. They are the most valuable tests in evaluating headaches of suspected organic etiology. The author feels that magnetic resonance imaging is even more accurate than CT in delineating abnormalities in the vicinity of the sella turcica, posterior fossa, cranial-cervical junction, and temporal lobe. MRI is better able to visualize vascular problems, neoplasms, white matter abnormalities, and congenital anomalies than is the CT scan. The additional modality of magnetic resonance angiography (MRA) has made MRI even more valuable in the diagnosis of vascular disorders and neoplasms.

Lumbar puncture is effective in determining the presence of an infectious process or increased intracranial pressure such as is seen in pseudotumor cerebri. With advanced studies of the globulin fractions, demyelinating disease can also be diagnosed. If an intracranial space-occupying lesion is suspected, lumbar puncture may be contraindicated, as it may cause herniation. It should be preceded in these instances by neuroimaging.

Psychological tests are useful in patients with stress-related headaches as well as those with migraine headaches thought to be precipitated by stressful circumstances (16). Included are tests of general intelligence such as the Wechsler Intelligence Scale for Children-3 and the Woodcock Johnson Achievement Battery. Personality tests such as the Minnesota Multiphasic Personality Inventory (MMPI), and projective testing such as the Rorshach and the Thematic Apperception tests may also be useful. An interview with an experienced psychologist or social worker is invaluable.

SPECIFIC HEADACHE SYNDROMES
Acute

An isolated acute headache may represent a difficult diagnostic problem. These headaches may be separated into those with generalized pain and those in which the pain is localized.

ACUTE GENERALIZED HEADACHE

Two to 6% of all emergency room visits are due to headache (17). Data relating to acute headaches in the emergency room in the pediatric and adolescent population are not available. In the general emergency room population, 40% of patients had non–central nervous system infections, 20% had tension headaches, 10% had traumatic headaches, 5% had vascular headaches, and 5% had headaches related to hypertension. The remaining patients had a variety of other disorders. The presence of altered consciousness, stiff neck, high fever, a shock-like state, or focal neurological abnormalities requires rapid evaluation. Acute illness, temperature elevation, hypertension, nuchal rigidity, papilledema, retinal hemorrhage, focal neurological signs, or a disturbed affect may direct the clinician to a specific diagnosis.

An unusual form of generalized acute headache related to exertion occurs in patients involved in weight lifting, running, or playing football (18). A generalized throbbing headache develops and lasts a few minutes to several hours. When transient neurological deficits occur, neuroimaging is necessary. When these headaches become recurrent, indomethacin is a useful prophylactic therapy. Laboratory evaluation of patients with acute headache depends upon their degree of illness and suspected diagnosis. If the patient is critically ill or has a stiff neck and subarachnoid hemorrhage or meningitis is suspected, hospital admission is necessary and neuroimaging will be needed.

ACUTE LOCALIZED HEADACHE

Sinusitis causes headaches in up to 13% of children with sinus disease (19). It is most frequently found in association with an upper respiratory tract infection or chronic allergies. Focal tenderness may be present. The diagnosis is best confirmed by CT or MRI scanning. Complications of sinusitis may include brain abscess, orbital cellulitis, and meningitis. Treatment with antibiotics and decongestants is usually needed; surgical drainage may be needed as well.

Otitis media is a common disorder of childhood. Its complications, hearing loss, mastoiditis, and (rarely) brain abscess, represent significant health hazards. Severe pain is localized to the ear. Examination reveals a hyperemic, bulging tympanic membrane with poor mobility. Antibiotics are the treatment of choice.

Astigmatism, refractory errors, exotropia, and esotropia are suspected of causing headaches but rarely do so (20). If frontal headaches are associated with reading, watching television, or doing homework, and occur in the late afternoon or evening, the patient should have an opthalmologic examination. If a specific abnormality is detected, its correction will bring relief. It should be stressed that most patients examined for eye strain or other ocular causes of headache have no abnormality.

Orbital cellulitis, an infection of the soft tissues around the eye, presents with fever, pain, swelling, and redness. An associated sinus infection is usually present, and *vigorous* parenteral antibiotic therapy is needed.

Optic and retrobulbar neuritis causing eye pain and decreased visual activity, are uncommon in younger children but become slightly more common in late adolescence. It may be idiopathic, postinfectious, or the initial symptom of multiple sclerosis.

Dental disorders and temporomandibular joint (TMJ) dysfunction may cause headaches. Pain localized to the jaw almost always predominates and suggests the proper diagnosis. When psychological factors seem to be important, the syndrome is called the myofascial pain syndrome; referral to a dental specialist and psychologist is indicated (21).

Acute headache associated with head trauma is related to the specific area of impact and usually resolves within a few days. Two forms of chronic protracted headache occur. The first is rare, is localized to the area of trauma, and may be related to the formation of a neuroma. Reassurance, analgesics, and time will usually result in improvement. If a fracture has occurred, a leptomeningeal cyst or growing skull fracture, must be ruled out. Reexamination is indicated if symptoms worsen, new symptoms appear, or new signs develop. The second form of protracted headache related to trauma is the postconcussion syndrome, which is considered in the discussion of chronic nonprogressive headaches.

Occipital neuralgia is a pain localized to the occipital and upper cervical areas. It is characterized by unilateral or bilateral acute or chronic occipital and suboccipital headaches. Scalp pain, local tenderness, and paresthesia in the distribution of the second cervical dermatome may be present. The normal cervical lordosis is lost. The pain may be related to congenital cervical spine abnormalities or trauma. There may be instability between the first and second cervical segments, with intermittent compression of the cervical roots. The pain is referred via the auricular, greater occipital, or lesser occipital nerves. Reflex spasm of the neck muscles reduces mobility and produces additional pain. Roentgenograms or MRI scanning of the cervical spine is necessary. Improvement is often achieved by using a soft cervical collar, muscle relaxants, analgesics, heat, massage, and cervical isometric exercises.

Acute Recurrent Headaches

MIGRAINE

Migraine is a specific genetic disorder characterized by episodic, periodic paroxysmal attacks of vasoconstriction and vasodilation (22). By age 15, 5% of adolescents have experienced a migraine attack. In 50% of all individuals who have migraine headaches, the attacks start before the age of 20. In early childhood, boys are affected more frequently, but with puberty, girls are affected more frequently. The family history is positive in 70% of cases. The disorder is inherited as an autosomal-dominant with greater penetrance in females. Episodes are precipitated by trigger phenomena such as anxiety, stress, fatigue, head trauma, excitement, exercise, menses, travel, illness, diet, and medication. In classic migraine the headache is preceded by an aura that usually consists of visual phenomena. The aura in common migraine is autonomic and includes irritability, fatigue, malaise, pallor, and nausea. The headache in either form may be unilateral or bilateral and is throbbing in nature. Anorexia, nausea and vomiting, abdominal pain, photophobia, phonophobia, and the desire to sleep are present in both forms of migraine. Attacks last an average of 2 to 6 hours and are briefer than those in adults. The usual frequency is one to two attacks per month. Less frequently, the disorder occurs once weekly or more.

Treatment is individualized depending on the age and reliability of the patients as well as the frequency and severity of attacks. Patients seem to have fewer and less severe attacks after they are reassured that no serious problem exists. In patients under age 14 years with occasional headaches, analgesics, antiemetics, and sedatives during the attack are useful. Narcotic analgesics are infrequently needed. If attacks occur several times per month or are particularly severe, prophylaxis using daily medication should be considered. Cyproheptadine and propranolol are the most commonly used medications. The supposed efficacies of phenytoin and phenobarbital are poorly documented. Methysergide and amitriptyline should not be used routinely. The usual dosage of cyproheptadine is 8 to 12 mg per day, and its major side effects are sedation and increased appetite. Propranolol has been used successfully in the prophylaxis of migraine in children and adolescents. It is contraindicated in patients with asthma, bradycardia, and depression. Doses of 80 to 320 mg per day for 4 to 6 months have been used with good results. Many patients will not experience a return of their problem when medications are discontinued. If attacks do recur and are severe, therapy may be resumed.

In older teenage patients with either frequent or infrequent attacks, and a well-defined aura, treatment includes the use of ergotamine or isometheptene mucate. The instructions are the same as those given for adults. If this approach is unsuccessful or if the attacks are frequent, prophylactic medication, using propranolol or amitriptyline is suggested.

COMPLEX MIGRAINE

Hemiplegic migraine is defined as recurrent unilateral weakness in association with headaches. In most patients, the weakness follows and outlasts the headache. The mechanism is thought to be vasoconstriction and resultant transient anoxia in the distribution of the internal carotid or middle cerebral arteries. The disorder may be familial. The hemiplegia may stay on one side or alternate sides during subsequent attacks. Intraarterial angiography should be avoided during the acute attack; an MRI-MRA to rule out a structural abnormality is needed. The treatment is similar to that for classic migraine. In recalcitrant cases, anticonvulsants calcium-channel blockers or rarely methysergide can be tried.

The presenting symptoms of ophthalmoplegic migraine are eye pain and complete or incomplete third-nerve palsy. Unilateral pupillary dilatation, outward deviation of the eye, and ptosis are common signs. The possible existence of an intracranial aneurysm is of concern. MRI-MRA is needed to rule out a vascular lesion. In many patients, the ocular abnormality lasts from days to weeks after the headache has disappeared. A short course of steroids may shorten the duration of the ophthalmoplegia. Most patients recover completely. This disorder may even occur in infants. Permanent sequelae are rare.

MIGRAINE VARIANTS

The symptoms of *acute confusional migraine* include an altered sensorium and agitation. Other causes of acute mental disturbance include encephalitis, psychosis, and toxic-metabolic disorders must be considered. The association with migraine is frequently appreciated in retrospect. Some patients have prolonged stupor preceding or following the episode of confusion. The evaluation of some of these patients includes toxicology screening, electroencephalography, and neuroimaging. When recurrent, the episodes can be treated as is migraine.

Basilar artery migraine is suggested by recurrent attacks of neurological dysfunction referable to the brainstem and cerebellum. Vasoconstriction in the distribution of the basilar artery is postulated. Episodes occur suddenly and clear completely. Symptoms include occipital headache, vertigo, nausea, vomiting, tinnitus, and facial or limb weakness. Signs include ataxia, alternating hemiparesis, and occasionally loss of consciousness. Basilar artery migraine is more common in children and adolescents.

Paroxysmal vertigo occurs in children between 2 and 7

years. The episodes are sudden and brief. The youngsters cannot stand. Consciousness is retained. They sit down and hold on tightly and are tearful during the attack. Nystagmus may be present. Typical migraine may develop in the future. This may be a variant of basilar artery migraine. Headache is usually absent, however; the prognosis is good. The administration of diphenhydramine daily for several months may be helpful if the attacks are frequent and disabling.

Paroxysmal torticollis is a self-limited, benign entity, characterized by recurrent episodes of head tilt, nausea, vomiting, pallor, agitation, and ataxia that last a few hours. Headache may or may not be present. This disorder is rare. One should consider other more serious posterior fossa problems when a child with head tilt or ataxia is evaluated.

The periodic syndrome and cyclic vomiting are episodes of unexplained abdominal pain and vomiting that occur paroxysmally in children. Headache may be absent. Structural intermittent obstruction of the GI tract must be ruled out prior to making this diagnosis. Classic or common migraine may coexist or develop later in some of these patients. Cyproheptadine, propranolol, or amitriptyline may be useful in preventing further attacks.

The diagnosis of the "epilepsy equivalent syndrome" is made too frequently in the author's opinion. Since both migraine and epilepsy are common, it is not uncommon for a patient to have both epilepsy and migraine headaches. The relationship between epilepsy and migraine has been reviewed by Basser (23). Episodes of headache, nausea, and vomiting in association with nonspecific electroencephalographic abnormalities or rolandic discharges should not be interpreted as seizure equivalents. My criteria for the diagnosis of the epilepsy equivalent syndrome include nausea, vomiting, and altered consciousness. A history of coexisting generalized or focal seizure supports the diagnosis, as does an EEG showing spikes or sharp waves other than rolandic spikes. A positive family history for epilepsy is frequently present. These spells respond to anticonvulsants. True epilepsy must be differentiated from migraine with an abnormal EEG (14).

Cluster headaches are not really a variant of migraine but are included here for purposes of discussion. They occur only rarely in children and adolescents (24). They consist of unilateral, periorbital pain, tearing, rhinorrhea, nasal stuffiness, and facial flushing. The pain is brief, lasting 20 to 60 minutes, and severe, recurring once or twice daily for weeks and then disappearing for months or years. A chronic form never disappears. Treatment is similar to that for migraine. The use of oxygen during an attack is helpful. The use of steroids or lithium in refractory cases has also been advocated.

Prognosis

There is a significant discrepancy in the literature concerning the outcome of migraine headaches in childhood. Bille stated that 50% of children became migraine-free and 34% improved 4 to 6 years after diagnosis (25). His criterion for recovery was freedom from attacks for 1 year. Hockaday questioned whether it was ever safe to say that migraine had remitted completely, since ten of her patients with migraine had been symptom-free for 4 to 10 years (5). The outcome in an individual case cannot be predicted.

Chronic Progressive Headaches

This group of disorders includes brain tumors, psuedotumor cerebri, hydrocephalus, brain abscess, and subdural hematoma, which cause headaches that are progressive both in severity and frequency over time. The rapidity with which the process progresses determines the rapidity of the evaluative process. Symptoms of increased intracranial pressure are common and include nausea, vomiting, ataxia, weakness, lethargy, personality change, intellectual deterioration, visual disturbances, sensory abnormalities, and seizures. The physical examination may be normal or show papilledema and a sixth-nerve palsy as nonlocalizing signs of increased intracranial pressure. The type of pathological process and its location may result in varying combinations of cortical, pyramidal, extrapyramidal, cerebellar, and cranial nerve abnormalities. If a structural abnormality of the central nervous system is suspected, an enhanced CT including the sinuses or an MRI scan is the diagnostic test of choice.

BRAIN TUMOR

Headaches caused by a brain tumor are progressive in both frequency and severity (26). There may be pain-free intervals. The headache may be caused by the mass itself or by hydrocephalus secondary to obstruction of cerebrospinal fluid flow. The location of the headache has limited localizing value. Exertion, change in position, coughing, and defecation may exacerbate the pain. The quality of the pain is variable and not diagnostic. The headache may be more severe in the morning and may be associated with and relieved by vomiting. Younger children unable to describe the pain may simply be irritable and restless. At least 70% of children with brain tumors have headache as a presenting symptom. The headache is diffuse in 50% of the patients, and awakens them or is present on awakening in approximately 65% of the patients. Treatment depends on the type and location of the neoplasm.

HYDROCEPHALUS

Hydrocephalus is associated with ventricular enlargement secondary to the obstruction of normal flow of cerebrospinal fluid from its point of origin to its site of absorption. There is an increased quantity of cerebrospinal fluid under increased pressure. It may be postmeningitic, posthemorrhagic, or caused by congenital abnormalities such as aqueductal stenosis. The symptoms and signs are those of increased intracranial pressure. In addition, macrocephaly, superficial cranial venous dilation, and the "sunset sign" may be present. Neuroimaging shows dilated ventricles. A ventriculoperitoneal shunt is the treatment of choice.

SUBDURAL HEMATOMA

Subdural hematomas result from head trauma, spontaneous rupture of vascular structures, or blood dyscrasia. They are frequently seen in the battered child syndrome, which may be associated with anemia and long-bone fractures. The symptoms and signs of increased intracranial pressure are usually present. Neuroimaging usually shows a rim of density in the subdural area that is distinct from the brain substance. Therapy includes drainage of the subdural collection by repeated subdural taps, external drainage, or shunting procedures.

BRAIN ABSCESS

Brain abscess is most commonly found in association with chronic ear infections or cyanotic congenital heart disease. It should also be suspected in patients who are immunosuppressed, such as patients receiving chemotherapy or those with HIV infection. The abscesses may be multiple. Fever and the usual symptoms and signs of increased intracranial pressure are present. A wide variety of focal neurological deficits may be present, depending on the location of the abscess. Neuroimaging is diagnostic. Treatment includes vigorous administration of antibiotics and surgical drainage.

PSEUDOTUMOR CEREBRI

Pseudotumor cerebri presents with symptoms and signs of increased intracranial pressure without evidence of CNS infection, mass lesion, or obstruction of cerebrospinal fluid flow. The most common symptoms are headache and visual dysfunction. The usual signs are papilledema and a sixth nerve palsy. Visual fields may show an enlarged blind spot and generalized constriction. Neuroimaging is normal. A lumbar puncture demonstrates increased pressure with normal chemistries and no cells. Among the many associated causes of this condition are outdated tetracycline, excessive vitamin A, obesity, menstrual irregularity, chronic otitis, and withdrawal from corticosteroid therapy. Most cases, however, are idiopathic. Treatment consists of repeated lumbar punctures, removing enough cerebrospinal fluid to return the pressure to normal. Diuretics as well as corticosteroids may be prescribed. If the vision is threatened or compromised, optic sheath decompression and/or shunting may be used.

Chronic Nonprogressive Headaches

Chronic nonprogressive headaches include muscle-contraction headaches, stress-related tension headaches, headaches that are depressive equivalents, conversion headaches, headaches as an expression of malingering, and protracted posttraumatic headaches (28). The combination of chronic nonprogressive headaches and migraine headache in the adolescent is not uncommon and is referred to as a mixed headache syndrome. It requires a combined psychological and pharmacological approach. The mechanism by which muscle-contraction headaches cause pain is not clear but may be related to prolonged muscle contraction and resultant muscle ischemia. In adults, nonorganic, nonvascular headaches are the most common types of headaches. In adolescents, this is probably true as well. Supportive epidemiologic evidence is lacking, however.

In Billie's study of a large series of schoolchildren, three times as many children at age 15 had frequent nonmigrainous headaches (16%) than had migraine headaches (5%). He stated that these frequent nonmigrainous headaches were stress-related. Data concerning the frequency, location, severity, quality, duration, precipitating factors, associated symptoms, family patterns, and psychological factors in chronic nonprogressive headaches in children and adolescents are not available. In reviewing "functional" headaches in adults, Friedman stated that they had no prodromata, were usually bilateral, and might be accompanied by nausea, vomiting, or both, in 15% of cases (29). The character of the pain and its frequency and duration were variable. Twenty percent of patients had constant headache, 30% had daily headaches, 35% had several headaches a week, and only 15% had headaches less than once a week. Most patients were women. A family history for any type of headache was present in 40% of the patients. Most adults began having symptoms between the ages of 20 and 40 years. My own experience suggests that stress-related headaches in children and adolescents follow clinical patterns similar to those in adults. Historically, these patients have had headaches for months to years prior to seeing a consultant. Although exacerbations and remissions are not uncommon, the course is usually prolonged, and the symptoms and signs nonprogressive. Patients may describe their symptoms in a vague and nonspecific manner. Common associated symptoms include blurred vision, fatigue, dizziness, and fainting; nausea and vomiting are uncommon. Frequent and prolonged absence from school despite an excellent academic record is quite common and suggests a stress-related disorder. It is important to ask specific questions concerning headaches in other family members, alcoholism, abuse, divorce, recent loss of a loved one, or departure of a sibling from the home. A past history of abdominal or limb pain for which no cause was found is occasionally noted. Other children have a history of psychological or behavioral problems. Anxiety, tension, and stress related to school performance, peers, or family are frequently apparent.

In these cases, the results of the general and neurological examination are normal. If one suspects a stress-related headache, laboratory testing can be limited. Some have advocated neuroimaging to rule out space-occupying lesions as well as to reassure the patient and the family that no organic abnormality exists. If this is to be done, scanning of the sinuses should be included. The psychologist or social worker is frequently able to add data supportive of a psychological etiology. In adolescents MMPI testing may be valuable. Intelligence testing and achievement testing may indicate that the youngster is incapable of meeting parental expectations of high scholastic performance. Projective testing may yield information concerning specific underlying anxieties, psychiatric disorders, or depression. The child psychologist and child psychiatrist are members of the headache evaluation unit and may confirm the diagnosis and suggest specific therapy. The patient and the family should be aided in accepting the concept of stress as the basis of the head pain.

Headaches may be a sign of depression. Manifestation of depression in childhood and adolescence include mood change, withdrawal, poor school performance, sleep disturbance, aggressive behavior, self-deprecation, lack of energy, somatic complaints, school phobia, and weight loss.

In conversion hysteria, anxiety is converted to a somatic symptom. Inappropriate lack of concern, *"LaBelle Indifference,"* about the symptom is usually present. The symptom usually provides secondary gain such as sympathy, attention, and relief from responsibilities. Often a precipitating but not causative factor is present, such as minor illness or minor trauma.

Malingering is a conscious simulation of illness used to avoid unpleasant situations. It is an uncommon cause of chronic-daily headache and usually occurs in individuals with preexisting personality disorders. Previous problems may have included emotional instability, excitable tendencies, over-reactivity, immaturity, and dependency.

The postconcussion syndrome consists of headache in association with insomnia, irritability, restlessness, personality change, lassitude, memory problems, school failure, and dizziness. A psychological problem should be suspected when the headaches have persisted longer than several months and clinical examination and laboratory studies are negative. The disorder may occur in patients in whom an underlying personality disorder predated the injury or in persons involved in litigation. Reexamination of the patient is indicated if symptoms change.

If the headaches have been present continuously or frequently for more than 6 weeks in the absence of neurological symptoms and signs, they are usually related to psychological factors. This is especially true when the headaches are coupled with prolonged absence from school. If this diagnosis is suspected during the initial interview, it should be discussed openly with both parents and child. The psychodynamics should be investigated, and a decision made quickly regarding treatment. Unfortunately, adequate data that support one therapeutic regimen over another are lacking. Treatment modalities include family counseling, individual counseling, and biofeedback, alone or in conjunction with pharmacological

agents (30). In our experience, treatment based solely on medication is rarely successful over the long term. A comprehensive treatment program must consider the patient's age, the family's responsiveness to the concept of a stress-related illness, and the availability of services in the community. Biofeedback in combination with individual counseling and amitriptyline may be useful in treating patients with stress-related headaches. Depression is best treated with antidepressants in association with counseling. If suicidal *ideations* are present, psychiatric referral is mandatory. Conversion headaches generally respond to family counseling. Malingering and the postconcussion syndrome are more complex problems, and the prognosis depends on the underlying personality disorder. Long-term psychotherapy may be necessary. No data concerning the prognosis of chronic nonprogressive headaches in children and adolescents are available. When a patient has migraine headaches superimposed upon chronic nonprogressive headaches, a combined psychological and pharmacological approach is useful. I find amitriptyline very useful in these patients.

Summary

The diagnosis and management of headache syndromes in children and adolescents have been reviewed. Deciding whether a child's headache is organic or stress-related may be difficult for even the experienced physician. A thorough and systematic history and examination coupled with selected laboratory tests will guide the practitioner to the correct diagnosis.

REFERENCES

1. Day WH. Essays on diseases of children. London: J & A Churchill, 1873.
2. Bille BS. Migraine in school children. Acta Paediatr Scand 1962;51(suppl 136):1–151.
3. Friedman AP, Harms E. Headaches in children. Springfield, IL; Charles C Thomas, 1967.
4. Barlow CF. Headaches and migraine in childhood. Philadelphia: Oxford Blackwell Scientific Publishers, 1984.
5. Hockaday JM, ed. Migraine in childhood. London: Butterworths, 1988.
6. Linet MS, Stewart WF, Celentano DD, Ziegler D, Sprecher M. An epidemiologic study of headache among adolescents and young adults, JAMA 1989;261:2211–2216.
7. Ray BS, Wolff HG. Experimental studies on headache. Pain-sensitive structures of the head and their significance in headache. Arch Surg 1940;41:813.
8. Lauritzen M, et al. Changes in regional blood flow during the course of classic migraine attacks. Ann Neurol 1983;13:633.
9. Headache Classification Committee of the International Headache Society. Proposed classification and diagnostic criteria for headache disorders, cranial neuralgias and facial pain. Cephalagia 1988;8(suppl 7):9–96.
10. Diamond S, Dalessio DJ. The practicing physician's approach to headache. 5th ed. Baltimore: Williams & Wilkins, 1992.
11. Rothner AD. Headaches in children: a review. Headache 1978; 18(3):169.
12. Paine RS, Oppe TE. Neurological examination of children. Clin Dev Med 1966;20/21.
13. Rothner AD. The diagnosis and treatment of headache syndromes in

children. In: Pediatrics update. New York: Elsevier Biomedical, 1983:55–77.

14. Kinast M, Luders H, Rothner AD, et al. Benign focal epileptiform discharges in childhood migraine (BFEDC). Neurology 1982;32:1 309–311.

15. Dooley JM, Camfield PR, O'Neill M, et al. The value of CT scans for children with headaches. Can J Neurol Sci 1990;17:309–310.

16. Harrison RH. Psychological testing in headache: a review. Headache 1975;14:177–185.

17. Dhopesh V, et al. A retrospective assessment of emergency department patients with complaint of headache. Headache 1979;19:37–42.

18. Diamond S. Prolonged benign exertional headache: its clinical characteristics and response to indomethacin. Headache 1982;22:96–98.

19. Faleck H, Rothner AD, Erenberg G, Cruse RP. Headache and subacute sinusitis in children and adolescents. Headache 1988;28:96–98.

20. Behrens MM. Headaches associated with disorders of the eye. Med Clin North Am 1978;62:507–512.

21. Belfer ML, Kaban LB. Temporomandibular joint dysfunction. Pediatrics 1982;69:564–567.

22. Rothner AD. The migraine syndrome in children and adolescents. Pediatr Neurol 1986;2:121.

23. Basser LS. The relation of migraine and epilepsy. Brain 1969;92:285–300.

24. Curless RG. Cluster headaches in childhood. J Pediatr 1982;101:393–395.

25. Hockaday JM. Late outcome of childhood onset migraine and factors affecting outcome, with particular reference to early and late EEG findings. Curr Concepts Migraine Res 1978:41–48.

26. The epidemiology of headache among children with brain tumor. Childhood Brain Tumor Consortium. J Neurooncol 1991;10:31–46.

27. Corbett JJ. Problems in the diagnosis and treatment of pseudotumor cerebri. Can J Neurol Sci 1983;10:221–229.

28. Ling W, Oftedal G, Weinberg W. Depressive illness in childhood presenting as severe headache. Am J Dis Child 1970;120:122–124.

29. Friedman AP, et al. Migraine and tension headaches—a clinical study of two thousand cases. Neurology 1954;4:773–778.

30. Fentress DW, Masek BJ, Mehegan JE, et al. Biofeedback and relaxation response to training in treatment of pediatric migraine. Dev Med Child Neurol 1986;28:139–146.

35

Headache in a Geriatric Population

ARTHUR H. ELKIND

Headache in the elderly presents many of the problems of diagnosis and treatment associated with younger individuals. Individuals over the age of 60 can be arbitrarily defined as elderly. With advancing age, numerous added difficulties arise to diagnose accurately and treat effectively without adverse events. Most of the headache types seen in younger individuals can occur in the elderly, but they often have concomitant illnesses. The complicating illnesses that exist in the geriatric patient may preclude certain therapies used successfully in younger patients. Headache sufferers will often continue with their headaches from an earlier age into the seventh and eighth decades of life or later. Symptoms of headache and characteristics of their particular type of headache may remain unchanged, but more often some gradual transition occurs so that the headache is altered in subtle ways when the patients describe their symptoms. The elderly patient with headache presents the clinician with more diagnostic possibilities that include a greater number of serious structural disorders in the differential diagnosis.

Therapeutic possibilities must include consideration of relative and absolute contraindications to treatment. Pharmacological agents that can be administered in younger patients are not as safe to use in the older patient or dosages have to be smaller and increased at a slower rate before reaching a maximum therapeutic level. However, nonpharmacological measures that were thought to be less effective in the elderly can be instituted, and my impression in recent years is that they can be safely and effectively adapted to the elderly. A recent report tends to confirm this impression (1). Biofeedback techniques are a form of nonpharmacological treatment that fits this category and may be considered in the elderly.

CLASSIFICATION OF HEADACHE IN THE ELDERLY

Table 35.1 lists the major and minor causes of headache in elderly patients. Alternate classifications include the recently proposed set provided by the International Headache Society and published in *Cephalalgia* (2). Omitted from Table 35.1 is the group of cranial typical and atypical neuralgias. Patients in the geriatric population often present with facial pains and an earlier history of migraine headaches. The source of the facial pain is not clear and is distinct from trigeminal neuralgia and other cranial neuralgic disorders.

DIAGNOSIS OF HEADACHE

A thorough history, and physical and neurological examinations are warranted for geriatric headache patients. Older individuals are more likely to have serious illnesses that mandate accurate therapy. The diagnosis must be precise if at all possible. A missed diagnosis can have immediate serious repercussions in all age groups, but the elderly are more likely to have structural disease, and therefore, an incorrect diagnosis of functional type of headache may have serious implications. In one study, tension headache was more common in older patients and migraine less common (3). In the same study, temporal arteritis occurred with the same frequency as migraine.

Several epidemiologic studies have been conducted to determine the frequency of headache in the population. The frequency is lower in individuals past the age of 55 than in those under the age of 55 (4). Migraine and tension headache may develop for the first time in later life. In one study (5), 1284 individuals past the age of 65 were questioned in an outpatient setting. Headache was reported by 11.2% of women and 5.4% of men. Women reporting numerous symptoms and diseases were more likely to report headache. Men reporting headache did not have associated symptoms or diseases. Few specific diseases were not found to relate to headache. Furthermore, glaucoma and hypertension were not significant risk factors for headache, although headache is frequently attributed to these diseases. Depression, which has long been suspected of a link to headache, was commonly associated with headache.

In addition to the history and physical examination, laboratory studies and radiologic and neuroimaging techniques must often be used in older individuals. Bruits over the carotid vessels should be sought; tonometry is important to rule out glaucoma, both to exclude the diagnosis and to establish the safety of using a tricyclic antidepressant. Elevated ocular pressures may contraindicate the use of tricyclic antidepressants in a patient with headache.

Table 35.1.
Headache Disorders in the Elderly

Major functional types
  Nonspecific for ages over 60
    Migraine
      Migraine without aura
      Migraine with aura
      Migraine with complications
    Tension-type headaches
    Tension-migraine and chronic daily headache
    Cluster headache
  Specific (although may occur over 50 as well)
    Transient migrainous accompaniments (TMA)
Structural-type disorders with a greater likelihood of occurring over 60
  Tumor, aneurysm, embolus, hemorrhage, subdural hematoma
  Atherosclerotic disease
  Cervical spondylosis
  Glaucoma
Associated with medical illnesses
  Hypertension and pheochromocytoma
  Renal disease
  Headache secondary to dialysis therapy
  Giant cell arteritis
    Temporal or cranial arteritis
  Subacute bacterial endocarditis
  Chronic obstructive pulmonary disease
  Primary and secondary polycythemia
  Infections of the central nervous system and extracranial structures
Metabolic disorders
  Hypoglycemia
  Hypercalcemia
  Endocrine disorders
  Dietary causes
Iatrogenic causes (medication)
  Nitrates: sublingual, oral, transdermal
  Caffeine abuse: as beverage and in analgesic preparations
  Ergot withdrawal
  Analgesic abuse: often combined in products with butalbital
  Antihypertensive medications: nifedipine, hydralazine
  Antiinflammatory agents: indomethacin
  Antilipidemic compounds: nicotinic acid, lovastatin

Routine chest x-rays may be indicated in individuals with a history of smoking or acute but progressive headaches suggesting neoplastic disease with metastasis to the brain. Electrocardiograms (ECGs) are also routinely indicated if a recent tracing is not available, particularly if cardiovascular agents are indicated for the treatment of migraine. An asymptomatic patient with subclinical cardiac disease may be easily detected with an ECG. The treating physician should be aware of the presence of cardiac disease if the clinician is planning to use β-adrenergic blockers or calcium entry blockers. Both groups of compounds contain agents that have negative inotropic action that can have a deleterious effect. Sedimentation rates are always advisable in elderly patients with headache, to aid in the diagnosis of temporal arteritis (discussed later).

SELECTED TYPES OF HEADACHE FOUND IN THE ELDERLY

Systemic Illnesses and Localized Disease

Headache may be a prominent symptom of systemic disease. Numerous diseases can present with headache, and headache may occur during the course of an illness al-

though not as a presenting symptom. The practitioner should attempt to elicit a history of headache during questioning about the present illness as well as during the review of systems. Individuals suffering from systemic disorders usually have physical and neurological abnormalities. Because headache may occur in so many systemic illnesses, a thorough history and physical examination is essential. Acute bacterial, rickettsial, or viral infections may result in headache. Collagen-vascular disorders can be associated with headache symptoms. Many of the acute infectious illnesses that occur in younger individuals may occur in the elderly.

A recent report by Jones and Siekert (6) comments on headache in subacute bacterial endocarditis (SBE). They note that headache may also occur with complications of SBE such as ruptured aneurysm and CNS infection. They found that 14 of 110 patients with SBE had severe headaches that led to the proper diagnosis. These individuals had no past history of headache but developed acute headache, often related to fever. Severe unremitting headache in SBE may suggest a mycotic aneurysm. New-onset headache in elderly individuals with fever should alert the physician to the possibility of SBE, particularly if a cardiac murmur is present. Diagnostic techniques including echocardiography should be employed and antibiotics withheld until blood cultures are obtained if the diagnosis is considered.

Diabetics or other patients with impaired immune responses may present with headache or facial pain and paranasal sinus symptoms. Mucormycosis is one of the more unusual infections seen in elderly patients with diabetes or those receiving immunosuppressive agents for neoplastic diseases. Urgent therapy with an antifungal agent may be lifesaving.

Headache is commonly attributed to hypertension. Mild degrees of hypertension are not usually associated with headache. Headache is more likely to be present in patients with hypertension and diastolic blood pressures in excess of 120 mm Hg. Headache is no more common in milder degrees of hypertension than in the normotensive population. Headache is described as occurring in the occipital and upper nuchal areas, and symptoms are most common upon arising in the morning. Lance reviews hypertension and headache in his text (7), which seems to bear out the impression of clinicians that diastolic levels of hypertension below 110 to 120 mm Hg are not associated with headache more often than headache is found in the normotensive age-matched population. Waters (8) also noted little difference in headache frequency between normotensive and hypertensive subjects. Probably treatment with antihypertensive medication has resulted in an increased number of patients with headache, since several of the compounds used may result in headache as an adverse effect.

Geriatric patients with hypertension may occasionally harbor a pheochromocytoma. Headache, palpitation, and diaphoresis may be associated with catecholamine excess. Recently improved techniques in diagnosis, including biochemical and imaging techniques, should lead to fewer missed diagnoses (9).

Patients with headache and hyptertension should be treated for the hypertension. Headache can be treated with symptomatic analgesic compounds. Acetaminophen or nonsteroidal antiinflammatory agents can be used if there is no contraindication. It is best to avoid the use of antihypertensive compounds that may further provide headache, specifically hydralazine and nifedipine. Many other drugs are available that are less likely to precipitate headache in an individual already suffering from such symptoms and hypertension.

Chronic obstructive pulmonary disease (COPD) with or without chronic bronchitis may be associated with headache and is more likely to be seen in a geriatric population. The frequently associated hypercapnia as well as secondary polycythemia as a result of chronic hypoxia may lead to headache. Theophylline is used often in the treatment of COPD and may result in headache as an adverse CNS effect. Measurement of serum theophylline is indicated to avoid a greater likelihood of adverse events. Increased intracranial pressure due to secondary polycythemia with increased blood volume and increased intracranial vasodilatation may lead to further headache. Primary polycythemia may also result in headache. Obese individuals with sleep apnea disorders occasionally awaken in the morning with dull headache that will subside as they become more active during their working hours.

Endocrine disorders are infrequent causes of headache. Hypoglycemia may be associated with headache, particularly in the elderly insulin-dependent diabetic individual. The use of oral hypoglycemic agents in diabetes may infrequently be associated with headache. The headache should be associated with a lower blood sugar in such instances.

Hypothyroidism and hyperthyroidism may occasionally result in headache accompanied by other symptoms suggestive of the illness. The use of rapidly acting replacement therapy if given rapidly or in excess can result in a vascular type of generalized headache.

Acute angle-closure glaucoma may present acutely with an irregular light reflex, a fixed mid-dilated pupil, and increased intraocular pressure. The headache is usually intense, localized in the eyeball and frontal areas. Referral to an ophthalmologist is required immediately. Specific medications such as amitriptyline and imipramine may precipitate an attack of acute angle-closure glaucoma, and individuals with narrow angles should not receive these agents nor should ophthalmologic patients with increased intraocular pressure.

GIANT CELL ARTERITIS

Temporal or cranial arteritis is a specific form of giant cell arteritis with involvement of the temporal arteries or their branches, which may present with headache in the elderly. The pathological picture is characterized by a predominance of mononuclear cell infiltrates or a granulomatous process with multinucleated giant cells. A necrotizing arteritis is present. The lumen of the vessel is nearly obliterated or at times completely obliterated.

The American College of Rheumatology has recently developed criteria for the classification of giant cell arteritis (10). The criteria were advanced from a comparison with other forms of vasculitis. The features include age greater than 50 years at disease onset, new onset of localized headache, localized temporal artery tenderness or diminished arterial pulsation, elevated erythrocyte sedimentation rate (Westergren) greater than 50 mm/hr, and a positive arterial biopsy specimen. The biopsy specimen should reveal a necrotizing arteritis. A further important feature that is helpful in diagnosis is claudication of the jaw with chewing. At times symptoms develop with chewing and may be referred to the temporomandibular joint area. The dentist may be the first to see the patient. Intermittent claudication of the jaw muscles may be considered pathognomonic. It is emphasized that a generous biopsy of the temporal artery is often necessary to establish the diagnosis. Five centimeters is recommended as the arterial biopsy length to confirm a diagnosis in suspected temporal arteritis (11). Skip lesions are not uncommon.

There may be symptoms that suggest polymyalgia rheumatica (12). The two disorders are interrelated, and a percentage of patients with polymyalgia rheumatica will have symptoms that overlap with temporal arteritis. Polymyalgia rheumatica is diagnosed by exclusion. The presenting symptoms are most often profound stiffness of the hip and shoulder muscles. An elevated sedimentation rate, anemia, and slightly abnormal liver enzymes are present. The disease is treated with smaller doses of corticosteroids than are required for giant cell arteritis. Corticosteroid therapy may have to be prolonged in both disorders; therapy may be required for as long as 2 years. A recent review estimates that 50% of patients with temporal arteritis will have the polymyalgia rheumatica syndrome (13).

Several features of temporal arteritis should be stressed. The headache may not affect the temporal arteries and in a small number of patients headache may not be present (14). The elderly individual presenting with headache of any type, location, or intensity should have temporal arteritis considered in the differential diagnosis.

Large artery involvement may occur in temporal arteritis and/or polymyalgia rheumatica. The subclavian and axillary arteries may be involved (15). Corticosteroids usually are effective in therapy, but involvement of major upper extremity vessels should be recognized as early as possible. Medium-sized arteries may also be involved. Coronary artery involvement with coronary arteritis and myocardial infarction may occur. The aorta and cerebral vessels may similarly be involved, leading to stroke (16).

A normal erythrocyte sedimentation rate is not common but can occur with temporal arteritis. In one study reviewing the literature (17), 35 cases of biopsy-positive giant cell arteritis in the temporal artery were identified, and the authors reported a 36th case. Headache (41%), temporal artery abnormalities (41%), and visual symptoms (36%) were the most common indications of temporal arteritis. Headache and jaw claudication were found less frequently in patients with a normal sedimentation rate.

Mehler and Rabinowich discuss the clinical neuro-ophthalmologic possibilities in temporal arteritis (18). Although bilateral blindness is the most dread complication of temporal arteritis, the authors point out that there is a wide spectrum of features involving the visual system. The loss of vision may occur rapidly or it may be insidious over weeks. Visual loss is estimated to occur in 17% of patients with temporal arteritis. Major neuroophthalmologic syndromes include visual loss, ophthalmoparesis, and autonomic dysfunction with a Horner's syndrome. Other rare syndromes are also discussed in this review of ocular involvement.

Treatment of temporal arteritis is considered emergency therapy if the diagnosis is strongly considered. Biopsy of the temporal artery can be performed on an outpatient basis and scheduled as an emergency procedure. Therapy should be started promptly, even prior to obtaining the results of the pathological specimen. If the diagnosis is confirmed by biopsy, therapy is continued, and if the diagnosis is not established, treatment can be discontinued. Corticosteroid dosage is usually in the range of 60 mg of prednisone a day, continued until the sedimentation rate falls to normal. Slowly tapering the dosage depending on the response is usual. Long-term therapy is frequent, and complications associated with long-term high-dosage corticosteroids is possible. Upper gastrointestinal complications including peptic ulcer disease and bleeding may be lessened with H_2-blocking agents, such as ranitidine or cimetidine. The use of concurrent sucralfate may be beneficial to prevent upper gastrointestinal disease.

Osteoporosis and diabetes mellitus should be considered complications, and appropriate measures are required to prevent or lessen their likelihood. Recently, with the increased incidence of tuberculosis in the population, the occult presence of tuberculosis should be considered in all patients who are to embark on long-term high-dosage corticosteroid therapy. A screening chest roentgenogram should be obtained. A tuberculin skin test may also be advisable, to be aware of the individual's previous exposure to tuberculosis.

The dosage of corticosteroids required for the treatment of temporal arteritis is very different from that used in the therapy of polymyalgia rheumatica, where a daily dose of 10 to 15 mg a day is usually adequate for control of signs and symptoms. The higher dose of 40 to 60 mg a day of prednisone may be required for weeks before tapering is begun. Symptomatic improvement and a decreased eryth-

rocyte sedimentation rate are usually good evidence of remission.

Progression of the disease during adequate therapy is unusual. However, a rare case is reported where massive intravenous methylprednisolone therapy in the range of 1000 mg every 12 hours was necessary to prevent retinal ischemia and deterioration of vision (in the second eye to be affected) during therapy with 60 mg a day of prednisone (19). Curiously, the authors reported that the sedimentation rate returned to normal when progression began in the second eye. The massive dose of methylprednisolone resulted in improvement in vision and resolution of the temporal arteritis.

In summary, the key points in temporal arteritis are the variable nature of the headache in elderly individuals, the need for measuring the erythrocyte sedimentation rate in all elderly patients with headache, considering jaw claudication to be pathognomonic, and the use of prompt biopsy followed by corticosteroid therapy in high dosages.

CERVICAL SPONDYLOSIS

Cervical spondylosis is often cited as the cause of headache in the elderly, and occasionally it may be. However, it is too often cited as the cause because cervical spondylosis deformans is noted on the cervical spine x-ray series. Many patients past the age of 50 will complain of headache and have cervical spine degenerative disease on x-ray. The x-ray findings may not be related to the headache. Instead, a muscle-contraction-type headache may occur in the patients with the x-ray abnormality. All too often, a mild depression and tension-type headache are responsible for the symptoms. If cervical spine disease is considered, more intensive radiologic confirmation with CT scanning or MR imaging studies should be considered.

MIGRAINE, CLUSTER, AND TENSION HEADACHE

Migraine in the elderly may include symptoms with transient migrainous accompaniments. Edmeads has thoroughly discussed this subject (20). Headache may no longer occur, only auras. Recurrent focal neurological symptoms occur in the elderly and have been designated transient migrainous accompaniments (TMA). TMA can be confused with cerebral vascular disease. Migraine may occur for the first time after the age of 50 with symptoms of TMA and must be distinguished from the more serious life-threatening cerebral vascular disease. Fisher (21) cites scintillations, paresthesias, aphasia, dysarthria, and paresis as symptoms of TMA. The buildup of symptoms with a "march" of paresthesias may occur. Symptoms may change from one type to another with an intervening delay. The similarity of symptoms may be helpful. There may be a "flurry" of symptoms with a benign course. Results of cerebral angiographic studies are normal, and no evidence of hypercoagulabiity is present.

The treatment of migraine, cluster, and tension headache in the elderly presents several added considerations. Table 35.2 outlines the acute and prophylactic treatment of these disorders. These entities are by no means rare, even in the very elderly. The headache and accompanying symptoms may change after many years. Chronic daily headache is often present in individuals with a past history of migraine and tension headache who have become dependent on daily ergotamine preparations or on other daily analgesic-sedative. It is extremely difficult to change the medication habits of these individuals. Some of the newer antimigraine agents can be used singly or in combination as prophylactic agents. Tricyclic antidepressants and β-adrenergic blocking agents may be used, or calcium entry blockers can be substituted for the β-blockers. Occasionally an older individual may respond to monoamine oxidase inhibitors. Slow withdrawal of the analgesic-sedative

combinations should be attempted in patients with chronic daily headache and drug dependency.

Elderly patients who develop an intercurrent illness, particularly a surgical problem or medical illness, and who are prohibited from using preparations containing ergotamine and caffeine will be amazed at their response to discontinuing the daily medication. There will be an improved sense of well-being and an absence of daily headache. The attending physician should promptly point out to them that they no longer require daily medication. Neither daily ergotamine or analgesics are necessary. If discussed immediately following recovery from intercurrent or acute illness, patients are less likely to resume their usual medication. Rebound headache following ergotamine use and chronic daily headache after prolonged analgesic ingestion are certainly important causes of headache in the elderly.

Table 35.2.
Therapy in a Geriatric Headache Population

Drug	Comments
Migraine: acute therapy	
Salicylates	Use metaclopramide if nausea is present
Ergotamine preparations with or without caffeine	Carefully check for contraindications; vascular disease, hypertension, and renal disease
Nonsteroidal antiinflammatory agents	Avoid if possible in presence of renal disease and watch for signs of gastrointestinal bleeding
Naproxen	
Naproxen sodium	
Ibuprofen	
Isometheptene mucate, acetaminophen, dichloralphenazone (Midrin)	Avoid in presence of cardiac, hypertensive, renal, and hepatic disease; also avoid in glaucoma and with concomitant MAO therapy
Migraine: prophylactic therapy	
β-Adrenergic blocking agents (without sympathomimetic action)	
Propranolol 40 to 160 mg a day	Other β-blocking agents may also be effective
Timolol 10 mg b.i.d.	
Calcium entry blockers	
Verapamil 40 mg t.i.d. to 240 mg a day	May be used with coexisting hypertension and/or angina pectoris
Nicardipine 20 mg to 30 mg t.i.d.	
Tricyclic antidepressants	Small doses may be effective
Monoamine oxidase inhibitors	
Phenelzine 15 mg t.i.d.	Prescriber should be aware of side effects and drug interactions
Trazodone 50 mg h.s. to 150 mg a day	Avoid in males because of risk of priapism
Aspirin 100 mg a day to 325 mg every other day	Some published reports suggest efficacy
Tension headache: symptomatic therapy	
NSAIDs	See migraine therapy
Acetaminophen or aspirin; also in combination with or without caffeine and butalbital	Avoid daily use
Midrin	See migraine therapy; limit therapy to 2 days a week
Tension headache: prophylactic therapy	
Tricyclic antidepressants	See migraine therapy
Trazodone	See migraine therapy
MAO inhibitors	See migraine therapy
Cluster headache: acute therapy	
Rapid-acting analgesics	Usually not effective
Oxygen therapy	High flow 6–8 liters/min
Ergotamine preparations	See migraine therapy
Cluster headache: prophylaxis for acute and chronic	
Methysergide	Avoid use over 6 months and similar precautions to ergotamine preparations
Lithium carbonate 300 mg t.i.d.	Check blood levels at regular intervals; watch for drug interactions
Calcium entry blocking agents	
Verapamil 80 mg to 120 mg t.i.d.	Constipation and cardiac adverse effects occur
Nicardipine 20 mg to 30 mg t.i.d.	Headache may be an adverse event; relatively safe with few serious adverse effects
Nifedipine 10 mg to 30 mg t.i.d.	
Prednisone	Use smallest effective dose possible; closely observe for adverse events
Combinations of calcium entry blocking agents, prednisone, and lithium	May be attempted in refractory chronic cluster headache patients; close follow-up is essential to avoid overlooking complications of treatment

The presence of hypertension and angina pectoris or other forms of coronary artery disease may preclude the use of ergotamine compounds, methysergide, and isometheptene mucate (Midrin). Physicians may wish to avoid tricyclic antidepressants in patients who are prone to cardiac arrhythmias. In the aforementioned instances, β-adrenergic blocking agents and calcium entry blockers are excellent substitutes for migraine prevention. Patients with mixed-type headaches may also show a salutary response. If congestive heart failure or chronic obstructive pulmonary disease is present, β-blocker therapy is to be avoided. Under these circumstances, verapamil, nifedipine, or nicardipine may be beneficial. If hypertension is of serious concern, clonidine may be helpful, and at times it may reduce the incidence of migraine headache and assist in weaning patients off narcotics. Clonidine has been marketed outside the United States for the treatment of migraine prophylaxis. Its efficacy in migraine prevention is questioned.

Cluster headache treatment in the elderly is similar to that of younger individuals except for omitting methysergide if coronary or peripheral atherosclerosis is present. Prednisone, lithium carbonate, and calcium entry blockers may be of value, and oxygen can be used for abortive treatment.

Recurrent tension headache in the elderly is often responsive to tricyclic antidepressants, trazodone, and (in refractory patients) monoamine oxidase inhibitors, particularly phenelzine. Experience with fluoxetine is limited, although it may also be shown to be effective.

Tricyclic antidepressants must be used with caution because of their atropine-like effects. Patients with prostatic enlargement with urinary retention and those with narrow angle-closure glaucoma or increased intraocular pressure may be at greater risk of provoking adverse events and worsening of their disease state.

Nonsteroidal antiinflammatory agents (NSAIDs) can be of help in abortive (22) and prophylactic (23) therapy. Naproxen or naproxen sodium can be used. Ibuprofen in dosages varying between 200 mg four times a day as an over-the-counter preparation or in larger doses of 400 to 800 mg repeated three to four times a day may be highly effective. Other compounds include fenoprofen, ketoprofen, mefenamic acid, and tolfenamic acid. Caution must be exercised, particularly in the elderly, with all NSIADs, because of the increased risk of renal failure even if used with mild renal impairment (24). Mild renal impairment is commonly found in elderly patients, because of concomitant hypertension and nephrosclerosis, decreased perfusion associated with congestive heart failure, and diabetes mellitus. Liver disease and chronic inflammatory bowel disease may also be associated with the use of NSAIDs. The use of shorter-acting NSAIDs is preferable, since the incidence of side effects is lower with a shorter half-life (25). Ibuprofen has one of the shortest elimination half-lives, 1 to 2 hours. Upper gastrointestinal bleeding is also a complication of NSAID use, and they should not be used in the elderly without a careful search for a history of peptic ulcer disease or previous upper gastrointestinal bleeding due to erosive gastritis. Sucralfate (26) or misoprotol (27) can be used concomitantly with NSAIDs in an attempt to prevent upper gastrointestinal complications from NSAID use. Misoprostol has been reported to cause a flare up of Crohn's disease (28). NSAIDs have also been reported to cause an aseptic meningitis (29) that may present with headache and complicate preexisting headache therapy.

A recent report in male physicians suggests that low-dosage aspirin therapy may prevent migraine (325 mg every other day), and this regimen may be of help in preventing recurrent migraine in elderly males (30).

CEREBROVASCULAR DISEASE IN THE ELDERLY

Headache occurs in cerebrovascular disease and stroke, and it may occur in 18% of patients with TIA or 33% of patients with partial nonprogressive stroke (31). It may occur on the side of the ischemic episode or, less often, on the opposite side. Usually the headache is mild and nonthrobbing, lasting minutes to hours. Some confusion can occur with preexisting migraine if headache occurs with other symptoms or signs, and one must be alert to the possibility of cerebrovascular disease or embolic episodes in patients with previous migraine. Cardiac sources of emboli should be sought, and carotid artery disease must also be excluded as a source of embolic or occlusive disease. Fisher (21) states that visual TMAs typically show a gradual buildup, and paresthetic TMAs march from region to region. A middle-life "flurry" of TMAs may be a special phenomenon.

An entity designated MELAS syndrome (32) is characterized by myopathy, encephalopathy, lactic acidosis, and stroke-like episodes with headache. Magnetic resonance imaging is more sensitive in demonstrating cortical lesions than CT scanning.

Gorelick and co-workers reported headache occurring in acute cerebrovascular disease (33). Their data suggested that some headache characteristics were more often associated with a particular type of stroke subtype. Onset headache and vomiting were direct predictors of subarachnoid hemorrhage. Their patients with subarachnoid hemorrhage had more sentinel headaches. Headache following carotid endarterectomy occurs in many patients (34) on the operative side. It may be associated with seizures, and the clinical picture resolves in all patients. It is thought to be due to a hyperperfusion syndrome with a preoperative loss of vascular autoregulation mechanisms caused by chronic cerebral ischemia.

PHARMACOLOGICAL AGENTS CAUSING HEADACHE

Due to the frequent use of medication in elderly patients, it is not uncommon to see individuals with headache (Table

35.1) that begins or is exacerbated by medication. Hypertensives treated with hydralazine and nifedipine or cardiacs treated with nitrates often complain of a new-onset headache. Estrogen started in the postmenopausal period may result in headache. Nonsteroidal antiinflammatory agents may cause headache, particularly indomethacin. Antilipidemic agents can also result in a headache not previously present. It is always advisable to review the medications of elderly patients to determine if their symptoms are exacerbated or induced by their medication. At times, drug interactions may elevate blood levels of compounds and increase the likelihood of adverse events including headache. An example is the effect of cimetidine on the microsomal enzyme system with decreased hepatic metabolism of theophylline products. Blood levels of theophylline may be increased, with a consequent increased incidence of side effects including headache. Physicians treat or see in consultation patients who are receiving a myriad of medications, including over-the-counter drugs. These patients are most frequently elderly, and headache is often present.

TREATMENT IN THE ELDERLY

Treatment may be similar to that used for younger patients. Contraindications and coexisting disease must be considered before instituting new drug therapy. At times, an increase in dosage may be adequate. An example is patients receiving propranolol at a dosage of 40 mg a day with control of hypertension or angina. An increase to a total daily dose of 120 mg or 160 mg may improve their migraine headaches. Switching to other classes of medication may initiate a response in headache symptoms. Emphasis is placed on a search for less apparent causes of headache in patients with tension or migraine if the headache changes. Increases in severity or frequency, alteration in the type of pain, or onset of associated signs and symptoms not previously present warrants a thorough evaluation.

Patients with tension, migraine, or mixed headaches may respond to nonpharmacological methods of treatment. Dietary causes of headache should be eliminated, including caffeine in excess of 250 mg a day in chronic daily headache sufferers. Relaxation, cognitive coping, and biofeedback therapy may be effective in geriatric patients (35). These methods should be considered in properly motivated individuals. Previous use of these techniques were less successful as nondrug therapy (36). One group suspects that cognitive stress coping should be added to the other techniques and may enhance the results (37).

SUMMARY

A list of the various causes of headache in the elderly is presented, with special attention to the more common types found in a geriatric population. Headaches, although less common in the elderly, still occur. Many of the head-

ache disorders treated earlier in life may continue in later decades. The greater likelihood of structural and concomitant disease requires a more diligent search by the physician for these disorders. Tension, mixed, and migraine headaches still occur in later life, and treatment is similar to the therapy in earlier decades but modified by the slower metabolism and other pharmacodynamics of older healthy individuals. Preexisting medical and surgical entities obviously modify treatment. Specific treatment or attention to a structural, medical, or iatrogenic cause will often ameliorate or resolve the headache symptoms.

REFERENCES

1. Arena JG, Hightower NE, Chong GC. Relaxation therapy for tension headache in the elderly: a prospective study. Psychol Aging 1988;3(1):96–98.
2. Headache Classification Committee of the International Headache Society. Classification and diagnostic criteria for headache disorders, cranial neuralgias and facial pain. Cephalalgia 1988;8(suppl 7):29.
3. Solomon GD, Kunkel RS Jr, Frame J. Demographics of headache in elderly patients. Headache 1990;30(5):273–276.
4. Waters WE. The Pontypridd headache survey. Headache 1974; 14:81–90.
5. Hale WE May FE, Marks RG, Moore MT, Stewart RB. Headache in the elderly: an evaluation of risk factors. Headache 1987;27(5):272–276.
6. Jones HR Jr, Siekert RG. Neurological manifestations of infective endocarditis. Brain 1989;112(Pt 5):1295–1315.
7. Lance JW. Chapter 8. In: Mechanism and Management of Headache, ed 4. Butterworth Scientific 1982:74–85.
8. Waters WE. Epidemiological data relevant to prognosis in migraine in adults. Int J Epidemiol 1975;2:189–194.
9. Krane NK. Clinically unsuspected pheochromocytomas. Experience at Henry Ford Hospital and a review of the literature. Arch Intern Med 1986;146(1):54–57.
10. Hunder GG, Bloch DA, Michel BA, Stevens MB, Arend WP, et al. The American College of Rheumatology 1990 criteria for the classification of giant cell arteritis. Arthritis Rheum 1990;33(8):1122–1128.
11. Kent RB 3rd, Thomas L. Temporal artery biopsy. Am Surg 1990;56(1):16–21.
12. Goodman BW. Temporal arteritis. Am J Med 1979;67:839–852.
13. Allen NB, Studenski SA. Polymyalgia rheumatica and temporal arteritis. Med Clin North Am 1986;70(2):369–384.
14. Solomon S, Cappa KG. The headache of temporal arteritis. J Am Geriatr Soc 1987;35(2)163–165.
15. Ninet JP, Bachet P, Dumontet CM, Colombier PB, Stewart MD, Pasquier JH. Subclavian and axillary involvement in temporal arteritis and polymyalgia rheuatica. Am J Med 1990;88:13–20.
16. Save-Sonderbergh J, Malmvall BE, Andersson R, Bengtsson BA. Giant cell arteritis as a cause of death. JAMA 1986;255(4):493–496.
17. Wons RL, Korn JH. Temporal arteritis without an elevated erythrocyte sedimentation rate: case report and review of the literature. Am J Med 1986;80(5):959–964.
18. Mehler MF, Rabinowich L. The clinical neuro-ophthalmologic spectrum of temporal arteritis. Am J Med 1988;85:839–844.
19. Rosenfeld SI, Kosmorsky GS, Klingele TG, Burde RM, Cohn EM. Treatment of temporal arteritis with ocular involvement. Am J Med 1986;80:143–145.
20. Edmeads J. Management of migraine in the elderly. In: Diamond S, ed. Migraine headache prevention and management. New York: Marcel Dekker, 1990:173–188.
21. Fisher CM. Transient migrainous accompaniments (TMAs) of late onset. Stroke 1979;10:96–97.
22. Andersson PG, Hinge HH, Johansen O, et al. Double-blind study of

naproxen vs placebo in the treatment of acute migraine attacks. Cephalagia 1989;9:29.

23. Ziegler DK, Ellis DJ. Naproxen in prophylaxis of migraine. Arch Neurol 1985;42:582.

24. Whelton A, Stout RL, Spilman PS, et al. Renal effects of ibuprofen, piroxicam, and sulindac in patients with asymptomatic renal failure. A prospective, randomized, crossover comparison. Ann Intern Med 1990;112:568.

25. Adams S. Nonsteroidal antiinflammatory drugs, plasma half-lives, and adverse reactions (letter). Lancet 1987;2:1204–1205.

26. Caldwell JR, Roth SH, Wu WC, et al. Sucralfate treatment of nonsteroidal anti-inflammatory drug-induced gastrointestinal symptoms and mucosal damage. Am J Med 1987;83:74.

27. Graham DY, Agrawal NM, Roth SH. Prevention of NSAID-induced gastric ulcer with misoprostol: multicentre, double-blind, placebo-controlled trial. Lancet 1988;11:1277.

28. Kornblutt A, Gupta R, Gerson CD. Life-threatening diarrhea after short term misoprostol use in a patient with Crohn ileocolitis. Ann Intern Med 1990;113:474–475.

29. Sylvia LM, Forienza SW, Brocavich JM. Aseptic meningitis associated with naproxen. Intell Clin Pharm 1988;22(5)399–401.

30. Buring JE, Peto R, Hennekens CH. Low-dose aspirin for migraine prophylaxis. JAMA 1990;264(13):1711.

31. Barnett HJM. Vertebral-basilar symptomatology. Clin Neurosurg 1976;23:543.

32. Rosen L, Phillips S, Enzmann D. Magnetic resonance imaging in MELAS syndrme. Neuroradiology 1990;32(2):168–171.

33. Gorelick PB, Hier DB, Caplan LR, Langenberg P. Headache in acute cerebrovascular disease. Neurology 1986;36(11):1445–1450.

34. Reigel MM, Hollier LH, Sundt TM Jr, Piepgras DG, Sharbrough FW, Cherry KJ. Cerebral hyperperfusion syndrome: a cause of neurologic dysfunction after carotid endarterecomy. J Vasc Surg 1987;5(4):628–634.

35. Colenda CC 3rd, Doughery LM. Positive ego and coping functions in chronic pain. J Geriatr Psychiatry Neurol 1990;3(1):48–52.

36. Blanchard EB, Andrasik F, Evans DD, Hillhouse J. Biofeedback and relaxation treatments for headache in the elderly: a caution and a challenge. Biofeedback Self Regul 1985;10:69–73.

37. Kabela E, Blanchard EB, Applebaum KH, Nicholson N. Self-regulatory treatment of headache in the elderly. Biofeedback Self Regul 1989;14(3):219–228.

36

Headache as a Symptom of Cerebrovascular Disease

EGILIUS L. H. SPIERINGS

The brain itself, like all other internal organs, is insensitive to pain and derives its protection with regard to nociceptive stimuli from the encapsulating membranes (1). The encapsulating membranes of the brain are the arachnoidea and dura mater, and they obtain their sensory innervation from nerve fibers that travel along with the blood vessels. This means, on the one hand, that the encapsulating membranes are sensitive to pain only where they are adjacent to blood vessels; and, on the other hand, that the blood vessels carry sensory nerve fibers and are, therefore, sensitive to pain only as long as they pass through these membranes. For the brain, this means that the major cerebral arteries are sensitive to pain as they pass through the arachnoidea, and the venous sinuses as they pass through the dura mater. The sensory innervation of the dural venous sinuses extends to a certain extent to the major cerebral veins that, like the major cerebral arteries, pass through the arachnoidea as well. The dura mater, on the other hand, also receives sensory innervation from nerve fibers that travel along with a vascular system that is not related to the circulation of the brain, i.e., the dural arteries.

As a result of this pattern of sensory innervation of the brain and its surrounding structures, only diseases that affect the larger blood vessels of the brain (i.e., the major cerebral arteries and dural venous sinuses and adjacent parts of the major cerebral veins) cause pain. Where the pain caused by diseases affecting these blood vessels is felt, depends on where the innervation of the blood vessels comes from; or, in other words, where in the central nervous system the nociceptive information coming from these blood vessels is processed and what other information is being processed there. In this regard, the division of the intracranial cavity by the dural sheets (i.e., the falx cerebri and tentorium cerebelli) is important as they form, to a great extent, the anatomical borders of the sensory innervation of the intracranial structures. The falx cerebri forms the border between the right and left sides of the intracranial cavity, and the innervation of the intracranial structures is lateralized accordingly. The tentorium cerebelli forms the border between the anterior and posterior parts of the intracranial cavity in which the anterior part contains the cerebrum and the posterior part, the cerebellum and brainstem.

The anterior part of the intracranial fossa is innervated by the ophthalmic division of the trigeminal nerve and the posterior part by the occipital nerves. Pain arising from diseases affecting the cerebral blood vessels will, therefore, be felt on the side of the affliction when it is unilateral, in the forehead and/or anterior vertex when the affected blood vessels lie in the anterior part of the intracranial cavity, and in the back of the head and/or posterior vertex when the affected blood vessels lie in the posterior part of the intracranial cavity. For example, pain caused by an arteriovenous malformation located in the left occipital lobe will be felt by the patient in the left forehead and/or anterior vertex.

The nerve fibers that travel along with the blood vessels of the brain and provide these blood vessels with sensory innervation coil around the blood vessels and are, like nociceptive sensory fibers in general, sensitive to mechanical, thermal, and chemical stimulation. As the nerve fibers travel along with the blood vessels and coil around them, they can be stimulated mechanically by stretching that occurs when a blood vessel expands, either actively (over-dilation) or passively (distension). Thermal stimulation generally does not occur with the pain fibers traveling along with the blood vessels of the brain unless they are exposed, such as with surgery. However, chemical stimulation, in addition to mechanical stimulation, is an important mechanism by which diseases affecting the blood vessels of the brain cause pain, in particular related to inflammation. As will be evident from what is to follow, diseases affecting the blood vessels of the brain often cause pain by stimulating the nerve fibers surrounding them, both mechanically and chemically.

To summarize, diseases affecting the blood vessels of the brain cause pain when they affect the **major** blood vessel, either arterial or venous, and generally do so by mechanical and/or chemical stimulation of the nerve fibers surrounding the blood vessels. The resulting pain, when it is unilateral, is felt on the same side as the affliction, in the forehead and/or anterior vertex when the involved blood vessels lie above the tentorium, and in the back of the head and/or posterior vertex when they lie below it. The diseases that affect the blood vessels of the brain in a way that causes pain have, in the headache classification of the International Headache Society (2), been divided into eight categories and will be discussed accordingly. These eight categories are acute ischemic cerebrovascular disease (6.1), intracranial hematoma (6.2), subarachnoid hemorrhage (6.3), unruptured vascular malformation (6.4), arteritis (6.5), carotid artery pain (6.6), venous thrombosis (6.7), and arterial hypertension (6.8).

ACUTE ISCHEMIC CEREBROVASCULAR DISEASE

It was not until the advent of computerized tomography in the middle of the 1970s that the diagnosis of ischemic cerebrovascular disease could be made with certainty unless the patient came to autopsy. Therefore, studies that can be relied on with regard to headache in relation to ischemic cerebrovascular disease must include diagnosis with computerized tomography or, more recently, with magnetic resonance imaging. The studies must be prospective to ensure reliable information about headache, as headache is generally a relatively minor and clinically insignificant symptom in acute cerebrovascular disease. Two studies qualify on the basis of both these criteria, the study by Portenoy et al. published in 1984 (3) and the one by Gorelick et al. published in 1986 (4).

The study by Portenoy et al. (3) included 165 patients with acute ischemic cerebrovascular disease, which was lacunar in 18 and transient (TIA) in 28. Of these 165 patients, 32 were unable to respond to the questions because of aphasia or altered mental status; none of these patients had either lacunar or transient ischemic cerebrovascular disease. This leaves 133 patients with acute ischemic cerebrovascular disease, which was lacunar in 18 and transient in 28. Headache in relation to the acute cerebrovascular disease was reported by 38 of these patients (29%). Patients with **transient** ischemic cerebrovascular disease reported a somewhat higher incidence of headaches (36%), and patients with **lacunar** cerebrovascular disease a somewhat lower incidence (17%). Half of the headaches reported by the 38 patients were unilateral, and of these, half were localized to the side of the cerebrovascular disease. Headaches were reported almost twice as frequently by women than by men, and more than half of the headaches occurred **before** the cerebrovascular event as opposed to during or after it.

The study by Gorelick et al. (4) included 160 patients with acute ischemic cerebrovascular disease, which was lacunar in 50. Patients with transient ischemic cerebrovascular disease were not included in this study. Headache in relation to the acute cerebrovascular disease was reported by 27 of the patients (17%). The headache was focal in 96%, unilateral in 74%, severe in 15%, and associated with vomiting in 7%. In the patients with acute ischemic cerebrovascular disease due to occlusion of a large artery as demonstrated by angiography, the headache was ipsilateral to the vascular lesion in 67%, bilateral in 26%, and contralateral in 7%. The size of the infarct, as determined by computerized tomography, did not show a relationship with the reported incidence of headache.

Portenoy et al. reported a higher incidence of headache in acute ischemic cerebrovascular disease than Gorelick et al. (29% vs. 17%). This difference, however, may be due to the fact that Gorelick's study included almost twice as many patients with lacunar disease as Portenoy's (31% vs. 14%), which is the group in which Portenoy et al. found the lowest incidence of headache.

On the basis of the studies reviewed above, it can be concluded that acute ischemic cerebrovascular disease is associated with headache in 20 to 25%. The headache is generally **not** severe and **not** associated with symptoms such as vomiting. It is unilateral in 50 to 75% and tends to lateralize to the side of the cerebrovascular disease. The mechanism by which the headache is caused relates to the affliction of the blood vessel involved rather than to the ischemia of the brain, and probably involves distension and inflammation of the blood vessel by the thrombus or embolus.

INTRACRANIAL HEMATOMA

Depending on its precise location, an intracranial hematoma can be either intracerebral, subdural, or epidural. Of these hematomas, it is the intracerebral (also called intraparenchymal) hematoma that relates to cerebrovascular disease and will be further discussed here; the sub- and epidural hematomas basically relate to head injury with rupture of a cerebral vein or dural artery, respectively. With regard to the diagnosis of intracerebral hematoma, the same applies as has been stated above for acute ischemic cerebrovascular disease, and computerized tomography or magnetic resonance imaging are also required for accuracy. Intracerebral hematoma can be primary, due to rupture of an intracerebral artery, or secondary, due to bleeding in an area of brain affected by ischemic cerebrovascular disease (i.e., hemmorrhagic infarct).

The above-reviewed studies by Portenoy et al. (3) and Gorelick et al. (4) also included patients with intracerebral hematoma, the first one 50, and the second 61. However, 20 of Portenoy's patients with intracerebral hematoma were nonresponders, while 60 of the patients in Gorelick's study were able to respond to the questions. Headache related to the intracerebral hematoma was reported by 17 of the 30 patients in Portenoy's study (57%) and by 33 of Gorelick's 60 patients (55%). In the study by Gorelick et al., the headaches were focal in 93%, unilateral in 70%, severe in 41%, and associated with vomiting in a little over 50%. It can, therefore, be concluded that intracerebral hematoma is associated with headache in 55%. This headache tends to be severe, unilateral, and associated with vomiting. Its mechanism is probably not related to the rupture of the blood vessel, which is generally a small intracerebral artery (not sensitive to pain), or to destruction of brain tissue. It is probably caused by the mass effect of the hematoma on the cerebral blood vessels, which causes stretching of the pain-sensitive major cerebral arteries and veins as they course over the cortex of the cerebral hemisphere.

SUBARACHNOID HEMORRHAGE

The diagnosis of subarachnoid hemorrhage can generally be made accurately without computerized tomography or magnetic resonance imaging, on the basis of the history (peracute onset of headache), physical examination (restriction of forward flexion of the neck with intact rotation to either side), and/or lumbar puncture (hemorrhagic spinal fluid that is xantochromic after centrifugation). Therefore, with headache in relation to subarachnoid hemorrhage, one can also rely on studies dating back to before the advent of computerized tomography.

Headache is reported by all patients with subarachnoid hemorrage, as was also observed in the study by Gorelick et al. (4), which included 51 patients with this disorder. In this study, the headache was severe in 94%, bilateral in 68%, and associated with vomiting in 58%. When a unilateral headache occurred, it was always ipsilateral when the aneurysm was either right- or left-sided.

Not fully resolved is the issue of the so-called sentinel headache. Sentinel headache is defined as any unusual headache that may be noted by the patient in the days or weeks before the occurrence of the subarachnoid hemorrhage. In the study by Gorelick et al., sentinel headache occurred in 31% of the patients with subarachnoid hemorrhage (as opposed to 14% in the patients with intracerebral hematoma and 10% in those with acute ischemic cerebrovascular disease). The sentinel headache in the patients with subarachnoid hemorrhage lasted longer than 24 hours in 93% and was bilateral in 67%. In a prospective study by Verweij et al. (5), published in 1988, sentinel headache was reported by 13 of 30 patients with subarachnoid hemorrhage (43%). The headaches occurred from 1 week to 1 month before the subarachnoid hemorrhage and lasted less than 2 days. No specific features to these headaches made it possible to recognize them as sentinel headache of subarachnoid hemorrhage.

The headache of subarachnoid hemorrhage is due to chemical inflammation of the arachnoidea. The mechanism involved in the sentinel headache is less clear. It has been suggested that the sentinel headache is in actual fact a true subarachnoid hemorrhage but with a very mild course or that the headache is due to expansion of the aneurysm or due to a small hemorrhage into the wall of the aneurysm. Aneurysms arise from the major cerebral arteries, mostly in the circle of Willis, and as these blood vessels are sensitive to pain, the aneurysms are likely to be sensitive to pain as well. Events happening to an aneurysm can, therefore, cause pain, again by stretching and/or causing inflammation of the wall of the aneurysm.

UNRUPTURED VASCULAR MALFORMATION

Arteriovenous malformation of the brain can rupture and, thereby, cause hemorrhage into the brain, subarachnoid space, and/or ventricular system. These are acute events in which headache is a prominent symptom caused by chemical inflammation of the arachnoidea (subarachnoid hemorrhage) or stretching of the major cerebral blood vessels in their course over the cerebral cortex (intracerebral and intraventricular hemorrhage). However, also without rupturing and causing hemorrhage, cerebral arteriovenous malformations can cause headache, sometimes mimicking migraine (6). The following case is an example.

The patient is a 37-year-old, right-handed man who related the onset of his headaches to the time he was in college. Until 5 years prior to consultation, the headaches had occurred once per month and after that 2 to 3 times per year. This infrequent occurrence of the headaches, however, changed 10 days prior to consultation, during which he had had 5 headaches. The patient described the headaches as coming during the day, usually in the afternoon. They built up to their maximum intensity relatively rapidly (i.e., within 5 to 10 minutes) and lasted a total of 6 to 12 hours. The headaches were located over the left forehead and behind the left eye as an intense pressure. More than 50% of the headaches were described as being severe, and they were associated with photophobia and occasionally also with vomiting. Prior to the onset of headache, the patient always experienced a visual disturbance that lasted 10 to 20 minutes. The visual disturbance consisted of colored spots in the right visual field, which persisted throughout the headache. Bright light and trying to concentrate or focus made the headaches worse. Bright light could also bring on headache as could glare or reflection, getting hot from exertion, red wine, monosodium glutamate, and drinking more than two cups of coffee.

The review of systems, past medical history, and family history were unremarkable, as were the physical and neurological examinations. However, because of the crossed occurrence of the visual disturbance and the headache and the lack of alternation (i.e., the fixed occurrence of these symptoms) magnetic resonance imaging of the brain was performed. This revealed a large arteriovenous malformation in the left occipital lobe with multiple, tubular, serpinginous structures containing flow voids, with the major feeding blood vessel being an enlarged left posterior cerebral artery.

Arteriovenous malformations are congenital abnormalities that develop at an early embryonic stage when the division of blood vessels into arteries, capilaries, and veins occurs. They are the result of an arrest in blood vessel development, which leads to the formation of direct artery-to-vein communications without the interposition of a capilary bed. Cerebral arteriovenous malformations occur at a frequency about one-tenth of that of intracranial aneurysms and most commonly manifest themselves in the second through fourth decades of life. They are almost always unilateral and located in a cerebral hemisphere, with equal distribution between the lobes (7).

Cerebral arteriovenous malformations most commonly manifest themselves through intracerebral, subarachnoid, and/or intraventricular hemorrhage (30 to 60%). The second and third most common manifestations of these arteriovenous malformations are seizures (20 to 40%) and headaches, respectively. These latter manifestations are more common in the large arteriovenous malformations, while the small and medium-size malformations more frequently hemorrhage (7).

Waltimo et al. (8) studied, by personal interviews, the occurrence of headache in 48 patients with intracranial arteriovenous malformations. Of these patients, 29 were men and 19 were women. The intracranial malformations were cerebral in 44 (92%), cerebellar in 1 (2%), and meningeal in 3 (6%). The cerebral malformations were all unilateral and located in the frontal lobe in 13 (30%), parietal lobe in 15 (34%), temporal lobe in 7 (16%), occipital lobe in 6 (14%), and centrally in 3 (6%). Of the malformations, 22 were large (i.e., 7 cm^3 or about 2.8 cm in diameter or larger) and 23 small.

All but 10 of the patients studied by Waltimo et al. (8) reported headaches, which makes the prevalence of headache in patients with intracranial arteriovenous malformations 79%. The headaches were unilateral in 18 of these 38 patients (47%), and in all but one (94%), the headaches occurred on the side of the malformation. In 15 of the 38 patients with headache (39%), the headaches were diagnosed as migraine, which was "classic" in 8 and "common" in 7. The headaches were more commonly diagnosed as "migraine" in women than in men. In addition, the occipital arteriovenous malformations had the highest occurrence of "migraine" (83%), followed by those located frontally (46%).

In a review article on intracranial arteriovenous malformation and migraine, Bruyn (9) concluded that the coincidental occurrence of the two conditions is more than a matter of chance. This means that intracranial arteriovenous malformations can probably manifest themselves as "migraine," which would be referred to as "symptomatic migraine." Waltimo et al. (8) found this to be most common with arteriovenous malformations located in the occipital lobe.

Cerebral arteriovenous malformations can also manifest themselves through transient neurological symptoms, and when located occipitally, these symptoms would be visual. Visual symptoms are also the most common transient neurological symptoms that occur with migraine, and this may be the reason for the confusion. On the other hand, the studies of large series of patients with occipital arteriovenous malformations (10, 11) show that when transient visual symptoms occur with these malformations, they are usually epileptic in origin. This means that these visual symptoms are generally short in duration (i.e., they last seconds rather than minutes), poorly formed without

definite shape, and possibly followed by a generalized seizure and/or headache. However, from the above-described case and the reports in the literature (6, 12), it must be concluded that transient visual symptoms that closely resemble those of migraine can occur with arteriovenous malformations as well. In such cases, the arteriovenous malformation may have initiated a phenomenon similar to Leao's spreading excitation and depression (13, 14), which has been postulated to be the mechanism involved in the migraine aura (15, 16). Different effects of the arteriovenous malformation on brain cell metabolism may be responsible for the initiation of epileptic activity versus spreading excitation and depression. The "crossed and fixed" occurrence of the symptoms (i.e., are the visual symptoms and headache **always** contralateral to each other and do they **always** occur on the same side?) are important features to look for in patients with classic migraine or migraine with aura.

As is the case with arteriovenous malformations, cerebral aneurysms can also cause headache without rupturing and causing hemorrhage into the subarachnoid space, brain, and/or ventricular system, although little information about this is available (17, 18). Cerebral aneurysms are generally located at the circle of Willis, and pain originating from there is referred behind the eye and/or to the forehead, ipsilateral to the aneurysm. Aneurysms probably cause pain by stretching the wall of the pain-sensitive artery as they develop out of a weak spot in the vessel wall and expand. The development and expansion of aneurysms may be a stepwise process and may be associated with recurrent headaches that may increase in intensity to culminate at the time of rupture of the aneurysm. When the aneurysm arises from the posterior communicating artery, during its development and expansion it may not only cause headache but also oculomotor nerve palsy with widening of the pupil, drooping of the upper eyelid, and double vision.

ARTERITIS

The most common form of arteritis affecting the cerebral blood vessels is giant cell arteritis, a condition that only affects the elderly. It is an autoimmune disease caused by the formation of autoantibodies against the elastine of the blood vessel wall. It was first described by Hutchinson (19) in 1890 and was defined by Horton et al. (20) in 1932 histologically as a chronic granulomatous arteritis, distinguishing it from Buerger's thromboangiitis obliterans and Kussmaul and Maier's periarteritis nodosa. In 1946 Cooke et al. (21) demonstrated that the condition, which by then had become known as "temporal arteritis," was in fact a generalized vascular disease. With regard to the cerebral blood vessels, it most commonly affects the ophthalmic artery and its branches, causing blindness in 20 to 30% of untreated cases (22). However other cerebral blood vessels can also be affected by giant cell arteritis, and ischemic stroke may occur as a complication of this condition.

Headache is almost always a symptom of giant cell arteritis, because of the predilection of the condition for the cranial arteries ("cranial arteritis"). Inflammation of the cranial arteries causes headache, which can be temporal but can also involve other areas of the head (23, 24). The headache is often moderate or severe and can be either intermittent or continuous. Pathognomonic for the condition is exercise ischemia of the jaw muscles, resulting in jaw pain on chewing (22). The sedimentation rate is almost always very high in giant cell arteritis, and the ultimate diagnosis is made through histological examination of an involved cranial artery, often the temporal artery.

Cerebral arteritis can (apart from giant cell arteritis) be caused by collagen-vascular diseases (lupus erythematosus, rheumatoid arthritis, etc.) and can also occur as an isolated condition. When it involves the major cerebral blood vessels, which are sensitive to pain, the condition is associated with headache due to the inflammation of these blood vessels. The diagnosis of cerebral arteritis is generally difficult to make and requires angiography, which will often show irregular narrowing and widening of the blood vessels (25). Small vessel disease of the brain is not considered to be a cause of headache, and the occurrence of headache in lupus erythematosus does not necessarily indicate involvement of the central nervous system in the disease process (26).

CAROTID ARTERY PAIN

In 1927, Fay (27) described a diagnostic sign for "atypical facial neuralgia," which consisted of aggravation of the pain in the face on pressure exerted upon the sympathetic chain in the neck. He called this sign "carotidynia" and looked upon it as an indication of a pathological process in the chest or abdomen causing pain in the face through the superior cervical ganglion. In 1932, Fay (28) redefined this sign as tenderness to pressure on the carotid arteries in cases of atypical facial neuralgia.

> If the thumbs are placed on the common carotid arteries, just below the bifurcation, and the structures are passed back against the transverse cervical processes with the rolling movement, a severe reaction of pain is produced on the side of the atypical neuralgia. This response I have termed "carotidynia," and it has been found present in almost every case where patients have complained of chronic, dull aching pain referred to the eye, deep in the molar region and traced back to the ear, behind the ear or down the neck.

In 1960, Lovshin (29) described a clinical syndrome of vascular neck pain, which he considered to be a variant of migraine. It occurred in all ages, but particularly in the fifth decade of life, and affected women four times more frequently than men. The pain was often unilateral but sometimes alternating or bilateral and usually centered about the carotid bulb, radiating upward along the course of the external carotid artery, behind the mandible, and up into the postauricular area. The neck pain was dull and deep-seated and usually not throbbing, although a throbbing component could be evoked by stooping, bending, or straining. Usually the pain was not severe, and it was sometimes associated with nausea but not with vomiting. In general, the duration of the neck pain was longer than that of vascular headaches, and an almost continuous aching from 2 to 8 weeks was usual. On physical examination, the carotid artery on the painful side was tender, with the tenderness being greatest at the carotid bifurcation or under the mandible. The sternocleidomastoid muscle on the same side was also often found to be tender, which was attributed to reflex muscle spasm. The treatment of the condition was considered to be the same as that of other painful vascular syndromes of the head, such as migraine. In 1977, Lovshin (30) referred to the syndrome of vascular neck pain as the most common form of carotidynia and related it to overdilation of the carotid artery. In the same year, Raskin and Prusiner (31) further emphasized the relationship of this syndrome to migraine and its response to antimigraine medications such as ergotamine, methysergide, and propranolol. A good response of the syndrome to pizotifen (32) and indomethacin (33) has also been described.

Carotidynia can also be caused by structural diseases of the carotid artery such as atherosclerosis (with subintimal hemorrhage), aneurysm formation, and fibromuscular dysplasia (34). The patients with these symptomatic forms of carotidynia tend to be older (i.e., over 45 years of age) and often have an associated carotid bruit. Treatment consisting of endarterectomy (atherosclerosis), resection (aneurysm), or denervation and dilation (dysplasia) has been reported to be often effective in relieving the pain (34). Dissection of the carotid artery can also be associated with vascular neck pain or carotidynia when it occurs in the proximal part of the cervical internal carotid artery. When it involves the distal part of the cervical internal carotid artery, headache may occur, usually located ipsilaterally in the frontal and orbital or sometimes temporal areas. The neck pain or headache of carotid artery dissection may precede the occurrence of stroke and may be associated with ipsilateral oculosympathetic paresis, resulting in narrowing of the pupil and drooping of the upper eyelid (34–38).

Headache following surgical endarterectomy of the internal carotid artery for occlusion of the artery was first described by Leviton (39, 40) in 1975. In a series of 50 patients in whom a total of 57 endarterectomies was performed, 24 complained of headache in the postoperative period (41). The headache following carotid endarterectomy usually has a delay of 1 to 3 days and is generally self-limiting over weeks or months. It can be either unilateral to the side of the endarterectomy or bilateral and is usually frontal. The headache has been attributed to cerebral hyperperfusion with distension of cerebral blood vessels due to the preoperative loss of cerebral autoregulation. The loss of autoregulation is due to the chronic cerebral ischemia caused by the carotid artery occlusion (42).

VENOUS THROMBOSIS

Thrombosis of cerebral veins and/or sinuses is a relatively rare condition that, especially in the milder cases, may be overlooked because it is difficult to diagnose clinically. With the advent of computerized tomography and, especially, magnetic resonance imaging (43), diagnosis of cerebral sinuvenous thrombosis has become easier, but it may still require angiography. Cerebral sinuvenous thrombosis basically manifests itself in two ways, depending on whether the accent lies on thrombosis of a sinus or vein (44). With sinus thrombosis, the clinical picture is very often that of "benign intracranial hypertension" with generalized headache, papilledema, and small ventricles on neurodiagnostic imaging. Venous thrombosis often manifests itself with focal signs such as hemiplegia and seizures, and neurodiagnostic imaging may reveal infarcts, ischemic and/or hemorrhagic. Headache is a common symptom accompanying sinuvenous thrombosis as the structures involved (i.e., the dural venous sinuses and the major cerebral veins) are sensitive to pain. The mechanisms involved are those of distension and inflammation due to the presence of the thrombus in the venous structure and the inflammation caused by the thrombus.

Cerebral sinuvenous thrombosis can occur "spontaneously" but can also be the result of minor head trauma, pregnancy, postpartum, oral contraceptive use, infection, or malignancy. The diagnostic method of choice is magnetic resonance imaging, which will show increased signal in the venous structures because of decreased flow velocity or cessation of flow (43). Treatment consists of anticoagulation with heparin, which seems to be beneficial even in patients who show evidence of hemorrhagic infarction on neurodiagnostic imaging (44). In contrast to the general belief, the outcome of cerebral sinuvenous thrombosis is generally favorable and without permanent sequelae, especially if focal signs are absent.

ARTERIAL HYPERTENSION

When arterial blood pressure increases abruptly and extends beyond the range of autoregulation, it distends the cerebral blood vessels and thus causes headache. The headache of generalized cerebral blood vessel distension is generally severe and throbbing or pounding. It may develop into a constant pain with persistence of the high blood pressure and development of cerebral edema, which may manifest itself by a decrease in the level of consciousness and/or the occurrence of seizures. Causes of an abruptly increasing blood pressure may be the use of a monoamine oxidase inhibitor, toxemia of pregnancy with (pre)eclampsia, malignant hypertension, pheochromocytoma, and autonomic dysinhibition in patients with a cervical cord lesion. The headache caused by arterial hypertension will resolve shortly after the blood pressure has been normalized, provided that the mechanism involved has not gone beyond distension of blood vessels.

REFERENCES

1. Ray BS, Wolff HG. Pain-sensitive structures of the head and their significance to headache. Arch Surg 1940;41:813–856.
2. International Headache Society. Classification and diagnostic criteria for headache disorders, cranial neuralgias and facial pain. Cephalagia 1988;8(suppl):1–96.
3. Portnoy RK, Abissi CJ, Lipton RB, Berger AL, Mebler MF, et al. Headache in cerebrovascular disease. Stroke 1984;15:1009–1012.
4. Gorelick PB, Hier DB, Caplan LR, Langenberg P. Headache in acute cerebrovascular disease. Neurology 1986;36:1445–1450.
5. Verweij RD, Wijdicks EFM, Van Gijn J. Warning headache in aneurysmal subarachnoid hemorrhage. Arch Neurol 1988;45:1019–1020.
6. Troost BT, Mark LE, Maroon JC. Resolution of classic migraine after removal of an occipital lobe AVM. Ann Neurol 1979;5:199–201.
7. Houser OW, Baker HL, Svien HJ, Okazaki H. Arteriovenous malformations of the brain. Radiology 1973;109:83–90.
8. Waltimo O, Hokkanen E, Pirskanen R. Intracranial arteriovenous malformations and headache. Headache 1975;15:133–135.
9. Bruyn GW. Intracranial arteriovenous malformation and migraine. Cephalagia 1984;4:191–207.
10. Troost BT, Newton TH. Occipital lobe arteriovenous malformations. Arch Ophthalmol 1975;93:250–256.
11. Maleki M, Kirkham TH. Arteriovenous malformations of the posterior cerebral hemispheres. Can J Opthalmol 1983;18:22–27.
12. Kattah JC, Luessenhop AJ, Kolsky M, Ferraz F. Removal of occipital arteriovenous malformations with sparing of visual fields. Arch Neurol 1981;38:307–309.
13. Leao AAP. Spreading depression of activity in the cerebral cortex. J Neurophysiol 1944;7:359–390.
14. Grafstein B. Mechanism of spreading cortical depression. J Neurophysiol 1956;19:154–171.
15. Milner PM. Note on a possible correspondence between the scotomas of migraine and spreading depression of Leao. EEG Clin Neurophysiol 1958;10:705.
16. Olesen J, Larsen B, Lauritzen M. Focal hyperemia followed by spreading oligemia and impaired activation of rCBF in classic migraine. Ann Neurol 1981;9:344–352.
17. Frankel K. Relation of migraine to cerebral aneurysm. Arch Neurol Psychiatry 1950;63:195–204.
18. Sugar O. Headache of intracranial vascular origin. Headache 1967;6:172–174.
19. Hutchinson J. Diseases of the arteries. On a peculiar form of thrombotic arteritis of the aged which is sometimes productive of gangrene. Arch Surg (London) 1890;1:323–331.
20. Horton BT, Magath TB, Brown GE. An undescribed form of arteritis of the temporal vessels. Proc Staff Meet Mayo Clin 1932;7:700–701.
21. Cooke WT, Cloake PCP, Govan ADT, Colbeck JC. Temporal arteritis: a generalized vascular disease. Q J Med 1946;15:47–75.
22. Horton BT. Headache and intermittent claudication of the jaw in temporal arteritis. Headache 1962;2:29–40.
23. Blaiss MS, Waxman J, Lange RK. Occipital headache as a manifestation of giant cell arteritis. South Med J 1982;75:887–888.
24. Solomon S, Cappa KG. The headache of temporal arteritis. J Am Geriatr Soc 1987;35:163–165.
25. Ferris EJ, Levine HL. Cerebral arteritis: classification. Radiology 1973;109:327–341.
26. Atkinson RA, Appenzeller O. Headache in small vessel disease of the brain: a study of patients with systemic lupus erythematosus. Headache 1975;15:198–201.
27. Fay T. Atypical neuralgia. Arch Neurol Psychiatry 1927,18:309–315.
28. Fay T. Atypical facial neuralgia, a syndrome of vascular pain. Ann Otology Rhinol Laryngol 1932;41:1030–1062.

29. Lovshin LL. Vascular neck pain—a common syndrome seldom recognized. Cleve Clin Q 1960;27:5–13.
30. Lovshin LL. Carotidynia. Headache 1977;17:192–195.
31. Raskin NH, Prusiner S. Carotidynia. Neurology 1977;27:43–46.
32. Murray TJ. Carotidynia: a cause of neck and face pain. Can Med Assoc J 1979;20:441–443.
33. Orfei R, Meienberg O. Carotidynia: report of eight cases and propsective evaluation of therapy. J Neurol 1983;230:65–72.
34. Mehigan JT, Olcott C. Carotidynia associated with carotid arterial disease and stroke. Am J Surg 1981;142:210–211.
35. Ehrenfeld WK, Wylie EJ. Spontaneous dissection of the internal carotid artery. Arch Surg 1976;111:1294–1301.
36. Mokri B, Sundt TM, Houser W. Spontaneous internal carotid dissection, hemicrania, and Horner's syndrome. Arch Neurol 1979;36:677–680.
37. Fisher CM. The headache and pain of spontaneous carotid dissection. Headache 1982;22:60–65.
38. Vanneste JAL, Davies G. Spontaneous dissection of the cervical internal carotid artery. Clin Neurol Neurosurg 1984;86:307–314.
39. Leviton A. Post carotid-endarterectomy "hemicrania." Headache 1975;15:13–17.
40. Leviton A, Caplan L, Salzman E. Severe headache after carotid endarterectomy. Headache 1975;15:207–209.
41. Messert B, Black JA. Cluster headache, hemicrania, and other head pains: morbidity of carotid endarterectomy. Stroke 1978;9:559–562.
42. Reigel MM, Hollier LH, Sundt TM, Piepgras DG, Sharbrough FW, Cherry KJ. Cerebral hyperperfusion syndrome: a cause of neurologic dysfunction after carotid endarterectomy J Vas Surg 1987;5:628–634.
43. Donohoe CD, Waldman SD, Resor LD. Magnetic resonance imaging in cerebral venous thrombosis, a case report. Headache 1987;27:155–157.
44. Bousser MG, Chiras J, Bories J, Castaigne P. Cerebral venous thrombosis—a review of 38 cases. Stroke 1985;16:199–213.

37

Uncommon Headache Disorders

GEORGE H. SANDS, LAWRENCE C. NEWMAN, and RICHARD B. LIPTON

The subject of this chapter is two groups of uncommon headache disorders classified, whenever possible, according to the nosology of the International Headache Society (IHS) (1). The first is a miscellaneous group comprised of idiopathic stabbing headache and several disorders triggered by ingestion, environmental factors, or sleep. Headaches related to ingestion include cold stimulus headache (ice-cream headache), nitrate/nitrite-induced headache, and monosodium glutamate–induced headache. The environmental headache disorders include high-altitude headache, hypoxic headache, and carbon monoxide headache. Finally, the sleep-related syndrome, hypnic headache, is discussed.

The second group includes headaches provoked by "exertional" triggers as manifested by coughing, lifting, and sexual activity. These have been classified by the IHS as benign cough headache, benign exertional headache, and headache associated with sexual activity. Throughout the text parenthetical numbers refer to the IHS codes (1).

MISCELLANEOUS HEADACHES

IDIOPATHIC STABBING HEADACHE (4.1)
(ICE-PICK HEADACHE)

Brief, sharp, jabbing pains occurring either as a single episode or in repeated volleys are referred to as idiopathic stabbing headache. Other terms used include jabs and jolts (2); sharp, short-lived head pain syndrome (3); needle-in-the-eye syndrome (3); and ophthalmodynia periodica (4). The pain is moderate. Episodes occur up to 50 times per day and typically last from 5 to 10 seconds (2). The IHS have established diagnostic criteria for the disorder (Table 37.1) (1).

Though this disorder is likely to appear with other headache types, it may be the primary problem. The sharp jabbing pains are most strongly associated with migraine (4, 7). Ice-pick pains were coincidental with the site of the patient's usual headache in 40% of migraineurs (8). This headache also occurs in patients with cluster headache, often presaging the termination of an attack (5, 6). Giant cell arteritis (9) and the cluster variant syndrome (10) have been associated with similar head pains.

To determine the prevalence of ice-pick headache and its association with migraine, 100 migraineurs and 100 con-trol subjects were questioned about their headaches (7). Sharp, jabbing head pains were reported at least once annually by 42 migraineurs and by only 3 patients in the control group. More than half of the migraineurs had the attacks more than monthly. A single jab of pain was usual (64%), but volleys of jabs (12%) also occurred. The pain was usually unifocal, occurring most frequently in the temple or orbital regions. When multifocal, the foci were usually ipsilateral. Seven of the migraineurs and 1 control subject reported at least one of the following precipitants to their sharp, jabbing pain: sudden postural change, physical exertion, transition from dark to light, and head motion during headache. These ice-pick pains preceded a migraine attack in seven patients.

When ice-pick headache is associated with migraine, it often improves with migraine prophylaxis. Indomethacin 50 mg three times daily dramatically decreased the number of attacks, in a small series (3).

INGESTION OF A COLD STIMULUS HEADACHE (4.3.2)
(ICE-CREAM HEADACHE)

Headaches are frequently precipitated by eating ice cream or other extremely cold foods. The pain is most often in the anterior temporal region, occasionally encompassing the orbit (11). It may also be experienced in the palate, throat, forehead, or ear (12). IHS criteria describe the clinical features of this syndrome (1) (Table 37.1).

Raskin and Knittle (13) interviewed 108 subjects without migraine regarding the presence of ice-cream headache and postural nonheadache symptoms. In this group, 31% had related ice-cream headache symptoms and 8% had postural symptoms. The authors postulated that there may be an excessive vascular reaction to cold in migraineurs because of an erratic modulation of vasomotor tone. They proposed that the presence of ice-cream headache or orthostatic symptoms may be a useful biological marker in suspected migraineurs.

Other theories have been suggested to account for ice-cream headache. Smith (11) implicated a vascular phenomenon, originating in vasoconstriction and requiring a significant stretching of the blood vessel wall. Wolff (14) theorized that the headache resulted from cold stimulation of the phar-

Table 37.1.
International Headache Society Classification and Diagnostic Criteria for Miscellaneous Headache Disorders [a]

(4.1) Idiopathic stabbing headache (ice-pick headache)
A. Pain confined to the head and exclusively or predominantly felt in the distribution of the first division of the trigeminal nerve (orbit, temple, and parietal area.)
B. Pain is stabbing in nature and lasts for a fraction of a second; it occurs as single stabs or series of stabs.
C. It recurs at irregular intervals (hours to days).
D. Diagnosis depends upon the exclusion of structural changes at the site of pain and in the distribution of the affected cranial nerve.

(4.3.2) Ingestion of a cold stimulus headache (ice-cream headache)
A. Develops during ingestion of a cold food or drink.
B. Lasts for less than 5 minutes.
C. Is felt in the middle of the forehead, except in people subject to migraine, in which case the pain may be referred to the area habitually affected by migraine headache.
D. Is prevented by avoiding rapid swallowing of cold food or drinks.
E. Is not associated with organic disease.

(10.1.1) High-altitude headache
A. Occurs within 24 hours after sudden ascent to altitudes above 3000 meters.
B. Is associated with at least one other symptom typical of high altitude
  1. Cheyne-Stokes respiration at night
  2. Desire to over breathe
  3. Exertional dyspnea

(10.1.2) Headache associated with hypoxia
  Headache associated with hypoxia (10.1.2) occurs within 24 hours after the acute onset of hypoxia with PaO_2 equal to or less than 70 mm Hg or in chronic hypoxic patients with PaO_2 persistently at or below this level.

[a]Modified from Headache Classification Committee of the International Headache Society. Classification and diagnostic criteria for headache disorders, cranial neuralgias and facial pain. Cephalalgia 1988;8(suppl 7).

ynx. He discovered that placing ice on the palate resulted in frontal headache. The application of ice to the fossa of Rosenmüller or the posterior fossa led to pain in and behind the ear. Ice in the stomach or esophagus did not produce pain.

Wolf and Hardy (15) noted that when the vertex of the head was placed in cold water, pain was engendered in the vertex and then spread down the back of the head and into the temples. Plum (16) showed that if a noxious stimulus, (e.g., cold air) was applied to structures innervated by one branch of the trigeminal nerve, pain was felt in areas supplied by another portion of the nerve, resulting in a severe headache.

Migraineurs seem to have an increased risk for ice-cream headache. Though the mechanism is uncertain, clearly a cold stimulus initiates a process that leads to pain. Perhaps migraineurs have a lower threshold for the initiation of this process. Pharmacological intervention is rarely required for this headache. The recommended treatment is to avoid the rapid ingestion of very cold food and drink.

NITRATE/NITRITE-INDUCED HEADACHE (8.1.1) (HOT DOG HEADACHE)

Sodium nitrite is added to meats such as hot dogs, salami, and bacon to ensure a homogenous red color. Data from surveys show that some of these foods may trigger migraine (17, 18). Henderson and Raskin (19) found a patient who developed bitemporal nonthrobbing headache within 30 minutes of eating cured meats. They tested this patient with identical solutions of sodium bicarbonate and sodium nitrite. Headache developed in 8 of 13 trials with sodium nitrite but in none of 8 trials with sodium bicarbonate. The headache was similar in duration and quality to those following eating cured meat.

This patient developed similar headache in 2 of 4 trials after ingesting tyramine. In 10 other volunteers without a history of food-induced headache, none of the solutions provoked a headache. The mechanism by which nitrite induces headache is unknown. It is conceivable that a mechanism similar to that operative in the headache triggered by nitroglycerin (i.e., vasodilation) is involved. Additional work is needed to clarify the importance of nitrates as a headache trigger. This disorder is recognized in the IHS classification (8.1.1), which requires that the headache occur within 1 hour after absorption of nitrate/nitrite (1).

MONOSODIUM GLUTAMATE–INDUCED HEADACHE (8.1.2)

Monosodium glutamate (MSG) is an additive commonly used for its flavor-enhancing properties in food. Ho Man Kwok (20) first described what later became known as the "Chinese restaurant" syndrome, in 1968. The syndrome consisted of numbness at the back, general weakness, and palpitation occurring 15 to 20 minutes after eating Chinese food. He thought that this syndrome might be partly caused by the MSG in the food. Following Kwok's article, other reports appeared in the literature (21–33). Approximately 30% of people who eat Chinese food experience headache, tightness of the face, dizziness, diarrhea, nausea, and abdominal cramps (34).

Schaumburg and Byck (35) and Ambos et al. (36) discovered that MSG was responsible for the syndrome. Schaumburg et al. (37) showed that 3 gm or less of MSG would lead to an attack. They gave 56 normal people MSG orally; all but one developed symptoms. Fifty milligrams of intravenous MSG produced symptoms in this patient. The authors also reported that in two subjects, 50 mg of diphenhydramine had no effect, decreasing the possibility that this was an allergy-related disorder.

Kenney and Tidball (38) and Kenney (33) found a dose-responsive relationship between the MSG administered and reported symptoms in placebo-controlled studies of normal volunteers. The authors postulated that MSG itself might not be responsible for this syndrome, since blood glutamine levels were not correlated with the symptomatology. They concluded that the "subcutaneous fine nerve endings of primitive chemical sense" may be involved because the symptoms are mostly peripheral. Another double-blind placebo-controlled trial by Gore and Salmon (39) tested 55 subjects who had not heard of the Chinese restaurant syndrome. The reaction to MSG was higher than that to placebo, although no one described the classic syndrome. These authors thought that MSG was not the sole cause of the syndrome; its interaction with another substance was responsible. Two other double-blind studies did not show a relationship between MSG ingestion and the Chinese restaurant syndrome (40, 41). However these studies used a large number of male subjects, previously reported to be less susceptible to the effects of MSG (24).

The available evidence suggests that MSG provokes a symptom complex, including headache, in susceptible individuals. This can be demonstrated in susceptible individuals but not in unselected subjects. Reif-Lehrer (42) postulated that the Chinese restaurant syndrome may result from a "benign" inborn error of metabolism. The susceptibility of migraineurs to MSG-evoked headache has not been evaluated.

Environmental Headaches

In this section we discuss high-altitude, hypoxic, and carbon monoxide headache.

HIGH ALTITUDE HEADACHE (10.1.1)

Increased air travel has hastened the rapid access of many sea-level residents to remote high mountain regions. This has led to an increased awareness of altitude illness or acute mountain sickness (AMS) (43–46). Jose De Acosta first recounted the headache of AMS, in 1569, when he became symptomatic riding his donkey, at approximately 12,500 feet elevation (43, 44, 46). The IHS diagnostic criteria for high-altitude headache and headache associated with hypoxia are detailed in Table 37.1.

Clinical Features. Hamilton et al. (44) have classified the clinical features of acute mountain sickness as benign or malignant. The earlier features are generally benign and include headache, nausea, vomiting, malaise, vertigo, anorexia, palpitations, insomnia, dim vision, and anxiety (44, 47, 48). AMS syndrome develops a malignant character as it progresses to high-altitude pulmonary edema (HAPE) or high-altitude cerebral edema (HACE), the more serious manifestations of AMS. Headache is the most frequent symptom of benign AMS and HACE (48, 49). Headache is uncommon below 8000 feet, although vigorous exercise can provoke acute effort migraine, as noted at the 1968 Mexico City Olympics (elevation 7000 feet) (43, 45, 47). Headache is more frequent at higher elevations. In the unacclimated person, headache is almost always present above 12,000 feet (43, 46, 47, 50).

The headache may be primarily frontal (43) or occipital (47, 48). The pain may be a generalized throbbing or pounding. Approximately 25% of patients have lateralized head pain (46). The pain is often augmented by coughing, straining, exertion, or sudden jolts to the head. The headache is increased by reclining and sleep. Cheyne-Stokes

respirations often occur during the latter. Taking cold fluids and carbohydrates seems to improve the headache (43, 46). Cerebral edema may be heralded by memory loss, irritability, retinal vein dilatation, and retinal hemorrhages (44). The latter are an accompaniment in over 50% of all persons ascending to high altitude (45). A constant headache, at high altitude, is frequently transformed into a pulsatile pain by exercise (47). The headache of AMS varies in severity and characteristics from person to person. However, it is usually triggered consistently at the same altitude in an individual at different times (47).

Exacerbation of the headache, with inadequate diuresis and growing breathlessness, portends severe papilledema, stupor, seizures, coma, and paralysis. These signs were only present in 24 of 840 symptomatic cases. Lumbar punctures performed in 34 patients during AMS and after established that the CSF pressure was 60 to 210 mm higher during the acute illness (48).

Pathophysiology. The delay of 6 to 96 hours between the time of achieving a high altitude and the onset of AMS symptoms suggests that the immediate cause of AMS is not hypoxia (44, 48). Early cerebral edema appears to result in early benign AMS. As the pathophysiology progresses, the malignant forms of AMS, HAPE and HACE, may follow. Continued hypoxia leads to pulmonary congestion, enhanced cerebral circulation, augmented CSF pressure, and cerebral edema. The change in cerebrovascular flow appears to be important in the development of HACE. Hypoxia-induced vasodilatation produces cerebral engorgement, with a resultant increase in cerebral blood volume. As the pCO_2 rises during sleep, cerebrovascular flow increases and headache results (47). It has been postulated that failure of cerebrovascular autoregulation may lead to cerebral edema with the transmission of increased pressure to the capillary vasculature, as found in hypertensive encephalopathy. Diffuse, congested, dilated cerebral capillaries with perivascular and petechial hemorrhages and advanced white matter edema have been seen at autopsy (44, 48). HACE's pathophysiology has been completely reviewed elsewhere (44, 45).

Prevention and Treatment. The rapidity of ascent and the magnitude of the elevation attained are directly related to the chances of acquiring AMS. Respiratory depressants such as drugs and alcohol are best avoided (45). The advantage of oxygen treatment for the headache is unclear (44–47).

Acetazolamide (250 mg) given every 8 hours, 1 to 2 days prior to ascent, may aide in preventing AMS (44, 50, 51). The headache is decreased when 250 to 500 mg of acetazolamide is taken prior to sleep (45). Acetazolamide acts as a mild diuretic that changes cerebral circulation, cerebrospinal fluid production, and acid-base balance (52). Its exact mode of action in treating these conditions is unknown.

Furosemide was effective in relieving AMS when used in 446 cases (48). Singh et al. used 80 mg every 12 hours for

2 days or longer. They treated 19 of their 24 cases, with neurological manifestations of HACE, with furosemide and betamethasone. Headache and vomiting became less prominent within 3 days (48). Other investigators found furosemide to be ineffective and perhaps even contraindicated in the treatment of AMS because climbers at high altitude are already volume-contracted (44).

Several other medications have also been reported to be helpful. Dexamethasone taken alone seems to be useful in preventing AMS. It has been prescribed prophylactically, in doses of 4 mg every 6 hours, 48 hours before climbing to 4300 meters elevation (53, 54). Dexamethasone has been used emergently, to allow safe descent, in patients with AMS (55). It was effective treating AMS in a hypobaric chamber at a simulated altitude of 3700 meters (56). Ergotamine gave some relief, after 6 of 9 injections, in 4 subjects. Its use has been accompanied by gastrointestinal upset almost routinely. This led some authors to advise that ergotamine not be used in this setting (51). There is suggestive evidence that phenytoin may be of use in AMS (57). Aspirin decreased headaches and enhanced sleep in 250 patients, when given 3 times daily for 2 days at a dosage of 0.6 gm (48). Some have warned that drugs interfering with platelet function, including aspirin, should not be used because of the high-altitude retinal hemorrhage syndrome (45). It is probably wise to avoid these medications, given that hemorrhages are commonly found at autopsy (44, 48). One case of HAPE was dramatically improved by treatment with sublingual nifedipine (20 mg) in a patient who had previously taken 500 mg of acetazolomide daily (58). The effect of the nifedipine makes it a possible future treatment for high-altitude headache. The best method for AMS prevention is gradual ascent, permitting adequate acclimatization. Protocols have been published for such acclimatization (44, 48).

Carbon Monoxide Headache. The headache produced by exposure to various levels of carbon monoxide (CO) is not distinctive. Both acute and chronic CO exposure will lead to headache, often associated with other symptoms. The IHS has not defined diagnostic criteria for this entity, although it is listed in the classification (1).

Acute and chronic exposure produce different syndromes. Acute exposure results in headache, dizziness, blurred vision, yawning, mydriasis, tremors, ataxia, anorexia, nausea, bradycardia, hypertension, and palpitation. Continued exposure induces stupor, confusion, and/or delirium (59). Chronic CO exposure most frequently causes a dull frontal headache associated with vertigo, nervousness, neuromuscular and chest pains, palpitations, decreased concentration, syncope, and dyspnea (60). The pain occasionally has a throbbing character but is more often described as a pressure (59).

The symptomatology seems to correlate to the degree of CO poisoning, as measured by carboxyhemoglobin (COHb) levels (60, 61). When the COHb level is 10 to 20%, the mild headache is frequently holocranial and suboccipital. There are no other neurological signs at this level. As the COHb level rises to 20 or 30%, the headache intensifies and may acquire a pounding character. The patient might exhibit faulty judgement, irritability, and fatigability. At levels of 30 to 40%, the headache further intensifies, becoming intolerable. Nausea, vomiting, dizziness, decreased vision and more confusion are also found at this level of CO intoxication. Above 40%, the patient develops more confusion with progressive obtundation and coma, preventing complaints of headache. Death may occur if the patient is not removed from the CO (60).

When considering the diagnosis of CO headache, the patterns of symptomatology over time and location may be useful. For example, if the patient is exposed to a faulty furnace overnight at home, symptoms may improve during the workday or after an overnight trip. Another strong clue is provided when several family members or work colleagues develop similar symptoms concurrently. Finally, associated symptoms such as cardiac arrhythmias or respiratory difficulties may suggest the diagnosis. Making a correct diagnosis is potentially lifesaving in this condition.

Hypnic Headache. The hypnic headache syndrome is a rarely recognized benign headache disorder of the elderly. To date, there have been 8 documented cases; 5 men and 3 women, ranging from 65 to 84 years of age (62, 63). Headache awakened patients from sleep at a consistent time each night, sometimes during a dream. The headache was global, often pulsatile, and it lasted from 30 to 60 minutes. They were occasionally associated with nausea but not by any other autonomic features. Two of the patients experienced more than 1 attack nightly, separated by a 2-hour interval. The periodicity of the attacks and the association of headache during dreaming suggest that this headache may be associated with rapid eye movement (REM) sleep. All 8 patients responded to therapy with lithium carbonate in doses from 300 to 600 mg at bedtime.

HEADACHES PROVOKED BY "EXERTION" IN ITS MANY FORMS

BENIGN EXERTIONAL HEADACHE (BEH)

In 1932, Tinel reported 4 patients with an intermittent headache accompanying effort, which he labeled "la céphalée à l'effort" (64, 65). Subsequently, Sir Charles Symonds, in the first English language description, reported 27 patients with similar transient intense head pain triggered by coughing, sneezing, laughing, stooping, or straining at stool (66). Symonds called these disorders "cough headache" and divided them into two groups. The first group was composed of patients with structural disease of the brain and skull. The second included 21 patients without any clinical manifestations of a mass lesion.

Rooke (67) used "benign exertional headache" to describe any headache provoked by exertion (e.g., "running, bending, coughing, sneezing, heavy lifting or straining at stool"), not associated with structural brain disease, which began rapidly and persisted seconds to minutes.

A recent approach to the classification of these disorders, as proposed by the IHS, is found in Table 37.2. We discuss benign cough headache and benign exertional headache (BEH) together because they share a similar clinical presentation, require a similar diagnostic evaluation, and have a similar treatment response.

Clinical Features. BEH has appeared infrequently in the literature. Approximately 180 cases have been reported in the English and French literature since 1932. Unfortunately, there are no data based on population surveys. A population-based survey using a careful history might establish that it occurs more frequently than currently appreciated. A history of an antecedent respiratory infection is obtained in up to 25% of cases (66–68). However, the etiology is unknown. The age of onset ranges from 19 to 73 years, with a mean of 55 years (66, 69). The headache is 4 times more frequent in men than women (67) and two times more common in patients older than 40 years of age (67). The pain has an immediate onset (66, 69) or occurs within seconds of the provocative event (64, 65, 70). Provocations include "muscular effort, cough, sneezing," and "lifting a burden, pushing to go to the toilet, blowing, crying, or singing"(65). Lowering the head or lying down may be impossible (3, 64–66). The severe pain has a bursting, explosive, or splitting character enduring for a few seconds or minutes (3, 64–66, 69, 71). Patients are generally pain-free between paroxysms. However, a dull ache may persist after the attack for several hours (66, 68, 71). Thirty-five percent of the time, the headache is unilateral (67). The most severe pain may be in the occipital, frontal, or temporal regions or at the vertex (3, 66, 69–72). Nausea and vomiting are generally unassociated with BEH (67). Vomiting suggests a structural basis for the headache. Vomiting has been correlated with posterior fossa meningiomas, basilar impression (66), and cerebellar tonsillar herniation (70).

Diamond expanded BEH's spectrum to include headache of more prolonged duration with vascular characteristics; several of his patients had histories of migraine or muscle-contraction headache (73). In Diamond's series, the headache ranged from 15 minutes to 16 hours in duration, with a mean of 4 hours. Nine patients had bilateral pain; one patient had it unilaterally.

A normal neurological examination is usually found in patients with the benign syndrome (66). Nevertheless, a number of provocative maneuvers have been published, particularly in the French literature. Tinel reported that a relatively tight rubber band around the patient's neck triggered the headache. The pain occurred simultaneously with facial congestion and disappeared soon after the compression was relieved (64, 65). Another test calls for patients to stand on their toes and quickly fall onto their heels (69). The "jolt" maneuver, which may elicit the pain, requires a swift rotary movement of the head to the side,

Table 37.2.
International Headache Society Classification and Diagnostic Criteria for Headache Disorders Associated with "Exertion"[a]

(4.4) Benign cough headache
A. Is a bilateral headache of sudden onset, lasting less than 1 minute, precipitated by coughing.
B. May be prevented by avoiding coughing.
C. May be diagnosed only after structural lesions such as posterior fossa tumor have been excluded by neuroimaging.

(4.5) Benign exertional headache
A. Is specifically brought on by physical exercise.
B. Is bilateral, throbbing at onset and may develop migrainous features in those patients susceptible to migraine.
C. Lasts from 5 minutes to 24 hours.
D. Is prevented by avoiding excessive exertion, particularly in hot weather or at high altitude.
E. Is not associated with any systemic or intracranial disorder.

(4.6) Headache associated with sexual activity
A. Is precipitated by sexual excitement.
B. Is bilateral at onset.
C. Is prevented or eased by ceasing sexual activity before orgasm.
D. Is not associated with any intracranial disorder such as aneurysm.
    4.6.1 *Dull type*—A dull ache in the head and neck that intensifies as sexual excitement increases
    4.6.2 *Explosive type*—A sudden severe ("explosive") headache at orgasm
    4.6.3 *Postural type*—Postural headache resembling that of low CSF pressure developing after coitus

[a]Modified from Headache Classification Committee of the International Headache Society. Classification and diagnostic criteria for headache disorders, cranial neuralgias and facial pain. Cephalalgia 1988;8(suppl 7).

followed by returning to midposition (66, 69, 74). These maneuvers cannot differentiate BEH from headache resulting from trauma, tumor, or lumbar puncture (69). It seems that these maneuvers are successful in eliciting pain when the intracranial vascular structures are distended or inflamed.

Rooke (67) followed 103 patients, without discernable intracranial disease at their initial examination, who presented with exertional headache. Ten developed structural lesions after 3 or more years of follow-up. The others improved or were free of headache after 10 years. Rooke, in this pre-CT report, emphasized the importance of carefully evaluating these patients for structural disease.

Etiology. When a patient presents with the picture of exertional headache, it must be determined whether the headache is benign or associated with intracranial disease. Five of 221 patients in one series reported exertional headache and subsequently had pathologically confirmed brain tumors (67, 75). As a result, high-quality brain imaging is necessary to appropriately evaluate patients with exertional headache.

Fifty-two of 232 cases of exertional and cough headache reported in the literature had identifiable structural etiology. Table 37.3 examines cases of cough and benign exertional headache, from several selected series, in etiologically related groups. The posterior fossa space-occupying lesion group also contains cases with the Arnold-Chiari deformity (67) and hindbrain herniation (70). Posttraumatic and postcraniotomy cases were also grouped together. Structural myocardial disease, producing ischemia, was found to be related to episodic headache similar to benign exertional headache (76–79).

Not all the cases of BEH in Table 37.3 meet the IHS diagnostic criteria (1). Many of these cases were collected before these criteria were published. Massey (80) described 3 runners with effort headache. Two of them had BEH by the IHS criteria. The third had effort migraine, not meeting the criteria for BEH or fitting any other IHS criteria. Indo and Takahashi (81) reported 2 cases of headache precipitated by swimming and one by diving. Their second case does not fulfill the IHS criteria for BEH, but it is clearly related to many published cases of benign cough headache. The other cases would meet IHS criteria if they had bilateral head pain. This is not clear from their description. We included weight-lifter's headache with the benign group, as we believe it to be part of the same spectrum of disease (73, 82–84).

Katchen reported two military pilots who complained of BEH triggered by antigravity straining maneuvers associated with flying high-performance jet aircraft (85, 86). The pain was "incapacitating," forcing the pilots to fly straight and level for several minutes until the pain abated. Interestingly, these two patients also complained of headache with orgasm.

Silbert et al. describe another patient who had an intense headache within 2 minutes of orgasm, which recurred 36 hours later when he chased and screamed at a dog (87). This patient also did not meet the IHS criteria but would fit into the "benign cough headache" appellation historically. A cerebral angiogram demonstrated arterial spasm of uncertain significance. This patient is included in the BEH group.

The various series we evaluated were not always comprised of consecutive patients. Some publications reported only nonorganic etiologies, while others only reported patients with structural disease. Therefore, it is difficult to precisely state the proportion of patients with exertional headache who have structural disease. It is likely that some patients with structural brain disease were undetected, since several of these series were collected in the pre-CT era. We may expect the frequency of cases with structural disease to increase as new series are compiled in the era of MRI. Special attention to the posterior fossa and foramen magnum with MRI is the preferred procedure for evaluating these patients.

Exertion may aggravate other types of headache. Coughing may exacerbate post-lumbar-puncture headache, severe migraine, and (infrequently) pseudotumor cerebri (71, 88, 89). There were no complaints of exertional headache among the 27 patients with an unruptured cerebral aneurysm or vascular anomaly in Rooke's collection of 303 patients with intracranial lesions (67). Third ventricular colloid cysts may produce paroxysmal headache by intermittent obstruction of the flow of CSF

Table 37.3.
Etiologies for Cough and Exertional Headache in Literature[a,b]

"Structural" (organic)	52(22.4%)
Posterior fossa space-occupying lesions	18 (35%)[c]
Postrauma or postcraniotomy	13 (25%)
Supratentorial space-occupying lesions	9 (17%)
Basilar impression/platybasia	6 (11%)
Syrinx	2 (04%)
Myocardial ischemia	4 (08%)
BEH	180(77.6%)
Total	232

[a]Modified after Sands GH, Newman L, Lipton R. Cough, exertional and other miscellaneous headaches. Med Clin North Am 1991;75:733–747.
[b]English and French literature including the following references: 3, 59, 61, 62, 64–66, 68, 79, 95–97, 104–113.
[c]Percentages calculated with the total number of patients with structural disease (n = 52) as the denominator.

through the foramen of Monro, resulting in a rapid increase in intracranial pressure (71, 90). Tumors of the lateral ventricles, cerebellum, and cerebrum; craniopharyngiomas; and pinealomas have produced similar headaches (68). Pheochromocytomas may lead to paroxysmal headache, especially with exercise (91–93). Hazelrigg reported thyrotoxicosis, hypoglycemia, chronic obstructive pulmonary disease, and essential hypertension as other possible causes of exertional headache (89).

Pathophysiology. A number of theories have been offered to explain exertional headache. Tinel (65) postulated a "thoracic block" causing jugular venous stasis with resultant intracranial venous hypertension. Symonds suggested that adhesions between mobile and immobile pain-sensitive structures might cause cough headache in some patients. Remissions of exertional headache has been induced occasionally by dissection of localized adhesions (66, 67). The disappearance of cough headache subsequent to extremely severe bouts of coughing or pneumoencephalography may also be explained by this mechanism (66, 67). Lichenstein (94) suggested that an elevation in subarachnoid pressure secondary to cough might result in the herniation of the arachnoid membrane and pacchionian bodies into the venous sinuses, somehow resulting in pain. Nick (69) thought that the increased intrathoracic pressure leads to intracranial venous hypertension with a resultant augmentation in the cerebral volume. The augmented volume results in cerebral herniation into the foramen magnum, with traction on the pain-sensitive dura and other mooring structures, engendering headache.

Williams researched the CSF pressure's response to coughing in patients with structural cerebral abnormalities (95). He documented an early CSF pressure wave that traveled into the cranium, followed by a reversal of the wave's direction down within the thecal sac, which could result in dural traction. Later, Williams established a pressure difference between the ventricles and the lumbar subarachnoid space during coughing in two patients with cough headache and cerebellar tonsillar herniation (96). The difference in pressure pushed the cerebellar tonsils further into the foramen magnum. Williams called this pressure difference "craniospinal pressure dissociation." He reported that headaches disappeared after surgical decompression of the cerebellar tonsils. Subsequently, four patients were reported with headache secondary to paroxysmal impaction of the cerebellar tonsils into the foramen magnum, after maneuvers causing craniospinal pressure dissociation (70). These mechanisms may be pertinent for patients with structural disease. However they do not solve the etiology of the pain in most benign cases.

Dental pathology may be invoked in some cases. Pain relief after dental extractions occurred in two of Symonds's 21 patients (66) and 4 of the 93 patients in Rooke's series (67). Searching for dental abscesses seems worthwhile. A study found that stimulating premolars or molar teeth may result in a severe pain radiating into the eye, the orbital ridge, and the temple (97). This pain frequently lasts from 5 to 20 minutes, although milder pain often persisted over 1 to 8 hours. This is a similar pattern to BEH. These pain patterns seem possible only when an upper tooth is involved.

Raskin (68) postulated that this disorder may be partly the result of heightened sensitivity of an unidentified receptor. He found that the cough headache syndrome may follow an electrode implantation into the periaqueductal gray matter. Raskin successfully treated 4 consecutive patients with this syndrome with intravenous dihydroergotamine. He thought that unstable serotonergic neurotransmission might be part of the pathophysiology of this disorder.

Treatment. One strives to eliminate as much pain as possible, for patients with benign etiologies. When the headaches are frequent or intense, prophylactic therapy is necessary, as the short duration often makes abortive therapy impractical. The prophylactic medication of choice is indomethacin, in doses from 25 mg to 150 mg daily (3, 73, 98). Treatment with misoprostol, sulcralfate, or antacids may be useful if there is gastrointestinal intolerance to indomethacin. Raskin states that naproxen, ergonovine, and phenelzine are helpful if indomethacin fails. Propranolol is not (68).

HEADACHE ASSOCIATED WITH SEXUAL ACTIVITY (4.6)

It is often believed that headache is an excuse to avoid sexual activity. In this section, we explore sexual activity and its role in provoking headache. Although we focus on benign headache, we also consider the organic differential diagnosis of sexual headache.

The IHS uses "headache associated with sexual activity" to include the disorders more colorfully called coital cephalgia, orgasmic cephalgia, and benign sexual headache. The IHS has published diagnostic criteria for all the headaches in this group (1) (Table 37.2).

There is an uncertain relationship between sexual and exertional headaches. Sexual headache is frequently dull during the initial phase of sexual excitement and intensifies

at orgasm, a type of exertion. Additionally, several patients with both exertional and sexual headache have been documented (72, 85, 86, 99, 100). However, Lance has written that physical exertion did not have a role in his patients with sexual headache (101).

Clinical features. Sexual headache is rare. It was discovered in approximately one of 360 headache patients seen in a general neurology clinic (72). Men are stricken four times more frequently than women. The second through sixth decades are the usual ages of onset. The headache is unpredictable, occurring in one instance and not another (101, 102). This variability renders the evaluation of the efficacy of therapy difficult.

Twenty-four percent of published cases are the dull or muscle-contraction type, also known as type I (101–103). The tightness or dull pain is often generalized or occipital and may last hours to days. It often starts early during sexual intercourse, intensifying at orgasm. The headache seems related to the quantity of sexual excitement and the degree of neck and facial muscular contraction. Some patients talked of "excessive muscular contraction" in the neck and jaw muscles. Relaxation of these muscles during intercourse or masturbation sometimes resulted in some relief (101).

The explosive or vascular-type headache is the most common subtype of headache associated with sexual activity. This subtype, previously known as type II, occurred in 69% of cases (101–103). The pain was very intense, described as "explosive" and "throbbing," often bilateral over the occipital or frontal regions (101–103). About one-quarter of these patients have a personal or family history of migraine.

Seven percent of cases are postural or low cerebrospinal fluid (CSF) pressure-type headache (101, 102). This postural, suboccipital, headache with nausea and vomiting was originally described as a type III headache (101). Two of the three described patients had CSF pressure under 20 mm H₂O. The authors proposed that intercourse somehow causes a meningeal tear resulting in a CSF leak producing headache. This headache may persist for 2 to 3 weeks and then resolve spontaneously.

Intracranial disorders must be excluded to make the diagnosis by the IHS criteria. A patient presenting with this headache needs evaluation to exclude structural brain disease including subarachnoid hemorrhage (SAH). Sexual headache presented as SAH in 3.3% (104), 4.5% (105), and 12% (106) of aneurysms and 4.1% of AVMs (104).

The acute onset of severe pain in the explosive type headache is suggestive of SAH. CT and CSF examinations must be done to exclude SAH. An explosive or "thunderclap headache" has been reported in one patient with an unruptured aneurysm and normal CT and CSF examinations (107). Day and Raskin proposed that cerebral angiography "is probably necessary" in this instance. More recently, other studies concluded that normal CT and CSF examinations in patients with thunderclap headache do not usually require cerebral angiography (108, 109). These evaluations are unlikely to be fruitful.

The differential diagnosis of sexual headache also includes other organic diseases. Embolic stroke and cerebrovascular accidents in general may have sexual headache as the initial complaint (72, 101, 110). Meningitis, hydrocephalus, encephalitis, and cerebral hemorrhage, including that into a tumor, are also part of the differential diagnosis (103, 111). The acute onset of an explosive headache is often provoked by a pheochromocytoma (91–93). This headache is sometimes associated with exertion.

Nonneurological diseases such as glaucoma, sinusitis, Cushing's disease, and acute anemia also need to be considered. Chronic obstructive pulmonary disease, myxedema, and any pathophysiology leading to hypoglycemia may also cause sexual headache as well as BEH (89). Recreational drugs, such as amyl nitrate, or birth control pills may be contributing factors (111).

One patient has been reported with coital cephalgia secondary to a total occlusion of the abdominal aorta a few centimeters below the origin of the renal vessels. The patient made a good recovery after an aortoiliac bypass was done (112).

Pathophysiology. There are speculative theories on the pathophysiology of this headache. The arguments discuss whether the dull (muscle contraction) and explosive (vascular) subtypes of sexual headache have a common pathophysiological substrate. Some believe there are distinct mechanisms, while other authors suggest that the headaches are cases on a continuum, with underlying commonalities (113). Lance had 10 patients with tension headache unrelated to sexual activity, leading to his proposal that muscle contraction accounts for the dull-type sexual headache (101). Seven of his patients experienced pain in a similar site and with a similar quality during sex. Some of Lance's patients do not meet the IHS criteria for headache associated with sexual activity because their headaches did not occur *only* with sexual activity. Raskin noted that propranolol and indomethacin seem to be effective treatments and therefore proposed that the dull-type headache is similar to the explosive type (68).

The pathophysiology of the explosive headache is unclear. One might invoke the autonomic and vascular changes accompanying sexual climax to explain this headache's pathogenesis. Simultaneous blood pressure augmentation with acute vasodilatation and enhanced cardiac output occur as orgasm approaches. Somehow these changes may lead to a transient augmentation in intracranial pressure via an acute failure of intracranial autoregulation and/or an elevated extracranial blood volume (111). Treatment with propranolol has been successful in uncontrolled studies, supporting a possible migrainous mechanism for this type of headache (68, 99, 100, 102, 103). A personal history of migraine was found in 23% of patients with the explosive type of sexual headache. Eleven percent had a family history and 28% had either a personal or family

history of migraine (102). The thesis that the explosive-type headache is a migraine variant is supported by these facts. The proposed etiology of the postural-type headache was previously discussed.

Treatment. Propranolol has been the most successful treatment, in doses of 40 to 200 mg per day (68, 100, 103). Bellergal S (100) and ergotamine tartrate (102) have also been used. The headache may be avoided or significantly decreased by taking ergotamine, either by oral or rectal routes, approximately 30 minutes before sexual orgasm (114). Indomethacin (50 mg) given after dinner, as needed, achieved "clear-cut success" in four of five patients with headache associated with sexual activity (68) (Neil Raskin, M.D., personal communication, 1990). Indomethacin has also been recommended, by Edmeads, for prophylaxis, in doses of 50 to 100 mg per day (114).

SUMMARY

We have discussed two groups of uncommon headache disorders. The first was a miscellaneous group including idiopathic stabbing headache and several disorders triggered by ingestions, environmental stimuli, or sleep. Idiopathic stabbing headache has no known precipitants but is common among migraineurs. Its development may presage the end of a cluster headache attack. Significant relief is achieved by indomethacin treatment.

Three headaches provoked by ingested substances were reviewed: cold stimulus headache, nitrate/nitrite-induced headache, and MSG-induced headache. Usually avoidance of the precipitant can prevent these headaches.

Several headaches triggered by environmental stimuli were also discussed. These included high-altitude, hypoxic, and carbon monoxide (CO) induced headaches. High-altitude headache is a part of the acute mountain sickness (AMS) syndrome during its initial benign stage and its later malignant stage of high-altitude cerebral edema (HACE). The headache is increased by exercise. Prevention via slow ascent and not using respiratory depressants is the best treatment. Acetazolamide and dexamethasone have a useful role in preventing this syndrome.

The headache associated with CO intoxication is not distinctive. The temporal pattern of the headache along with the identification of several affected individuals helps to suggest the diagnosis. It is important to make the diagnosis to prevent possible brain injury or death of the patient and his family or work colleagues. Hypnic headache is a rare disorder of the elderly, coming on during sleep. It has been successfully treated with lithium carbonate at bedtime.

The second group of headaches discussed herein are triggered by "exertional" precipitants such as coughing, lifting, and sexual activity. Benign cough headache, benign exertional headache, and headache associated with sexual activity are part of this group. The classification and diagnostic criteria of the IHS were discussed. BEH and benign cough headache were discussed at the same time because of the major similarities between them. Generally, BEH presents with an intense short-lived pain after coughing, sneezing, lifting a burden, sexual activity, or other similar quick effort. Structural disease of the brain or skull is the most important differential diagnosis for these headaches. Posterior fossa space-occupying lesions were the most common organic etiology. MRI is the preferred method of neuroimaging, with special emphasis on the posterior fossa and foramen magnum. Structural disease of the myocardium may also have a similar presentation. Indomethacin is the treatment of choice for the benign variety of this headache.

The headache associated with sexual activity is often dull at onset. It intensifies at orgasm. The occurrence of this headache is unpredictable. The headache associated with sexual activity may be a symptom of structural disease, as in BEH. These headaches seem to be related to high-altitude headache and benign exercise headache, as the various types often occur together. CT scanning and examination of the cerebrospinal fluid must be done initially to exclude the diagnosis of SAH. Patients with the benign headache have benefitted from treatment with indomethacin and β-blockers.

REFERENCES

1. Headache Classification Committee of the International Headache Society. Classification and diagnostic criteria for headache disorders, cranial neuralgias and facial pain. Cephalalgia 1988;8(suppl 7).
2. Sjaastad O, Apfelbaum R, Caskey W, et al. Chronic paroxysmal hemicrania (CPH). The clinical manifestations. A review. Ups J Med Sci 1980;31:27–35.
3. Mathew NT. Indomethacin responsive headache syndromes. Headache 1981;21:147–150.
4. Lansche RK. Ophthalmodynia periodica. Headache 1964;4:247–249.
5. Ekbom K. Some observations on pain in cluster headache. Headache 1975;14:219–225.
6. Lance JW, Anthony M. Migrainous neuralgia or cluster headache? J Neurol Sci 1971;13:401–414.
7. Raskin NH, Schwartz RK. Ice pick-like pain. Neurology 1980;30:203–205.
8. Drummond PD, Lance JW. Neurovascular disturbances in headache patients. Clin Exp Neurol 1984;20:93–99.
9. Russell RWR. Giant cell arteritis: a review of 35 cases. Q J Med 1959;8:471–489.
10. Medina JL, Diamond S. Cluster headache variant, spectrum of a new headache syndrome. Arch Neurol 1981;38:705–709.
11. Smith RO. Ice cream headache. In: Vinken PJ, Bruyn GW, eds. Headaches and cranial neuralgias. (Handbook of clinical neurology, vol 5). Amsterdam: North-Holland Publishing, 1968:188–191.
12. Diamond S, Prager J, Freitag FG. Diet and headache is there a link? Postgrad Med 1986;79:279–286.
13. Raskin NH, Knittle SC. Ice cream headache and orthostatic symptoms in patients with migraine. Headache 1976;16:222–225.
14. Wolff HG. Headache and other head pain. 2nd ed. New York: Oxford University Press, 1963:36–37.
15. Wolf S, Hardy JD. Studies on pain. Observations on pain due to local cooling and on factors involved in the "cold pressor" effect. J Clin Invest 1941;20:521–553.
16. Plum F. Personal communication. In: Wolff HG. Headache and other head pain. 2nd ed. New York: Oxford University Press, 1963:36–37.
17. Blau IN, Diamond S. Dietary factors in migraine precipitation: the physician's view. Headache 1985;25:184–187.
18. Perkin JE, Hartje J. Diet and migraine: a review of the literature. J Am Diet Assoc 1983;83:459–463.
19. Henderson WR, Raskin NH. "Hot-dog" headache: individual susceptibility to nitrite. Lancet 1972;2:1162–1163.
20. Kwok RHM. Chinese-restaurant syndrome. N Engl J Med 1968;278:796.
21. Beron EL. Chinese-restaurant syndrome. N Engl J Med 1968;278:1123.
22. Davies NE. Chinese-restaurant syndrome. N Engl J Med 1968;278:1124.
23. Gordon ME. Chinese-restaurant syndrome. N Engl J Med 1968;278:1124.
24. Himms-Hagen J. Chinese-restaurant syndrome. Nature 1970;228:97.
25. Kandall SR. Chinese-restaurant syndrome. N Engl J Med 1968;278:1123.
26. McCaghren TJ. Chinese-restaurant syndrome. N Engl J Med 1968;278:1123.
27. Menken M. Chinese-restaurant syndrome. N Engl J Med 1968;278:1123.
28. Migden W. Chinese-restaurant syndrome. N Engl J Med 1968;278:1123.
29. Rath J. Chinese-restaurant syndrome. N Engl J Med 1968;278:1123.
30. Rose EK. Chinese-restaurant syndrome. N Engl J Med 1968;278:1123.
31. Sauber WJ. What is Chinese-restaurant syndrome? Lancet 1980;1:721–722.
32. Schaumburg H. Chinese-restaurant syndrome. N Engl J Med 1968;278:1122.
33. Kenney RA. Placebo-controlled studies of human reaction to oral monosodium glutamate. In: Filer LJ Sr, Garrantini S, Kare MR, et al., eds. Glutamic acid: advances in biochemistry and physiology. New York: Raven Press, 1979:363–373.
34. Kerr GR, Wu-Lee M, El-Lozy M, et al. Objectivity of food symptomatology questionnaires. J Am Diet Assoc 1977;71:263–268.
35. Schaumburg HH, Byck R. Sin Cib-Syn: Accent on glutamate. N Engl J Med 1968;279:105.
36. Ambos M, Leavitt NR, Marmorek L, et al. Sin cib-syn: accent on glutamate. N Engl J Med 1968;279:105.
37. Schaumburg HH, Byck R, Gerstle R, et al. Monosodium L-glutamate: its pharmacology and role in the Chinese-restaurant syndrome. Science 1969;163:286–288.
38. Kenney RA, Tidball CS. Human susceptibility to oral monosodium L-glutamate. Am J Clin Nutr 1972;25:140–146.
39. Gore MME, Salmon PR. Chinese restaurant syndrome: fact or fiction? Lancet 1980;1:251–252.
40. Morselli PL, Grattini S. Monosodium glutamate and the Chinese restaurant syndrome. Nature 1970;227:611–612.
41. Rosenblum I, Bradley JD, Coulston E. Single and double blind studies with oral monosodium glutamate in man. Toxicol Appl Pharmacol 1971;18:367–373.
42. Reif-Lehrer L. Possible significance of adverse reactions to glutamate in humans. Fed Proc 1976;35(1):2205–2212.
43. Appenzeller O. Cerebrovascular aspects of headache. Med Clin North Am 1978;62:467–480.
44. Hamilton AJ, Cymmerman A, Black PM. High altitude cerebral edema. Neurosurgery 1986;19:841–849.
45. Meehan RT, Zavala DC. The pathophysiology of acute high-altitude illness. Am J Med 1982;73:395–403.
46. Raskin NH. Headache: an overview. In: Headache. 1st ed. New York: Churchill Livingstone, 1988:16–17.
47. Appenzeller O. Barogenic headache. In: Vinken PJ, Bruyn GW, Klawans HL, et al., eds. Headache, (Handbook of clinical neurology, vol 48). New York: Elsevier, 1986:395–404.

48. Singh I, Khanna PK, Srivastava MC, et al. Acute mountain sickness. N Engl J Med 1969;280:175–184.
49. King AB, Robinson SM. Vascular headache of acute mountain sickness. Aerosp Med 1972;43:849–851.
50. Larson EB, Roach RC, Schoene RB, et al. Acute mountain sickness and acetazolamide. JAMA 1982;248:328–332.
51. Carson RP, Evans WO, Shields JL, et al. Symptomatology, pathophysiology and treatment of acute mountain sickness. Fed Proc 1969;28:1085–1091.
52. Meyer JS, Dalessio DJ. Toxic vascular headache. In: Dalessio DJ, ed. Wolff's headache and other pain. 5th ed. New York: Oxford University Press, 1987:136–171.
53. Johnson TS, Rock PB, Fulco CS, et al. Prevention of acute mountain sickness by dexamethasone. N Engl J Med 1984;310:683–686.
54. Rock PB, Johnson TS, Cymerman A, et al. Effect of dexamethasone on symptoms of acute mountain sickness at Pikes Peak, Colorado (4,300 m). Aviat Space Environ Med 1987;58:668–672.
55. Ferrazzini G, Maggiorini M, Kriemler S, et al. Successful treatment of acute mountain sickness with dexamethasone. Br Med J 1987;294:1380–1382.
56. Levine BD, Yoshimura K, Kobayashi T, et al. Dexamethasone in the treatment of acute mountain sickness. N Engl J Med 1989;321:1707–13.
57. Wohns RN, Colpitts M, Clement T, et al. Phenytoin and acute mountain sickness on Mount Everest. Am J Med 1986;80:32–36.
58. Oelz O. A case of high altitude pulmonary edema treated with nifedipine. JAMA 1987;257:780.
59. Beck HG. Slow carbon monoxide asphyxiation. JAMA 1936;107:1025–1029.
60. Ellenhorn MJ, Barceloux DG. Carbon monoxide. In: Ellenhorn MJ, Barceloux DG. Medical toxicology. New York: Elsevier, 1988:820–829.
61. Couch JR. Toxic and metabolic headache. In: Vinken PJ, Bruyn GW, Klawans HL, et al., eds. Headache, (Handbook of clinical neurology, vol 48). New York: Elsevier, 1986:395–404.
62. Raskin NH. The hypnic headache syndrome. Headache 1988;28:534–536.
63. Newman LC, Lipton RB, Solomon S. The hypnic headache syndrome: a benign headache disorder of the elderly. Neurology 1990;40:1904–1905.
64. Tinel J. Un syndrome d'algie veineuse intracranienne. La céphalée à l'effort. Prat Med Fr 1932;13:113–119.
65. Tinel J. La céphalée à l'effort. Syndrome de distension douloureuse des veines intracraniennes. Médecine (Paris) 1932;13:113–118.
66. Symonds C. Cough headache. Brain 1956;79:557–568.
67. Rooke ED. Benign exertional headache. Med Clin North Am 1968;52:801–808.
68. Raskin NH. The indomethacin-responsive syndromes. In: Headache, 1st ed. New York: Churchill Livingstone, 1988:255–268.
69. Nick J. La céphalée d'effort. A propos d'une série de 43 cas. Sem Hop Paris 1980;56:525–531.
70. Nightingale S, Williams B. Hindbrain hernia headache. Lancet 1987;1:731–734.
71. Ekbom K. Cough headache. In: Vinken PJ, Bruyn GW, Klawans HI, et al., eds. Headache, (Handbook of clinical neurology, vol 48). New York: Elsevier, 1986:367–371.
72. Nick J, Bakouche P. Headache related to sexual intercourse (in French). Sem Hop Paris 1980;56:621–628.
73. Diamond S. Prolonged benign exertional headache: its clinical characteristics and response to indomethacin. Headache 1982;22:96–98.
74. Dalessio DJ. Pain sensitive structures within cranium. In: Dalessio DJ, ed. Wolff's headache and other head pain. 4th ed. New York: Oxford University Press, 1980.
75. Rushton JG, Rooke ED. Brain tumor headache. Headache 1962;2:147–152.
76. Blacky RA, Rittelmeyer JT, Wallace MR. Headache angina. Am J Cardiol 1987;60:730.
77. Fleetcroft R, Maddocks JL. Headache due to ischaemic heart disease. J R Soc Med 1985;78:676.
78. Lefkowitz D, Biller J. Bregmatic headache as a manifestation of myocardial ischemia. Arch Neurol 1982;39:130.
79. Vernay D, Deffond D, Fraysse P, et al. Walk headache: an unusual manifestation of ischemic heart disease. Headache 1989;29:350–351.
80. Massey EW. Effort headache in runners. Headache 1982;22:99–100.
81. Indo T, Takahashi A. Swimmer's migraine. Headache 1990;30:485–487.
82. Ibbotson S. Weight-lifter's headache. Br J Sports Med 1987;3:138.
83. Paulson GW. Weightlifters headache. Headache 1983;23:193–194.
84. Powell B. Weight lifter's cephalgia. Ann Emerg Med 1982;11:449–451.
85. Katchen MS. Cases from the aerospace medicine residents' teaching file. Case #28. An aviator with exertional migraines. Aviat Space Environ Med 1988;59:1203–1204.
86. Katchen MS. Exertional headaches with multiple triggers. Aviat Space Environ Med 1990;61:49–51.
87. Silbert PL, Hankey GJ, Prentice DA, et al. Angiographically demonstrated arterial spasm in a case of benign sexual headache and benign exertional headache. Aust N Z J Med 1989;19:466–468.
88. Silberstein S, Marcelis J. Pseudotumor cerebri without papilledema. Headache 1990;30:304.
89. Hazelrigg RL. Discussion: exertional headache. Headache Q Curr Treat Res 1990;1:244–250.
90. Raskin N. Headaches associated with organic diseases of the nervous system. Med Clin North Am 1978;62:459–466.
91. Lance JW, Hinterberger H. Symptoms of pheochromocytoma with particular reference to headache correlated with catecholamine production. Arch Neurol 1976;33:281–288.
92. Paulson GW, Zipf RE, Beekman JF. Pheochromocytoma causing exercise-related headache and pulmonary edema. Ann Neurol 1979;5:96–99.
93. Thomas JE, Rooke ED, Kvale WF. The neurologist's experience with pheochromocytoma, a review of 100 cases. JAMA 1966;10:100–104.
94. Lichtenstein BW. So-called "cough headache". Arch Neurol (Chicago) 1961;4:112–113.
95. Williams B. Cerebrospinal fluid pressure changes in response to coughing. Brain 1976;99:331–346.
96. Williams B. Cough headache due to craniospinal pressure dissociation. Arch Neurol 1980;37:226–230.
97. Howell FV. The teeth and jaws as sources of headache and facial pain. In: Dalessio DJ, ed. Wolff's headache and other head pain. 5th ed. New York: Oxford University Press, 1987:255–259.
98. Diamond S, Medina JL. Benign exertional headache: successful treatment with indomethacin. Headache 1979;19:249.
99. Edis RH, Silbert PL. Sequential benign sexual headache and exertional headache. Lancet 1988;1:993.
100. Paulson GW, Klawans HL. Benign orgasmic cephalgia. Headache 1974;13:181–187.
101. Lance JW. Headaches related to sexual activity. J Neurol Neurosurg Psychiatry 1976;39:1226–1230.
102. Johns DR. Benign sexual headache within a family. Arch Neurol 1986;43:1158–1160.
103. Porter M, Jankovic J. Benign coital cephalalgia. Differential diagnosis and treatment. Arch Neurol 1981;38:710–712.
104. Locksley HB. Natural history of subarachnoid hemorrhage, intracranial aneurysms and arteriovenous malformations based on 6368 cases in the cooperative study. J Neurosurg 1966;25:219–239.
105. Fisher CM. Headache in cerebrovascular disease. In: Vinken PJ, Bruyn GW, eds. Headaches and cranial neuralgias, (Handbook of clinical neurology, vol 5). Amsterdam: North-Holland Publishing, 1968:124–156.
106. Lunberg PO, Osterman PO. The benign and malignant forms of orgasmic cephalgia. Headache 1974;14:164–165.

107. Day JW, Raskin NH. Thunderclap headache: symptom of unruptured cerebral aneurysm. Lancet 1986;2:1247–1248.
108. Harling DW, Peatfield RC, Van Hille PT, et al. Thunderclap headache: is it migraine? Cephalalgia 1989;9:87–90.
109. Wijdicks EF, Kerkhoff H, Van Gijn J. Long-term follow-up of 71 patients with thunderclap headache mimicking subarachnoid haemorrhage. Lancet 1988;1:68–70.
110. Levy RL. Stroke and orgasmic cephalgia. Headache 1981;21:12–13.
111. Braun A, Klawans HL. Headaches associated with exercise and sexual activity. In: Vinken PJ, Bruyn GW, Klawans HL, et al., eds. Headache (Handbook of clinical neurology, vol 48). New York: Elsevier, 1986:373–382.
112. Staunton HP, Moore J. Coital cephalgia and ischaemic muscular work of the lower limbs. J Neurol Neurosurg Psychiatry 1978;41:930–933.
113. Raskin NH. Tension headaches. In: Headache. 1st ed. New York: Churchill Livingstone, 1988:215–227.
114. Edmeads J. The worst headache ever: 2 innocuous causes. Postgrad Med 86:107–110, 1989.

38

Integrating Pharmacological and Nonpharmacological Treatments

KENNETH A. HOLROYD

Although both pharmacological and nonpharmacological treatments have been intensively studied and applied widely in clinical practice for over two decades, little attention has been devoted to determining how to best integrate these two treatment modalities in a multidimodal treatment strategy. The first research priority has been to establish the effectiveness of specific pharmacological or nonpharmacological treatments; the task of determining the relative effectiveness or combined effects of different treatment modalities has been left for later research efforts. Thus, the effectiveness of just two widely used migraine treatments—propranolol and thermal biofeedback training—has been evaluated in well over 100 separate studies; in contrast, the comparative or combined effects of these two types of treatment have been evaluated in only three studies. Similarly, clinical textbooks address either pharmacological or nonpharmacological treatment, or, at best, place unrelated chapters on pharmacological and nonpharmacological treatment side by side. Guidelines that would assist the clinician in choosing pharmacological or nonpharmacological treatment, or in deciding when to combine these two treatment modalities, are thus unavailable.

The time may have come, however, to begin formulating a more integrative treatment strategy. Information about both pharmacological and nonpharmacological treatments has grown dramatically in the last two decades, so the benefits and limitations of different treatment modalities can now be examined empirically. Among clinicians there is also frustration with the need to make everyday decisions about the integration of pharmacological and nonpharmacological therapies without adequate guidelines from relevant scientific evidence.

The present chapter is an initial effort to address the problem of integrating pharmacological and nonpharmacological treatments. First, studies that provide information about the relative effectiveness or combined effects of widely used pharmacological and nonpharmacological treatments are reviewed. Then, professional, ideological, and scientific obstacles to the development of a integrative treatment strategy are identified. Finally, preliminary clinical guidelines for integrative treatment are offered. The goal is to draw attention to the lack of a coherent multimodal treatment strategy for recurrent headache disorders and, hopefully, to interest both clinicians and researchers in developing such a strategy.

WHAT DOES RESEARCH TELL US?

Interest in an approach to treatment that integrates pharmacological and nonpharmacological interventions will depend on the various professionals who are involved in the treatment of the recurrent headache sufferer acknowledging the value of both types of treatments. If either treatment modality is seen as having little to offer, interest in an integrative strategy will be minimal. Information on the comparative effectiveness of these treatments and on the benefits and limitations of combining them is evaluated first. Because only the effectiveness of specific treatments (not whole classes of treatments) can be accurately compared, the effectiveness of the most widely used and intensively evaluated pharmacological and nonpharmacological treatments is examined.

Adult Migraine

PROPHYLACTIC TREATMENT

Comparative Effectiveness. The best estimate of the comparative effectiveness of pharmacological and nonpharmacological treatments can be obtained by comparing the outcomes achieved with propranolol and with relaxation/thermal biofeedback training. These treatments are the most intensively evaluated interventions within each treatment class; outcomes obtained with these two treatments thus can be compared more accurately than can outcomes obtained with less intensively evaluated pharmacological and nonpharmacological treatments. Also, there do *not* appear to be more effective interventions within each treatment class; alternate prophylactic medications generally have not proven more effective than propranolol (1), and alternate nonpharmacological interventions have not proven more effective than relaxation/biofeedback

Table 38.1.
Average Percentage Improvement in Migraine Headache for Treatment and Control Groups Using Daily Headache Records as Outcome Measures

	Treatment Conditions			
	Relaxation/ Biofeedback	Propranolol	Placebo	Untreated
Average patient improvement[a] (%)	43.3	43.7	14.3	2.1
Range of scores (%)	11 to 87	26 to 65	−23 to 32	−30 to 33

[a]Average improvement in headache activity weighted by sample size

training (2–4), at least when comparisons are made in general samples of migraine sufferers. Finally, propranolol is the most widely used pharmacological treatment and relaxation/biofeedback training the most widely used nonpharmacological treatment; information about the relative effectiveness of these two treatments thus may have practical implications for practice.

Percentage reductions in migraine activity achieved with propranolol and with relaxation/biofeedback training are presented in Table 38.1. These figures are from a meta-analytic (i.e., statistical) review that averaged results from 25 clinical trials of propranolol and 35 clinical trials of combined relaxation/thermal biofeedback training (2445 patients collectively) (5). Only trials that used *daily headache recordings* to assess treatment outcome are included in the calculations presented in Table 38.1; trials that used less conservative outcome measures (e.g., physician/therapist ratings of improvement, patient retrospective reports) report improvements with each treatment that are about 20% larger than the figures in Table 38.1.

It can be seen that propranolol and relaxation/ biofeedback training produced almost identical results in clinical trials of these two treatments—approximately a 43% reduction in migraine activity in the average patient. Improvements observed with either treatment have been significantly larger than improvements observed with placebo or in untreated migraine sufferers. Available clinical trials thus provide empirical support for the effectiveness of both propranolol and relaxation/biofeedback training, but provide no indication that these two treatments differ in effectiveness.

Results from the three studies that have directly compared the effectiveness of propranolol and relaxation/biofeedback training, for the most part, are consistent with results reported in Table 38.1. Two studies (6, 7) report findings that are quite similar to those summarized in Table 38.1: that is, equivalent improvements with propranolol and relaxation/ biofeedback training that are similar in magnitude to the mean improvement scores reported in Table 38.1. In the third study (8), substantially larger improvements were reported with propranolol than with relaxation/biofeedback training. However, better propranolol results and poorer relaxation/biofeedback training results were reported in this study than in other similar studies. Thus, results obtained in

this latter study may not be representative of results that can typically be expected (5).

Combined Effects. Little is known about the advantages and disadvantages of combining pharmacological and nonpharmacological treatments, despite the fact that these two types of treatments are frequently administered conjointly in specialized headache clinics. Interactions might take at least four forms (9): (*a*) additive, where the combined effects are equal to the sum of the contributions from the individual treatments; (*b*) potentiation, where the combined treatment effect is greater than the sum of the individual treatment effects; (*c*) inhibition, where results achieved with the combined therapy is less than achieved with the individual therapies; or (*d*) reciprocation, where results achieved with the combined therapy is equal to the results achieved with the most effective treatment.

Observed interactions also may reflect a number of distinct facilitative or inhibitive mechanisms. Nonpharmacological treatment might enhance the effectiveness of drug therapy through its effects on behavior; for example, by improving compliance with concurrently prescribed drug therapy. Alternatively, drug therapy might inhibit the effectiveness of nondrug therapy through its physiological effects; for example, propranolol might inhibit the acquisition of the handwarming response during biofeedback training by blocking peripheral adrenergic receptors in the finger (10). Understanding the effects of combined pharmacological and nonpharmacological treatments thus requires an understanding not only of the effects of combined treatment on headache activity but also of how these combined treatment effects are achieved.

Unfortunately, only two studies have examined the interaction of pharmacological and nonpharmacological treatments in the prevention of recurrent migraine. The larger of these studies (8) examined the benefits obtained by combining relaxation/thermal biofeedback training with each of three prophylactic regimens (propranolol, amitriptyline, or propranolol plus amitriptyline). The three combined treatments yielded only slightly better results than were attained with the corresponding drug therapies alone; however, two of the three combined treatments yielded better results than relaxation/biofeedback training alone. This study provides strong support for drug therapy but only limited support for combining drug and nondrug therapies. The second study (11) reported that amitriptyline initially enhanced the effectiveness of biofeedback training; however, beginning at month 8 and continuing through the 24-month observation period, results achieved with biofeedback training alone were superior to results obtained with the combination of amitriptyline and biofeedback training. It is not clear why poorer results were observed with the combined treatment than with biofeedback alone; however, several investigators have cautioned that patients who receive combined pharmacological/nonpharmacological treatment might attribute their improvement to drug therapy, and cease or reduce use of self-regulation skills, thereby reducing the effectiveness of the combined treatment (12). In any case, these latter findings highlight the need for information about long-term treatment effects of combined treatments.

Long-Term Treatment Effects. For the most part the above studies only provide information about relatively short-term (less than 1 year) treatment effects; considerably less information is available about longer-term treatment results. The only propranolol study that has examined long-term treatment effects (13) reported good maintenance of improvements in most propranolol responders for evaluation periods that ranged (for individual patients) from 8 to 16 months. Unfortunately, the extent to which treatment gains were maintained can not be determined precisely, because levels of migraine activity at follow-up were not reported.

The eight relaxation/biofeedback studies that have examined long-term maintenance of improvements have reported one-half to two-thirds of contacted patients maintained improvements (i.e., without continuing treatment) at 1-year follow-up (14–16). However, in a review of six of these studies, Blanchard (14) suggested there may be a greater loss of treatment gains over longer (3 to 5 years) time periods.

The only study that has examined the long-term effects of combined pharmacological and nonpharmacological treatment reported better results with biofeedback training alone than with the combination of biofeedback and amitriptyline (11).

Summary. Available studies suggest that, in unselected migraineurs, propranolol and relaxation/biofeedback training yield similar short-term treatment effects, with each treatment yielding just under a 50% reduction in migraine activity in the average patient. Unfortunately, conclusions about long-term treatment effects are more problematic. Only a handful of studies have provided information about long-term treatment results, and almost all of these studies have evaluated nonpharmacological treatments. Nonetheless, the substantial support available for the short-term effectiveness of both pharmacological and nonpharmacological treatments raises the possibility that the management of recurrent migraine would be improved if we were able to identify the patients most likely to benefit from each treatment, and if the advantages and disadvantages of combining these two treatment modalities were better understood.

ABORTIVE TREATMENT

While pharmacological treatments can usefully be classified as either prophylactic or abortive, nonpharmacological treatments share characteristics of both categories of agents. It is thus not surprising that two studies have compared the effectiveness of relaxation/biofeedback training and abortive medication with adult migraineurs.

Holroyd et al. (17) found relaxation/biofeedback training and ergotamine tartrate equally effective at 2-month

and 6-month evaluations (mean reductions in migraine activity of 52% and 41%, respectively). However, long-term follow-up results suggested that for most patients, ergotamine was not an effective long-term treatment: At 3-year follow-up, patients who had received ergotamine were significantly less likely than patients who had received relaxation/biofeedback training to be still using the treatment they had been provided (either ergotamine or relaxation/handwarming exercises) to manage their headaches (15). In the second study, Mathew (8) found a 10-session relaxation/biofeedback training intervention significantly more effective than ergotamine with both migraine (35 vs. 20% reduction in headache activity) and mixed-headache sufferers (48 vs. 18% reduction). One explanation for the discrepant short-term results reported in these two studies is that the ergotamine treatment protocol used in the Holroyd et al. study (but not in the Mathew study) incorporated an adjunctive educational intervention that has been shown to help patients effectively use abortive medication; this adjunctive intervention may well have increased the effectiveness of ergotamine.

Pediatric Migraine

Pharmacological and nonpharmacological therapies for pediatric migraine have been compared in only one study. In this study (18) with classical migraine sufferers aged 6 to 12 years, combined relaxation and self-hypnosis training (5 treatment sessions) yielded significantly better results than propranolol (3 mg/kg/day). In fact, while combined relaxation/self-hypnosis produced better results than placebo, results achieved with propranolol and placebo did not differ. This is an excellent study, with carefully diagnosed patients and good patient compliance with both treatment protocols. Consequently, these findings raise the possibility that nonpharmacological interventions may prove to be the preferred treatment for pediatric migraine.

Other studies also suggest that nonpharmacological treatments deserve greater attention in the management of pediatric migraine. Results reported in clinical trials of propranolol appear to be poorer in children than in adults. Two (18, 19) of three (18–20) available double-blind trials of propranolol found that propranolol and placebo did not differ in effectiveness, while propranolol has consistently been found to be superior to placebo with adults (Table 38.1). On the other hand, relaxation and biofeedback treatments have yielded improvements with pediatric migraine that equal or exceed improvements reported with adult migraine (21–24).

For the most part, research with pediatric migraine has focused on evaluating interventions that have proven effective with adult migraineurs. However, a study by McGrath et al. (25) suggests that interventions that yield unimpressive results with adults may prove to be cost-effective treatments for children. McGrath et al. (25) reported that in children aged 9 to 17 years, a one-session treatment that focused on managing migraine triggers (headache diary recordings were reviewed and strategies for coping with migraine triggers offered) yielded moderate improvements (34% reduction in migraine activity) in children suffering from severe migraines. Although improvements observed with a more intensive six-session relaxation treatment tended to be larger (55% reduction), the single-session intervention produced sufficient improvement to warrant its inclusion in other pharmacological or nonpharmacological treatment packages.

In summary, the limited available data raise the possibility that behavioral interventions may prove to be the treatment of choice for pediatric migraine. Clinical trials that compare the effectiveness of pharmacological and nonpharmacological interventions for pediatric migraine are needed to further explore this possibility. Where pharmacological treatment is required, the usefulness of nonpharmacological treatment to reduce the dose or length of required pharmacological treatments also deserves attention. If we are to accurately gauge the comparative impact of pharmacological and nonpharmacological treatments, however, more information will be needed about the natural course of this disorder. High remission rates have been noted for pediatric migraine (26, 27), and children may be particularly likely to be brought to treatment during a temporary worsening of migraine attacks (27). It is thus important to determine the impact of treatment not just on the immediate cluster of migraine episodes, but on the long-term course of this disorder.

Tension Headache

The most commonly used agent for the prevention of recurrent tension headaches is amitriptyline HCl. The literature on the effectiveness of amitriptyline is surprisingly sparse, given the widespread use of this drug throughout the world (28). While two double-blind placebo-controlled evaluations of amitriptyline provide evidence that amitriptyline is superior to placebo, they also reveal only a moderate amitriptyline treatment effect. Thus, Lance and Curran (29) reported about half (55%) of patients were judged improved with amitriptyline (in the placebo-controlled portion of their study); in the Diamond and Baltes study (30), differences between amitriptyline and placebo were nonsignificant on a number of physician ratings. A recent double-blind multicenter comparison of amitriptyline and doxepin (31) also found no reduction in headache-free days with either agent (although headache intensity was reduced), leading the authors to conclude that "as a rule monotherapy with these substances is not sufficient" (p 223).

The effectiveness of nonpharmacological interventions has been more intensively evaluated. Thus, a recent meta-analytic (i.e., statistical) review summarized results from 33 studies that evaluated relaxation training, EMG biofeedback training, or the combination of the two (32). Results averaged across clinical trials indicated these three treatments produced similar improvements, with each

yielding about a 50% reduction in tension headache activity. All three treatments also produced significantly better results than have been observed with the most commonly used pseudotherapy control procedure (noncontingent or "fake" biofeedback training). Other research further suggests that the addition of stress-management procedures to relaxation training or EMG biofeedback training may enhance the effectiveness of relaxation/biofeedback treatments (33, 34).

The effectiveness of pharmacological and nonpharmacological treatments in the management of recurrent tension headaches has been compared in only two studies. Holroyd et al. (35) compared the effectiveness of combined relaxation/stress management training (administered in a minimal therapist contact treatment format that required three office visits) and amitriptyline (individualized dose of 25 to 75 mg/day). Both relaxation/stress management training and amitriptyline yielded clinically significant improvements in tension headache activity, both when improvement was assessed with patient daily headache recordings (56% and 27% reduction in headache index, respectively) and when improvement was assessed with neurologist ratings of clinical improvement (94% and 69% of patients rated at least moderately improved, respectively). Where significant differences were observed (headache index, somatic complaints, treatment side effects, perceptions of control of headache activity), relaxation/stress management training yielded better results than amitriptyline.

In the second study, Pavia et al. (36) compared the effectiveness of EMG biofeedback training (12 sessions) and diazepam (dose unspecified) using an interesting double-blind design. Patients were randomized to one of four treatment conditions: true (contingent) or false (noncontingent) EMG biofeedback and diazapam or placebo. Significant reductions in headache frequency were observed with true (but not with false) biofeedback and with diazepam (but not with placebo). However, the time course of both improvement and relapse were different with diazepam and biofeedback training. With diazepam, improvement was evident immediately, but patients relapsed in month 2 when diazapam was discontinued. With biofeedback training, improvement was not observed until the 1-month training period was completed, but patients maintained improvements after training was discontinued. This study points up the limitations of diazapam therapy. However, diazapam is not recommended for general use in managing recurrent tension headaches because of its abuse potential, so this study provides little information about the comparative effectiveness of currently accepted pharmacological and nonpharmacological treatments. Relapse rates following the discontinuation of more widely accepted pharmacological agents such as amitriptyline are unknown, but it is likely that they are lower than with diazepam.

Despite clinically significant reductions in headache activity, Holroyd et al. (35) noted that at least half the patients treated with either amitriptyline or relaxation/ stress management therapy continued to record at least some tension headache activity 3 or more days a week. This suggests that a significant number of patients could benefit from the development of more powerful treatments. Research is thus needed to determine if (*a*) the combined use of amitriptyline and relaxation/stress management therapies yields better results than either treatment by itself; and (*b*) if patients who have failed to improve, or have shown only limited improvement with one treatment are likely to benefit when subsequently treated with the other treatment modality.

Improving Medication Adherence

Poor adherence limits the effectiveness of drug therapy for many recurrent headache sufferers. Packard and O'Connell (37) concluded on the basis of 100 patient interviews that over 50% of headache sufferers fail to properly adhere to drug treatment regimens. Fitzpatrick, Hopkins, and Havard-Watts (38) similarly found that 1 year after initiating drug therapy only 24% of patients reported they had used headache medications exactly as instructed. These observations suggest that psychological interventions might be used to facilitate patients' effective use of prescribed medications.

The one study evaluating an intervention designed to improve adherence with drug therapy attempted to address adherence problems encountered with ergotamine (39). Ergotamine may present special problems for patients because the effective use of this medication requires complex self-management skills: accurate identification of migraine onset, a method of keeping medication readily available, correct timing of medication intake, and the control of intake to prevent overuse. Patients who received a brief adherence intervention (a meeting with an allied health professional following the neurologist's prescription of ergotamine, three telephone calls to identify and remedy problems with ergotamine use, and a workbook to help identify and correct adherence problems) attempted to abort 70% of migraine attacks and showed clinically significant reductions in migraine activity (40% reduction). In contrast, patients who received standard ergotamine therapy attempted to abort only about 40% of their migraine attacks and showed smaller reductions in migraine activity (26% reduction). These results suggest that interventions to facilitate the chronic headache sufferer's effective use of medication deserve more attention than they have received to date. For many patients, brief interventions that successfully improve adherence with existing medical regimens could yield greater benefits than new pharmacological agents.

Conclusion

Existing research provides convincing support for the effectiveness of both pharmacological and nonpharmacologi-

cal treatment modalities. Additional findings raise the intriguing possibility that treatments could be rationally selected on the basis of a limited number of patient characteristics or by comparing treatment effect profiles. For example, headache variables or psychological test scores have shown some promise in predicting patient response to both pharmacological and nonpharmacological treatments (17, 40). Thus, patient variables might be identified that would allow the most appropriate treatment for a given patient to be identified. Pharmacological and nonpharmacological treatments are also likely to have different treatment effect profiles. Nonpharmacological treatments may produce improvement more slowly than pharmacological treatments (11, 17), yield fewer side effects than pharmacological treatment (but require more time and effort to complete), and produce psychological effects not observed with pharmacological treatments (35, 41). Even where treatments are equally likely to be effective, it thus might be possible to rationally select treatments on the basis of treatment effect profiles. These findings, as well as the positive initial results reported in the nonpharmacological treatment of pediatric migraine and in the use of brief interventions to improve compliance with drug regimens, argue that the clinical management of recurrent headache disorders could be improved if strategies for rationally integrating pharmacological and nonpharmacological treatments were developed.

Unfortunately, to date, little research attention has been devoted to this problem. It thus may prove worthwhile to examine obstacles that may have impeded progress in this area.

INTEGRATIVE TREATMENT: OBSTACLES

At least three obstacles appear to have impeded the development of integrative pharmacological/nonpharmacological treatment strategies. First, clinical trials of pharmacological treatments and clinical trials of nonpharmacological treatments are often conducted by investigators from different professions. Thus, investigators who evaluate pharmacological treatments often have little first-hand knowledge of nonpharmacological treatments, while investigators who evaluate nonpharmacological treatments often have equally little first-hand knowledge of pharmacological treatments. These two groups of investigators also are likely to conceptualize treatment phenomena at different levels of analysis—one focusing on the relatively molecular biological processes that underlie the therapeutic action of pharmacological agents and the other on more molar psychological processes that underlie the acquisition of self-regulation skills. These differences probably have impeded the establishment of a productive dialogue on integrative treatment strategies.

Second, the different cultures that evolve in settings that emphasize pharmacological or nonpharmacological treatment can present an obstacle to the development of integrative treatment strategies. Because positive results obtained with nonpharmacological treatments are likely to depend on the patient actively engaging in self-regulatory activities, clinicians often must convince patients to take an active role in the management of their headaches and to devote time and effort, first to learning and then to using self-regulation skills. Clinical settings where nonpharmacological treatments are emphasized tend to evolve a culture that emphasizes the active involvement of patients in the management of their disorder. Because pharmacotherapy is likely to be less dependent on the patient's active involvement in treatment (beyond compliance with the drug regimen), less emphasis may be placed on patient activity in clinical settings that emphasize pharmacological therapy. In the latter settings, patients referred for nonpharmacological treatment may already have adopted a compliant, rather than actively involved, stance toward therapy, making nonpharmacological treatment more difficult.

Finally, both the professional literature and professional associations focus primarily on intraprofessional communication and pay relatively little attention to facilitating the interprofessional interactions that might stimulate interest in integrative pharmacological/nonpharmacological treatment strategies. Cross-disciplinary dialogue between clinicians and researchers thus has been limited, and when it occurs, this dialogue has often been more ideological than scientific. Excellent textbooks and monographs in neurology, even those that carefully evaluate the available scientific evidence for pharmacological treatments, often draw summary conclusions about nonpharmacological treatments without reference to relevant clinical trials. In much the same manner, monographs and textbooks that focus on nonpharmacological treatments typically ignore, or pay only cursory attention to pharmacological treatments. Conventions attended primarily by neurologists (e.g., American Association for the Study of Headache) frequently devote only limited and cursory attention to the role nonpharmacological treatments might play in the management of recurrent headache disorders, and presentations on headache at conventions attended primarily by psychologists (e.g., Society of Behavioral Medicine, Applied Psychophysiology and Biofeedback) typically ignore or treat pharmacological interventions in only a cursory fashion.

If an empirically based treatment strategy that effectively integrates pharmacological and nonpharmacological treatments is to be developed, clinicians and researchers who have focused exclusively on one of these two treatment modalities will have to join efforts to collaborate in both their clinical work and research. This will require that clinicians/investigators transcend the confines of professional disciplines and of the informal cultures that evolve in settings where they work. In spite of the difficulties inherent in such an endeavor, the potential advantages are likely to be many, including, for patients, the develop-

ment of more effective and flexible treatment approaches, and, for clinicians and investigators, the intellectual rewards of truly cross-disciplinary collaboration.

INTEGRATIVE TREATMENT: RESEARCH ISSUES
Choosing a Research Design

A number of problems must be addressed when designing studies that compare the effectiveness of pharmacological and nonpharmacological treatments or evaluate combined pharmacological/nonpharmacological treatment. Two problems immediately confront the investigator familiar with research designs used in clinical trials of pharmacological treatments: the inability to use crossover designs (because new skills taught during nonpharmacological treatment cannot be withdrawn) and the inability to double-blind the administration of nonpharmacological treatments (because the patient's informed cooperation is required if self-regulation skills are to be successfully acquired and used). Some efforts have been made to address the latter difficulty in evaluations of EMG and thermal biofeedback training (42–44). It may not be possible, however, to construct a "placebo" that incorporates all the nonspecific elements of a nonpharmacological treatment but none of the treatment's active ingredients (45,46).

Studies to date have tended to use parallel-groups designs to compare the effectiveness of the most widely used pharmacological and nonpharmacological treatments (7, 8, 17, 35). (An interesting exception is Olness et al.'s (18) use of a crossover design that incorporates the evaluation of nonpharmacological treatment into a double-blind placebo-controlled crossover evaluation of propranolol.) In an influential example of a parallel-group design, Mathew (8) used a reference treatment (ergotamine) to calibrate the effectiveness of two prophylactic pharmacological treatments and one nonpharmacological treatment, administered alone and in combination. While this design fails to incorporate placebo or no-treatment control groups, thereby limiting the conclusions that can be drawn concerning the absolute effectiveness of the individual treatments, it does permit an evaluation of the relative effectiveness of pharmacological and nonpharmacological treatments with reference to an alternate and widely used comparison treatment. No study yet has employed the highly desirable, but relatively complex, parallel-group design depicted in Figure 38.1. This design allows the investigator to examine the effectiveness of selected pharmacological and nonpharmacological treatments (with reference to placebo and no-treatment comparison groups) as well as examine results achieved when these two treatment modalities are administered conjointly.

Other types of research designs are necessary if questions of specific relevance to the development of integrative pharmacological/nonpharmacological treatment strategies are to be addressed. For example, clinical decision making

		Nonpharmacological Treatment	
		Present	Absent
Pharmacological	Drug	Nonpharmacological plus pharmacological treatment	Pharmacological treatment
	Placebo	Nonpharmacological treatment plus placebo	Placebo
	No pill	Nonpharmacological treatment and no pill	No treatment

Figure 38.1. Nonpharmacological treatment. Six-group design for evaluating separate and combined treatment effects.

would be facilitated if more information were available concerning the most effective treatment for patients who fail to respond to one of the standard initial therapies. Propranolol is widely used as the initial step in the management of recurrent migraines (1); however, little is known about the most effective intervention for propranolol nonresponders. To address this question, a two-step design is required. A large number of migraine sufferers first must be treated with propranolol, with propranolol nonresponders subsequently randomized to alternative treatment conditions: for example, to flunarizine, placebo, or relaxation/biofeedback training. This design permits the investigator to determine if patients who fail to respond to one (pharmacological or nonpharmacological) treatment do better when subsequently treated with the same, or a different treatment modality.

Clinical decision making also would be facilitated if we were able to identify the patients most likely to benefit from pharmacological treatment and the patients most likely to benefit from nonpharmacological treatment. This problem has not received sufficient attention, possibly because it is widely believed such efforts are likely to be unfruitful (47, 48). However, little additional effort is required to determine if variables can be identified that are predictive of a positive (or negative) patient response to treatment when analyzing data from clinical trials. Investigators conducting clinical trials of nonpharmacological treatments have had some initial success in identifying patient characteristics that predict a poor response to nonpharmacological treatment (17, 37, 49). This issue deserves greater attention in future clinical trials of pharmacological treatments. In fact, editors probably should require that all clinical trials (with sufficient number of patients) report the results of statistical analyses that examine patient variables as predictors of treatment response. Information thus could be cumulated about patients most likely to benefit from specific treatments across clinical trials; if no predictor variables were identified, little would be lost.

Assessing Treatment Outcome

Because improvements in headache activity produced by pharmacological and nonpharmacological treatments may differ along a number of dimensions, studies that compare or combine these two treatment modalities should examine multiple outcome indices. Useful indices include (12): *magnitude*, or the amount of change in headache activity observed in the typical patient treated with a particular treatment modality; *universality*, or the proportion of treated patients evidencing clinically significant reduction in headache activity; *generality*, or the pattern of effects observed across different dimensions of headache activity; *time course*, or how rapidly improvements in headache activity occur; *acceptability*, or the likelihood that a given treatment will be accepted and/or completed; *safety*, or the likelihood of negative treatment effects or complications; and *stability*, or the likelihood of relapse if treatment is successful.

Because pharmacological and nonpharmacological treatments may affect different aspects of the patient's functioning (17, 35, 41), clinical trials that compare or combine these two treatment modalities should use a wide range of outcome measures. Unfortunately, only patient recordings or patient reports of headache activity are collected in many studies. Valuable information about the impact of treatment on psychological symptoms and physical complaints that frequently accompany recurrent headache problems, headache-related disability, or use of medical care services is thus often not obtained. (Exceptions to this generalization include individual studies in which efforts were made to evaluate the impact of headache-related disability on work, family, and occupational functioning (30), and studies in which psychological tests are used to evaluate the impact of treatment on psychological symptoms and the patients' beliefs concerning their headaches (17, 35, 50). More information would be obtained from future clinical trials if a broader range of measures were assessed than have been assessed in past trials.

INTEGRATIVE TREATMENT: CLINICAL GUIDELINES

Information is lacking that might guide the clinician in deciding whether to initiate treatment with pharmacological, nonpharmacological, or the combination of these treatments; as we noted above, surprisingly little research attention has been devoted to this topic. In practice, the treatment patients receive is typically determined by accidental factors: primarily by the beliefs and training of the clinician the individual consults. In this section, the limited information that might guide the clinician's choice of treatment is reviewed.

General Considerations

DIAGNOSIS

The number of pharmacological or nonpharmacological treatment alternatives available varies with the patient's diagnosis. The available, adequately evaluated, preventative therapies include a greater number of drug therapies than nondrug therapies for migraine, while the reverse may be true for tension headache. If pharmacological and nonpharmacological treatments are similarly effective and the choice of treatment modality were to be based solely on diagnosis, it could be argued that pharmacological intervention would be advantageous for migraine sufferers and nonpharmacological intervention advantageous for tension headache sufferers: in both cases, this decision permits the greatest number of treatment alternatives to be offered the patient who is nonresponsive to the initial treatment. Basing initial treatment decisions solely on the potential number of interventions that might be offered the nonresponsive patient is, of course, unsatisfactory. Such a strategy not only fails to take into account the likelihood that individual patients will respond to these interventions, but it fails to take into account the possibility that switching to a different treatment modality (rather than a different intervention within the same treatment modality) would be preferable.

PATIENT BELIEFS AND PREFERENCES

Patients often have treatment preferences. Patients self-select themselves into certain treatments simply by choosing to seek help at one facility rather than at another. Preferences for different treatments are related to patients' beliefs about their headaches (51): patients who believe that headache episodes are influenced primarily by chance factors (e.g., genetics, weather) tend to prefer pharmacological treatment, while patients who believe headache episodes are primarily influenced by factors that are potentially within their control (e.g., stress, self-care) tend to prefer nonpharmacological treatment. These beliefs, which vary widely among patients with the same headache disorder, can be expected to influence patients' perceptions of the treatment they are offered and their compliance with treatment regimens. Patients' beliefs about their headaches have yet to be studied as a predictor of treatment response; however, such beliefs can be easily assessed via tests designed for this purpose (51) or by interview, and they deserve consideration in choosing treatment.

SELF-MANAGEMENT SKILLS

In an interesting study that may have relevance for the treatment of recurrent headache sufferers, Simmons and colleagues (52) reported that depressed patients with high scores on the Self-Control Schedule (which assesses skills necessary to monitor and regulate feelings, thoughts, and behavior (53)) were most likely to benefit from psychological treatment; in contrast, patients who scored low on this measure (and thus were lacking in these skills) were most likely to benefit from pharmacological treatment. These self-management skills also can easily be assessed and deserve attention as a possible predictor of differential

patient response to pharmacological and nonpharmacological treatment.

Empirically Based Criteria

Some attention has been devoted to identifying patients who are not likely to respond to the most commonly used nonpharmacological treatments. Although only a handful of predictor variables have been replicated across studies, the three patient characteristics discussed below appear to be predictive of a poor response to nonpharmacological treatment. Unfortunately, similar patient variables have not been examined as predictors of patient response to pharmacological treatments, so it is often unclear if these variables identify patients who are only unresponsive to nonpharmacological treatment or patients who are also unresponsive to pharmacological treatments.

CONTINUOUS HEADACHES

Patients with near continuous, often intense headaches frequently do not benefit from nonpharmacological treatments (17, 34, 54–56). Blanchard et al. (55), for example, found that only 13% of patients who recorded almost continuous (one or fewer headache-free days during a 1-month baseline) and frequently painful headaches showed clinically significant reductions (50% or greater) in headache activity with brief nonpharmacological treatment. In contrast, more than 50% of patients with 2 or more headache-free days per week showed clinically significant improvements. (Only about 10% of these near continuous headache sufferers also met criteria for excessive medication use, so continuous headache activity in these patients did not appear to be a function of excessive medication use.) Information about the response of these patients to pharmacotherapy is unavailable. Nonetheless, the treatment of such patients probably should be initiated with pharmacotherapy or combined pharmacological and nonpharmacological treatment.

EXCESSIVE MEDICATION USE

The observation that regular, especially daily, use of analgesic or abortive medications can produce paradoxical increases in headache activity was made several decades ago (57, 58). It is only with the recognition that excessive medication use limits the benefits obtained from both pharmacological and nonpharmacological treatments, however, that this problem has begun to receive serious attention (59, 60). While clear quantitative criteria for excessive medication use have yet to be specified (61), the Second International Workshop on Drug Related Headache (62) has taken an important step in this direction. Medication withdrawal frequently confers clear benefits and, in fact, is likely to be necessary for the effective treatment of patients whose headaches are aggravated by high levels of analgesic or abortive medication use (63–65). Studies that evaluate the effectiveness of pharmacological and nonpharmacological treatments in retaining patients in medication-withdrawal protocols and in controlling headache activity in patients who have reduced or eliminated problematic medication use are not currently available but are needed. However, positive results have been reported from uncontrolled clinical series where medication-withdrawal protocols are combined with prophylactic pharmacotherapy, nonpharmacological treatment, or both (60, 64–66). Clearly, more information is needed about the benefits and limitations of both pharmacological and nonpharmacological treatment options for patients who excessively use analgesic or abortive medications. Clinical impressions suggest that these multiple-problem patients may require treatment programs that combine education with both pharmacological and nonpharmacological therapies.

CONCURRENT PSYCHIATRIC DISORDER

Little information is available about the differential effectiveness of various treatment options for recurrent headache sufferers with concurrent psychiatric disorders or those who show elevated levels of psychological symptoms. Patients with elevated scores on the Beck Depression Inventory (BDI)(67) or on certain Minnesota Multiphasic Personality Inventory (MMPI)(68) subscales have been observed to do poorly in some studies (69), but not in other studies (70), where nonpharmacological treatments have been evaluated. Unfortunately, information about the response of similar patients to pharmacological treatments is not available. A recent epidemiological study reports that both anxiety disorders (including panic disorder) and major depression occur in recurrent migraine sufferers with significantly greater frequency than in individuals who do not suffer from migraine (71). Greater attention thus may need to be paid to the effects of psychopathology on treatment outcome, as well as to the development of effective treatment strategies for recurrent headache sufferers who suffer from concurrent psychiatric disorders.

Patients seen in specialized headache treatment centers who exhibit high levels of psychological symptoms or frank psychiatric disorders often are referred for nonpharmacological treatment and receive combined pharmacological/nonpharmacological treatment. Compliance with treatment regimens can be a significant problem in this patient population, and clinical impressions suggest that brief psychotherapy directed at the management of acute psychiatric symptoms can be useful with at least some of these patients. Until research that evaluates alternate treatments for this population is available, these patients probably should be considered for joint pharmacological/nonpharmacological treatment.

CONCLUSION

The value of preventive pharmacological and nonpharmacological treatments for recurrent headache disorders has been established in separate clinical trials over the last two decades. The handful of studies that have directly compared the effectiveness of pharmacological and nonpharmacological treatments or have evaluated combined treatments further suggest that a treatment strategy that integrates pharmacological and nonpharmacological interventions can offer benefits not available with either alone. For example, initial findings from these later studies raise at least three promising possibilities: that patient variables or treatment effect profiles might be used to select the most effective treatment modality for individual patients, that brief educational intervention might be used to improve adherence with drug regimens, and that nonpharmacological treatments might reduce or eliminate the need for drug therapy in managing pediatric migraine. Such findings suggest that methods of optimally integrating pharmacological and nonpharmacological treatments deserve increased attention.

Studies that evaluate strategies for integrating pharmacological and nonpharmacological interventions also present special methodological and practical challenges. A number of these methodological difficulties were identified, and where feasible, suggestions for coping with these difficulties were offered. Practical obstacles to productive cross-disciplinary collaboration that arise from differences in the training, dominant ideologies, and work settings of physicians and psychologist also were identified and discussed. Despite these methodological and practical challenges, the potential benefits and rewards of developing a strategy that effectively integrates pharmacological and nonpharmacological treatments are likely to be many. These include, for patients, the development of more effective and flexible treatments, and, for clinicians and investigators, the intellectual rewards of truly cross-disciplinary collaboration. Hopefully, the next decades will see not only a continued interest in the development of more powerful pharmacological and nonpharmacological treatments but also a new interest in methods of optimally integrating these two types of interventions in managing recurrent headache disorders.

Acknowledgements. Support for this chapter was provided (in part) by an Academic Challenge Award from the State of Ohio.

REFERENCES

1. Holroyd KA, Penzien DB, Cordingley GE. Propranolol in the management of recurrent migraine: a meta-analytic review. Headache 1991;31:333–340.
2. Blanchard EB, Andrasik F. Psychological assessment and treatment of headache: recent developments and emerging issues. J Consult Clin Psychol 1982;50:859–879.
3. Blanchard EB, Andrasik F. Biofeedback treatment of vascular headache. In: Hatch JP, Rugh JD, eds. Biofeedback: studies in clinical efficacy. New York: Plenum Press, 1987:1–79.
4. Penzien DB, Holroyd KA, Hursey KG, Holm JE, Wittchen HU. Behavioral treatment of recurrent migraine: a meta-analysis of over five-dozen group outcome studies. Paper presented at the meeting of

the Association for Advancement of Behavior Therapy, Houston, 1985.

5. Holroyd KA, Penzien DB. Pharmacological versus nonpharmacological prophylaxis of recurrent migraine headache: a meta-analytic review of clinical trials. Pain 1990;42:1–13.

6. Penzien DB, Johnson CA, Carpenter DE, Prather RC, Beckham JC, et al. Home-based behavioral treatment vs. propranolol for recurrent migraine: preliminary findings. Paper presented at the meeting of the Society of Behavioral Medicine, San Francisco, CA, 1989.

7. Sovak M, Kunzel M, Sternback R, Dalessio DJ. Mechanism of the biofeedback therapy of migraine: volitional manipulation of the psychophysiological background. Headache. 1981;21:89–92.

8. Mathew NT. Prophylaxis of migraine and mixed headache. A randomized controlled study. Headache 1981;21:105–109.

9. Klerman GL. Drugs and psychotherapy. In: Garfield SL, Bergin AE, eds. Handbook of psychotherapy and behavior change. 3rd ed. New York: John Wiley & Sons, 1986:777–818.

10. Freedman RR, Sabharwal SC, Ianni P. Nonneural beta-adrenergic vasodilating mechanism in temperature biofeedback. J Psychosom Med 1988:394–401.

11. Reich BA. Photoplethysmograph biofeedback combined with tricyclic medication: a two-year assessment. Headache 1990:313.

12. Hollon SD, DeRubeis J. Placebo-psychotherapy combinations: inappropriate representations of psychotherapy in drug-psychotherapy comparative trials. Psychol Bull 1981;90:467–477.

13. Diamond S, Kudrow L, Stevens J, Shapiro DB. Long-term study of propranolol in the treatment of migraine. Headache 1982;22:268–271.

14. Blanchard EB. Long-term effects of behavioral treatment of chronic headache. Behav Ther 1987;18:375–385.

15. Holroyd KA, Holm JF, Penzien DB, Cordingley GE, Hursey KG, et al. Long-term maintenance of improvements achieved with (abortive) pharmacological and nonpharmacological treatments for migraine: preliminary findings. Biofeedback Self Regul 1989;14:301–308.

16. Sorbi M, Tellegen B, DuLong A. Long-term effects of relaxation and stress-coping in patients with migraine: a 3-year follow-up. Headache 1989;29:111–121.

17. Holroyd KA, Holm JE, Hursey KG, Penzien DB, Cordingley GE, et al. Recurrent vascular headache: home-based behavioral treatment vs. abortive pharmacological treatment. J Consult Clin Psychol 1988;56:218–223.

18. Olness K, MacDonald JT, Uden DL. Comparison of self-hypnosis and propranolol in the treatment of juvenile migraine. Pediatrics 1987;79:593–597.

19. Forsythe WI, Gillies D, Sills MA. Propranolol (inderal) in the treatment of childhood migraine. Develop Med Child Neurol 1984;26:737–741.

20. Ludvigsson J. Propranolol used in prophylaxis of migraine in children. Acta Neurol Scand 1974;50:109–115.

21. Guarnieri P, Blanchard E. Evaluation of home-based thermal biofeedback treatment of pediatric migraine headache. Biofeedback Self Regul 1990;15:179–184.

22. Labbe EE, Williamson DA. Treatment of childhood migraine using autofenic feedback training. J Consult Clin Psychol 1984;52:968–976.

23. Richter JL, McGrath P, Humphrey PJ, Goodman JT, et al. Cognitive and relaxation treatment of pediatric migraine. Pain 1986;25:195–203.

24. Werder DS, Sargent JD. A study of childhood headache using biofeedback as a treatment alternative. Headache 1984;24:122–126.

25. McGrath PJ, Humphreys P, Goodman JT, Keene D, et al. Relaxation prophylaxis for childhood migraine: a randomized placebo-controlled trial. Dev Med Child Neurol 1988;30:626–631.

26. Congdon PJ, Forsythe WI. Migraine in childhood: a study of 300 children. Dev Med Child Neurol 1979;21:209–216.

27. Prensky AL, Sommer D. Diagnosis and treatment of migraine in children. Neurology 1979;29:506–510.

28. Raskin NH. Headache. New York: Churchill Livingstone, 1988.

29. Lance JW, Curran DA. Treatment of chronic tension headache. Lancet 1964;7345:1236–1239.

30. Diamond S. Baltes BJ. Chronic tension headache treated with amitriptyline: a double-blind study. Headache 1971;11:110–116.

31. Wörz R, Scherhag R. Treatment of chronic tension headache with doxepin or amitriptyline: results of a double-blind study. Headache Q 1990;1:216–223.

32. Holroyd KA, Penzien DB. Client variables and the behavioral treatment of recurrent tension headache: a meta-anlaytic review. J Behav Med 1986;9:515–536.

33. Blanchard EB, Appelbaum KA, Radnitz CL, Michultka D, Morrill B, et al. Placebo-controlled evaluation of abbreviated progressive muscle relaxation and of relaxation combined with cognitive therapy in the treatment of vascular headache. J Consul Clin Psychol 1990;58:210–215.

34. Tobin DL, Holroyd KA, Baker A, Reynolds R, Holm JE. Development and clinical trial of a minimal contact, cognitive-behavioral treatment for tension headache. Cogn Ther Res 1988;12:325–339.

35. Holroyd KA, Nash JM, Pingel JD, Cordingley GE, Jerome A. A comparison of pharmacological (amitriptyline HCl) and nonpharmacological (cognitive-behavioral) therapies for chronic tension headaches. J Consult Clin Psychol 1991;59:387–393.

36. Pavia T, Nunes JS, Moreira A, Santos J, Teixeira J, Barbosa A. Effects of frontalis EMG biofeedback and diazepam in the treatment of tension headache. Headache 1982;22:216–220.

37. Packard RC, O'Connell P. Medication compliance among headache patients. Headache 1986;26:416–419.

38. Fitzpatrick RM, Hopkins AP, Harvard-Watts O. Social dimensions of healing: a longitudinal study of outcomes of medical management of headaches. Soc Sci Med 1983;17:501–510.

39. Holroyd KA, Cordingley GE, Pingel JD, Jerome A, Theofanous AG, et al. Enhancing the effectiveness of abortive therapy: a controlled evaluation of self-management training. Headache 1989;29:148–153.

40. Blanchard EB, Andrasik JG, Neff DF, Jurish SE, Teders SJ, Barron KD, Rodichok LD. Nonpharmacologic treatment of chronic headache: prediction of outcome. Neurology 1983;33(12):1596–1603.

41. Penzien DB, Johnson CA, Carpenter DE. Home-based behavioral treatment vs. long-acting propranolol for recurrent migraine. Paper presented at the meeting of the Society of Behavioral Medicine, Chicago, April, 1990.

42. Budzynski TH, Stoyva JM, Adler CS, Mullaney DJ. EMG biofeedback and tension headache: a controlled outcome study. Psychosom Med 1973;35:484–496.

43. Holroyd KA, Andrasik F, Noble J. Comparison of EMG biofeedback and a credible pseudotherapy in treating tension headache. J Behav Med 1980;3:29–39.

44. Holroyd KA, Penzien DB, Hursey KG, Tobin DL, Rogers L, et al. Change mechanisms in EMG biofeedback training: cognitive changes underlying improvements in tension headache. J Consult Clin Psychol 1984;52(6):1039–1053.

45. O'Leary KD, Borkovec T. Conceptual, methodological, and ethical problems of placebo groups in psychotherapy research. Am Psychol 1978;33:821–830.

46. Wilkins W. Placebo problems in psychotherapy research. Am Psychol 1986;41:551–556.

47. Cleveland SE. Personality factors in the mediation of drug response. In: Fisher S, Greenberg RP, eds. The limits of biological treatments for psychological distress. Hillsdale, NJ: Lawrence Erlbaum, 1989:235–262.

48. Dance KA, Neufeld RWJ. Aptitude-treatment interaction research in the clinical setting: a review of attempts to dispel the "patient uniformity" myth. Psychol Bull 1988;104(2):192–213.

49. Blanchard EB, Andrasik F, Neff DF, Arena JG, Ahles TA, et al. Biofeedback and relaxation training with three kinds of headache: treatment effects and their prediction. J Consult Clin Psychol 1982;50(4):562–575.

50. Blanchard EB, Andrasik F. Management of chronic headaches: a psychological approach. New York: Pergamon Press, 1985.

51. Martin NJ, Holroyd KA, Penzien DB. The headache-specific locus of control scale: adaptation to recurrent headaches. Headache 1990; 30(11):729–734.

52. Simons AD, Lustman PJ, Wetzel RD, Murphy GE. Predicting response to cognitive therapy: the role of learned resourcefulness. Cognit Ther Res 1985;9:79–89.

53. Rosenbaum M. A schedule for assessing self-control behaviors: preliminary findings. Behav Ther 1980;11:109–121.

54. Bakal DA, Demjen S, Kaganov JA. Cognitive behavioral treatment of chronic headache. Headache 1981;21:81–86.

55. Blanchard EB, Appelbaum KA, Radnitz CL, Jaccard J, Dentinger MP. The refractory headache patient—I. Chronic, daily, high-intensity headache. Behav Res Ther 1989;27:403–410.

56. Jacob RG, Turner SN, Szekely BC, Edelman BH. Predicting outcome of relaxation therapy in headaches: the role of "depression." Behav Ther 1983;14:457–465.

57. Isler H. Headache drugs provoking chronic headache: historical aspects and common misunderstandings. In: Diener HC, Wilkinson M, eds. Drug induced headache. New York: Springer-Verlag, 1988:87–94.

58. Wolfson W, Graham J. Development of tolerance to ergot alkaloids in a patient with unusually severe migraine. N Engl J Med 1949;241:296–298.

59. Michultka DM, Blanchard EB, Appelbaum KA, Jaccard J, Dentinger MP. The refractory headache patient—II. High medication consumption (analgesic rebound) headache. Behav Res Ther 1989;27:441–420.

60. Kudrow L. Paradoxical effects of frequent analgesic use. In: Critchley M, Friedman AP, Gorini S, Scuteri F, eds. Advances in neurology: headache: physiopathological and clinical concepts. New York: Raven Press, 1982:33.

61. Scholz E, Diener HC, Geiselhart S. Drug-induced headache—does a critical dosage exist? In: Diener HC, Wilkinson M, eds. Drug induced headache. New York: Springer-Verlag, 1988:29–43.

62. Diener HC, Wilkinson M, eds. Drug induced headache. New York: Springer-Verlag, 1988.

63. Rapaport N. Headaches associated with substances and substance withdrawal. This volume.

64. Baumgartner C, Wessely P, Bingol C, Maly J, Holzner F. Long-term prognosis of analgesic withdrawal in patients with drug-induced headaches. Headache 1989;29:510–514.

65. Deiner HC, Dichgans J, Scholz E, Geiselhart S, Gerber WD, Bille A. Analgesic-induced chronic headache: long-term results of withdrawal therapy. J Neurol 1989;236:9–14.

66. Wittchen HA. A biobehavioral treatment program (SEP) for chronic headache patients. In: Holroyd KA, Scholote B, Zenz H, eds. Perspectives in research on headache. Toronto: CJ Hogrefe, 1983:183–197.

67. Beck AT, Steer RA. Beck depression inventory manual. New York: Psychological Corp, 1987.

68. Hathaway SR, McKinley JC. Minnesota multiphasic personality inventory: manual for administration and scoring. Minneapolis: University of Minnesota Press, 1983.

69. Blanchard EB, Andrasik F, Evans DD, Neff DF, Applebaum KA, Rodichok LD. Behavioral treatment of 250 chronic headache patients: a clinical replication series. Behav Ther 1985;16:308–327.

70. Ford MR, Strobel CF, Strong P, Szarek BL. Quieting response training: predictors of long-term outcome. Biofeedback Self Regul 1983;8:393–408.

71. Merikangas KR, Angst J, Isler H. Migraine and psychopathology. Arch Gen Psychiatry 1990;47:849–853.

39

Headache Diary

MICHAEL G. MCKEE

The patient with the headache and the doctor treating the headache will have many questions about the severity of pain. How much does it hurt? How much does the headache vary during the day, week, month? What makes it worse? What makes it better? Has the suffering changed even if the sensory pain hasn't? Has the treatment been effective in reducing pain?

Barlow (1) notes that historians writing in the year 2000 will comment on the fact that the science of human behavior developed during the 1900s, but that objective measurement of feelings had been slighted, that most clinicians would continue to ask patients with pain, "How do you feel?" He comments that it would seem very strange if physicians evaluated the progress of someone with pneumonia by simply asking patients how they were doing. The historical problem in evaluating subjective complaints is that most practitioners never learned how to evaluate the phenomena objectively, how to use measuring instruments for feelings (1). The headache diary fills the gap; it enables clinicians and researchers to measure headache pain.

Because pain is a subjective experience, some behaviorally oriented psychologists have emphasized the importance of evaluating pain behaviors as distinct from the subjective experience of pain (2, 3). Their argument is that the only objective measures of how much impact pain is having on one's life derive from direct observations of behavior. Actions influenced by pain include taking of medication, time in bed, complaints of pain, both verbal and nonverbal (e.g., grimacing and groaning). Other pain behaviors include, but are not limited to, asking for help, avoidance of responsibilities such as work or school (measured in hours and days missed from such activities), deficit in performance in important activities at time of reported pain (such as fall-off in grades at school), changes in social behavior (amount of time spent in socializing), change in individual hobbies (measured in amount of time spent), decrease in sexual behavior, amount of time spent in family interaction, including time spent in verbal communication (4).

Evaluating subjective complaints of pain and evaluating objective behaviors related to pain are both invaluable in understanding the person with a headache. Evaluating pain complaints is like evaluating complaints of emotional distress. In evaluating emotional disorders, DSM-III (5) cites disability or distress as both representing legitimate grounds for diagnosing a mental disorder, with both to be evaluated. Sometimes people simply feel bad—anxious, depressed, etc. Sometimes they function badly, as in withdrawal from activities, avoidance of people or situations. Many psychometrically sophisticated devices have been developed to measure such inner experiences as anxiety and depression. In evaluating pain, many devices are aimed at evaluating location of pain, qualitative nature of the pain, and its impact on one's life (6).

Observations of pain behavior can be rated by family members in real-life situations or rated in a structured environment in which patients engage in designated activity with specific pain behaviors being rated. The McGill pain questionnaire (7) breaks the pain experience down into sensory, affective, and evaluative components.

The primary self-report methods are visual analog scales and ratings of magnitude. Psychophysical scaling methods can also be used to identify intensity of pain (8). Psychological tests, such as the MMPI, are used to assess personality characteristics related to pain experience and expression. Physiological assessment is particularly important for headache, with EMG especially relevant to tension headaches and digital peripheral temperature measured by biofeedback equipment particularly relevant to vascular headaches. Ideally, all methods of evaluating pain are used in research studies, including psychological testing, physiological evaluation, reports from observations by outsiders, and self-monitoring (9).

What clinicians want most is what the headache diary provides—a quick, direct, and easy way to measure pain intensity. The headache diary has been developed to meet this need. It is not a diary in the conventional sense of the term, not a narrative of the sort many patients already volunteer. Rather, the headache diary is a self-anchoring scale (10). When you want to know the degree to which someone experiences a feeling or a sensation or a perception, the self-anchored scale is the quick and easy way to get the answer, and in some cases, the only way. Measuring intensity of pain is a requirement perfect for the self-anchored scale, which can be completed as frequently as needed. In the ideal development of a self-anchored scale, the patient and doctor work together to make sure there is shared understanding about what each point on the scale indicates. The scale from 0 to 10 or 1 to 9 is a common scale, with the lowest number representing no pain, and the highest number representing the most intense experience of pain (10). If these two extremes and midpoints can be anchored to specific experiences of pain, it is easier for the patient to fill out the scale, and the meaning is clearer. When scales are being used with many people, it is more common to attach verbal descriptors to points on the scale. An example of a headache scale without attached adjectives is in Figure 39.1. It allows for recording finger temperature as well as headache severity.

In evaluating severity of tension headaches, a 6-point scale was introduced by Budzynski et al. when they first used the diary format (11, 12). A 0–10 scale, more common in self-anchored instruments, was introduced by Haynes et al. (13) and used by Holroyd et al. (14). Sargent et al. (15) introduced a 4-point scale for evaluating intensity of migraine. The SUNYA Headache Project, reported in detail by Blanchard and Andrasik (16), uses a 6-point scale, with the numbers corresponding to the following verbal descriptors: 0, no headache; 1, very mild headache, aware of it only when attending to it; 2, mild headache, could be ignored at times; 3, moderate headache, pain is noticeably present; 4, severe headache, difficult to concentrate, can do undemanding tasks; 5, extremely intense headache, incapacitated.

How often and when recordings are made varies from study to study. Budzynski et al. (12) asked patients to make hourly ratings over a 24-hour period. In marked contrast, Sargent et al. (15) asked only for the maximum intensity of the migraine headache during a 24-hour period. Bakal (17) asked for readings made every 2 hours from 6 AM until midnight. Blanchard and Andrasik (16) and Epstein and Abel (18) use a four-times-a-day rating schedule, without precise times specified, but with rough correspondence to breakfast, lunch, dinner, and bedtime. In one sense, the more ratings the better, but in actual clinical practice, it proves difficult to get people to make hourly ratings.

Various measures can be derived from the headache ratings in the diary. Sargent et al. (15) only asked for one rating of intensity for the day. In contrast, Budzynski et al. (12) averaged the 24 hourly ratings to derive what was termed the "headache index," the average hourly rating of headache severity. Omitting the hours of sleep, excluding the 0 ratings, was a procedure followed by Philips (19) to get an average rating, which seems more representative of headaches than a rating derived by averaging many 0's obtained during time of sleep. The headache index of Blanchard and Andrasik (16) is the average of all 28 ratings for a week. These investigators also calculate a peak headache rating, which is the highest rating of the week, and calculate the number of headache-free days. The latter

rating has particular meaning for the patient; the most intense headache rating seems useful in evaluating treatment procedures that can reduce but not eliminate headaches.

Many variables other than headache severity or intensity can be recorded in a diary. Self-monitoring is a powerful way to record correlates of behavioral or subjective experiences. For example, in attempting to modify eating behavior, people are often asked to record not only exactly what they eat and when, but the circumstances, where they are, who they are with, and what their mood is. Similarly, with headache diaries it is possible to record mood, degree of stress experienced, where one is, how much sleep was obtained the night before, who one is with, and how much exercise was obtained during the day. Amount of medication taken is of particular relevance. Some investigators simply record number of pills. Some assign a potency index to medications and calculate overall medication by the potency index (20). Recording medication seems particularly important, since various studies indicate that simply going off medication will help a large percentage of headache sufferers and since reduction in medication is one index of positive outcome. In rating pain, there is increasing attention to rating the two dimensions of pain identified by research. These are the sensory discriminative aspect and the motivational-affective component (the suffering). Some individuals appear to experience a reduction in suffering as a result of various treatment procedures, but with the sensory discriminative aspect of pain relatively unaffected (21).

Self-anchored scales have advantages and disadvantages, and they certainly have great variability. Client diaries, or client logs as they are often called, come in great variety (22). The ratings are made by the patient's experience and have face validity; that is they make sense to the patient. There is probably a positive side effect to that, with the patient feeling that he or she counts, is part of the treatment program, is taken seriously, and that the doctor really wants to know in detail what the patient's experience is. The disadvantage is that, no matter how much you try to have the scales have the same meaning for each person, checkpoints such as "too intense to bear," in fact probably differ from person to person. Psychometrically, it is difficult to get reliability and validity data on self-anchored scales. Blanchard et al. (23) provide some information about validity in a study in which a "significant other" evaluated improvement in the patient using a visual analog scale reading from 0 for unimproved or worst to 100 for completely cured. The patient also used a visual analog scale for self-rating of improvement, as well as completing the headache diary. The correlation of .44 between headache diary improvement score and ratings by the significant other indicated validity for the headache diary, but it should be noted that the obtained correlation still leaves much variance to be accounted for. Another finding of this study was that the patient's rating on the visual analog

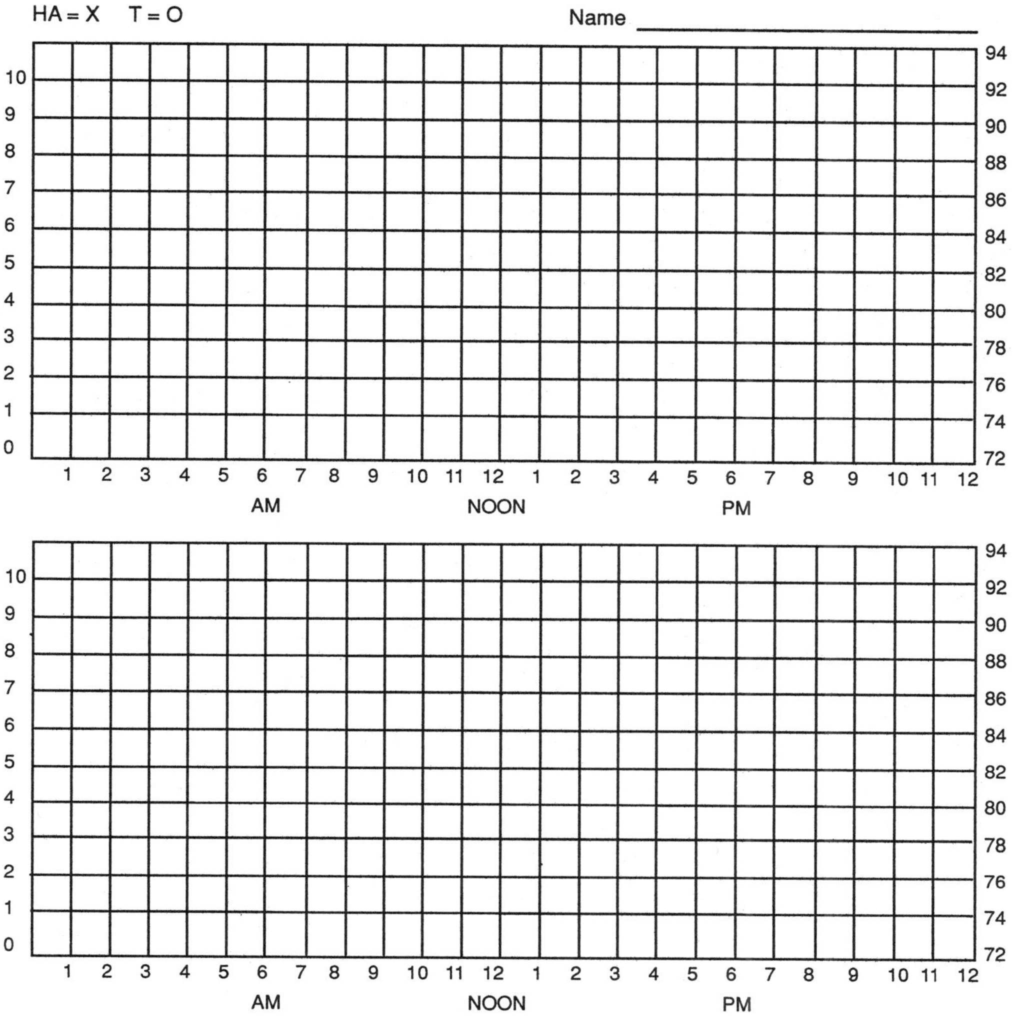

HA = X   T = O   Name _____

Figure 39.1. Example of headache scale without adjectives.

scale showed about 35% more improvement than did the headache diary, suggesting distortion in a global rating.

Some patients may want to distort answers on the headache diary, either to try to please the doctor by indicating improvement in pain and reduction in medication or to make the pain seem worse, so that treatment is legitimate and chances for getting medication are increased. Secondary gain factors, such as asking for letters for relief from work or other responsibilities can also influence distortion of self-ratings.

Compliance is a major problem in obtaining headache diary ratings. Ideally, ratings would be obtained for several weeks prior to treatment for migraine patients and at least 2 weeks prior to treatment for tension headache patients. Realistically, it is very difficult to get even 2 weeks of ratings prior to treatment in a clinical practice and probably not feasible to ask for a baseline period longer than 2 weeks. Many studies using headache diaries have had research subjects who are more highly motivated to complete forms than are patients in a standard clinical

practice. It seems likely that even when ratings are made, many of them are not made at the specified time; one study found 40% of them in this category (24). When you do get compliance with ratings, you probably get more compliance with the overall treatment protocol; diaries can be motivating by involving the patient.

To facilitate compliance, you want a system that is easy to follow. More than one system is advised, so the patient can pick. Some prefer 8″ × 11″ pages, some like 3″ × 5″ cards, and others, notebooks. The person explaining the diary and asking the patient to keep records must be personally convinced of the importance and feasibility of it, or else there will be subtle communication that undermines compliance. Explaining the reasons for obtaining the information and how the patient might benefit from this will help increase motivation. As in any clinical situation, however, it is not sufficient for you to persuasively, confidently, and logically explain why you want the patient to provide data. It is particularly important to be sensitive to any resistances, to allow the patient an opportunity to express those resistances, so that there is an opportunity to change beliefs or feelings, which will make behavioral compliance more likely.

Shelton and Levy (25) have emphasized steps in gaining compliance. Elicit resistances, listen to them, and acknowledge them, or else you may have someone agreeing with you out loud and silently deciding not to cooperate. Ask too little rather than too much; start small. Be specific and detailed and don't rely on memory; give written instructions. Practice in imagery by having the patient go through the steps in imagination, and practice in reality by having the patient fill out a form for right now. Compliment and reward cooperation.

Keeping headache diaries can have therapeutic value for the patient as well as research value for the investigator and informational value for the clinician. Self-monitoring in itself often produces behavior change because it forces awareness, so that habitual patterns don't operate outside of consciousness. Thus, a headache diary becomes a therapeutic homework task for the patient, as well as providing data for quality assurance and research purposes (26). When data about antecedents and consequences are also gathered, as when looking at stressful circumstances that might precede headache and changes in activity that might follow its onset, a broader understanding of the context of the headache, possible causes, and effects is also facilitated. In clinical biofeedback therapy, where physiological retraining and psychotherapy intended to change patterns of thought, feeling, and action are inextricably intertwined, such patient awareness facilitates progress. Additionally, simply recording, provided there is progress in the treatment regimen, provides a record of improvement, which itself has therapeutic value and contributes to further improvement. Fordyce (27) has pointed out that we are always communicating with our patients, and homework assignments constitute a particular form of communication. The message is that the problem is taken seriously, that we believe change can take place, that the pattern of headache can be better understood, and that it can be changed. The message is further that the patient is an active part of the treatment program, that his or her opinions and experiences are highly valued. When separate records are kept for the sensory discriminative aspect of pain and the motivational affective part of pain and the evaluative aspect, there is also an important message: that even if the sensory discriminative part of pain doesn't change, the emotional feelings associated with it, the judgment about it, and the effect on one's daily life can change.

In summary, the headache diary, by giving those of us who diagnose and treat headache a simple and realistic measure of pain, gives us a tool to enhance compliance, further therapeutic progress, research our efforts (as in recent studies of psychophysiology of headache (28), which help clarify diagnostic (29) and cognitive correlates of headaches (30)) and have routine measures for quality

assurance needs. The headache diary, like the lever, is simple and powerful.

REFERENCES

1. Barlow D. In: Corcoran K, Fischer J, eds. Measures for clinical practice: a source book. New York: Free Press, xxi–xxiii, 1987.
2. Keefe FJ. Behavioral assessment and treatment of chronic pain: current status and future directions. J Consult Clin Psychol 1982;50:896–911.
3. Kaplan RM. Behavior as the central outcome in healthcare. Am Psychol 1990;45:1211–1220.
4. McKee MG. Behavior techniques and pain modification. Cleve Clin J Med 1989;56:502–508.
5. American Psychiatric Association Diagnostic and Statistical Manual, 3rd ed. Washington, D.C., 1980.
6. Williamson DA, Davis CJ, Prather RC. Assessment of health related disorders. In: Bellack AS, Hersen M, eds. Behavioral assessment: a protocol handbook. 3rd ed. New York: Pergamon, 1988.
7. Melzack R. The McGill pain questionnaire: major properties and scoring methods. Pain 1975;I:277–299.
8. Tursky B. The development of a pain perception profile: a psychophysical approach. In: M Weisenberg, B Tursky, eds. Pain: new perspectives in therapy and research. New York: Plenum, 1976:171–194.
9. Feuerstein M, Labbé EE, Kuczmierczyk AR. Health psychology: a psychobiological perspective. New York: Plenum, 1986.
10. Corcoran K, Fischer J. Measures for clinical practice: a source book. New York: Free Press, 1987.
11. Budzynski TH, Stoyva J, Adler CS. Feedback induced muscle relaxation: application to tension headache. J Behav Ther Exp Psychiatry 1970;1:205–211.
12. Budzynski TH, Stoyva J, Adler CS, Mullaney DJ. EMG biofeedback in tension headache: a controlled outcome study. Psychosom Med 1973;6:509–514.
13. Haynes SN, Griffin P, Mooney D, Parise M. Electromyographic biofeedback and relaxation instructions in the treatment of muscle contraction headaches. Behav Ther 1975;6:672–678.
14. Holroyd KA, Andrasik F, Noble J. Comparison of EMG biofeedback, and acredible pseudotherapy in treating tension headache. J Behav Med 1980;3:29–39.
15. Sargent JD, Green EE, Walters ED. Preliminary report on the use of autogenic feedback training in the treatment of migraine and tension headaches. Psychosom Med 1973;35:129–135.
16. Blanchard EB, Andrasik F. Management of chronic headaches: a psychological approach. New York: Pergamon, 1985.
17. Bakal DA. The psychobiology of chronic headache. New York: Springer, 1982.
18. Epstein LH, Abel GG. An analysis of biofeedback training affects for tension headache patients. Behav Ther 1977;8:37–47.
19. Philips C. The modification of tension headache pain using EMG biofeedback. Behav Res Ther 1977;15:119–129.
20. Coyne L, Sargent J, Segerson J, Abourn R. Relative potency scale for analgesic drugs: use of psychophysical procedures with clinical judgments. Headache 1976;16:70–71.
21. Hilgard ER, Hilgard JR. Hypnosis in the relief of pain. Los Altos, CA: William Kaufman, 1975.
22. Bloom M, Fischer J. Evaluating practice: guidelines for the accountable professional. Inglewoods Cliffs, NJ: Prentice-Hall, 1982.
23. Blanchard EB, Andrasik F, Neff DF, Jurish SE, O'Keefe DM. Social validation of a headache diary. Behav Ther 1981;12:711–715.
24. Collins FL, Thompson JK. Reliability and standardization in the assessment of self-reported headache pain. J Behav Assess 1979;1:73–86.
25. Shelton JL, Levy RL. Behavioral assignments and treatment compli-

ance: a handbook of clinical strategies. Champaign, IL: Research Press, 1981.

26. Russell ML. Behavioral counseling in medicine: strategies for modifying at risk behavior. New York: Oxford University Press, 1986.

27. Fordyce WE. Pain and suffering: a reappraisal. Am Psychol 1988;43:276–283.

28. Lichstein KL, Fischer SM, Gabin TL, et al. Psychophysiological

parameters of migraine and muscle-contraction headache. Headache 1991;31:27–34.

29. Headache Classification Committee of the International Headache Society: Classification and diagnostic criteria for headache disorders, cranial neuralgias and facial pain. Cephalalgia 1988;8(suppl 7).

30. Demjen S, Bakal DA, Dunn BE. Cognitive correlates of headache intensity and duration. 1990;30:423–427.

40

Drug Detoxification Protocols

DAVID A. FISHBAIN

SUBSTANCE ABUSE DEFINITIONS

Substance abuse definitions are a major problem. There is no agreement between researchers on terms such as drug abuse, drug dependence, psychological drug dependence, and drug addiction (1). Often, drug dependence, psychological drug dependence, and drug addiction are used interchangeably. Because of this, psychiatric operational diagnostic criteria for these groups of disorders have been difficult to develop.

In an attempt to rectify this confusing situation, Rinaldi (1) developed a standardized list of substance abuse terms. Six definitions important to this chapter are taken from this list and presented in Table 40.1: tolerance, physical dependence, psychological dependence, drug dependence, drug addiction, and drug withdrawal syndrome. The following is to be noted in reference to these six terms (1–3):

1. They are distinct concepts in themselves.
2. They should not be used interchangeably.
3. Physical and psychological dependence are encompassed within drug dependence.
4. Drug addiction includes the concept of "compulsive" drug use.
5. Psychological dependence is distinct from tolerance and physical dependence.
6. Tolerance and physical dependence develop on parallel time courses, but the rate of development of tolerance varies greatly between individuals.

Following long-term use of opiates or sedative drugs, psychological dependence, physical dependence, and tolerance can develop. It is estimated that of those who use opiates sporadically on a nondaily basis, 25% will become dependent or addicted (2). Physical dependence is a function of the dosage schedule of the opiate, but it can be produced by very little opiate exposure, can persist for a long time after drug cessation, and will develop in every patient so exposed. In general, of those who advance to twice-daily use, the majority may become physically dependent within 6 to 8 weeks.

Psychological dependence is a behavior pattern characterized by continued craving for opiates, and it *does not occur in every patient* exposed to opiates. Compulsive drug-seeking behavior leading to overwhelming involvement in drug use and obtainment is a manifestation of this craving. In some individuals, compulsive drug-seeking behavior can occur *before* true physical dependence develops.

Addiction has been defined as an "atypical behavioral pattern of drug use, characterized by overwhelming involvement with the use of drug (compulsive use), the securing of its supply, tendency towards progressive drug intake (loss of control), and the high tendency of relapse after drug withdrawal, and reversal of physical dependence" (1–4). This definition tends to equate drug addiction and psychological dependence; however, this is not the case. Ludwig (4) believes that compulsive drug use derives its strength from three sources of pharmacological reinforcement: physical dependence (drug-engendered changes), tolerance (metabolic and behavioral neuroadaption to the drug effect), and psychological dependence (personality-linked factors).

Several points apply to the interrelationships between these various concepts (3, 4).

1. One can be physically dependent without being drug addicted.
2. One can be drug addicted without being physically dependent or drug tolerant.
3. Those who are drug addicted are likely to be physically dependent.
4. Not all drugs produce physical dependence, psychological dependence, and tolerance; some drugs produce one manifestation only.
5. Drug-addicted patients who are physically dependent are usually drug tolerant.

Drug withdrawal syndrome will appear after abrupt withdrawal or drop in blood level of the drug to which the patient is physically dependent (4). The severity of the withdrawal syndrome will reflect the degree of physical dependence. In the case of opiate drugs, a withdrawal syndrome can also be precipitated by the administration of an opiate antagonist (4). The lowest dose and shortest duration of action of opiates and sedatives that may predispose to withdrawal is unknown. Severity of withdrawal is a function of the dose and duration of administration of the

Table 40.1.
Substance Abuse Terminology Definitions[a]

(Drug) Addiction: A chronic disorder characterized by the compulsive use of a substance resulting in physical, psychological, or social harm to the user and continued use despite that harm

(Drug) Dependence: A generic term that relates to physical or psychological dependence, or both. It is characteristic for each pharmacological class of psychoactive drugs. Impaired control over drug-taking behavior is implied

Physical dependence: A physiological state of adaptation to a drug or alcohol, usually characterized by the development of tolerance to drug effects and the emergence of a withdrawal syndrome during prolonged abstinence

Psychological dependence: The emotional state of craving a drug either for its positive effect or to avoid negative effects associated with its absence

Tolerance: Physiological adaptation to the effect of drugs, so as to diminish effects with constant dosages or to maintain the intensity and duration of effects through increased dosage

Drug withdrawal syndrome: The onset of a predictable constellation of signs and symptoms involving altered activity of the central nervous system after the abrupt discontinuation of, or rapid decrease in, dosage of a drug

[a]Adapted from Rinaldi RC, Steindler EM, Wilford BB, Goodwin D. Clarification and standardization of substance abuse terminology. JAMA 1988;259:577–561.

discontinued drug. However, physical dependence itself does not impede rapid tapering. The elimination half-life of the opiate or sedative determines when the withdrawal syndrome will begin (4). Withdrawal will appear in 6 to 12 hours for short half-life drugs (such as morphine) and peak in 24 to 72 hours. For long half-life drugs (such as methadone), withdrawal will begin in 36 to 48 hours.

WHAT PERCENTAGE OF CHRONIC PAIN PATIENTS ARE DRUG/ALCOHOL ADDICTED?

Before addressing this question, we should review what is known about drug-addicted groups. The DSM-III-R (5) and Ludwig (4) describe two different addicted populations: street addicts and licit drug scammers. Street addicts are patients who became involved in drug use in their teens or early twenties, use opiates obtained illegally, and have histories of polysubstance abuse and IV opiate use. Licit drug scammers are patients who focus on illegitimate procuring of opiates from physicians for many physical complaints. These patients originally obtained an opiate by prescription from a physician for a legitimate medical reason but have gradually increased the dose and frequency of the opiate on their own. Substance-seeking behavior is prominent here, although the patient justifies use on the basis of symptoms. There may also be street addicts within this latter group. Therefore, to place chronic pain patients into either of these groups, researchers must assess psychological dependence and compulsive use. The author has reviewed 20 relevant studies in this area (6–25), trying to assess whether chronic pain researchers use this concept of addiction, and has concluded the following:

1. Most studies did not use appropriate definitions for drug abuse, physical dependence, psychological dependence, and addiction.

2. Only 7 studies attempted to make a drug misuse diagnosis by some means: three by DSM-III criteria, one by NIMH-DIS criteria, two by urine toxicology, and one (11) by its own criteria. There appears to be a major problem with the criteria used in this last study, as anyone who lacked an adequate medical reason for pain was given a drug abuse diagnosis.

3. Of these seven studies, only four (19–22) had usable percentages.

4. Not one study adequately addressed the concept of addiction, although according to DSM-III criteria (5), addicted patients would be encompassed within the drug-dependent group.

5. Current drug/alcohol abuse/dependence in chronic pain patients has been reported to be approximately 15 and 30%, while current illicit drug use has been reported to be 6 and 12%.

6. The percentage of chronic pain patients who could be diagnosed according to the definition of addiction is unknown.

7. It is likely that chronic pain patients who use illicit drugs are addicted to other substances.

These observations and conclusions are supported by one large study that has demonstrated that addiction is rare in medical patients treated with opiates (26). This view is also supported by Portenoy (3). Through his review of the literature of published reports of *chronic opiate therapy for chronic nonmalignant pain and cancer*, he has concluded the following:

1. There is a subpopulation of patients that may obtain partial analgesia without opiate toxicity or clinically significant tolerance.

2. Drug abuse behavior occurs but is uncommon.

3. Patients with a prior history of substance abuse appear to be at increased risk for management problems.

4. Concern that opiates cannot relieve pain related to "psychological factors" is not confirmed.

5. Dose escalation (tolerance) is observed in those cancer patients with advancing painful lesions and is not a problem with patients with stable pain.

6. Some patients with chronic pain after opiate tapering may relapse, not because they are addicted, but because of their chronic pain.

7. Opiate craving in chronic pain patients may not be a symptom of addiction, but may represent an appropriate search for pain relief. The term, "pseudoaddiction" has been applied to this syndrome in the cancer population (27). Here, because of iatrogenic undertreatment of pain, the patient develops addictive behavior.

8. There may be fundamental epidemiological and genetic differences between chronic pain patients and addicts.

9. Patients *without* a prior history of substance abuse are at low risk for abuse behavior in short-term opiate treatment for painful medical conditions.

Portenoy (3) has attempted to define "addiction" as it relates to the chronic pain patient. He believes it is characterized by

1. Psychological dependence: intense desire for the drug and overwhelming concern about availability;
2. Evidence of compulsive drug use (unsanctioned dose escalation, use for other symptoms, etc.);
3. Associated behavior: manipulation of physicians to obtain additional drugs, obtaining drugs from multiple physicians, drug sales, drug hoarding, and unapproved use of other drugs, such as alcohol.

The author's clinical experience supports Portenoy's views. Few chronic pain patients display addictive behavior, and the vast majority are easily detoxified from opiates. This is in strong contrast to street addicts, who are extremely difficult to detoxify from opiates and relapse in a large percentage of cases. This last point has been made by Halpern (28), who believes that more systematic research is needed on the response of chronic pain patients to detoxification. The ease of detoxification of the vast majority of pain patients indicates that these patients do not fall within the definition of "addiction."

WHY DETOXIFY CHRONIC PAIN PATIENTS FROM OPIATES AND SEDATIVES?

Since their early development, pain centers have maintained the position that all chronic pain patients should be detoxified from potentially addictive substances as a part of treatment. This position has been based on two beliefs: most chronic pain patients are addicted and p.r.n. medication schedules contribute to drug-seeking behavior (29); medication contributes to the dysfunction found in chronic pain (28). Portenoy (3) has demonstrated that some chronic pain patients can be maintained on opiates without displaying addictive behavior. In addition, this chapter has demonstrated that the evidence for addiction in chronic pain patients is slim, if not nonexistent. Halpern (28), in his review, has pointed out that there is a paucity of rigorous evidence for the belief that medications contribute to the dysfunction found in chronic pain. However, the author believes that there are *other* reasons for detoxifying chronic pain patients. These are as follows:

1. Some detoxified chronic pain patients experience a sense of well-being with abstinence (16).
2. Methadone-maintained addicts do not differ from drug-free ex-addicts in pain threshold and pain tolerance (30). This indicates that chronic opiate use may not ameliorate pain.
3. Chronic pain patients who are drug abusing and/or dependent, may have deficits in their neuropsychological function secondary to the drugs (31).
4. Opiates may have no analgesic effect on chronic neuropathic and idiopathic pain (32). This, in fact, is frequently stated by chronic pain patients.
5. Although chronic pain patients may not display addictive behavior, nevertheless, they will become drug tolerant and dependent. Therefore, a proportion of them may seek the drug to prevent physical discomfort and the psychological distress of the withdrawal syndrome (4).
6. Snyder (33) has postulated that opiate receptors become overloaded with enkephalins when there is a chronic exogenous supply of opiates. A feedback loop conveys a message to the enkephalin-producing cells to stop enkephalin release. In this way, a chronic exogenous supply of opiates disrupts the body's natural pain-control system.
7. Chronic headache patients may experience what has been labeled "analgesic-rebound headache" or "analagesic-abuse headache" (34). This refers to the worsening of the headache 3 to 4 hours after medication wears off and a withdrawal syndrome after medication is discontinued. This headache improves simply with detoxification in about 50% of patients (34). Although the rebound phenomena have not been described for other chronic pain patients, an improvement in pain with detoxification has been (10). Evidence suggests that drug-induced headache may be restricted to those with primary headache disorders, especially migraineurs (34). There could be such a subgroup in other chronic pain patients.

The above points demonstrate many potentially valid scientific reasons for pain center detoxification other than addiction. The concept that pain centers detoxify because of patient addiction should be abandoned for all but a small select group of chronic pain patients with addictive behavior. When this concept is misapplied, as often is the case, it is pejorative to the patient.

WHERE SHOULD CHRONIC PAIN PATIENTS BE DETOXIFIED?

Because of the misconception concerning the "addiction" status of chronic pain patients, many pain centers have taken the position that these patients should be treated in drug facilities first, and then in pain centers. These centers routinely refer any chronic pain patient who is on large doses of opiates to a drug facility first. There is no scientific evidence for this position. However, one study indicates that chronic pain patients would do better if detoxification occurred in a pain center. In this study, from a drug facility, no patient initially perceived that chronic pain, due to a medical condition, would be an impediment to withdrawal from opiates. However, pain masked by opiate dependency emerged during detoxification and proved to be an insurmountable barrier to total withdrawal in most patients (35). This study supports the author's clinical impression that chronic pain patients with drug dependence are best detoxified in a chronic pain setting. The reasons for this are as follows:

1. Pain centers can provide the chronic pain patient with adjunct pain relief during detoxification, at a time when the patient's pain usually dramatically increases. Drug facilities are unable to do this.
2. Chronic pain patients are alienated by the drug facility's milieu, as they do not see themselves as "addicted," and believe that they have a legitimate reason to be on medication (i.e., chronic pain). However, chronic pain patients respond well to the pain center milieu, which assists them with pain control during detoxification.
3. Chronic pain patients feel they have nothing in common

with the drug facility "street addicts," whom they view pejoratively.

4. Chronic pain patients are insulted by the "addiction" label placed on them by the drug facility. Therefore, they are unwilling to accept the kind of treatment these facilities offer.

5. Often, the chronic pain patient is involved in litigation, which can be affected by the addiction label. Thus the patient is very sensitive to this type of approach.

6. Lastly, chronic pain patients with drug dependence can be thought of as dual-diagnosis patients (discussed below). However, the primary diagnosis is "chronic pain" and not "drug dependence." Because patients view it this way, treatment is most successful when it is directed at what the patients view as their primary problem.

What about the truly addicted patient with chronic pain? These patients are generally failures in drug treatment facilities and can be treated within pain centers. However, drug detoxification protocols for these patients may need to be individually tailored, and these patients may require drug facility follow-up.

DIAGNOSIS OF DRUG ABUSE, DRUG DEPENDENCE, DRUG ADDICTION, POLYSUBSTANCE DEPENDENCE

Operational psychiatric diagnostic criteria for drug dependence (psychoactive substance dependence) and drug abuse (psychoactive substance abuse) were developed for the DSM-III-R (5). These psychiatric diagnostic criteria are presented in Tables 40.2, 40.3, and 40.4. There are no DSM-III-R (5) criteria for drug addiction. Instead, the operational diagnosis of psychoactive substance dependence appears to incorporate the concept of compulsive use in criteria 1, 2, 3, and 6. Psychoactive substance abuse is then a residual category for maladaptive patterns of drug use that have never met the criteria for drug dependence. These DSM-III-R (5) diagnosis then may not assist in distinguishing the "addicted" patient from the patient who is psychologically and physically dependent, or simply physically dependent.

If a patient has repeatedly consumed at least three categories of psychoactive substances (not including caffeine and nicotine) for the last 6 months, no single substance has predominated, and criteria for dependence have been met as a group, that patient fulfills DSM-III-R (5) diagnostic criteria for polysubstance dependence. This category is important because it appears that 50% of the patients in outpatient alcohol clinics have this problem (5). Here one drug is the primary drug of abuse (e.g., cocaine (euphoria)); while a secondary (e.g., alcohol) is used to control the negative side effects of the primary drug (e.g., anxiety).

CLUES TO THE DIAGNOSIS OF DRUG ABUSE

For those patients who admit to drug abuse/dependence, a drug history should be taken (Table 40.5) to answer the following questions:

1. Is the patient physically dependent?
2. Is the patient psychologically dependent?

Table 40.2.
DSM-III-R Diagnostic Criteria for Psychoactive Substance Dependence

A. At least three of the following:
 1. Substance often taken in larger amounts or over a longer period than the person intended.
 2. Persistent desire or one or more unsuccessful efforts to cut down or control substance use.
 3. A great deal of time spent in activities necessary to get the substance (e.g., theft), taking the substance (e.g., chain smoking), or recovering from its effects.
 4. Frequent intoxication or withdrawal symptoms when expected to fulfill major role obligations at work, school, or home (e.g., does not go to work because hung over, goes to school or work "high," intoxicated while taking care of his/her children), or when substance use is physically hazardous (e.g., drives when intoxicated).
 5. Important social, occupational or recreational activities given up or reduced because of substance use.
 6. Continued substance use despite knowledge of having a persistent or recurrent social, psychological or physical problem that is caused or exacerbated by the use of the substance (e.g., keeps using heroin despite family arguments about it, cocaine-induced depression, or having an ulcer made worse by drinking.
 7. Marked tolerance: Need for markedly increased amounts of the substance (i.e., at last a 50% increase) in order to achieve intoxication or desired effect, or markedly diminished effect with continued use of the same amount.
   Note: The following items may not apply to cannabis, hallucinogens or phencyclidine (PCP):
 8. Characteristic withdrawal symptoms (see specific withdrawal syndromes under psychoactive substance-induced organic mental disorders).
 9. Substance often taken to relieve or avoid withdrawal symptoms.
B. Some symptoms of the disturbance have persisted for at least one month, or have occurred repeatedly over a longer period of time.

Table 40.3.
DSM-III-R Diagnostic Criteria for Psychoactive Substance Abuse

A. A maladaptive pattern of psychoactive substance use indicated by at least one of the following:
 1. Continued use despite knowledge of having a persistent or recurrent social, occupational, psychologic, or physical problem that is caused or exacerbated by use of the psychoactive substance.
 2. Recurrent use in situations in which use is physically hazardous (i.e., driving while intoxicated).
B. Some symptoms of the disturbance have persisted for at least 1 month or have occurred repeatedly over a longer period of time.
C. Never met the criteria for psychoactive substance dependence for this substance.

3. Is the patient addicted?
4. What drug is the patient physically dependent on and in what doses?
5. Will the patient develop a withdrawal syndrome?
6. How severe will the withdrawal syndrome be?
7. What doses of medication will be required to prevent or minimize the withdrawal syndrome?
8. Is the patient a polysubstance abuser?
9. What kind of drug rehabilitation will the patient require?

Because of the "denial" of some drug abuse patients, the physician will not be able to elicit a history readily or that history will be unreliable. Under those circumstances, other historical clues may lead the physician to suspect potential drug abuse (Table 40.6). The physician should also look for drug abuse clues in the physical examination (Table 40.7) and the laboratory workup. In addition, the drug abuser may manifest a number of ocular manifestations (38). The laboratory workup for patients suspected of drug abuse is presented in Table 40.8. Physicians who request drug urine toxicologies must be aware of the following (5, 39, 40):

1. In most laboratories, the urine toxicology screen is performed in two steps:

a. The first procedure is a screening test with great sensitivity and therefore few false-negative results but many false-positive results. This first procedure is usually thin-layer chromatography or an immunoassay.

b. Urines positive on the first test are then subjected to a second test. The second test is much more specific for the substance detected on the first test and is usually gas chromatography, high-performance liquid chromatography, or mass spectrometry.

2. Positive results must be interpreted in relationship to the specificity of the method used. All positive results in the first test should be checked by the more specific method.

3. Negative test results can be interpreted as follows:

a. Patient is not using a drug that can be detected by the test.

b. Patient may be taking the drug detected by the test but:

(1) Is not taking large enough dose;

(2) Is not taking the drug frequently enough to be detected;

(3) Urine is collected too long after the drug is ingested;

(4) Urine sample is tampered with.

Table 40.4.
DSM-III-R Criteria for Polysubstance Dependence

A. A period of at least 6 months during which the person was repeatedly using at least 3 categories of psychoactive substances (not including nicotine and caffeine), but no single psychoactive substance predominated.

B. During this period, the dependence criteria were met for psychoactive substances (as a group) but not for any specific substance.

Table 40.5.
Outline of Drug History[a]

1. *Reason for referral*
Type of help sought
2. *First exposure*
Age
Which drug
Mode of administration
Circumstances
Where
Who/how initiated
Source of drug
Reaction to drug
3. *Subsequent use*
Which drug(s)
Dose
Frequency of administration
Route
Date and age of becoming a regular user
Periods of heavy use
Reasons for continuation
Circumstances of drug taking: solitary/with friends
Preferred drug(s)
Periods of abstinence:
Voluntary
Enforced
4. *Recent-use drug(s)*
Dose
Frequency
Route
Any withdrawal symptoms
Evidence of increasing tolerance: escalating dose
Source of supply
Price paid
5. *Method of self-injection*
Route: subcutaneous/intramuscular/intravenous
Site
Source of injection equipment
Sharing of injection equipment
Sterilization procedures

6. *Consequences and complications of drug use*
Physical illness: malnutrition; hepatitis; jaundice; abscesses; septicemia; deep vein thrombosis; overdose; road, traffic, and other accidents; symptoms of abstinence syndrome
Mental illness: episodes of drug-induced psychosis; intoxication leading to drowsiness; confusion; dementia
Social problems associated with drug use: amount spent weekly on drugs; source of this money
7. *Contact with other treatment agencies or sources of help* (e.g., DDTUs; doctors; probation services; local authorities; voluntary agencies–religious organizations, self-help groups, etc.)
8. *Legal history*
Number of arrests, court appearances, convictions
Periods in detention center, approved school, reformatory, prison
Periods of probation
Nature of offenses
Outstanding court cases
Disqualification from driving
Drug-related offenses
9. *Developmental history* with review of family of origin, significant relationships, familial history of substance abuse or psychological disorders or problems
10. Current status of relationships with significant others and family, occupational status and issues, legal concerns, hobbies, leisure-time use, support systems, and community resources
11. Treatment history, including nature of past treatment of substance abuse disorders or psychological problems and results of treatment, with attention given to the use of follow-up or aftercare and involvement in self-help or other support groups in the community
12. Patient's perception of problem and expectations of hospitalization and treatment
13. Family's perception of problem and expectations of hospitalization and treatment

[a]Adapted from Ghodse H. Drugs and addictive behavior, a guide to treatment. Oxford: Blackwell Scientific Publications, 1990.

Table 40.6.
Other Historical Clues to Potential Drug Abuse[a]

A change in performance at work or at school
Abrupt change in behavior or personality
Multiple medical illnesses in a person under the age of 40
A history of overdose or prior suicide attempts
The patient's friends are substance abusers
Poor self-care
Weight loss
Oversensitivity to questions about drinking or drugs
Sudden changes in friends
Loss of communication with family
Obvious signs of intoxication noted by significant other
Denial of use even with drug paraphernalia
Deterioration of moral values
Truancy

[a]Adapted from Fauman BJ, Fauman MA. Emergency psychiatry for the house officer. Baltimore: Williams & Wilkins, 1981.

(5) Assay used was not sensitive enough to detect the drug.

4. Some drugs, like cocaine (40) and canabinoids, may be taken up by the tissues and slowly released into the body. Thus, these patients may continue to demonstrate positive urine test results, even though they may be in an environment where drug use is prohibited, (e.g., a pain center). Therefore, a decision for terminating a patient from treatment based on a positive toxicology should be finalized cautiously.

DRUGS OF ABUSE CLASSIFICATION SCHEME

Common drugs of abuse can be classified according to their action on the nervous system and their pharmacological properties. There are eight basic groups: hypnotic-sedatives, opiates, stimulants, psychotomimetics, muscle relaxants, antidepressants, vasoconstriction α-adrenergic blocking agents and others (Table 40.9). These eight groups are further subclassified as shown.

Ludwig (4) has outlined six laws that pertain to this drug classification scheme:

1. The classification reflects the drug's *primary* action; e.g., in the vast majority of cases, depressants will produce a sedating effect.
2. Drugs within the same category (e.g., sedatives) will or will not produce physical dependence and tolerance.
3. Patients becoming tolerant of one drug in a category (e.g., sedatives), will be cross-tolerant to *all* other drugs in the same category. Thus, drugs within the same category may substitute for each other in maintaining physical dependence and preventing the withdrawal syndrome.
4. Generally, withdrawal will be *the reverse* of the physiological effects of the drug to which the patient is physically dependent.
5. Drugs in the same class, if administered together, will act synergistically.
6. The shorter the half-life of the drug, the faster the withdrawal syndrome. Because the withdrawal syndrome can itself reinforce drug addiction, drugs with short half-lives provide many more episodes of reinforcement within a unit of time than do drugs with long half-lives.

Table 40.7.
Physical Examination Clues to Drug Abuse[a]

I. *General appearance*	
General neglect	(drug lifestyle)
Poor nutrition	(drug lifestyle)
Fever	(septicemia secondary to IV drug use)
II. *Gait*	
Ataxic	(drug intoxication)
III. *Eyes*	
Watery	(opiate withdrawal)
Nystagmus	(sedative intoxication)
Pin-point pupils	(opiate use)
Dilated pupils	(opiate abstinence)
	(use of amphetamines, cocaine, hallucinogens, anticholinergics)
Jaundice	(inhalant abuse)
Red conjunctiva	(cannabis use, inhalant use)
IV. *Nose*	
Congestion nasal mucosa	(snorted drugs)
Ulceration nasal mucosa	(snorted drugs, cocaine or heroin)
Rhinorrhea	(opiate abstinence)
Nose Rash	(inhalant abuse)
V. *Mouth*	
Breath odor	(Inhalants, eth)
Caries	(Opiate dependence)
VI. *Skin*	
Abscesses	(IV drug use)
Healed abscesses	(IV drug use)
Skin necrosis	(IV drug use)
Thrombophlebitis	(IV drug use)
Pigmentation of the skin over veins (tracking)	(IV drug use)
Tattoos	(IV drug use)
Gangrene	(IV drug use)
Goose flesh	(Opiate abstinence)
VII. *Cardiovascular system*	
Tachycardia	(Withdrawal or intoxication)
High blood pressure	(Stimulant use)
Low blood pressure	(Opiate and sedative use)
Orthostatic hypotension & increase in H.R. of 15 or greater	(Sedative withdrawal)
Heart murmur (Changing) (fever)	(Endocarditis secondary to IV drug use)
VIII. *Respiratory system*	
Pulmonary embolism	
Pulmonary infarction	
Pulmonary hypertension	
Chest infections	
Asthma	
IX. *Abdomen*	
Hepatomegaly	
Lower bowel distended with feces	(opiates)
X. *Neuromuscular*	
Tremor	(opiate abstinence)
Muscle twitching	(opiate abstinence)
Muscle wasting	(pentazocine & Demerol injection)
Muscle fibrosis	(pentazocine & Demerol injection)
Muscle calcification	(pentazocine & Demerol injection)
XI. *Lymphatic system*	
Enlarged lymph nodes	(IV drug use)
Puffy hands	(IV drug use)
Brawny edema	(IV drug use)

[a]Compiled from Ghodse H. Drugs and addictive behavior, a guide to treatment. Oxford: Blackwell Scientific Publications, 1990.

Table 40.8.
Laboratory Workup[a]

Hemoglobin
Erythrocyte sedimentation rate
White blood count
Blood urea nitrogen
Liver function tests**
VDRL, FTA-ABS
Hepatitis screen
HIV
Chest x-ray
Urine for toxicology
Blood alcohol level[b]
Elevated mean corpulscular volume[b]
Elevated SGOT, SGPT, and LDH[b]
Elevated SGGT (serum γ-glutamyl transpeptidase)[b]
Decreased albumin, B_{12}, folic acid[b]
Increased uric acid[b]
Increased serum amylase[b]

[a]Compiled from Ghodse H. Drugs and addictive behavior, a guide to treatment. Oxford: Blackwell Scientific Publications, 1990.
[b]May indicate alcohol abuse.

Closer inspection of Table 40.9 indicates that some unusual therapeutic drugs can be abused; e.g., tricyclic antidepressants (41, 42) and MAO inhibitors (43). This is because the patient uses these drugs for their side effects (e.g., anticholinergic effect of the tricyclic or the stimulant effect of the MAO inhibitor).

ORGANIC MENTAL SYNDROME ASSOCIATED WITH PSYCHOACTIVE SUBSTANCES

Table 40.10 lists the organic mental syndromes associated with various types of psychoactive substances. Pain physicians may encounter any of these organic mental syndromes in chronic pain patients who abuse drugs. If they are uncertain of the etiology or diagnosis of the psychopathology, a psychiatric consultation should be requested. However, most of these syndromes are rarely encountered within the chronic pain setting. Drug withdrawal and withdrawal delirium would occur with much greater frequency if drug detoxification protocols were not carried out. Drug detoxification protocols can prevent or minimize withdrawal and withdrawal delirium for the drug groups listed in Table 40. 10. This is why drug detoxification protocols and their correct use are important to the treatment of the chronic pain patient. The balance of this chapter is devoted to delineating these protocols and methods for their use.

Although a number of drug groups can be associated with withdrawal, only alcohol and sedative/hypnotics/anxiolytics are associated with withdrawal delirium (Table 40.10). Withdrawal can be uncomfortable, but it is not life-threatening; withdrawal delirium can result in death. It is therefore necessary to adequately prevent and treat potential withdrawal delirium. Table 40.11 presents the signs of withdrawal for the various drug groups. The reader should refer to the DSM-III-R (5) for the diagnostic criteria for delirium.

Table 40.9.
Drugs of Abuse[a]

A. *Hypnotic-sedatives*
  Alcohol
  Barbiturates: e.g., pentobarbital (Nembutal)
  Nonbarbiturates: e.g., methaqualone (Quaalude)
  Antianxiety agents: e.g., diazepam (Valium)
B. *Opiates*
  Agonists: e.g., hydromorphine (Dilaudid)
  Agonist/antagonist: e.g., pentazocine (Talwin)
C. *Stimulants*
  Amphetamines: e.g., *d*-amphetamine (Dexedrine)
  Amphetamine congeners: e.g., methylphenidate (Ritalin)
  Anoretic agents: e.g., fenfluramine (Pondimin)
  Others: e.g., caffeine, cocaine
D. *Psychotomimetics*
  Psychedelic: e.g., D-lysergic acid diethylamide (LSD), cannabis (marijuana)
  Anticholinergic: e.g., benzotropine (Cogentin)
  Inhalants-solvents: e.g., nitrous oxide, amyl nitrite
  Unclassified: e.g., phencyclidine (PCP)
E. *Antidepressants*
  Tricyclics: e.g., amitriptyline (Elavil)
  MAO inhibitors: e.g., tranylcypromine
F. *Muscle relaxants:* e.g., baclofen (Lioresal), methocarbamal (Robaxin), orphenadrine (Norflex)
G. *Vasoconstriction* α-adrenergic blocking agents: e.g., ergotamine
H. *Other drugs:* e.g., nicotine, anabolic steroids

[a]Adapted from Ludwig AM. Principles of clinical psychiatry. New York: Free Press, 1980.

DUAL DIAGNOSIS

In addition to the organic mental syndromes caused by psychoactive substances presented in Table 40.10, drugs of abuse through chronic intoxication can cause the following psychiatric syndromes: schizophrenia, acute psychosis, major depression, manic depressive illness, personality changes, and panic disorder. The other potential relationships between substance abuse and psychopathology can be summarized as follows:

1. Psychiatric disorders may serve as risk factors for substance abuse disorders.
2. Psychopathology may modify the course of outcome of a substance abuse disorder.
3. Long-term substance abuse may lead to the development of certain psychiatric disorders that may remain even after remission of the substance abuse.
4. A substance abuse disorder and a psychiatric disorder may occur in the same individual without being related.

Patients in whom the interrelationships between psychiatric pathology and psychoactive substance abuse appear to be important are called "dual-diagnosis" patients (44).

Prevalence rates of dual diagnosis in alcohol- and drug-dependent patients range from 20 to 80% of patients surveyed, depending upon the study sample and diagnostic criteria used (44). Currently, there is no agreement on the length of time a patient should be alcohol/drug-free before another disorder can be confidently diagnosed. The possible presence of protracted withdrawal syndrome, charac-

Table 40.10.
Organic Mental Syndromes Associated with Psychoactive Substances[a]

	Intoxication	Withdrawal	Delirium	Withdrawal Delirium	Delusional Disorder	Mood Disorder	Other Syndromes
Alcohol	x	x		x			x[b]
Amphetamine & related substances	x	x	x		x		
Caffeine	x						
Cannabis	x				x		
Cocaine	x	x	x		x		
Hallucinogen	x (hallucinosis)				x	x	x[c]
Inhalant	x						
Nicotine		x					
Opiate	x	x					
Phencyclidine (PCP) & related substances	x		x		x	x	x[d]
Sedative, hypnotic, or anxiolytic	x	x		x			x[e]

[a]From American Psychiatric Association Diagnostic and Statistical Manual of Mental Disorders (Third Edition, Revised). Washington, D.C., 1987
[b]Alcohol idiosyncratic intoxication, alcohol hallucinosis, alcohol amnestic disorder, dementia associated with alcoholism.
[c]Posthallucinogen perception disorder.
[d]Phencyclidine (PCP) or similarly acting arylcyclohexylamine organic mental disorder not otherwise specified.
[e]Sedative, hypnotic, or anxiolytic amnestic disorder.

terized by anxiety, depression, and drug craving, can confound the correct diagnosis of other disorders.

Despite the above, researchers have agreed on the following:

1. The vast majority of alcohol/drug-dependent patients are depressed at entry into treatment programs.
2. Most patients recover during treatment, but a significant percentage will continue to be depressed with some fulfilling criteria for major depression.
3. Bipolar and cyclothymic disorders are discovered more frequently than in the general population, especially cocaine abusers.
4. Panic and anxiety disorders may be linked with sedative-hypnotic abuse.
5. Alcohol- and drug-dependent patients will have a 15 to 30% prevalence of antisocial personality disorder.
6. Overall level of psychiatric impairment is the single most important factor in predicting prognosis in alcoholics and drug addicts.
7. The co-occurrence of major depression and substance abuse can be an independent and interactive risk factor for suicidal ideation and suicide attempts (45).
8. Dual-diagnosis patients need a different form of treatment than other substance abuse patients. These patients are not readily treated in a drug facility because of the major psychiatric co-morbidity problems.

The dual-diagnosis concept has not been intensely investigated in chronic pain patients. However, convergent lines of evidence in related chronic pain research indicates that the dual-diagnosis concept may be extremely important in chronic pain work. Chronic pain patients who use narcotics and sedatives are more likely to have elevated MMPI hypochondriasis and hysteria scores (14) than patients who do not use narcotics and sedatives. Chronic pain patients with substance dependence demonstrate signifi-

Table 40.11.
Opiate Withdrawal Syndrome Graded Symptoms and Signs[a]

Grade 0	Drug craving
	Anxiety
	Drug-seeking behavior
Grade 1	Yawning
	Sweating
	Running eyes and nose
	Restless sleep
Grade 2	Dilated pupils
	Gooseflesh (cold turkey)
	Muscle twitching
	Hot and cold flushes; shivering
	Aching bones and muscles
	Loss of appetite
	Irritability
Grade 3	Insomnia
	Low-grade fever
	Increased pulse rate
	Increased respiratory rate
	Increased blood pressure
	Restlessness
	Abdominal cramps
	Nausea and vomiting
	Diarrhea
	Weakness
	Weight loss

[a]Compiled from Ghodse H. Drugs and addictive behavior, a guide to treatment. Oxford: Blackwell Scientific Publications, 1990.

cant elevations on almost every MMPI scale, compared with general medical patients without substance dependence (15). A significant percentage of veterans with chronic pain and posttraumatic stress disorder have had alcohol and/or drug use disorders (18). Because a significant percentage of chronic pain patients could be abusing drugs (20–22), psychiatric dual diagnosis could be extremely important to the pain physician. Therefore, the pain physician should maintain a high index of suspicion for the presence of psychiatric dual diagnosis in any chronic pain patient abusing psychoactive substances.

OPIATE DETOXIFICATION
Opiate Withdrawal Syndrome

Abrupt termination of opiates leads to the development of the opiate withdrawal syndrome. This syndrome usually begins approximately two to three half-lives after the last opiate dose. The plasma half-lives of the various opiates are presented in Table 40.12. Generally, the syndrome begins with 6 to 8 hours of the last opiate dose, peaks in 48 to 72 hours, and lasts for 7 to 14 days. However, lingering physical effects of opiate withdrawal can appear up to 6 months after resolution of acute symptoms (4). Ludwig (4) believes that these physical symptoms may contribute to relapse in some patients. The severity of the opiate withdrawal syndrome depends on which opiate is being taken, the dose, and for how long. As demonstrated in Table 40.12, each opiate has its own capacity for inducing physical dependence. The severity of the withdrawal syndrome depends upon the degree of physical dependence.

Signs and symptoms of opiate withdrawal are presented in Tables 40.11 and 40.13. Ghodse (36) has attempted to grade the severity of withdrawal from 0 to 3 (Table 40.11). In our experience with opiate detoxification of approximately 2000 chronic pain patients, grades 1, 2 and 3 withdrawal are rarely seen.

Diagnostic criteria for opiate withdrawal syndrome can be found in the DSM-III-R (5). These criteria concentrate on the physiological symptoms of withdrawal, which are the most reliable. However, there appears to be little correlation between the patient's subjective ratings, objective nurse ratings, and physical parameters of severity of withdrawal (49). Thus, clinicians should not base their assessment of the severity of opiate withdrawal syndrome solely on physical parameters. Rating scales for opiate withdrawal symptoms are available (50). These should be used if the amount of opiate that the patient will receive is to be determined by the presence or absence of withdrawal symptoms and signs.

Opiate Detoxification Protocols

The primary purpose of any opiate detoxification protocol is to *minimize* or *eliminate* the signs and symptoms associated with the opiate withdrawal syndrome. Major principles for the management of opiate withdrawal (4, 46) are

1. Opiate withdrawal can be associated with major patient discomfort, both psychological and physiological, but has no serious medical consequence (such as death) if untreated. This is not the case for sedative/hypnotic withdrawal.

Table 40.12.
Opiate Analgesics, Equidoses, Peak Time of Analgesia, Duration of Analgesia, and Plasma Half-Life[a]

Name	Route	Equianalgesic Dose (mg)	Peak of Analgesia (hr)	Duration of Analgesia	Plasma Half-Life (hr)	Physical Dependence Liability (compared with morphine)
Morphine-like Agonists						
Morphine	Intramuscular	10	0.5–1	4–6	2–3.5	—
	Oral	60	1.5–2	4–7		
Meperidine	Intramuscular	75	0.5–1	4–5	3–4	
	Oral	300	1–2	4–6		
Methadone	Intramuscular	10	0.5–1	4–6	15–30	Similar
	Oral	20	1.5–2	4–7		
Levorphanol	Intramuscular	2	0.5–1	4–6	12–16	Similar
	Oral	4	1.5–2	4–7		
Oxycodone	Oral	30		4–6		
Heroin	Intramuscular	5	0.5–1	4–5	0.05	Similar
	Oral	60	1.5–2	4–7		
Hydromorphone	Intramuscular	1.5	0.5–1	4–5	2–3	Similar
	Oral	7.5	1.5–2	4–7		
Codeine	Intramuscular	130	0.5–1	4–6	3	Less
	Oral	200				
Mixed Agonists/Antagonists						
Pentazocine	Intramuscular	60	0.5–1	4–6	2–3	Less
	Oral	180	1/5–2	4–7		
Nalbuphine	Intramuscular	10	0.5–1	4–6	5	Less
Butorphanol	Intramuscular	2	0.5–1	4–6	2.5–3.5	Less
Partial agonist						
Buprenorphine	Intramuscular	0.4	0.5–1	4–6		
	Sublingual	0.8	2–3	5–6		Less
Opiate-like Agonists						
Propoxyphene	Oral	12				
Norpropoxyphene	Oral	40–40				
Antagonists						
Naloxone						
Nalorphine						
Naltrexone						

[a]Adapted from Inturrisi CE. Role of opioid analgesics. Am J Med 1984;(Sep 10):27–36.

2. Opiate withdrawal can be treated with any opiate, but if a long-acting opiate is used (long half-life, Table 40.11), withdrawal symptoms are milder and there is less patient distress.
3. Dosage equivalencies (Table 40.12) can be used to withdraw patients from methadone or any opiate.
4. Titration of methadone or any opiate should be based on objective withdrawal signs (dilation, stuffy nose, and gooseflesh).
5. Some patient discomfort is inevitable, as signs and symptoms of withdrawal can rarely be entirely abolished, unless the detoxification process is much prolonged.
6. Number 5 (above) and the procedure of detoxification should be explained to the patient beforehand.
7. Detoxification can be blind (cocktail) or open (pills), depending on patient preference.
8. Usual daily dose *required to prevent withdrawal is equal to 25% of the previous daily dose.* Therefore, daily tapers can be from 75 to 5%, depending on preference. However, the usual figure used is 50%.
9. At higher dose levels, the daily dose reduction can be greater because it represents a smaller percentage of the total.
10. As daily dose falls, reduction should be more gradual.
11. An opiate with a short half-life, such as meperidine or codeine, can be detoxified in 5 to 7 days.
12. Opiates with intermediate half-lives, such as nalbuphine, may require 10 to 14 days for detoxification.
13. Opiates with long half-lives, such as methadone, may require 14 to 21 days, depending on the original dose.

All opiate detoxification protocols generally use the above principles. Presently, protocols can be characterized by the type of opiate that is used in the detoxification process. The following protocols have appeared in the literature: methadone substitution/detoxification, nonmethadone opiate substitution/detoxification, nonmethadone opiate detoxification, propoxyphene substitution/detoxification, and buprenorphine opiate substitution/detoxification.

Methadone is an opiate with an extremely long half-life (Table 40.12). It has negligible euphoria, it plateaus in 2 hours, and its onset of action is one-half hour. It cannot be used to detoxify patients dependent on mixed agonist/antagonist opiates. Additionally, it may accumulate between the 24th and 48th hour, and therefore patients on this drug must be assessed for toxicity. Because of its long half-life, methadone has been used in a number of opiate detoxification protocols. The best example is a protocol presented by Halpern (51) (Table 40.14). In this protocol there is an initial 48-hour time span during which the patient is on an opiate PRN demand schedule; a pain cocktail is used; adjunct medications are used in the cocktail, and the time required to complete this protocol from 50 mg of methadone at 20% reduction is 17 days. Two alternatives to this protocol are presented in Table 40.15. Alternative (A) still takes 20 days, while alternative (B) would require 11 days to complete from 50 mg of methadone.

A nonmethadone opiate substitution/detoxification protocol is presented in Table 40.16. There are a number of reasons for considering this protocol over a methadone

Table 40.13.
Other Symptoms and Signs of Opiate Withdrawal Including Laboratory Findings[a]

Symptoms
  Severe sneezing
  Muscle spasms
  Severe bone pain in lower back and upper legs (monkey on my back)
  Depression
  Hypochondriasis
  Irritability
  Negative mental attitude
  Increase extraversion
  Increase excitability
Signs
  Spontaneous ejaculation
  Spontaneous orgasm (women)
  Dehydration
Laboratory Tests
  Increased excretion of urinary 17-ketosteroids and epinephrine
  Leukocytosis
  Acid-base imbalance
  Decreased urinary creatinine

[a]Compiled from Ludwig AM. Principles of clinical psychiatry. New York: Free Press, 1980; Ghodse H. Drugs and addictive behavior, a guide to treatment. Oxford: Blackwell Scientific Publications, 1990; Madden C, Ong B, Singer G. Mood state of heroin-dependent persons undergoing methadone detoxification. Int J Addict 1989;22(1):93–102; and Haertzen CA, Hooks NT. Changes in personality and subjective experience associated with chronic administration and withdrawal of opiates. J Nerv Ment Dis 1969;148(6):606–614.

Table 40.14.
Methadone Opiate Substitution/Detoxification Protocol

1. Patients given any and as much medication as they need for 24–48 hours.
2. From the amount of drug taken in #1 (above), calculate equivalent daily dose of methadone (Table 40.11) required.
3. If unable to determine above, give methadone 15 mg q4h until respiratory rate decreases to 16 breaths/minute.
4. The total daily substitution dose of methadone is the total dose given to reduce the respiratory rate to 16.
5. This dose is given in 4 divided doses for 24 hr.
6. Methadone dose is reduced daily by 15–20% in a "pain cocktail" (drug plus masking vehicle to blind patient to detoxification).
7. Doxepin 50–100 mg is added to cocktail if sleep is a problem.
8. Hydroxyzine 50 mg t.i.d. added to cocktail if anxious.

[a]Compiled from Halpern L. Substitution-detoxification and its role in the management of chronic benign pain. J Clin Psychiatry 1982;43(8 pt2):10–14.

Table 40.15.
Alternative Methadone Opiate Substitution/Detoxification Protocols[a]

A. As in Table 40.5, except decrease methadone at 7 mg/day over 20 days.
B. As in Table 40.5, but as follows:
  1. If taking more than 30 mg/day, drop at 10 mg/day to 30 mg/day, then
  2. Drop at 5 mg/day to 20 mg/day, then
  3. Drop at 2.5 mg/day to zero.
  4. If taking less than 30 mg/day, start at step #2.

[a]Compiled from Frances RJ, Franklin JE. Alcohol and other psychoactive substance use disorders. In: Talbott JA, Hales RE, Yudofsky SC, eds. The American Psychiatric Press textbook of psychiatry. Washington, D.C.: American Psychiatric Press, 1988.

Table 40.16.
Nonmethadone Opiate Substitution/Detoxification Protocol[a]

1. Patient given as much opiate of choice as he/she requires for 24–48 hours.
2. Total intake of opiate over the 48 hours is calculated and translated into opiate of doctor's choice, e.g., codeine (Table 40.1).
3. This total dose of codeine is divided into four doses and given over 24 hours (q6h).
4. This dose is given for 2 days.
5. Then this dose is decreased by 50% every 2 days.
6. When a dose equivalent to 10 mg methadone is reached, that dose is given for 2 days.

[a]Compiled from Inturrisi CE. Role of opioid analgesics. Am J Med 1984;(Sep 10):27–36.

Table 40.17.
Nonmethadone Opiate Detoxification Protocol

1. Patient is given as much opiate of choice as he/she requires for 3 days (i.e., a p.r.n. demand schedule).
2. No intramuscular or IV opiates are allowed, and these routes are immediately switched to p.o., according to Table 40.1.
3. At the end of 3 days, total dose of opiate is calculated and is translated into a daily opiate dose.
4. If the patient is taking two or three opiates (as is often the case), the opiates taken less frequently are translated into the opiate taken most frequently (Table 40.1), and the daily opiate dose is calculated.
5. Detoxification proceeds with the opiate taken most frequently.
6. The daily opiate dose is split over the day according to the original demand schedule of the patient. For example, if the patient was taking Percodan q2h, the daily opiate dose is given q2h.
7. Patient is maintained on the q2h schedule for 2 days. This is not a demand schedule, and the patient is brought the medications.
8. Detoxification then proceeds by decreasing the dosage by 25–50% per day. For example, a patient taking three Percodans every 2 hours would be detoxified to 2 every 2 hours, then 1 every 2 hours.
9. Once dosage detoxification is complete (i.e., patient is taking *one* pill at the time interval), then *time detoxification* begins. An example of this is
  (a) one tab q4h × 1 day, then
  (b) one tab q6h × 1 day, then
  (c) one tab q8h × 1 day, then
  (d) one tab q12h × 1 day, then
  (e) one tab q.h.s. × 1 day, then
  (f) D/C
10. No adjunct medications (doxepin, hydroxyzine) are given unless indicated (i.e., other reasons than detoxification problems).
11. Clonidine is given if patient has major difficulties in withdrawal.
12. This protocol requires the cooperation of the patient, who is therefore advised of the following:
  (a) During the first 3 days, patients should take as much medication as they require; if they take less, their detoxification may be more difficult than necessary.
  (b) Although we will try to minimize patient detoxification discomfort, many times this is not possible.
  (c) Once the detoxification schedule is written, it will not be changed, no matter how much discomfort the patient experiences.
  (d) During detoxification, no p.r.n. opiates will be administered.
  (e) Patients are advised not to worry about their schedules during detoxification, as it is now nursing's responsibility to bring the medications to the patients.
  (f) Patients may refuse a dosage; however, this is not advisable and they will not be able to have any medication until the next scheduled dosage.
  (g) If patients are asleep when they should receive an opiate dose, they will not be awakened.

opiate substitution/detoxification protocol. First, most chronic pain patients are taking opiates that have short or intermediate half-lives. Generally, the longer the half-life of the opiate, the longer the detoxification protocol required. Thus, it does not make any sense to transfer patients from short half-life drugs to long half-life drugs and prolong detoxification if the goal is rapid detoxification. Second, many drug addicts believe (although there is little evidence for this) that methadone may be more difficult to detoxify from than other opiates. In support of this, methadone detoxification protocols with true opiate addicts generally are extremely long. Third, because few chronic pain patients demonstrate true opiate addiction, it may not be necessary to use the same detoxification techniques with this group as with the opiate addict. It may be that this patient group can tolerate a very rapid detoxification protocol. The protocol presented in Table 40.16 will take 8 to 9 days to complete from an equivalent dose of 50 mg of methadone.

A nonmethadone detoxification protocol is presented in Table 40.17. This is the type of protocol used by the University of Miami Comprehensive Pain Center. It has a number of advantages over other protocols: It is simple; it does not use methadone; it does not use cocktails; it can be very rapid (most patients are detoxified within 10 days); patients are detoxified with the opiate of their choice and preference (i.e., the one they are most familiar with); and for patients taking one opiate only, there is no need for conversions to other opiates. The major disadvantage to this protocol is that, in most cases, detoxification proceeds with an opiate that has a short or intermediate half-life, thereby potentially permitting more patient discomfort than with methadone. However, this is minimized to some extent by first dose- then time-detoxification, since patients using short half-life opiates generally take them frequently. There is one literature report of the successful use of this protocol (53). At our center, we have used this protocol for about 10 years, without major problems.

Propoxyphene is a structural analogue of methadone, has cross-tolerance with other opiates, and has a long half-life (Table 40.12). A propoxyphene substitution/detoxification protocol has been described (Table 40.18). This protocol generally requires levels of drug administra-

tion in excess of the maximum advised for analgesia. Therefore, it should be used with caution, if at all. In addition, toxic doses of propoxyphene produce central nervous system respiratory depression and central nervous system excitation that can be manifested as convulsions.

Buprenorphine is an opiate with mixed agonist/antagonist properties and a long duration of action, which may be a function of slow disassociation from opioid receptors and not a long half-life (as for methadone) (55, 56). Buprenorphine can also block the effects of exogenously used opiates and therefore reduce heroin self-administration (55). The drug is also associated with a very mild withdrawal syndrome that can be prolonged (55, 56). These properties suggested that this drug could be used in an opiate detoxification protocol, and buprenorphine was demonstrated to be as effective as methadone using such a protocol (55) (Table 40.19).

Pyschopharmacological Tests for Opiate Dependence

When working with true opiate addicts, it is important to determine if the addict in alleged opiate withdrawal is indeed physically opiate dependent. To make this determination, a test using naloxone, an opiate antagonist, has been developed (Table 40.20). To the author's knowledge, this procedure has not been used in chronic pain patients to determine what percentage are physically opiate dependent.

In addition to determining if the patient is physically opiate dependent, opiate antagonists such as naloxone can be used to reduce the time required for opiate detoxification (57). This is called "opiate-antagonist-precipitated withdrawal." The opiate withdrawal is compressed into as short a time as possible, with the hope that a short period of very severe symptoms may be easier to cope with than a prolonged period of milder symptoms. This technique is demonstrated in Table 40.21; however, because of the potential severity of the withdrawal symptoms precipitated by this protocol, it is not recommended for chronic pain patients.

As a final point, the naloxone challenge test appears to predict treatment outcome in opiate addicts (58). High naloxone-challenge-test scores at intake (high levels of opiate dependence) predict poor program retention (58). It is unclear if this is the same for chronic pain patients, but, clinically, there is a perception that addicted patients are more difficult to treat.

Clonidine Opiate Detoxification Protocols

Clonidine is an α_2-adrenergic agonist that appears to suppress the acute dysphoric state associated with opiate withdrawal. Opiate withdrawal is a state of adrenergic hyperactivity in which neurons of the locus ceruleus become markedly activated. Clonidine appears to inhibit the firing of the locus ceruleus by opening potassium channels (59).

Clonidine has some opiate-like properties, but it does not bind to the opiate receptor and does not produce euphoria. Most signs and symptoms of withdrawal are reversed or prevented by 5 to 30 μg/kg oral clonidine (60). However, it cannot be precisely titrated, and higher doses may be limited by side effects like hypotension. As a result, clonidine has limitations in its ability to suppress withdrawal manifestations, as compared with methadone (61), and opiate addicts being detoxified with clonidine are more likely to fail at detoxification (62). However, with the addition of clonidine, the percentage of narcotic addicts who achieve a symptom-free state in inpatient studies is greater than with methadone alone; the same is true in outpatients (60). It is also claimed that clonidine can decrease the time required for opiate detoxification to 3 to 5 days for short-acting opiates, 5 to 7 days for intermediate-acting opiates, and 7 to 10 days for long-acting ones (36). Clonidine can be used to detoxify from mixed agonist/antagonist opiates, which is a major plus. As described above, clonidine appears to offer an additional option in the amelioration of the opiate withdrawal syndrome. However, physicians must remember that abrupt discontinuation of clonidine can result in a withdrawal syndrome. Therefore, patients placed on clonidine detoxification regimes should be tapered off this drug (36).

Clonidine opiate detoxification protocols can be classified as follows: clonidine alone, clonidine plus opiate-

---

Table 40.18.
Propoxyphene Opiate Substitution/Detoxification Protocol[a]

1. Initial first day dosage 800 mg/day split over q6h intervals.
2. Add 100 mg q12h p.r.n. for withdrawal symptoms.
3. Reevaluate patient after first 24 hours for withdrawal symptoms and/or propoxyphene toxicity.
4. If withdrawal symptoms are mild, continue on 800 mg/day.
5. If withdrawal symptoms are severe, increase to 200 mg/q4h or 1200 mg/day.
6. If toxic, reduce by 200 mg/day.
7. Reevaluate on third day; if withdrawal symptoms are still severe, can increase to a maximum dose of 1.500 mg/day.
8. Once stabilized, may decrease at a rate of 200 mg/day.

[a]Compiled from Schmalsteg WJ, Hayden JM, Comstock EG. Propoxyphene napsylate detoxification. Tex Med 1975;71:70–76.

Table 40.19.
Buprenorphine Opiate Substitution/Detoxification Protocol[a]

1. 2 mg buprenorphine is equivalent to 30 mg methadone.
2. Determine patient's opiate stabilization dose in mg methadone.
3. Buprenorphine is prepared in 20% aqueous alcohol and given once daily sublingually.
4. Buprenorphine detoxification proceeds for 4 weeks, with cuts of 25% in the first week and 50% thereafter.

[a]Compiled from Bickel WK, Stitzer ML, Bigelow GE, Liebson IA, Jasinski DR, Johnson RE. A clinical trial of buprenorphine: comparison with methadone in the detoxification of heroin addicts. Clin Pharmacol Ther 1988;43(1):72–78.

Table 40.20.
Naloxone Opiate Physical Dependence Test[a]

1. Administer naloxone 0.4–0.6 mg IM.
2. Watch for signs of opiate withdrawal syndrome.
3. If no effect, not physically dependent.
4. To relieve withdrawal syndrome, give morphine 15–30 mg.

[a]Compiled from Kosten TR, Krystal JH, Charney DS, el al. Rapid detoxification from opioid dependence. Am J Psychiatry 1989;146:1349.

Table 40.21.
Clonidine Plus Opiate Antagonist (Naloxone) Detoxification Protocol[a]

1. Clonidine 0.1 mg t.i.d. first day.
2. Clonidine 0.2–0.3 mg t.i.d. (monitor B.P.) and naloxone 0.2 mg IM, then 0.4 mg IM q2h for four doses, on second day.
3. Clonidine same dose as on day 2; naloxone 0.8 mg IM; 5 doses at 2-hour intervals on third day.
4. Demonstrate completeness of detoxification by a naloxone challenge: 0.4 mg IM should cause no withdrawal, then follow with 0.8 mg IM 1 hour later, also no withdrawal should be noted; this is day 4.

[a]Compiled from Ghodse H. Drugs and addictive behavior, a guide to treatment. Oxford: Blackwell Scientific Publications, 1990.

antagonist (naloxone or naltrexone), methadone followed by clonidine, clonidine alone–transdermal patch, and adjunct clonidine. These detoxification protocols are presented in Tables 40.21 to 40.26. The following observations apply to these protocols:

1. There is major variability in how much clonidine is given initially. The doses vary from 0.1 to 1.6 mg per day.
2. With the clonidine/antagonist protocol, one can detoxify a patient in 3 days. However, the author believes that there is no need for such dramatic steps in chronic pain patients.
3. The methadone/clonidine protocol does not contain a clonidine detoxification step. The author believes this step is necessary.
4. Transdermal clonidine offers the advantage of weekly application and even blood levels of clonidine (63). However, this protocol requires 2 days of oral clonidine and continues for 21 days.
5. The adjunct clonidine protocol is only used if there are difficulties in detoxification, and it is the protocol used by our pain center. Patients are placed on clonidine until the opiate detoxification is complete, at which point they are detoxified from clonidine.

Table 40.22.
Clonidine Alone Opiate Detoxification Protocol[a]

1. At first sign of withdrawal, 0.3–0.4 mg p.o. (5 μg/kg body wt) stat of clonidine.
2. Then 0.1–0.25 mg q4h for a total of 0.9–1.6 mg (or 15–20 mg/kg) on the first day.
3. Monitor vital signs hourly first day, every 2 hours on the second, and every 4 hours thereafter.
4. Hold clonidine if B.P. less than 90/50 combined with a bradycardia of 50 beats or less per minute. Hold until vital signs are acceptable.
5. When vital signs are acceptable, reinstate clonidine q4h.
6. On second day and each day thereafter, reduce clonidine dosage by 50%.

[a]Compiled from Cuthill JD, Beroniade V, Salvatori VA, Viguie F. Evaluation of clonidine suppression of opiate withdrawal reactions: a multidisciplinary approach. Can J Psychiatry 1989;35:377–382.

Table 40.23.
Variants of Clonidine Alone Opiate Detoxification Protocol[a]

1. Calculate amount of daily opiate required from history or observe intake.
2. Translate into methadone equivalents.
3. If required, 25 mg methadone or less, begin at 0.05 mg clonidine b.i.d.
4. If required, more than 25 mg methadone, use 0.1 mg clonidine b.i.d.
5. Maintain on this dose for 3 days.
6. Then decrease clonidine by 25% per day.

[a]Compiled from Ghodse H. Drugs and addictive behavior, a guide to treatment. Oxford: Blackwell Scientific Publications, 1990.

Table 40.24.
Methadone Followed by Clonidine Detoxification Protocol[a]

1. Stabilize patient on methadone.
2. Taper methadone to 20 mg/day.
3. Then switch to clonidine 0.1–0.3 mg t.i.d. for 2 days.
4. Then clonidine 0.2–0.7 mg t.i.d. for 8–14 days.
5. Then D/C.

[a]Compiled from Frances RJ, Franklin JE. Alcohol and other psychoactive substance use disorders. In: Talbott JA, Hales RE, Yudofsky SC, eds. The American Psychiatric Press textbook of psychiatry. Washington, D.C.: American Psychiatric Press, 1988.

Nonopiate Detoxification Protocols for Opiate Dependence and Adjunct Medications and Procedures

Nonopiate detoxification protocols for opiate dependence are presented in Table 40.27. These protocols will ameliorate opiate withdrawal syndrome but less successfully than opiates and clonidine. The protocols mainly affect anxiety generated by the syndrome.

Often, in opiate withdrawal syndrome, the patients note restless anxiety that sounds like akasthisia. Propranolol, at doses of 20 to 40 mg/day, has been used successfully for this problem during detoxification (64). Propranalol can therefore be an adjunct medication in the detoxification process.

Another adjunct medication used successfully during opiate detoxification is doxepin. Doxepin appears to augment methadone opiate withdrawal (65). It is generally administered in doses from 50 to 100 mg. p.o. h.s. during detoxification and is maintained for 6 weeks. It is not clear by what mechanism doxepin augments opiate withdrawal. It may simply increase the levels of methadone, or it may combat anxiety and/or depression. Considering that tricyclic antidepressants have some analgesic properties, doxepin may be the ideal adjunct to opiate detoxification in chronic pain patients.

Naltrexone is an opiate antagonist that is claimed to be nonaddicting. It is taken in the AM three times per week, and it will block all euphoriant effects of additional opiates (66). It is postulated that if the opiate addict no longer

Table 40.25.
Clonidine Alone Transdermal Patch Detoxification Protocol[a]

1. Test dose oral clonidine 0.1 mg administered and B.P. measured 1 hour later. If B.P. systolic is less than 90, patient does not get patch.
2. Place 2 #2 transdermal clonidine patches or 3 patches (if patient weighs more than 150 lbs) on hairless area of upper body.
3. For first 24 hours after patch application, give oral clonidine 0.2 mg q6h.
4. For the next 24 hours, give oral clonidine 0 1 mg q6h.
5. Change patches weekly.
6. After 2 weeks of 2 patches, switch to 1 #2 patch or 2 #2 patches, if patient weighs more than 150 lbs.
7. After 1 week of #6 (above), D/C patches.

[a]Compiled from Spencer L, Gregory M. Clonidine transdermal patches for use in outpatient opiate withdrawal. J Subst Abuse Treat 1989;6:113–117.

Table 40.26.
Adjunct Clonidine Detoxification Protocol

1. Only start clonidine if patient demonstrates signs of withdrawal syndrome and/or exhibits major behavioral problems with detoxification (e.g., inability to handle the increased pain off opiates).
2. Clonidine 0.1–0.4 mg per day in divided doses to start.
3. Increase gradually to a maximum of 1.2 mg per day (divided in 3 doses), according to symptoms.
4. Blood pressure is taken lying and standing q.i.d. If less than 90 systolic, clonidine is held for the next dose.
5. Stop increases as soon as symptoms decrease.
6. Maintain on this dose until completion of opiate detoxification.
7. Then begin clonidine detoxification at 25–50% decrease per day.
8. Space clonidine detoxification over 1 week.

Table 40.27.
Nonopiate Detoxification Protocols for Opiate Dependence[a]

I. *Neuroleptics*
   (1) Thioridazine 25 mg p.o., b.i.d. and 75 mg h.s. for 2 weeks
   (2) Then tapered for 1 week
II. *Diphenoxylate (Lomotil)*
   (1) Two tabs q.i.d. for 4 days
   (2) Then slowly tapered
   (3) Can be combined with thioridazine
III. β-Adrenoreceptor blocking drugs
   (1) Reduces craving after heroin withdrawal
   (2) May be helpful if high somatic anxiety, as indicated by raised pulse rate and high blood pressure
   (3) Propranolol, 80–160 mg in divided doses for 2–3 weeks
   (4) Then slowly tapered
IV. *Sedative protocol for opiate detoxification*
   (1) Does not relieve opiate withdrawal syndrome, only the anxiety
   (2) Not the treatment of choice
   (3) Use diazepam as follows:
     (a) 10 mg q.i.d. × 3 days; then
     (b) 10 mg t.i.d. × 1 day; then
     (c) 10 mg b.i.d. × 1 day; then
     (d) 5 mg b.i.d. × 1 day; then
     (e) 5 mg h.s. × 1 day; then
     (f) D/C

[a]Compiled from Ghodse H. Drugs and addictive behavior, a guide to treatment. Oxford: Blackwell Scientific Publications, 1990.

Table 40.28.
Barbiturate Withdrawal Syndrome Symptoms and Signs[a]

Clinical Phenomenon	Frequency (%)	Time of Onset	Duration (days)
Apprehension	100	1st day	3 to 14
Muscle weakness	100	1st day	3 to 14
Tremors	100	1st day	3 to 14
Postural faintness	100	1st day	3 to 14
Anorexia	100	1st day	3 to 14
Twitches	100	1st day	3 to 14
Seizures	80	2nd to 3rd day	8
Psychoses and/or delirium	60	3rd to 8th day	3 to 14

[a]Adapted from Shader RI, Caine ED, Meyer RE. Treatment of dependence on barbiturates and sedative-hypnotics. In: Shader RI, ed. Manual psychiatric therapeutics. Boston: Little, Brown & Co., 1989.

experiences the opiate euphoria, then drug-seeking behavior will diminish and eventually extinguish. Data indicate that opiate addicts who receive naltrexone are more likely to complete detoxification and less likely to relapse (66). Thus, naltrexone has been added to some opiate detoxification protocols, used much like naloxone. Patients should be placed on naltrexone only when the physician is convinced that the patient is opiate-addicted and there is a good chance of relapse.

Lastly, there have been reports of the use of auricular acupuncture to augment opiate detoxification (67). In this study, auricular electrical stimulation acupuncture was provided to the Shen Men and lung points. The current used was 1 to 3 Hz pulses alternating with 600 to 1000 Hz pulses. Patients received acupuncture a mean of 3 to 9 hours per day during detoxification. Acupuncture appeared to speed opiate detoxification, with few side effects from naloxone-precipitated withdrawal.

SEDATIVE DETOXIFICATION

Hypnotic-Sedative (Barbiturate and Nonbarbiturate) Dependence and Withdrawal Syndrome

Barbiturate/nonbarbiturate dependence and withdrawal syndromes are well-described phenomena. The signs and symptoms of this withdrawal syndrome are presented in Table 40.28. Generally, barbiturates/nonbarbiturates can result in a severe withdrawal syndrome, much like alcohol. The DSM-III-R (5) criteria for this syndrome indicate that the severe type of withdrawal reaction is characterized by delirium, which can result from any sedative-hypnotic, including alcohol and/or anxiolytic agents.

Because of their abuse potential, the barbiturate and nonbarbiturate drugs have fallen out of favor with physicians and are rarely administered. Patients who are addicted or dependent within the hypnotic-sedative group are now usually addicted/dependent on alcohol or antianxiety agents.

Drugs in the hypnotic-sedative group are cross-tolerant to each other. Thus, any drug within this group can be detoxified by using any other drug within this group (4). However, some drugs, because of their properties (e.g., long half-life), appear to be more efficacious in preventing withdrawal syndrome than others. Dosage equivalences and half-lives of the hypnosedatives are presented in Table 40.29.

Antianxiety Agents and the Benzodiazepines

Antianxiety agents are equated with the benzodiazepine group. Until recently, there was much controversy about how addictive this group is and the type of withdrawal syndrome that can develop on abrupt cessation of benzodiazepines. This group is now believed to have the following psychopharmacological properties relevant to this chapter:

1. Benzodiazepine use is extremely widespread, with about 1.8% of total population being long-term users; yet few of these patients exceed prescribed dosage, i.e., risk of dependence and addiction is extremely low (70).
2. Benzodiazepine abuse occurs in those who abuse other substances; the benzodiazepine is a *secondary* drug of abuse. These patients often take high doses (70). Benzodiazepines differ in abuse liability (i.e., attractiveness as drugs of abuse). This abuse liability is rated as follows (highest to lowest): diazepam, lorazepam, alprazolam, chlorazepate, oxazepam, and chlordiazepoxide (71). Abuse potential does not appear to depend upon the half-life of the drug.
3. Physical dependence can occur even with doses in the clinical range, but it requires 6 to 8 months. Interestingly, tolerance to the therapeutic effect *does not* develop (70). Three types of dependence syndromes have been described (72). The patient takes several times the normal therapeutic dose: primary high-dose dependency. The patient takes therapeutic doses: primary low-dose dependency. The patient takes benzodiazepines to treat alcohol or opiate withdrawal: secondary dependency.
4. Rebound is the return of a symptom for which the drug was

Table 40.29.
Dosage Equivalences of the Hypnosedatives[a]

Generic Name	Trade Name	Half-Life (hr)	Equivalent Dose	Short-acting (S) vs Long-acting (L) vs Intermediate (I)
Phenobarbital	Luminal	24–140	30 mg	L
Pentobarbital	Nembutal	15–48	100 mg	S
Secobarbital	Seconal	19–34	100 mg	S
Butalbital	Butisol	34–42	60 mg	I
Meprobamate	Miltown, Equanil	6–17	400 mg	S
Ethchlorvinol	Placidyl	10–25	350 mg	L
Glutethimide	Doriden	5–22	250 mg	L
Methyprylon	Noludar	4–15	100 mg	S
Chloral hydrate	Noctec	4–10	500 mg	S
Alprazolam	Xanax	12–15	0.5 mg	S
Chlordiazepoxide	Librium	10–24	10 mg	L
Clorazepate	Tranxene	30–200	7.5 mg	L
Diazepam	Valium	26–55	5 mg	L
Flurazepam	Dalmane	23–100	15 mg	L
Lorazepam	Ativan	10–20	1 mg	S
Oxazepam	Serax	5–10	15 mg	S
Temazepam	Restoril	10	15 mg	S
Triazolam	Halcion	2–4	0.5 mg	S
Clonazepam	Klonopin	18–50	1 mg	L
Quazepam	Doral	75	15 mg	L
Alcohol	—		10–14 oz	L

[a]Adapted from Wartenberg AA. Detoxification of the chemically dependent patient. RI Med J 1989;72(12):451–456.

originally prescribed, to a degree that is worse than before the drug (72). The benzodiazepine drugs are associated with rebound, especially the short-acting hypnotic benzodiazepine triazolam, which produces prompt and severe rebound.

5. The difficulties in determining if a benzodiazepine withdrawal syndrome existed, occurred because of the difficulty in separating withdrawal syndrome from rebound, or simply the return of anxiety in a patient being treated for anxiety (73). It is now clear that some form of withdrawal syndrome can be observed in about half the patients discontinuing benzodiazepines (74).
6. The tendency to experience the benzodiazepine withdrawal syndrome is a function of dosage and duration of treatment (73).
7. Withdrawal syndrome occurs more rapidly in patients taking short half-life benzodiazepines(73).
8. Duration of withdrawal reaction is variable, lasting 5 to 20 days (73).
9. The more rapid the fall in benzodiazepine blood levels, the more likely is a withdrawal to occur (73).
10. Short-acting benzodiazepines may have a stronger potential for physical dependence (73).
11. Severity of withdrawal may be related to benzodiazepine potency, with high-potency drugs like lorazepam producing more severe withdrawal than medium-potency drugs, such as diazepam, and low-potency drugs, such as chlordiazepoxide (72). In addition, individuals with a psychobiological predisposition to addiction (often with a past history or family history of alcoholism) may manifest severe benzodiazepine withdrawal symptoms on abrupt benzodiazepine cessation. The two types of benzodiazepine withdrawal symptoms are presented in Table 40.30. The major withdrawal symptoms resemble those of sedative hypnotic withdrawal.
12. It is alleged that unless a sedative-hypnotic has been

Table 40.30.
Types of Withdrawal Symptoms after Withdrawal from Benzodiazepines[a]

Major Withdrawal Symptoms (20% of cases)	Minor Withdrawal Symptoms (50% of cases)
Epileptic fits	Increased anxiety
Confusional state	Insomnia
Abnormal perception of movement	Iritability
Depersonalization or derealization	Palpitations
Muscle twitchings	Headache and muscle tension
Lowered perceptual threshold to sensory stimuli	Dysphoria
"Psychosis"	

[a]Adapted from Owen RT, Tyrel P. Benzodiazepine dependence. A review of the evidence. Drugs 1983;25:385–398.

administered daily for more than 1 month in amounts equivalent to 400 to 600 mg of a short-acting barbiturate, a severe withdrawal syndrome will not develop (74).
13. Severe sedative-hypnotic-type withdrawal syndrome will occur from the 2nd to the 14th day after drug cessation (74).
14. Recent evidence indicates that the signs and symptoms of the benzodiazepine withdrawal syndrome outlined in Tables 40.30 and 40.31 rarely reach the severity of sedative-hypnotic withdrawal (75). The DSM-III-R (5) calls any type of withdrawal uncomplicated if it does not involve delirium. Criteria for uncomplicated sedative, hypnotic, or anxiolytic withdrawal can be found in the DSM-III-R (5). Most anxiolytic withdrawal syndromes would fall into *this* diagnostic category.
15. A benzodiazepine withdrawal syndrome will develop even when a gradual taper of *25% per week* is undertaken (Table 40.32) (76). In this type of taper, a large percentage (approximately 36%) of patients treated for anxiety syn-

Table 40.31.
Benzodiazepine Withdrawal Syndrome Symptoms and Signs on Abrupt Withdrawal[a]

Anxiety
Restlessness
Agitation
Loss of appetite
Diaphoresis
Nausea
Loss of drive
Lethargy
Increased acuity for sound and smell
Weakness
Insomnia

[a]Adapted from Rickels K, Schwerzer E, Case WG, Greenblatt DJ. Long-term therapeutic use of benzodiazepines. I. Effects of abrupt discontinuation. Arch Gen Psychiatry 1990;47:899–907.

Table 40.32.
Benzodiazepine Withdrawal Syndrome: Percentage of Symptoms and Signs on Gradual Discontinuation[a]

Adrenergic	
Anxiety, nervousness	56%
Diaphoresis	32%
Restlessness	27%
Agitation	27%
Loss of appetite	21%
Nausea	14%
Lethargy	
Irritability	46%
Fatigue	37%
Dysphoric mood	32%
Lethargy	22%
Loss of drive	19%
Constipation	6%
Disequilibrium	
Light-headedness	29%
Dizziness	21%
Tinnitus	14%
Perceptual distortions	11%
Poor coordination	11%
Confusional	
Difficulty with concentrating	21%
Increased acuity for sound and smell	17%
Nightmares	13%
Depersonalization	11%
Confusion	5%
Difficulty with expressing thoughts	3%
Neurasthenia	
Tremor, tremulousness	52%
Weakness	25%
Muscular	
Muscle fasciculations	14%
Muscle cramps	13%
Individual	
Insomnia	52%
Diarrhea	25%
Headaches	24%
Delusions, hallucinations	2%

[a]Adapted from Schwerzer E, Rickels K, Case WG, Greenblatt DJ. Long-term therapeutic use of benzodiazepines. II. Effects of gradual taper. Arch Gen Psychiatry 1990;47:908–915.

dromes will not complete detoxification because of the withdrawal syndrome, rebound, and reemerging anxiety symptoms (76). Patients on long half-life benzodiazepines achieve detoxification in greater numbers (76). This last point indicates that it may be foolish for pain programs to attempt to detoxify pain patients from benzodiazepines, if these patients have preexisting anxiety syndromes.

16. In summary, after benzodiazepine drug reduction or cessation, the patient could experience the following syndromes: none, return of preexisting disorder, rebound, major withdrawal symptoms, minor withdrawal symptoms, combination of rebound and withdrawal, disturbed social/behavioral problems, mood disturbance (major depression), and new anxiety symptoms, e.g., panic and emotional reaction to anticipated drug withdrawal (77). It is difficult to make a distinction between these syndromes. However, the pain physician detoxifying a patient from benzodiazepines should be aware of the possibility of the development of these syndromes.

What Percentage of Chronic Pain Patients Are Sedative/Hypnotic Dependent and/or Addicted?

To date, only one study (78) has addressed the issue of potential benzodiazepine abuse by chronic pain patients. This study reported the following:

1. At evaluation, 38% of their chronic pain patients were taking benzodiazepines.
2. In 93%, the benzodiazepine was initiated after onset of chronic pain.
3. In 60.4%, the medication was taken for longer than 1 year.
4. In 86%, benzodiazepine was administered to improve sleep, but most still had sleep problems.
5. Tolerance *was not* reported by the patients in this study.
6. The issue of whether these patients were dependent and/or addicted was not addressed.

Based on this one study and evidence from other sources, this author (78, 79) has listed some reasons why chronic pain patients should not be placed on benzodiazepines and, therefore, some reasons for detoxification:

1. Lack of evidence that benzodiazepines are of benefit in chronic pain (78).

2. Benzodiazepines cause dependency (78).
3. Benzodiazepines cause cognitive impairment (78).
4. Benzodiazepines may contribute to depression (78).
5. Drug dependency may interfere with rehabilitation (78).
6. Benzodiazepines may exacerbate chronic pain (79).
7. Chronic pain patients who abuse drugs are at greater risk for developing additional dependence, if placed on benzodiazepines (79).
8. Recent anxiety research indicates that for patients with anxiety syndromes, benzodiazepines should be prescribed in intermittent courses, confined to periods of stress (78).

However, the situation is not clear-cut. First, chronic pain patients have major sleep difficulties that are pain-related. Because of this, the clinician is almost forced to place the patient on benzodiazepines. Second, there is a high prevalence, 62.5% (20), of anxiety syndromes in chronic pain patients. Lastly, recent evidence indicates that benzodiazepines may be efficacious for chronic pain (80, 81) in some patients. Therefore, this author would not recommend that every patient be detoxified from benzodiazepines; rather, the pain physician should make this decision on clinical grounds. Based on the above, the following patients should be detoxified from benzodiazepines:

1. Any patient who is intoxicated or cognitively impaired on the current dose of benzodiazepines.
2. Any patient who is abusing alcohol and/or other drugs.
3. Any patient who escalates dose above therapeutic dose without the physician's knowledge.
4. Any patient exhibiting any drug-seeking behavior.
5. Severely depressed patients who appear to be unresponsive to antidepresants.
6. Patients with a history of alcohol abuse/dependence.
7. Any patient taking large doses of benzodiazepines for a sleep problem, with less than 4 hours sleep per night.
8. Any patient taking benzodiazepines as muscle relaxants.
9. Patients who are taking benzodiazepines for anxiety require a diagnostic interview to determine the type of anxiety syndrome and if this syndrome preexisted the onset of chronic pain. If the syndrome preexisted the pain condition, that patient is less likely to be successfully detoxified and may not be a candidate for detoxification. However, efforts should be made, according to the anxiety syndrome diagnosed, to place the patient on other agents that may control the anxiety syndrome (i.e., buspirone, MAO inhibitors, tricyclics, β-blockers, etc.). Patients who do not have preexisting anxiety syndromes but have current anxiety problems should be detoxified *if possible*, although detoxification may not be successful, secondary to rebound and anxiety reemergence.

Benzodiazepine Detoxification Protocols

There are three major types of benzodiazepine detoxification protocols. All three, together with their indications, are presented in Table 40.33. Selection of the technique depends upon a variety of factors, including severity of dependency, interaction with other drugs, setting for detoxification, and M.D. expertise (83).

There is disagreement on the speed of detoxification. Some authors advocate a 25% reduction every 3 days, which should be titrated according to severity of withdrawal symptoms (83). Other authors advocate a 6 to 12 week detoxification schedule, where the dose reduction is no greater than 5 mg of diazepam per week (84). The manufacturer of alprazolam has recommended that for this drug, dosage should be reduced *weekly*. If taking over 3 mg/day of alprazolam, the dosage reduction should be 0.5 mg/week, while for patients taking less than 3 mg, the reduction should be 0.25 mg/week. Some authors, however, allege that alprazolam can be detoxified much faster, and they advocate a reduction of 1 mg every 3 days, or 0.5 mg every 3 days, with a gradual reduction over 3 to 12 weeks (85). Again, the pain physician will need to decide between a slow taper and an expeditious taper on clinical grounds. Patients with preexistent anxiety syndromes (prepain), intense anxiety, trouble coping with current anxiety, and increased anxiety with increased pain and

Table 40.33.
Acute Benzodiazepine Detoxification Methods[a]

Detoxification Method	Indications	Drugs Used
Graded reduction of the benzodiazepine of dependence	Primarily used in medical setting for therapeutic range dependency	Drug used
Substitution of long-acting benzodiazepine	Primarily used for alcohol and/or alcohol-benzodiazepine combination dependency; also now used for therapeutic range dependency	Chlordiazepoxide, diazepam Clonazepam
Phenobarbital substitution	Primarily used for benzodiazepine-polydrug use; also useful for high-dose benzodiazepine dependency; this method has the broadest utility for all sedative-hypnotics	Phenobarbital

[a]Adapted from Smith DE, Wesson DR. Phenobarbital technique for the treatment of barbiturate dependence. Arch Gen Psychiatry 1971;24:56–60.

those who have dependent personality features are candidates for a slow taper. Problems encountered in the detoxification process can be due to a number of factors, some of which are presented in Table 40.34.

Shorter-acting benzodiazepines, such as alprazolam, may be associated with more withdrawal symptomatology than the longer-acting agents, such as clonazepam (86). Thus, to make detoxification more tolerable, four long-acting agents have been used in substitution detoxification: chlordiazepoxide, diazepam, clonazepam, and phenobarbital.

The following protocols have been advocated for benzodiazepine detoxification:

1. The dosage of diazepam equivalent to the patient's total benzodiazepine daily dose is calculated from Table 40.29. For high-dose benzodiazepine abuse, a loading dose of diazepam which is 40% of the patient's total benzodiazepine daily dose is given. Diazepam is then reduced at 10% per day for a probable 14-day taper (87). A slower variant of this technique is to estimate total daily dose by history. Divide this dose into 4 equivalent doses and administer for 2 days. Then, decrease by 10% per day. If required, give 5 mg Valium p.r.n. for signs of withdrawal syndrome. When the remaining diazepam dose reaches 10%, reduce over 4 days. Although slower, the author recommends this latter method.
2. Using clonazepam to substitute for alprazolam (88):
   a. First day, transfer to clonazepam at a mg to mg equivalency (this is higher than shown on Table 40.29).
   b. Divide clonazepam into b.i.d. dosage.
   c. Taper clonazepam at 1 to 1.5 mg every 2 days.
   d. Taper completed in 7 to 10 days.
3. Using phenobarbital (82):
   a. To calculate the amount of sedative-hypnotic required

Table 40.34.
Factors Involved in Benzodiazepine Detoxification Problems

Taper too rapid
Dosage decrease too large
Fear of tapering, patient was not sufficiently prepared
Caffeine use
Alcohol use
Illicit drug use
Menstrual syndrome (PMS) symptoms
Medical condition problem (e.g., increased pain)
Life stressors
Difficulties in handling tapering problems in a flexible manner
Return of preexisting disorder
Rebound
Major and minor withdrawal symptoms
Mood disorder
New anxiety symptoms

per day, the patient is given the pentobarbital challenge test (82).

   b. The amount of pentobarbital in mg required for 24 hr is calculated from the test.

   c. This dose is translated into phenobarbital equivalency from Table 40.29.

   d. Phenobarbital is divided in q8h doses.

   e. Detoxification proceeds at 1/10 the starting dose per day (68).

For some patients, substitution to long-acting benzodiazepines for alprazolem withdrawal has not been effective, but phenobarbital has been (83).

Adjunct Medications for Benzodiazepine Detoxification Protocols:

Based on research for opiate and alcohol withdrawal syndrome, clonidine has been recommended for benzodiazepine withdrawal. Unfortunately, it is only partially effective at dose (0.1 to 1.2 mg/day) (72). Propranalol in doses of 20 mg q.i.d. is also only partially effective, but it should be used for rebound and symptom reemergency (72, 83). Because carbamazepine demonstrated some efficacy in alcohol withdrawal, it was tried for benzodiazepine withdrawal. Carbamazepine was initiated at 200 mg p.o., b.i.d. at the onset of detoxification, and increased to 800 mg/day, depending upon symptoms. It was then discontinued in 3 to 14 days after completion of benzodiazepine detoxification (89). Of these three agents, carbamazepine may have the greatest effectiveness as an adjunct medication for benzodiazepine withdrawal.

Recently, a new nonbenzodiazepine anxiolytic has been developed: Buspirone. This drug has been used in one study of alprazolam detoxification and has demonstrated that it can decrease the manifestations of withdrawal (90). Buspirone was initiated 2 weeks before beginning the taper, at a dosage of 5 mg t.i.d. Because buspirone appears not to have any abuse liability, it could be very useful in this area.

A final approach could be the addition of an antipanic agent, e.g., imipramine (TCA) or phenalzine (MAO), be-

fore beginning detoxification. Such an approach could minimize rebound and symptom reemergence problems.

Acknowledgements Acknowledgement is made to Ms. Stella Mitnick and Ms. Barbara Hubschman for their assistance in the preparation of this manuscript.

REFERENCES

1. Rinaldi RC, Steindler EM, Wilford BB, Goodwin D. Clarification and standardization of substance abuse terminology. JAMA 1988;259:557–561.
2. Newman RG. The need to redefine "addiction." N Engl J Med 1983;18:1096–1098.
3. Portenoy RK. Chronic opioid therapy in normalignant pain. J Pain Symp Manage 1990;5(1,suppl):S46–S58.
4. Ludwig AM. Principles of clinical psychiatry. New York: Free Press, 1980.
5. American Psychiatric Association Diagnostic and Statistical Manual of Mental Disorders (Third Edition, Revised). Washington, D.C., 1987.
6. Khatame M, O'Brien C. Chronic pain and narcotic addiction: a multitherapeutic approach—a pilot study. Compr Psychiatry 1979;20(1):55–60.
7. Ready LB, Hare B. Drug problems in chronic pain patients. Anesthesiol Rev 1979;6(12):28–30.
8. Ziesat HA. Drug use and misuse in operant pain patients. Addict Behav 1979;4:263–266.
9. Ready LB, Sarkis E, Turner JA. Self-reported vs actual use of medications in chronic pain patients. Pain 1982;12:285–294.
10. Barr Taylor C, Zlutnick SF, Curley MS, Flora J. The effects of detoxification relaxation and brief supportive therapy on chronic pain. Pain 1980;8:319–329.
11. Maruta T, Swanson DW, Finlayson RE. Drug abuse and dependence in patients with chronic pain. Mayo Clin Proc 1979;54:241–244.
12. Maruta T, Swanson DW. Problems with the use of oxycodone compound in patients with chronic pain. Pain 1981;11:389–396.
13. Portenoy RK, Foley KM. Chronic use of opioid analagesics in non-malignant pain: report of 38 cases. Pain 1986;25:171–186.
14. Turner J, Calsyn DA, Fordyce WE, Ready LB. Drug utilization patterns in chronic pain patients. Pain 1982;12:357–363.
15. Finlayson-Richard E, Maruta-Toshihiko, Morse RE, Swenson WR, et al. Substance dependence and chronic pain: profile of 50 patients treated in an alcohol and drug dependence unit. Pain 1986;26(2):167–174.
16. Finlayson-Richard E, Maruta-Toshihiko, Morse-Robert M, Martin-Mary A. Substance dependence and chronic pain: experience with treatment and follow-up results. Pain 1986;26(2):175–180.
17. Swanson DW, Maruta T, Wolff VA. Ancient pain. Pain 1986;25(3)383–387.
18. Benedikt-Richard A, Kolb-Lawrence C. Prelinary findings on chronic pain and posttraumatic stress disorder. Am J Psychiatry 1986;143(7):908–910.
19. Katon W, Egan I, Miller D. Chronic pain: lifetime psychiatric diagnoses and family history. Am J Psychiatry 1985;142(10):1156–1160.
20. Fishbain DA, Goldberg M, Meagher B, Steele R, Rosomoff H. Male and female chronic pain patients categorized by DSM-III psychiatric diagnostic criteria. Pain 1986;26:181–197.
21. Steele-Rosomoff R, Fishbain DA, Goldberg M, Rosomoff H. Chronic pain patients who lie in this psychiatric examination about current drug/alcohol use. Pain Suppl 1990;5:S299.
22. Rafii A, Haller DL, Poklis A. Incidence of recreational drug use among chronic pain clinic patients. American Pain Society Ninth Annual Meeting, St. Louis, MO. Abstract: 1990;33.
23. Medina JL, Diamond S. Drug dependency in patients with chronic headache. Headache 1977;17:12–14.

24. Evans PJD. Narcotic addiction in patients with chronic pain. Anaesthesia 1981;36:597–602.

25. Langemark M, Olesen J. Drug abuse in migraine patients. Pain 1984;19:81–86.

26. Porter J, Jick H. Addiction rare in patients treated with narcotics. N Engl J Med 1980;302:128.

27. Weissman DE, Haddox JD. Opioid pseudoaddiction—an iatrogenic syndrome. Pain 1989;36:363–366.

28. Halpern-Lawrence M, Robinson-James. Prescribing practices for pain in drug dependence: a lesson in ignorance. Adv Alcohol Subst Abuse 1985–1986;5(1–2):135–162.

29. Fordyce WW. Behavioral methods for chronic pain and illness. St. Louis: Mosby, 1976.

30. Ho A, Dole VP. Pain perception in drug-free and in methadone-maintained human ex-addicts. Proc Soc Exp Biol Med 1979; 162(3):392–395.

31. McNairy SL, Maruta T, Ivnik RJ, Swanson DW, Ilstrup DM. Prescription medication dependence and neuropsychologic function. Pain 1984;18(2):169–177.

32. Arner S, Meyerson BA. Lack of analgesic effect of opiods on neuropathic and idiopathic forms of pain. Pain 1988;33:11–24.

33. Snyder SH. Opiate receptors and internal opiates. Sci Am 1977;236(3):44–56.

34. Mathew NT, Kurman R, Perez F. Drug induced refractory headache-clinical features and management. Headache 1990;30:634–638.

35. Tennant FS, Rawson RA. Outpatient treatment of prescription opioid dependence. Comparison of two methods. Arch Intern Med 1982;142:1845–1847.

36. Ghodse H. Drugs and addictive behavior, a guide to treatment. Oxford: Blackwell Scientific Publications, 1990.

37. Fauman BJ, Fauman MA. Emergency psychiatry for the house officer. Baltimore: Williams & Wilkins, 1981.

38. McLane NJ, Carroll DM. Ocular manifestations of drug abuse. Surv Ophthalmol 1986;30(5):298–313.

39. Hawks RH, Chiang CN. Urine testing for drugs of abuse. NIDA Res Monogr 1986;73:43–61.

40. Burke WM, Ravi NV, Dhopesh V, et al. Prolonged presence of metabolite in urine after compulsive cocaine use. J Clin Psychiatry 1990;51:145–148.

41. Delisle J. A case of amitriptyline abuse. Am J Psychiatry 1990;147:1377–1378.

42. Wilcox JA. Abuse of fluoxetine by a patient with anorexia nervosa. Am J Psychiatry 1987;144(8)1100–1101.

43. Briggs NC, Jefferson JW, Koenecke FH. Tranylcypromine addiction: a case report and review. J Clin Psychiatry 1990;51(10):426–428.

44. Rose HE, Glaser FB, Germanson T. The prevalence of psychiatric disorders in patients with alcohol and other drug problems. Arch Gen Psychiatry 1988;45:1023–1032.

45. Levy JC, Deykin EY. Suicidality, depression, and substance abuse in adolescence. Am J Psychiatry 1989;146(11):1462–1467.

46. Inturrisi CE. Role of opioid analgesics. Am J Med 1984;(Sep 10):27–36.

47. Madden C, Ong B, Singer G. Mood state of heroin-dependent persons undergoing methadone detoxification. Int J Addict 1989;22(1):93–102.

48. Haertzen CA, Hooks NT. Changes in personality and subjective experience associated with chronic administration and withdrawal of opiates. J Nerv Ment Dis 1969;148(6):606–614.

49. Turkington D, Drummon DC. How should opiate withdrawal be measured? Drug Alcohol Depend 1989;24(2):151–153.

50. Cuthill JD, Beroniade V, Salvatori VA, Viguie F. Evaluation of clonidine suppression of opiate withdrawal reactions: a multidisciplinary approach. Can J Psychiatry 1989;35:377–382.

51. Halpern L. Substitution-detoxification and its role in the management of chronic benign pain. J Clin Psychiatry 1982;43(8 pt 2):10–14.

52. Frances RJ, Franklin JE. Alcohol and other psychoactive substance use disorders. In: Talbott JA, Hales RE, Yudofsky SC, eds. American Psychiatric Press textbook of psychiatry. Washington, D.C.: American Psychiatric Press, 1988.

53. Goldstein E, Pollack R, Weiner B, Lazoritz R: Rapid treatment of percodan addiction: a case report. Int J Addict 1978;13(6):1003–1007.

54. Schmalsteg WJ, Hayden JM, Comstock EG. Propoxyphene napsylate detoxification. Tex Med 1975;71:70–76.

55. Bickel WK, Stitzer ML, Bigelow GE, Liebson IA, Jasinski DR, Johnson RE. A clinical trial of buprenorphine: comparison with methadone in the detoxification of heroin addicts. Clin Pharmacol Ther 1988;43(1):72–78.

56. Kosten TR, Krystal JH, Charney DS, et al. Rapid detoxification from opioid dependence. Am J Psychiatry 1989;146:1349.

57. Clarney DS, Riordan CE, Kleber MD, et al: Clonidine and naltrexone: a safe, effective, and rapid treatment of abrupt withdrawal from methadone therapy. Arch Gen Psychiatry 1982;39:1327–1332.

58. Jacobsen LK, Kosten TR. Naloxone challenge as biological predictor of treatment outcome in opiate addicts. Am J Drug Alcohol Abuse 1989;15(4):355–366.

59. Aghajanian GK, Vander Mallen CP. Alpha-2-adreno-receptor-induced hyperpolarization of locus coeruleus neurons: intracellular studies in vivo. Science 1982;215:1394–1396.

60. Kleber HD, Riordan CE, Rounsaville B, Kosten T, Charney D, et al. Clonidine in outpatient detoxification from methadone maintenance. Arch Gen Psychiatry 1985;42(4):391–394.

61. San L, Cami J, Peri JM, Mata R, Porta M. Efficacy of clonidine, guanfacine and methadone in the rapid detoxification of heroin addicts: a controlled clinical trial. Br J Addict 1990;85(1):141–147.

62. Kosten TR, Rounsaville BJ, Kleber HD. Comparison of clinician ratings to self reports of withdrawal during clonidine detoxification of opiate addicts. Am J Drug Alcohol Abuse 1985;11(1–2)1–10.

63. Spencer L, Gregory M. Clonidine transdermal patches for use in outpatient opiate withdrawal. J Subst Abuse Treat 1989;6:113–117.

64. Roehrich HJ, Gold MS. Propranolol as adjunct to clonidine in opiate detoxification. Am J Psychiatry 1987;144(8):1099–1100.

65. Dufficy RG. Use of psychotherapeutic drugs in the acute detoxification of heroin addicts. Milit Med 1973;133:748.

66. Rawson RA, Washton AM, Resnick RB, Tennant FS Jr. Clonidine hydrochloride detoxification from methadone treatment—the value of naltrexone aftercare. Adv Alcohol Subst Abuse 1984;3(3):41–49.

67. Kroening RJ, Oleson TD. Rapid narcotic detoxification in chronic pain patients treated with auricular electroacupuncture and naloxone. Int J Addict 1985;20(9):1347–1360.

68. Shader RI, Caine ED, Meyer RE. Treatment of dependence on barbiturates and sedative-hypnotics. In: Shader RI, ed. Manual psychiatric therapeutics. Boston: Little, Brown & Co., 1989.

69. Wartenberg AA. Detoxification of the chemically dependent patient. RI Med J 1989;72(12):451–456.

70. Uhlenhuth E, DeWit H, Balter MB. Risks and benefits of long-term benzodiazepine use. J Clin Psychopharmacol 1988;8:161–167.

77. Griffiths RR, Wolf B. Relative abuse liability of different benzodiazepines in drug abusers. J Clin Psychopharmacol 1990;10(4):237–243.

72. Lader M. Long-term anxiolytic therapy: the issue of drug withdrawal. J Clin Psychiatry 1987;48(12 suppl):12–16.

73. Owen RT, Tyrel P. Benzodiazepine dependence. A review of the evidence. Drugs 1983;25:385–398.

74. Noyes R, Garvey MN, Cook BL, et al. Benzodiazepine withdrawal: a review of the evidence. J Clin Psychiatry 1988;49:382–389.

75. Rickels K, Schwerzer E, Case WG, Greenblatt DJ. Long-term therapeutic use of benzodiazepines. I. Effects of abrupt discontinuation. Arch Gen Psychiatry 1990;47:899–907.

76. Schwerzer E, Rickels K, Case WG, Greenblatt DJ. Long-term therapeutic use of benzodiazepines. II. Effects of gradual taper. Arch Gen Psychiatry 1990;47:908–915.

77. Burrows GD, Norman TR, Judd FK, et al. Short-acting versus

long-acting benzodiazepines: discontinuation effects in panic disorders. J Psychiatric Res 1990;24(suppl 2):65–72.

78. King SA, Strain JJ. Benzodiazepine use by chronic pain patients. Clin J Pain 1990;6:143–147.

79. King SA, Strain JS. Benzodiazepines and chronic pain. Pain 1990;41:3–4.

80. Westbrook L, Cicala RS, Wright H. Effectiveness of alprazolam in the treatment of chronic pain: results of a preliminary study. Clin J Pain 1990;6:32–36.

81. Ferretti T, Fishbain DA, Goldberg M, Steele-Rosomoff R, Rosomoff HL. Open clinical trial of clonazepam for chronic pain patients with myofascial pain syndrome. Pain Suppl 1990;5:S163.

82. Smith DE, Wesson DR. Phenobarbital technique for the treatment of barbiturate dependence. Arch Gen Psychiatry 1971;24:56–60.

83. Smith DE, Landry MJ. Benzodiazepine dependence discontinuation: focus on the chemical dependency detoxification setting and benzodiazepine-poly-drug abuse. J Psychiatric Res 1990;24(suppl 2):145–156.

84. DuPont RL. A practical approach to benzodiazepine discontinuation. J Psychiatric Res 1990;24(suppl 2):81–90.

41

Manipulation and Mobilization

PHILIP E. GREENMAN

Headache is one of the most common presenting complaints to the health care delivery system. Many headache sufferers self-treat themselves, making it difficult to identify the total extent of the impact of the condition on society. Headache appears to have its origins in antiquity. Archeological findings have shown skulls with evidence of trephination. Despite the rapid accumulation of new medical knowledge in the last half of the 20th century, many aspects of the etiology and cause of headache, as well as headache treatment, defy our understanding.

The discipline of manual medicine is quite similar to headache. It has its origins in antiquity (1) and was part of the health care delivery system prior to Hippocrates. Hippocrates did use forms of manual medicine as part of his holistic patient care. Manipulation and mobilization are terms that describe some of the components of the manual medicine discipline. Dorland's 26th Edition Medical Dictionary definition of manipulation is "skillful or dextrous treatment by the hand." "Manipulation" is also a term long-used in the European medical community for high-velocity, low-amplitude, direct-action thrust procedures. Mobilization is defined as "the process of making a fixed or ankylosed part movable." There are a wide variety of different manual medicine approaches (2–7) that accomplish increased mobility in the structures of the human body by the skillful use of the hands.

To address the role of manipulation and mobilization in the management of patients suffering from headache, one needs as much clarity as possible in defining the type of headache, as well as the type of manual medicine procedure used as part of the treatment plan.

HEADACHE CLASSIFICATION

There are many diverse classifications for the presenting complaint of headache (8, 9). Other chapters in this book refer to the wide variety of headache types and their multiple causes. For our purposes, a simple classification of three types of headache will be used: (*a*) vascular, (*b*) muscle-contraction, and (*c*) traction/inflammatory (organic). The vascular group is represented by migraine, both with and without aura; migraine variants; cluster headache; and temporal arteritis. Muscle contraction head-

ache (10) includes those related to alteration of muscle tone, particularly in the suboccipital and cervical regions, which may be related to altered biomechanical function or disease of the musculoskeletal system. They are also described as "tension headaches" and accompany other symptoms of anxiety, depression, and tension response to stress. Traction/inflammatory headaches, or organic headaches, are related to specific pathologies of the central nervous system or of the anatomical structures of the skull and face itself. Cranial neuralgias, allergy, CNS tumors and infectious disease are all within this part of the classification.

This simple classification is useful in defining the role of manual medicine, either as a primary or as an adjunctive treatment modality in the headache patient. It is not uncommon to have more than one type of headache pathology (11) ongoing in the patient. It is also not uncommon to have more than one therapeutic approach to deal with the problems of the headache patient. In the use of manual medicine procedures, it is not uncommon to use more than one type as part of the management plan.

MANUAL MEDICINE: DEFINITIONS

The discipline of manual medicine has two component parts. The first is the diagnostic process, termed structural diagnosis, using a combination of hand and eye coordination in the observation and palpation of the function of the total musculoskeletal system. Structural diagnosis should be a component part of the physical examination and viewed within the context of total patient evaluation. Structural diagnosis is a three-stage process in identifying the entity amenable to manual medicine treatment. That entity, called somatic dysfunction, is defined as impaired or altered function of related components of the somatic (body framework) system; skeletal, arthrodial, and myofascial structures; and related vascular, lymphatic, and neural elements (Hospital Adaptation of International Classification of Disease Adapted (HICDA), edition 2, 1973). This is the current codable diagnosis for the "manipulable lesion." The three-stage diagnostic process includes a screening examination, scanning examination, and specific segmental definition. The screening examination evaluates the total musculoskeletal system and attempts to identify alteration of function within the musculoskeletal system that appears to be significant within the context of the patient's total evaluation. One evaluates not only the presence of significant altered function but also the location(s) of the areas of dysfunction. The scanning examination further evaluates the region(s) appearing to be significantly dysfunctional. If that region is the cervical spine (commonly seen in headache sufferers), the specific segmental definition phase of the diagnostic process locates the dysfunction in the cervical spine and identifies the structures that are specifically dysfunctional.

Throughout this three-phase diagnostic process, the structural diagnostician is looking for the classic diagnostic triad of somatic dysfunction. The mnemonic for the diagnostic triad is ART. *A* stands for *a*symmetry of form or function of related component parts of the musculoskeletal system; *R* stands for alteration in *r*ange of motion of the components of the musculoskeletal system, primarily hypomobility; and *T* stands for *t*issue texture abnormality. Tissue texture abnormalities are altered palpable characteristics of the tissues of the musculoskeletal system including the skin, subcutaneous fascia, deep fascia, musculature, ligaments, tendons, and pericapsular and joint structures. Frequently, the area of somatic dysfunction is also tender to palpation. When one or more areas of somatic dysfunction are identified, the physician must decide whether it is significant in the pain syndrome presented by the patient or whether it is an incidental and nonsignificant finding.

Types of Manual Medicine

Within the discipline of manual medicine, there are a variety of treatment procedures and techniques, similar to the pharmacological armamentarium of the physician. There is more than one type of antibiotic, and there is more than one type of manual medicine. Within the armamentarium of manual medicine are the following procedures:

1. Soft tissue;
p2. Articulatory (mobilization without impulse);
3. High-velocity, low-amplitude thrust (mobilization with thrust);
4. Muscle energy technique;
5. Myofascial release;
6. Functional and release by position;
7. Craniosacral.

The soft tissue procedures include massage, effleurage, pétrissage, and traction, which deal with the direct mechanical effect on soft tissues, as well as reflex effect upon muscle physiology. Other soft tissue procedures include lateral stretch, longitudinal stretch, separation of origin and insertion, and inhibition of musculotendinous junction; procedures that have also been described as peripheral stimulating therapies (such as acupressure). Areas of

tissue texture abnormality treated by soft tissue techniques have been described differently by various authors. These include the acupuncture point, Travell's trigger point, and Jones' tender point. Soft tissue procedures can be used in acute and chronic conditions and provided singly or in concert with other manual medicine techniques. Soft tissue procedures are frequently used to prepare the tissues of the musculoskeletal system for other types of procedures.

Articulatory procedures, or mobilization without impulse, are procedures widely practiced by physical therapists as well as manual medicine physicians. These techniques use oscillatory repetitive motions in the direction of motion loss, with gradations in the amount of force used. They are extensions of the diagnostic process of range-of-motion testing. When an area appears to be restricted, a series of repetitions of operator force in the direction of motion loss occurs. These procedures appear to influence the mechanical behavior of the articulation and its articular tissues, as well as influencing the behavior of the variety of mechanoreceptors associated with the articulation (s) involved.

High-velocity, low-amplitude, thrusting procedures (mobilization with impulse) are those most frequently visualized by patients when they think of manipulation. These procedures are some of the most widely used in the manual medicine armamentarium. They have historically been described as "manipulation" in the European community. These procedures are directed primarily toward an articulation and related periarticular structures. A rapidly accelerating, high-velocity operator force is induced into a joint in the direction of restriction and is frequently associated with a "popping" sound. This sound accompanies the cavitation phenomenon within the articulation. These procedures not only affect the joint mechanics but also influence associated paravertebral musculature.

Muscle energy techniques have been used by manual medicine for the past 30 years. They are also described as postisometric technique and neuromuscular treatment (4, 7). They use patient muscular activity to achieve a variety of treatment outcomes. The restricted joint can be mobilized, muscle physiology restored to more normal, and circulation enhanced by these procedures. The muscle activity can be isometric, concentric, or eccentric isotonic. When using isometric technique, the physiological principle operative is the ability to stretch a short, tight, hypertonic muscle to a new resting length following an isometric contraction. Isotonic procedures function on the principle of reciprocal inhibition, as well as sequential muscle fiber firing, to strengthen a muscle that is physiologically inhibited. Of prime importance in successful use of these procedures is the ability of the physician to appropriately engage the areas of restriction of motion present in the articulation(s).

Myofascial release procedures (12) are relatively new to manual medicine, and they focus upon the biomechanical and reflex behavior of the fascial tissues of the musculoskeletal system. They include all of the soft connective tissues of the body, skin, fascia, muscle, ligament, and tendon, and their relationship to the hard connective tissue, bone. The examiner looks for areas of symmetry or asymmetry in tightness and looseness within the musculoskeletal system. When asymmetry of tightness and looseness is identified, procedures are applied to enhance return of symmetrical tissue function. The physician applies tension, traction, and twisting loads to the soft tissues to overcome the tightness within the tissues and achieve more symmetrical balance. These procedures appear to function by biomechanical effect on the soft tissue, as well as neuroreflexive change in the tone of the musculature, and they can be used in broad regions or at a single vertebral segmental level.

Functional techniques, including those described as release by positioning, address areas of dysfunction of the musculoskeletal system in a different fashion. Instead of putting a force in the direction of motion restriction, the physician attempts to identify a position of the body part that puts the joint and its associated tissues in a position of maximum ease. The procedure involves palpating areas of dysfunction with one hand and introducing motion with the other hand and/or giving instructions, constantly searching for a point of maximum ease under the palpating hand. The structures are held at this point of maximum ease for 1 to 90 seconds. Sequential applications of body positioning, often with small increments of change, are used until the area of dysfunction is improved. These procedures include the use of both a dynamic, constantly changing process and a sequence of balance-and-hold positions.

A variation of functional technique is described as release by positioning, or strain/counterstrain. The physician palpates one of a large number of tender points on the anterior and posterior surfaces of the body, which correlate with areas of dysfunction within the spinal complex and extremities. The patient is placed in the body position that is most pain-free with the tender point less tender to palpation. Holding the patient's body in that position for some 90 seconds and then reexamining is quite effective in overcoming both acute and chronic areas of somatic dysfunction.

The craniosacral system of manual medicine (13, 14) functions through the small amount of inherent mobility found within the skull and spinal column. The small amount of motion includes the inherent mobility of the brain and spinal cord, the fluctuation of the cerebral spinal fluid, the mobility of the sutures of the skull, the mobility of the sacrum between the two innominates, and the mobility of the intercranial and intraspinal membranes. The diagnostic process includes evaluation of the cranial rhythmic impulse (which averages 8 to 14 cycles per minute in normal, average patients) and the symmetry of articular mobility within the numerous sutures of the osseous cranium. When alteration of the cranial rhythmic impulse or sutural mobility is identified, the craniosacral treatment procedures include the application of extrinsic force to the musculoskeletal system, particularly the skull and sacrum, to enhance the normal physiological mobility of the skull and sacrum and restore appropriate amplitude to the cranial rhythmic impulse.

Manipulative Prescription

As in all other disciplines of medicine, the appropriate use of the therapeutic modality must be prescribed. Manual medicine procedures need to be viewed in the same fashion as medications. In using a pharmacological agent, a physician identifies the type, strength, frequency, and the length of drug treatment necessary. Manual medicine is no different. A physician needs to identify the type of manual medicine procedure, the length of application at each visit, the frequency of visits, and the length of treatment plan. Several different types of manual medicine are frequently applied during one treatment session. Different factors influence the manipulative prescription, including the patient age, acuteness or chronicity of the problem, general physical condition of the patient, and other forms of therapy being given to the patient. The manual medicine procedure may be the only treatment for the headache patient, but more frequently, it is used in combination with other therapeutic techniques.

MODELS AND MECHANISMS OF MANUAL MEDICINE

In using manual medicine procedures, one identifies the effect and physiological mechanism anticipated from the manipulative intervention. Model is a term used to describe the approach to the patient.

One of the more commonly used models is called biomechanical. In this model, the physician approaches the patient from the perspective of the body being formed by a number of bones, joined together at joints, stabilized by ligaments, and moved by muscles. This primarily functional anatomical model begins with the feet and ascends to the head. The manual medicine approach restores the biomechanical relationship of each bone, joint, and muscle group, resulting in maximal symmetrical mobility.

A second model, the neurological, begins with the concept that all functions of the human body are under some form of neural control. The musculoskeletal system is viewed not only as an expression of nervous system activity but also as the point of afferent stimulation transmitted to the central nervous system for processing. There are several different neurological models. The reflex model includes the effect of afferent mechanoreceptor musculoskeletal system activity manifesting itself in different ways through different neurological mechanisms. One output is on the somatic structures in the form of altered muscle activity. Frequently this is manifest as hypertonicity of skeletal muscle. A second output is through the visceral structures, the internal organs, and the skin viscera, through the vasomotor, secretomotor, or pilomotor systems. These skin visceral changes are manifested as the tissue texture abnormality found during structural diagnosis. Altered reflex activity may involve both somatic and visceral structures. Of particular importance to the headache patient is the reflex control of the vasculature through the sympathetic division of the autonomic nervous system. Restoration of more normal afferent mechanoreceptor activity appears to have a positive influence on vasomotor tone through a somatovisceral reflex arc involving the sympathetic nervous system. Another and different neurological model is that of neural entrapment. Small nerves and nerve fibers may be entrapped by elements of the musculoskeletal system resulting in pain manifestations along the course of the entrapped nerve. It is postulated that much of the occipital pain associated with muscle contraction headache is a function of entrapment of the greater occipital nerve by the suboccipital musculature. Reduction in muscle hypertonicity potentially reduces the amount of neural entrapment and therefore is efficacious in managing the headache symptom.

A third model is the circulatory model, which approaches the patient from the perspective of the influence of the musculoskeletal system on body circulation. Manual medicine approaches the patient to enhance the normalcy of arterial, venous, and lymphatic circulation. Arterial influence is through reflex influence on neural control of vasomotor tone via the sympathetic division of the autonomic nervous system. Manual medicine uses this mechanism to assist in the management of vascular headaches. The vasomotor tone for the head is controlled through the superior cervical ganglion. The preganglionic fibers to the superior cervical ganglion come from the upper four thoracic segments, ascending in the cervical sympathetic trunk. It is postulated that some fibers also come from adjacent cervical nerves. Maximizing biomechanical function of the cervical and upper thoracic spine to normalize afferent stimulation provides more normal neurological control of cerebral vasculature through the superior cervical ganglion. The musculoskeletal system has a different manner of influence on venous and lymphatic circulation. Venous and lymphatic circulation is almost totally dependent upon activity of the musculoskeletal system, particularly the thoracolumbar diaphragm and the major muscles of the extremities. Contraction of somatic musculature compresses the venous and lymphatic vessels and enhances circulation centrally. The diaphragm, through its influence on negative interthoracic pressure, works as a pump of the low-pressure venous and lymphatic systems, enhancing centripetal fluid flow. In headache patients, venous circulation is influenced by the cervical musculature and the function of the osseous cranial base on the internal and external jugular vein systems. Any restriction of mobility in or around the jugular foramen can reduce the venous outflow from the head, and any change in cervical muscle function could involve the external jugular circula-

tion. Maximum function of the cervical spine and osseous cranial base would certainly be of value in preventing venous congestion within the head and neck.

The manual medicine practitioner makes use of one or more of these models to positively influence the overall capability of the patient. Although these models are described individually, manual medicine interventions influence all of them. Certain types of manual medicine seem to influence more significantly either the biomechanical, neurological, or circulatory mechanism. If one uses manual medicine with the therapeutic goal of obtaining maximum biomechanical function of the musculoskeletal system in postural balance, this should positively influence the neurological and circulatory systems as well.

CLINICAL APPLICATIONS IN HEADACHE

In the clinical application of manual medicine to the headache patient, the practitioner must know the functional anatomy (15, 16) of the areas involved in somatic dysfunction and the potential effects on the patient's physiology. Of particular importance is an understanding of the anatomy of the cranium, cervical spine, cervical thoracic junction, thoracic inlet, and upper thoracic spine.

In the use of structural diagnosis and manual medicine procedures in a headache patient, there are both general and specific approaches. All headache patients can be approached the same in a general sense, that is, identify any areas of dysfunction within the musculoskeletal system and attempt to restore maximum possible functioning to assist the patient in coping with the headache syndrome. Depending upon the specific headache diagnosis, a more specific manual medicine approach might be indicated (17, 18).

Since tension/muscle-contraction headache is so common, a biomechanical approach to the patient is a good first step. Beginning with the screening examination of the musculoskeletal system, the physician looks for the presence or absence of symmetrical function of the musculoskeletal system. Beginning with the gait, one looks for symmetry of length of stride, symmetry of lumbar sidebending, cross-pattern arm swing with equal excursion, and head carriage. The location of altered mobility and asymmetry is noted. Static evaluation of posture includes the position of the feet, the status of the arches, level of the greater trochanters and iliac crests, presence or absence of altered AP and lateral curvatures of the thoracic and lumbar spine, level of the shoulder girdle at the acromion process and inferior angle of the scapula, symmetry of arm posture, and head and neck carriage. In addition to looking at the relationship of anatomical parts in the coronal plane, both from in front and behind, evaluation is made of the postural plumb line beginning at the ear, through the tip of the acromion, the greater trochanter, and anterior to the lateral malleolus. When area(s) of dysfunction are identified, specific segmental diagnostic definition is made, and a decision is made about how to approach the patient using manual medicine procedures and which type of procedure(s) to use.

Despite the presenting complaint being in the head and neck, it is usually advisable to start by evaluating the lower extremities for significant biomechanical dysfunction. Altered gait from foot, ankle, knee, and hip changes can affect the overall postural balance, culminating in stress at the craniocervical junction. Of particular importance is the effect of a short lower extremity, resulting in the pelvic tilt syndrome (19). Unleveling of the base of the skull of the occiput has been shown (20) to strongly correlate with unleveling of the weight-bearing surface of the sacral base. It is postulated that this finding results in a number of compensatory postural changes within the musculoskeletal system. Leveling the sacral base plane by appropriate lift therapy is frequently of great assistance in managing a patient with intractable headache.

Attention is then directed toward the "crossover" areas of the vertebral complex, the areas of greatest biomechanical stress. They are the lumbosacral junction, the thoracolumbar junction, the cervicothoracic junction, and the cranial occipital junction. Each of these areas is evaluated for difficulty, and if found, appropriate manipulation or mobilization is provided. The change in biomechanical behavior of the spine at the thoracolumbar junction results from the change in facet facings as well as the myofascial relationships between the upper and lower halves of the body. The quadratus/lumborum attachments respond to alterations in the lower half of the body, and the trapezius/latissimus dorsi fascias respond to the upper half of the body. Combinations of myofascial imbalance influence the thoracolumbar diaphragm and rib cage function, which negatively influence the patient's respiratory and circulatory capacity.

The cervicothoracic junction is of major significance because of the influence on vascular and neural structures to the upper extremity, manifested as thoracic outlet syndrome, and the intimate relation of the myofascial attachments of the head and neck, through the scalenes, sternocleidomastoid, and the superficial and deep long vertebral muscles on the cervical spine and base of the cranium. Altered cervicothoracic function strongly influences the efficiency of venous and lymphatic return and is strongly related to the sympathetic trunk as it ascends into the cervical area.

Altered biomechanical craniocervical function (21) is extremely important because of the negative impact on the motor function of the suboccipital musculature, the postulated entrapment of the occipital nerves (22, 23), and the relation to the superior cervical ganglion. A second significant factor is the observation that the density of mechanoreceptors to area of articular surface is the greatest in the upper cervical portion of the vertebral column. Altered motion increases aberrant afferent stimulation to the spinal cord and central brain structures. Restoration of appropriate symmetrical afferent stimulation from these mechanoreceptors clearly aids in the management of the headache patient. The biomechanics of the upper cervical complex are quite atypical, with the integrated mobility of the occipitoatlantal, atlantoaxial, and C2, 3 articulations. Ligamentous and muscular relationships link the axis directly to the occiput, as well as relating the atlas to both the occiput above and the axis below (24). Understanding the anatomy and biomechanics of this area is of major importance to the physician managing the headache patient (15, 16, 22, 23).

The use of specific manipulation or mobilization techniques depends greatly upon the knowledge and experience of the clinician (3). However applied, the role of manual medicine procedures is to restore maximum, painless, movement of the musculoskeletal system in postural balance (2). Fortunately, some of the simplest procedures can be the most effective. Soft tissue and articulatory procedures applied to the cervical spine are quite effective in reducing muscle tension and enhancing symmetrical articular mobility. These procedures can then be amplified by other techniques, examples of which are described below.

Soft tissue procedure: The operator cradles the occiput in the hand, with the tips of the fingers bilaterally contacting the nuchal line. Inhibitory pressure is given symmetrically to the musculotendinous junction at the attachment to the occiput, with particular emphasis on areas of muscular tension. Cephalic traction is applied with both hands contacting the occiput, with greater force on the side of major restriction (Fig. 41.1).

Myofascial release: The patient's skull is grasped with one hand on the occiput and the other on the frontal region. Flexion, sidebending right or left, and rotation right or left, are introduced, looking for areas of most restriction (tightness). Increased loading of the tissues is applied by further traction against the area of tightness and is held until "release" of the tissue is felt. The release phenomena can be enhanced by asking the patient to inhale/exhale deeply, move eyes in multiple directions, clench the teeth, or make other maneuvers that increase the afferent stimulation to the central nervous system. Sequential applications of load are frequently necessary to restore the balance of tissue tone (Fig. 41.2).

Release by positioning: The head and neck are controlled by the operator's hands, with the right hand palpating over an area of specific tissue texture abnormality and tenderness (Jones' tender point). Combined activity of both hands positions the head and neck to where the patient reports reduction in pain and the palpating right hand feels a decrease in tissue texture abnormality and tenderness. This posture is held for 90 seconds or until marked reduction of the tender tissue texture occurs (Fig. 41.3).

Muscle energy technique: To overcome restriction of extension, right sidebending, and right rotation of a typical cervical segment, the operator's right hand contacts the pillar of the inferior vertebra involved in the dysfunction, to stabilize that segment. The operator's left hand introduces extension, right sidebending, and right rotation to the first motion barrier

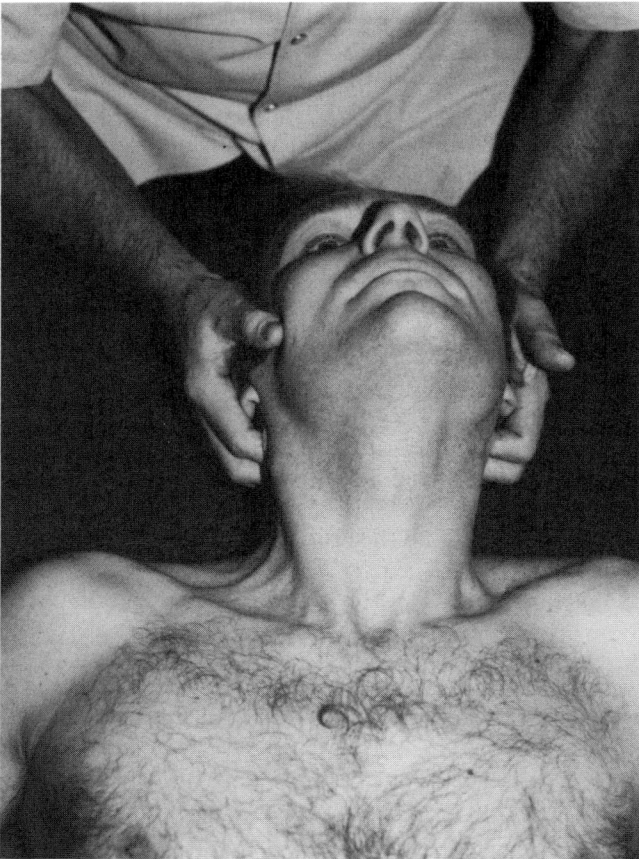

Figure 41.1. Soft tissue technique: inhibitory pressure.

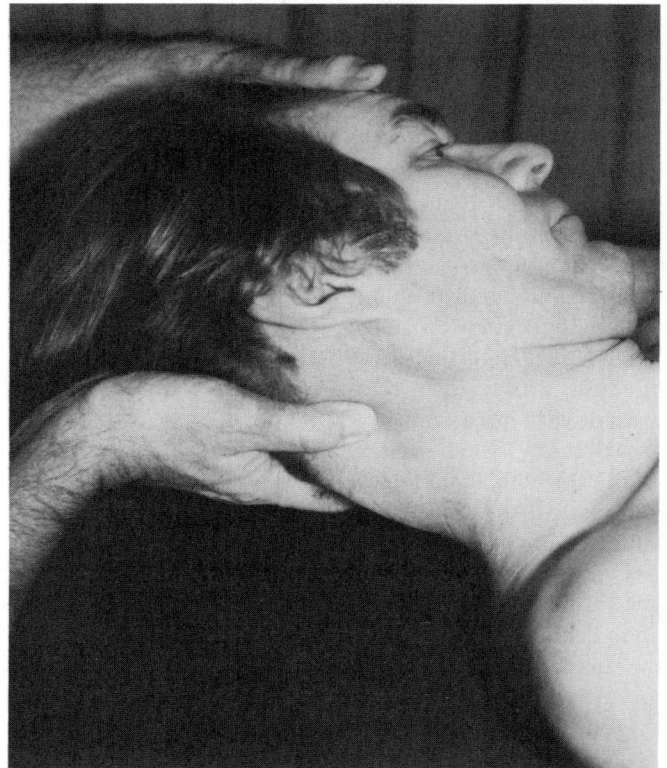

Figure 41.2. Myofascial release technique.

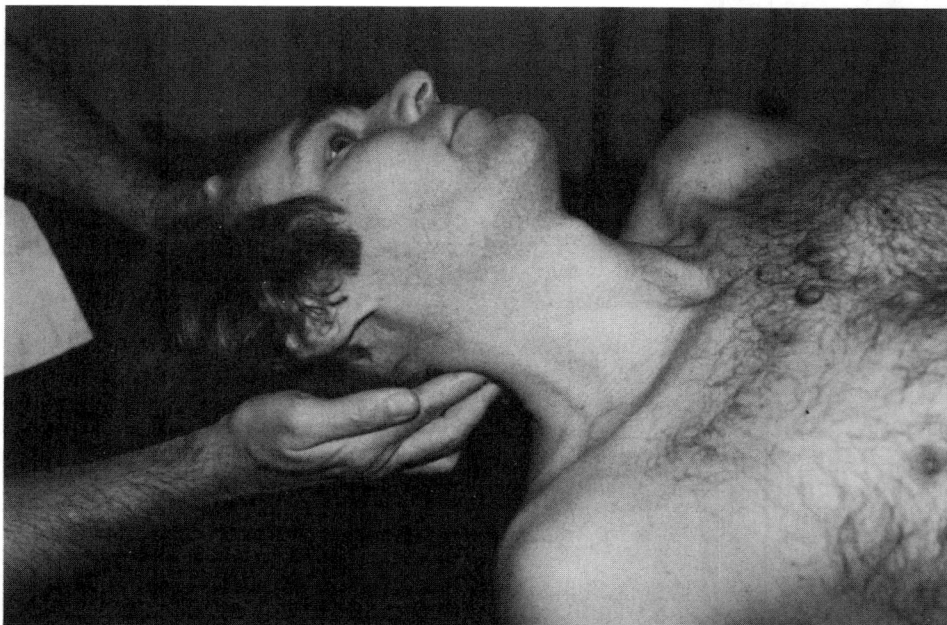

Figure 41.3. Release by positioning technique (counterstrain).

palpated by the right hand. In this position, the patient is instructed to exert an isometric contraction of either left sidebending or flexion for 3 to 5 seconds. Following the contraction and complete relaxation of the patient, the operator increases the amount of extension, right sidebending, and right rotation to the next motion barrier, and the patient is in-

structed to again provide a 3- to 5-second isometric contraction, either in the direction of left sidebending or flexion. This process is repeated from three to five times or until maximum motion is restored at the dysfunctional segment (Fig. 41.4).

High-velocity, low-amplitude technique (mobilization with impulse): To restore function to a typical cervical segment on the right side that resists extension, right sidebending, and right rotation, the operator places a contact point of the proximal interphalangeal or metacarpophalangeal joint on the pillar of the superior vertebra of the dysfunctional segment. The operator's left hand controls the position of the head on the neck, and the barrier of motion is engaged by sidebending the cervical spine to the right while rotating the head to the left at the upper cervical spine. When all slack motion is taken up by the position, the operator provides a thrust through contact with the right hand in the direction of the spinous process of T1. This results in increase of mobility in the directions of extension, right sidebending, and right rotation at the involved segment (Fig. 41.5).

Regardless of the manual medicine procedure to be applied, it should be appropriately prescribed to meet the requirements of the patient at that particular time.

PATIENT MANAGEMENT

Manual medicine procedures have been found to be clinically useful in headaches from a wide variety of causes (25). They need to be appropriately used in conjunction with regular medical treatment (26). They are most useful with tension/muscle-contraction headache and have a major contribution to vascular headache problems. Manual medicine procedures have little role in the traction/inflammatory (organic) group. Frequently, the structural diagnostic process alerts the clinician to serious organic pathology, when the biomechanical dysfunctions do not correlate with the rest of the history and physical findings.

Manual medicine can be used both to treat the acute attack and to prevent subsequent occurrences. The use of myofascial release and craniosacral technique in the early

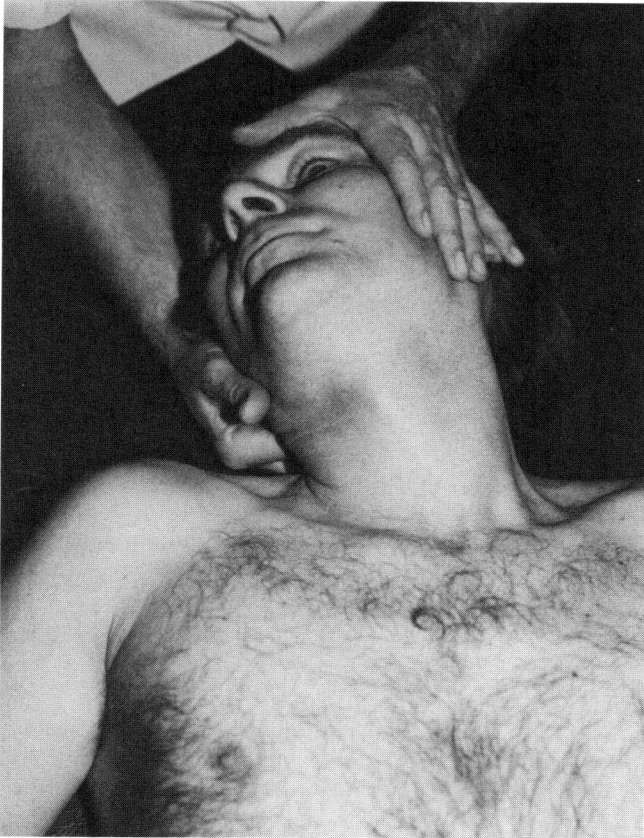

Figure 41.4. Muscle energy technique: postisometric relaxation.

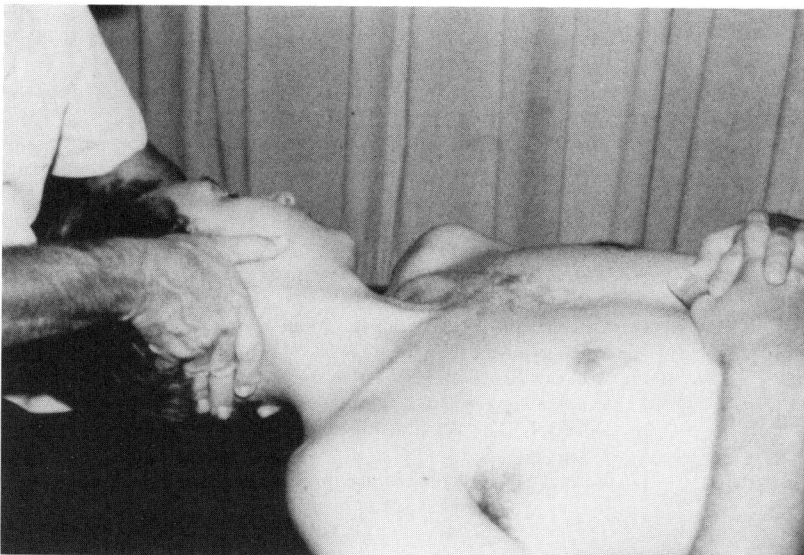

Figure 41.5. Mobilization with impulse technique (high-velocity, low-amplitude thrust).

phases of a migraine attack may effectively abort the attack (27–29). It is postulated that the mechanism of action is through restoration of more normal vasomotor tone. Soft tissue, myofascial release, release by positioning, and muscle energy technique have all been found to be useful in the management of the acute excerbation of the tension/ muscle-contraction headache syndrome. For prevention, it is useful to provide appropriate manual medicine to the entire musculoskeletal system enhancing musculoskeletal symmetry and postural balance. Used in conjunction with appropriate exercise programs, there appears to be a reduction in the adverse effects of muscle tension and tone.

When the clinician uses manual medicine, in addition to the regular medication program, occasionally, appropriate drug therapy is needed to cover the reactions to the manipulation/mobilization intervention. It is occasionally necessary to increase the nonsteroidal antiinflammatory medication to cover the posttreatment reaction occuring when initially addressing a chronic postural problem. It is seldom necessary to use specific muscle relaxants to cover the reaction to manual medicine; if it is necessary, Valium is most effective for this purpose.

Appropriately prescribed exercises are uniformly given to the patient to maintain the beneficial effect of the manual medicine. While a wide variety of exercise programs is available, the exercise principles useful in manual medicine are directed in a three-stage plan. The goal is to maximize and maintain the overall posture. The first phase is to assure balance capability. Exercises are prescribed to maximize proprioceptive balance with the eyes both open and closed. This assists in restoration of more normal muscle firing patterns within the musculoskeletal system. When this is achieved, the next phase is stretching all tight myofascial tissues to symmetry. A wide variety of stretching programs can be used, but symmetry is the goal, not necessarily maximum range. Once symmetry of length is achieved, then a strengthening program can be implemented, again with the goal of symmetrical strength in postural balance.

Complications and Contraindications

Complications of manual medicine procedures have their highest incidence in the cervical spine. The complications usually involve deleterious effects upon the vertebral basilar artery system. Most frequently, the complications follow high-velocity, low-amplitude thrust, but they have been reported for other procedures as well. The important element is for the clinician to recognize the unique anatomy of the vertebral basilar system and know what body positions put it at maximum risk. Normal vertebral arteries can be physiologically narrowed by marked extension and rotation of the head on the neck. In the presence of disease or a developmental variant to the vertebral artery system, the impact of extension and rotation is multiplied exponentially. Therefore, regardless of the technique

used, avoidance of marked extension and rotation of the head on the neck is appropriate. Obviously, in the presence of developmental variations (such as Down's syndrome) and organic disease (such as rheumatoid arthritis of the upper cervical spine), extreme caution must be used when employing any manual medicine procedure. As in all other phases of the practice of medicine, appropriate and complete diagnosis, followed by appropriate and complete treatment, should avoid complications from manual medicine procedures. Despite the severity of complications from manual medicine procedures, their frequency is still extremely low and compares favorably with the incidence of anaphylactic reaction to aspirin.

CONCLUSION

Manipulation and mobilization in the treatment of the patient suffering from headache can be most useful and effective when used in the context of total patient evaluation and care. Knowledge, skill, and experience in the field is necessary for its appropriate use. Whether given by the attending physician or prescribed for implementation by other clinical practitioners, an appropriate manipulative prescription needs to be identified. The manual medicine armamentarium is quite broad and must be specifically and appropriately applied.

REFERENCES

1. Schiotz EH, Cyriax J. Manipulation—past and present. London: Heinemann Medical Books, 1975.
2. Dvorak J, Dvorak V, Schneider W. Manual medicine 1984. Berlin: Springer-Verlag, 1984.
3. Fisk JW. Medical treatment of neck and back pain. Springfield, IL: Charles C Thomas, 1987:168–171.
4. Greenman, PE. Principles of manual medicine. Baltimore: Williams & Wilkins, 1989.
5. Maigne R. Orthopedic medicine. Springfield, IL: Charles C Thomas, 1972.
6. Mennell, J.McM. Back pain. Boston: Little, Brown & Co., 1960.
7. Schneider W, Dvorak J, Dvorak V, Tretschler. Manual medicine— therapy. Stuttgart: Georg Thieme Verlag, 1988.
8. Anderson CD, Franks RD. Migraine and tension headache: is there a physiological difference? Headache 1981;21:63–71.
9. Silberstein SD, Silberstein MM. New concepts in the pathogenesis of headache. Part I. Migraine versus tension-type headache. Pain Manage 1990;297–303.
10. Gallagher RM, Freitag FG. Muscle contraction headache: diagnosis and treatment. J Osteopath Med 1987;1(6):8–17.
11. Tfelt-Hansen P, Louis I, Olesen J. Prevalence and significance of muscle tenderness during common migraine attacks. Headache 1981;21:49–54.
12. Ward RC. Headache: an osteopathic perspective. J Am Osteopath Assoc 1982;81:458–469.
13. Magoun HI. Osteopathy in the cranial field. Kirksville, MO: Journal Printing Co., 1966.
14. Upledger JE, Vredevoogh JD. Management of autogenic headache. Osteopath Ann 1979;7:232–241.
15. Arbuckle BE. The cranio-cervical area. Ann Arbor: Yearbook American Academy of Osteopathy 1953;26–33.
16. Dove CI. The occipito-atlanto-axial complex. Manuelle Medizin 1982;20:11–15.
17. Vernon H. Chiropractic manipulative therapy in the treatment of

headaches: a retrospective and prospective study. J Manipulative Physiol Ther 1982;5:109–112.

18. Vernon HT. Spinal manipulation and headaches of cervical origin. J Manipulative Physiol Ther 1989;12:455–468.

19. Greenman PE. Lift therapy: use and abuse. J Am Osteopath Assoc 1979;79:238–350.

20. Greenman PE. Roetgen findings in the craniosacral mechanism. J Am Osteopath Assoc 1970;70:24–35.

21. Lewit K. The craniocervical syndrome. In: Lewit K, ed. Manipulative therapy in rehabilitation of the locomotor system. London: Butterworths, 1985(chap 7):322–325.

22. Dugan MC, Locke S, Gallagher JR. Occipital neuralgia in adolescents and young adults. N Engl J Med 1962;267:1166–1172.

23. Ng SY. Upper cervical vertebrae and occipital headache. J. Manipulative Physiol Ther 1980;3:137–141.

24. Lewit K. Pain arising in the posterior arch of the atlas. Eur Neurol 1977;16:263–269.

25. Hoyt WH, Shaffer F, Bard DA, Benesler JS, Blankenhorn GD, et al. Osteopathic manipulation in the treatment of muscle-contraction headache. J Am Osteopath Assoc 1979;78:322–325.

26. Solomon S, Elkind A, Freitag FG, Gallagher RM, Moore K, et al. Safety and efficacy of cranial electrotherapy in the treatment of tension headache. Headache 1989;29:445–450.

27. Beckwith CG. Migraine—physiopathology and manipulative treatment. Ann Arbor Yearbook American Academy of Osteopathy 1953;5–9.

28. Mountjoy MG. Migraine mitigated by manipulation. Clin Trends Osteopath Med 1977;4:1–3.

29. Vernon H. Vertebrogenic migraine. J Can Chiropract Assoc 1985;29:20–24.

42

Nerve Blocks and Invasive Therapies

ROGER S. CICALA and JEFFREY R. JERNIGAN

For the purposes of this chapter, invasive procedures are considered to be those that are performed percutaneously using a needle or trochar, without requiring a surgical incision to be made. Perhaps no subject in the headache literature has been met with more extreme points of view than that of invasive therapy. Some practitioners claim that there is no indication for invasive therapy in any headache patient. Others are so aggressive that invasive therapies become the mainstay of their headache management practice. As is so often the case when extremely opposed convictions are expressed, both sides have legitimate arguments and an intermediate approach is probably more realistic.

Invasive procedures should always be considered as one aspect of the overall multidisciplinary management of such patients and not a complete therapy by themselves. The use of invasive therapies for the treatment of patients with headache should be reserved for that minority of patients who both have a specific type of headache that is amenable to such therapy and have failed more conservative treatments. Invasive procedures are most likely to benefit patients whose diagnosis is in classifications XIV or XV of the National Institutes of Health classification of headache; that is, patients with cranial neuritides or neuralgias. These syndromes may involve the sensory cranial nerves (especially the trigeminal nerve), the autonomic nervous system, or the 2nd and 3rd cervical spinal nerves. Occasionally, patients with vascular or tension headaches may also benefit from some forms of invasive treatment.

Neural blockade with local anesthetics (perhaps containing corticosteroids) can be an invaluable aid for both diagnosis and treatment of these specific types of headache. Other invasive procedures such as neurolysis and gangliolysis have produced dramatic relief in carefully selected patients. It must be pointed out that some of these procedures require specialized equipment that may not be readily available. Fluoroscopy is usually required to accurately place needles near the proper structures. In many cases, these procedures are best performed in the surgery suite, since heavy sedation (or even general anesthesia) may be necessary.

Patients must be carefully informed of the expected benefits and risks involved prior to performing invasive procedures. Far too often, the term "nerve block" has a magical connotation. Patients and even some practitioners wrongly assume that permanent total relief of pain will be obtained by such a procedure. The effects and side effects of these procedures vary greatly, depending on the specific nerve or ganglion injected and the type of agent used.

OCCIPITAL AND CERVICAL NEURALGIA
Anatomy

The greater occipital nerve is the largest purely afferent nerve in the body (1), innervating the posterior skull from the suboccipital area to the vertex. It is formed from the posterior division of the 2nd cranial nerve. Within the substantia gelatinosa of the spinal cord, the afferent fibers from this nerve lie in close approximation to the nucleus and spinal tract of the trigeminal nerve (2–4). Rather than exiting through a discrete spinal foramen, the nerve leaves the bony spinal column between the arch of the atlas and axis. It travels inferolaterally toward the area of the C2-3 zygapophyseal (facet) joint and then curves around the inferior oblique capitis muscle to ascend toward the occiput deep to the semispinalis capitis muscle. It pierces either through the tendinous insertion of the trapezius muscle (5) or between the trapezius and semispinalis muscle (6, 7) to reach the subcutaneous tissue of the occipital area. The site of perforation through these muscles is located just medial to the occipital artery (Fig. 42.1).

The lesser occipital nerve forms from the anterior divisions of the 2nd and 3rd cervical nerves. It ascends along the posterior margin of the sternocleidomastoid muscle and provides sensory fibers to the area of the scalp lateral to the greater occipital nerve (Fig. 42.1).

Pathophysiology

While most practitioners agree that greater occipital neuralgia is a common cause of posterior headaches, the condition has received limited attention in the literature and is frequently neglected as part of the differential diagnosis of headache. In one series of 92 patients successfully treated for occipital neuralgia, the diagnosis had previously been considered in fewer than 5% of patients (3).

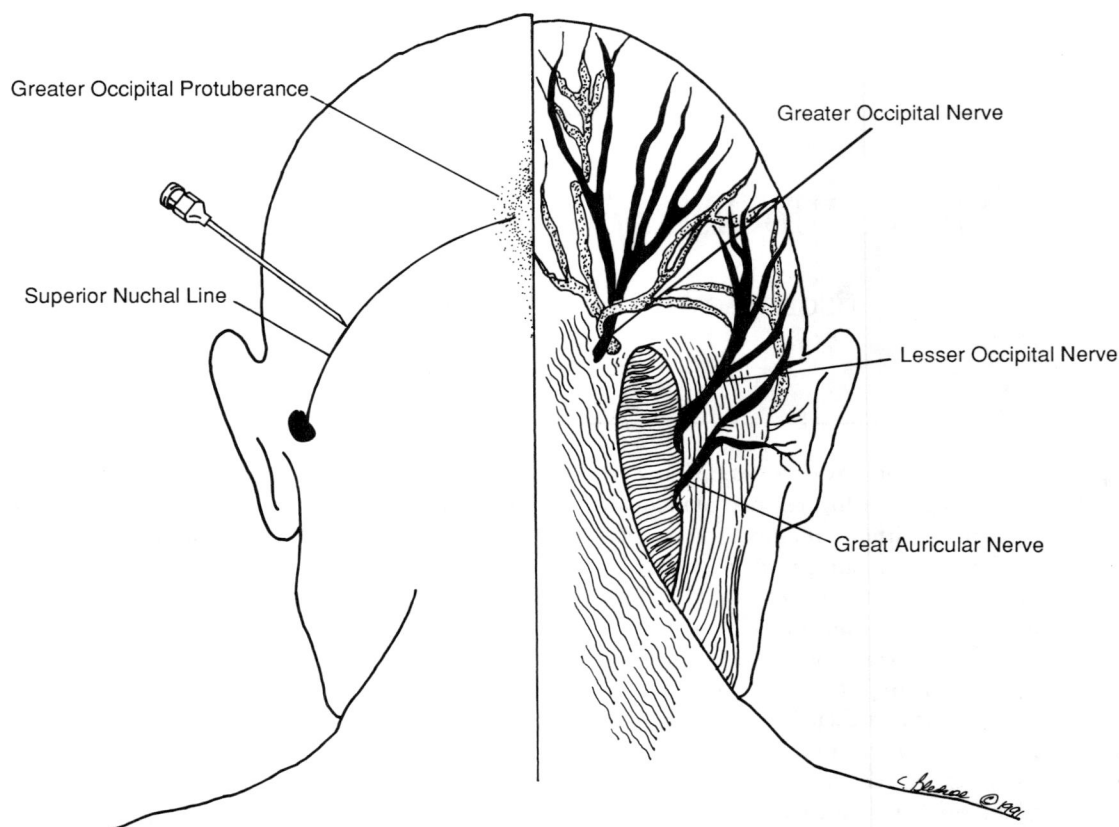

Figure 42.1. The distal course of the *greater occipital nerve*. When injecting the nerve at this location, the needle should be inserted just medial to the palpation of the occipital artery at the *superior nuchal line*. At this location the nerve and artery are in close approximation.

There is much argument about the causes of occipital neuralgia. The mechanism originally proposed by Hunter and Mayfield (8) was entrapment of the occipital nerve between the posterior arch of the atlas and the lamina of the axis, but this has been proven to be anatomically inaccurate by several authors (5–7). The occipital nerve would appear to be particularly vulnerable to traumatic injury, since it rests upon the arch of the axis and atlas rather than passing laterally through a vertebral foramen. However, occipital neuralgia secondary to direct injury to the nerve itself is probably rare (9). Entrapment neuropathy is much more common and may occur in either of two areas. The first location is near the origin of the nerve root as it exits the spine, where entrapment may occur by compression of the nerve root either as it turns around the inferior oblique capitis muscle or as it passes near the C2-3 facet joint (10). Compression at this location is usually associated with degenerative disease of the C2 facet joint, which is best visualized by open-mouth cervical radiographs or by bone scan (11, 12). Additionally, abnormally tight connections between the occiput and the atlas have been described in some patients (13). Such immobility of the occipitolatlantoid joint causes a secondary hypermobility of the C1-C2 joint on flexion of the cervical spine. This may cause irritation of the occipital nerve at this level,

secondary to chronic stretching of the nerve when the neck is flexed. While such patients will appear to have normal cervical spines radiographically, if flexion views are obtained the lack of occipital-atlas movement and hypermobility of C1-C2 will become apparent (13).

The second area in which the occipital nerve may become compressed is in the suboccipital region. Because of the tortuous course of the nerve through the various muscles of the suboccipital area, it may be compressed and irritated by any condition that causes spasm of these muscles. Since somatic efferent innervation to these muscle groups is supplied by the posterior rami of the third to sixth cervical nerve roots, any condition that irritates these nerves (such as a ruptured cervical disc, cervical spondylosis, or scalenus anticus syndrome) may initiate muscle spasms that cause a secondary occipital neuralgia (1).

Diagnosis

The first modern description of occipital neuralgia was provided by Hunter and Mayfield (8) in 1949, and their description remains valid today. Patients with occipital neuralgia usually complain of suboccipital pain that radiates to the back of the head and occasionally down the back of the neck. Often, patients can give a clear description of pain radiating in the distribution of one of the greater occipital nerves to the vertex of the skull. Retroorbital radiation of pain often occurs during severe episodes, apparently because of the close proximity of the afferent connections of the occipital nerve with the spinal nucleus of the trigeminal nerve (4). Secondary radiations to the temporal areas are also common. The pain may be bilateral, but usually one side predominates. Attacks are usually intermittent, but last for up to several days at a time. They may be initiated by sustained awkward positioning of the head and neck, which might occur during prolonged reading or sleeping in an abnormal position (14). Palpation or percussion over the course of the occipital nerve will usually exacerbate symptoms and may even initiate a headache in patients who are temporarily asymptomatic. Occasionally, there is hypesthesia or dysesthesia in the distribution of the occipital nerve. Occipital neuralgia can be extremely difficult to differentiate from muscle-tension headache, headache caused by myofascial trigger points (15), and even vascular headaches. Diagnostic nerve blocks with local anesthetic may be required to obtain a definitive diagnosis.

Entrapment of the nerve near the cervical spine should result in increased symptoms during extension or rotation of the head and neck. Compression of the skull on the neck (Spurling maneuver), especially with extension and rotation of the neck to the affected side, may reproduce or increase the patient's pain if cervical degenerative disease is the cause of the neuralgia. Pressure over both the occipital nerve at the superior nuchal line and near the C2-C3 facet joints should cause an exacerbation of pain in such patients (4), at least when the headache is present. Often, a previous history of cervical or occipital trauma or of arthritic disease of the cervical spine is obtained (4, 14). Cervical radiographs with an open-mouth view to evaluate the C2 facet joints, and flexion views to determine if hypermobility of C1-C2 is present may help determine the cause of the nerve entrapment.

Entrapment of the nerve as it passes through the tendinous insertion of the trapezius muscle on the skull is less likely to exacerbate symptoms during extension or compression of the head on the neck, and more likely to demonstrate symptomatology during flexion of the neck and on palpation of the nerve at the superior nuchal line (5). Even if the actual pathology is in the cervical spine, tenderness over the occipital nerve at the superior nuchal line is usually present (12). This is of prognostic importance when attempting to determine where a nerve block should be performed.

Procedures

Local anesthetic nerve blocks are valuable, both as an aid to diagnosis and as a treatment in themselves. The location of compression of the nerve must be determined accurately to properly select the type of procedure that should be performed. If the entrapment is in the suboccipital muscle groups, a classic occipital nerve block should be performed. If the cause of the occipital neuralgia is compression by degenerative changes in the cervical spine, occipital nerve blocks will be of limited value. In such cases, cervical facet injections (16) or cervical epidural steroid injections (17) may provide superior relief. When hypertrophic facet joints are present at C2 without diffuse degenerative disease of the cervical spine, a cervical facet injection is more likely to give relief. When diffuse cervical degenerative disease is present, a cervical epidural injection may provide superior benefit.

Classic occipital nerve block is performed using a small (22- to 25-gauge) needle. The occipital nerves exit through the tendinous muscular insertions at the base of the skull and are located approximately 3 cm lateral to the occipital protuberance. Careful palpation at this location along the superior nuchal line will usually elicit distinct tenderness, localizing the nerve. The pulsation of the occipital artery can usually be palpated in this area and serves as an additional landmark, since the nerve is located just medial to it. Care should be taken not to direct the needle medially, or inadvertant dural puncture could occur. Careful aspiration and injection of a 1-ml test dose should be performed to ensure both that the subarachnoid space has not been entered and that the occipital artery has not been punctured. The injection of 6 to 10 ml of 0.25% bupivacaine in this area will effectively anesthetize the nerve within a few minutes. We recommend depositing the agent deep to the facial aponeurosis of the trapezius muscle, since theoretically this is the site of potential nerve irritation. Following occipital nerve block, posterior headache pain is relieved within minutes. Radiating retroorbital pain may not resolve for an additional 15 minutes or more, however (1). Pain relief consistently outlasts the duration of action of the local anesthetic, as might be expected with a spasm-pain-spasm cycle. The addition of a long-acting corticosteroid agent such as 40 mg of Depo-medrol (Upjohn Co, Kalamazoo, Michigan) to the local anesthetic should theoretically decrease any inflammatory changes at this location and is advocated by most practitioners (3). However, we know of no controlled studies that demonstrate additional benefit from including corticosteroids in occipital nerve blocks.

Cervical facet injections may be performed using either a lateral or a posterolateral approach. Excellent descriptions of the lateral approach are available in many texts, but we prefer the posterolateral approach for several reasons. Using this approach, the vertebral artery is less likely to be punctured, avoiding a potentially catastrophic intraarterial injection or the development of a deep cervical hematoma. The posterolateral approach would also seem more appropriate for patients with occipital neuralgia, since it would place the agent in the vicinity of the occipital nerve near the atlantoaxial joint and the inferior oblique capitis muscle. Additionally, in our experience, patients have less pain both during and following the procedure when the posterolateral approach is used.

The posterolateral cervical facet injection is performed by inserting a 22-gauge B-bevel needle at the lateral margin of the thick paracervical musculature. The needle should be directed slightly caudad, to minimize the chance of entering the spinal canal. The needle is advanced anteriorly and slightly medially until the lamina of the cervical vertebra is reached and then "walked" caudally and laterally until the facet joint is encountered. Radiographic visualization is useful to confirm proper position at the facet joint, but is not absolutely required. It has been our practice to inject both the C1-C2 and the C2-C3 joints on the affected side, but again, there are no studies to confirm the necessity of injecting both areas. Usually, pain relief is obtained within 5 to 7 minutes following the injection of 2 to 4 ml of 0.25% bupivacaine containing 20 to 40 mg of Depo-medrol into the affected joint.

Cervical epidural steroid injections may be the most efficacious therapy for patients with degenerative disease of the cervical spine causing occipital headache (17) and may also relieve the pain of refractory muscle-tension headache (18). Cervical epidural injections are best performed at the C7-T1 interspace, since the epidural space is larger at this level than at more cephalad levels (19). A midline approach is recommended because the epidural space is thicker in the midline. The procedure may be performed with the patient sitting, but we prefer to place the patient prone, with the chest supported on 1 or 2 pillows and the neck flexed forward. With the patient in this position, a 17- or 18-gauge blunt epidural needle is inserted between the C7 and T1 spinous processes and directed 10 to 20° cephalad. Entrance into the epidural space may be confirmed with either a hanging drop or loss of resistance technique. The injection of 10 ml of 0.5% lidocaine containing 1 mg/kg of Depo-medrol will spread sufficiently to reach the C2 level. While the usual complications of epidural injection (including inadvertant dural puncture, nerve irritation, or actual nerve damage, and infection) can occur, they do not appear to be more common with cervical than with lumbar epidural injections (20, 21).

When patients do not respond with at least temporary symptomatic relief to properly performed local anesthetic blocks, the diagnosis of occipital neuralgia should be discarded and an alternative diagnosis explored. In cases in which the headaches are episodic, intermittent local anesthetic blocks can totally abort the pain, often providing prolonged relief. Patients who report continuous discomfort are unlikely to benefit from a single procedure for more than a week or so (4). Overall, approximately 50% of patients with occipital neuralgia will obtain relief with occipital nerve block therapy alone (1). However, most patients with classic occipital neuralgia also demonstrate high levels of anxiety and stress on psychological profiles (2), and these factors must be addressed. Even in these cases, the use of occipital nerve injections to provide temporary relief while psychotherapy is undertaken, oral medications become effective, and other factors are addressed can certainly be beneficial.

Neurolytic blocks using alcohol or other agents should not be performed near the occipital nerve because of the likelihood of developing deafferentation neuralgia (3, 22); however, cryoneurolysis (freeze destruction) of the occipital nerve has been used effectively (23). For maximum effectiveness, cryoneurolysis requires surgical exposure of the occipital nerve.

TRIGEMINAL NEURALGIA

Anatomy

The trigeminal nerve (cranial nerve V) originates from the ventrolateral surface of the pons and passes through the temporal bone. The nerve expands in the trigeminal cistern prior to exiting the skull, forming the gasserian ganglion in which the cell bodies of sensory nerve fibers are located. The three main divisions of the trigeminal nerve exit the skull shortly after leaving the gasserian ganglion. The ophthalmic nerve exits through the lateral wall of the cavernous sinus and the superior orbital fissure. It provides purely sensory fibers to the globe, the mucosa of the sinuses and nose, and the skin of the forehead and periorbital areas. The maxillary nerve exits through the foramen rotundum and provides sensory fibers to the face, nasopharynx, and maxillary gums and teeth. The mandibular nerve exits through the foramen ovale and is both motor and sensory. Sensory fibers from this nerve innervate the mandibular skin, gums, and teeth as well as the internal auditory meatus.

Pathophysiology

Trigeminal neuralgia (tic douloureux) is characterized by paroxysms of severe lancinating pain in the distribution of the fifth cranial nerve, often triggered by nonnoxious stimuli. Any branch of the trigeminal nerve may be involved, but the pain most often occurs in the distribution of the maxillary branch. Stimuli that trigger painful paroxysms may be initiated in areas of the face other than the affected division. Chewing, temperature change, or light touch are common triggers of painful attacks. There is little or no sensory deficit associated with the condition, and pain-free intervals usually occur. Trigeminal neuralgia usually presents in the 5th to 7th decades of life and affects females (60%) somewhat more frequently than males (22). Atypical facial pain can be differentiated from typical trigeminal neuralgia on the basis of several characteristics. Atypical facial pain may be bilateral, often occurs in younger patients, may be constant, and usually is not triggered by afferent stimuli.

The most common cause of trigeminal neuralgia is vascular compression of the intracranial portion of the trigeminal nerve (24). Degenerative arterial elongation and atherosclerosis cause blood vessels in close proximity to the trigeminal nerve to compress the root entry zones of the nerve itself. Various patterns of vascular compression have been described and have been shown to correlate with different presentations of the syndrome (25). The superior cerebellar artery is most commonly involved in this process, although other vessels (including the anterior and posterior cerebellar arteries and even some veins) have also been reported to cause trigeminal compression (26). Nonvascular pathology, such as compression from tumors (27) or demyelination secondary to multiple sclerosis (28), has also been demonstrated to cause tic douloureux. For a more thorough discussion of the symptomatology and pathophysiology of trigeminal neuralgia see Chapter 31.

Procedures

Primary medical therapy for trigeminal neuralgia is usually successful to some degree and should be thoroughly explored before invasive therapy is undertaken. Definitive therapy can be provided by surgical microvascular decompression of the trigeminal nerve root, but many patients with the condition are poor surgical candidates because of their age and other factors. Percutaneous invasive procedures are appropriate for patients who have failed medical therapy and who are poor surgical candidates.

Local anesthetic blockade is useful as a diagnostic tool, to demonstrate the expected effects of neurolytic procedures to the patient, and occasionally to provide palliation until oral medications become effective. Many approaches to injection of the gasserian ganglion have been described, but the most widely used is the anterolateral transcutaneous approach. A 10-cm 22-gauge needle is inserted 2 to 3 cm lateral to the corner of the mouth, at the level of the second upper molar (Fig. 42.2). It is advanced superiorly and posteriorly at an angle that will pass beneath the midpoint of the zygomatic arch, while at the same time it is also directed medially at an angle that points toward the pupil of the ipsilateral eye. At a depth of 6 to 7 cm, the needle point will come in contact with the infratemporal plate. The needle is then withdrawn about 1 cm, redirected slightly more posteriorly, and advanced an additional centimeter. At this point it should pass through the foramen ovale (which can be confirmed radiographically) and lie in close proximity to the gasserian ganglion. The injection of 2 ml of local anesthetic is sufficient to provide temporary anesthesia of the trigeminal nerve. It must always be remembered that inadvertant dural puncture and subarachnoid injection into the cranium is possible when performing gasserian ganglion block. Hematoma may occur from accidental puncture of the maxillary artery. Additionally, in 4% of humans the foramen ovale is fused with the foramen lacerum, which would predispose to puncture of the carotid artery. In cases where carotid artery puncture has occurred, the creation of carotid-cavernous sinus fistulas has been reported (29).

Both 90% ethyl alcohol (30, 31) and 5% pheno (32) in

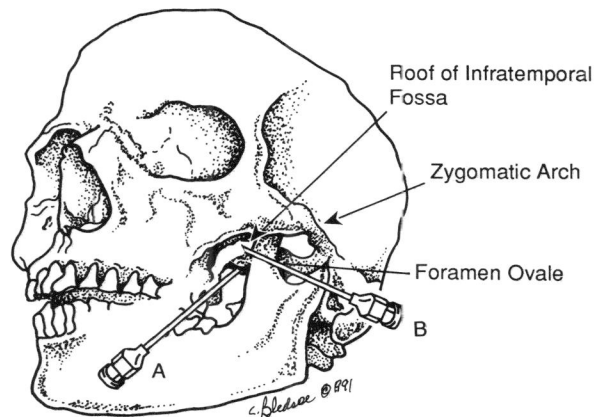

Figure 42.2. The general location and approach for performing injections of the gasserian ganglion (*A*) and the sphenopalatine ganglion (*B*).

small volumes (0.2 to 0.3 ml) have been injected in the same location to provide a more permanent neurolytic block of the gasserian ganglion. Very careful aspiration for cerebrospinal fluid must be performed when injecting neurolytic agents, since paresis of other cranial nerves has been reported following accidental subarachnoid injection. Approximately 70% of patients obtain long-term relief following chemical neurolysis, but major complications frequently occur following the procedure. Sensory deficits in one or more branches of the trigeminal nerve are to be expected, although their severity may be quite variable. Corneal anesthesia is particularly bothersome and leads to keratitis with corneal ulceration in up to 5% of patients (30). As with other procedures causing partial destruction of the trigeminal nerve, anesthesia dolorosa (deafferentation pain of the trigeminal nerve) may also occur. This complication is particularly devastating, and patients who develop it universally suffer pain that is more severe than that of tic douloureux. Because of the frequency with which such complications occur, alcohol and phenol neurolysis of the trigeminal nerve has generally been replaced by other therapeutic modalities for the treatment of tic douloureux.

Using the same approach described above, further advancement of the needle through the foramen ovale will result in puncture of the trigeminal cistern, with free flow of cerbrospinal fluid. Pure glycerol may be injected to fill the trigeminal cistern, causing neurolysis of the gasserian ganglion and its central rootlets (percutaneous retrogasserian glycerol rhizolysis or PRGR) (33, 34). The procedure must be performed with the patient in a sitting position and the neck flexed, to allow the hyperbaric glycerol to pool in the cistern. Radiography with the injection of contrast media for confirmation of needle placement should be performed before the actual injection of glycerol is made. Since the trigeminal cistern contains only about 0.6 ml of CSF (35), the total volume of injectate required is usually quite small. The injection is usually performed in

0.05-ml increments. Following each incremental injection, paresthesias are assessed until the patient perceives a sensory loss in the affected area. An average total injection of 0.2 to 0.4 ml is required (34, 35). It has been claimed that this procedure causes less severe sensory losses than either peripheral neurolytic blocks or thermocoagulation lesions (36). Nevertheless, some authors have reported that uncomfortable sensory deficits occur in over 1/3 of patients treated with PRGR (37–39) (Table 42.1). Severe reactions have been reported if any glycerol accidentally flows out of the trigeminal cistern (37). Additionally, hypertension, tachycardia, and possible coronary vasospasm have been reported to occur during the procedure (40).

A high rate of pain recurrence has been reported following PRGR by some authors (41), while others find recurrence no more likely than following other forms of trigeminal neurolysis. In a very well controlled study, North et al. (42) determined that a long-term successful outcome following PRGR was more likely in patients who had a positive response to carbamazepine, in female patients,

and if good CSF return was obtained at the time of the procedure. Patients with atypical facial neuralgia and those who had some cluster symptoms had lower success rates, and their symptoms tended to recur earlier than those of patients with classic trigeminal neuralgia (42).

The use of radiofrequency electrodes to produce thermal lesions of the ganglion and nerve rootlets is an alternative therapy for patients with tic douloureux (43, 44). Since the smaller unmyelinated nerve fibers associated with pain transmission are more sensitive to thermal lesions, it was initially hoped that selective destruction of these fibers might be obtained while motor and sensory functions were preserved (45, 46). Clinically, however, sensory loss in the distribution of pain usually occurs. In fact, the presence of a sensory loss in the affected area correlates well with successful long-term results (47). For this reason, the usual practice is to attempt to produce a localized sensory deficit in the division(s) of the trigeminal nerve affected by the neuralgia (44). Since the central rootlets of the ganglion are arranged with the fibers of the third division most lateral

Table 42.1.
Results of Various Percutaneous Procedures for Trigemina Neuralgia

Author (Date)	No. of Patients	Initial Success	Recurrence	Complications
Retrogasserian glycerol injection				
Sweet (1985)	77	83%	22%	Dysesthesia (37%) Corneal anesthesia (9%)
Spaziante (1987)	50	94%	24%	Zoster (78%) Corneal anesthesia (6%)
Sweet (1981)	27	89%	NA	Corneal anesthesia (18.5%) Dysesthesia (18.5%)
North (1990)	85	90 + %	2-year av	Corneal anesthesia (3%) Dysesthesia (4%)
Saini (1987)	469	NA	41% 2 year	Dysesthesia (13.5%) Anesthesia dolorosa (5%) Keratitis (5%) Paresis (3.4%) Zoster (3%)
Fujimaki (1990)	122	90 + %	60%	Dysesthesia (29%) Anesthesia dolorosa (3%)
Radiofrequency neurolysis				
Fraioli (1989)	533	97%	10%	Dysesthesia (17%) Keratitis (2%) Anesthesia dolorosa (1.5%) Paresis (3%)
Piquer (1987)	98	68%	46%	Corneal anesthesia (19%) Corneal keratitis (3%) Anesthesia dolorosa (2%)
Broggi (1990)	1000	95%	18%	Paresis (11%) Dysesthesia (5%) Anesthesia dolorosa (1.5%) Corneal anesthesia (19%)
Siegfried (1977)	500	98%	6%	Corneal anesthesia (3.6%) Keratitis (1%) Anesthesia dolorosa (0.3%) Paresis (15%)
Balloon microcompression				
Fraioli (1989)	159	90%	10%	Dysesthesia (7%) Anesthesia dolorosa (0.6%)
Lichtor (1990)	100	97%	17% at 5 years	Dysesthesia (2%)
Lobato (1990)	144	94%	10%	Zoster (11%) Hematoma (3%) Dysesthesia (19%)
Meglio (1987)	47	91.5%	42%	Dysesthesia (8.5%) Paresis (4.2%)

and inferior and those of the first division most medial and superior, selective lesions can usually be produced with a fair degree of accuracy. Once the proper location is reached (determined by paresthesia produced by a stimulating current), a thermal lesion is produced at about 60°C for 60 seconds. Hypesthesia following the production of this lesion is assessed, and if it appears to overlap the zone of neuralgia properly, the thermocoagulation is repeated at 70 to 80°C. Higher-temperature lesions are associated with a denser sensory loss but a lower incidence of recurrence (48, 49). Although excellent initial results and low incidences of recurrence have been obtained with this method (50), some persistent sensory loss is generally present, and residual corneal anesthesia occurs in 5% of cases (46). Anesthesia dolorosa has been reported to occur in as many as 12% of patients (51), although most series report a much lower frequency (Table 42.1). As with glycerol injection, hypertension and tachycardia often accompany the production of the lesion in the gasserian ganglion (52). Pretreatment with an anticholinergic agent is recommended prior to performing thermocoagulation, since bradycardia and asystole have also been reported to occur in some cases (52).

Percutaneous balloon microcompression of the gasserian ganglion has also been described as an effective treatment for tic douloureux (53, 54). For this technique, a large needle (14-gauge) or trochar is introduced in the same manner as for PRGR. A number 4 Fogarty catheter is passed through the needle, and the balloon is inflated with 0.7 to 1 ml of fluid to a pressure of 1200 mm of Hg for 1 minute (55), compressing the ganglion. Initial success rates are comparable to those seen with glycerol injection and thermocoagulation (53–55). This procedure also appears to result in less sensory loss than do the other procedures (54, 55). Recurrence rates following balloon microcompression are similar or slightly higher than those for the other procedures (56) (Table 42.1), but the incidence of untoward side effects, especially dysesthesia and anesthesia dolorosa, is quite low (57). As with the other procedures involving the gasserian ganglion, hypertension and bradycardia occur commonly during balloon compression (58), and an anticholinergic should usually be administered prior to performing the procedure.

Thermocoagulation, glycerol injection, and balloon microcompression make up the bulk of percutaneous procedures currently performed for the treatment of trigeminal neuralgia. Fraioli et al. recently compared the results of these procedures over a 10-year period and recommended a protocol for their use (41). Because of their low incidence of associated sensory loss, PRGR and balloon microcompression were recommended as the first choice for most patients with trigeminal neuralgia who have failed conservative therapy. Of the two, balloon compression had a higher overall initial success rate and seemed both easier and safer for less-experienced practitioners to perform. For this reason, they recommended that microcompression

should be the initial treatment for most patients with trigeminal neuralgia refractory to medical therapy. PRGR was considered to be an acceptable alternative therapy. If microcompression or PRGR was unsuccessful, radiofrequency thermocoagulation could often give beneficial results (59). Patients with trigeminal neuralgia caused by extrinsic compression from tumors, those with trigeminal neuralgia secondary to multiple sclerosis, and patients with other atypical presentations of trigeminal neuralgia were less likely to improve with balloon compression and glycerol injection and more likely to require radiofrequency coagulation of the gasserian ganglion (41, 42). Additionally, patients with trigeminal neuralgia involving the 3rd division are more likely to require thermocoagulation.

Percutaneous placement of electrical stimulating devices near the gasserian ganglion has also been attempted as a treatment for both trigeminal neuralgia and anesthesia dolorosa (60). Techniques of percutaneous insertion of electrical stimulation devices near the gasserian ganglion have been developed, but the procedure has generally yielded poor results (61).

SPHENOPALATINE NEURALGIA AND CLUSTER HEADACHES
Anatomy

The sphenopalatine ganglion (also known as the pterygopalatine ganglion) is the largest collection of neurons located in the head, with the exception of the brain itself (62). The ganglion is approximately 5 mm in length and is located in the pterygopalatine fossa 2 to 3 mm inferior to the maxillary nerve (Fig. 42.3). The pterygopalatine fossa is located in the lateral wall of the nasopharynx, directly posterior to the middle turbinate. The ganglion is readily accessible to therapeutic intervention from the nasopharynx, since it is separated from it only by the nasal mucosa.

The sphenopalatine ganglion contains both sympathetic and parasympathetic fibers. Postganglionic sympathetic fibers from the carotid plexus form the deep petrosal nerve, which joins the greater petrosal nerve to form the nerve of the pterygoid canal (vidian nerve). The sympathetic fibers pass through the sphenopalatine ganglion without synapsing and innervate the pharynx, nasal cavity, palate, and lacrimal glands. Preganglionic parasympathetic fibers leave the brain via the nervus intermedius of the facial nerve and pass through the geniculate ganglion, greater petrosal nerve, and the nerve of the pterygoid canal to synapse in the sphenopalatine ganglion (Fig. 42.3). The sphenopalatine branches of the maxillary nerve (pterygopalatine nerves) are two short trunks connecting the ganglion with the maxillary nerve. These nerves contain primarily somatic afferents that do not synapse within the ganglion, but rather are distributed with the peripheral nerves that leave the ganglion (63). Additionally, postgan-

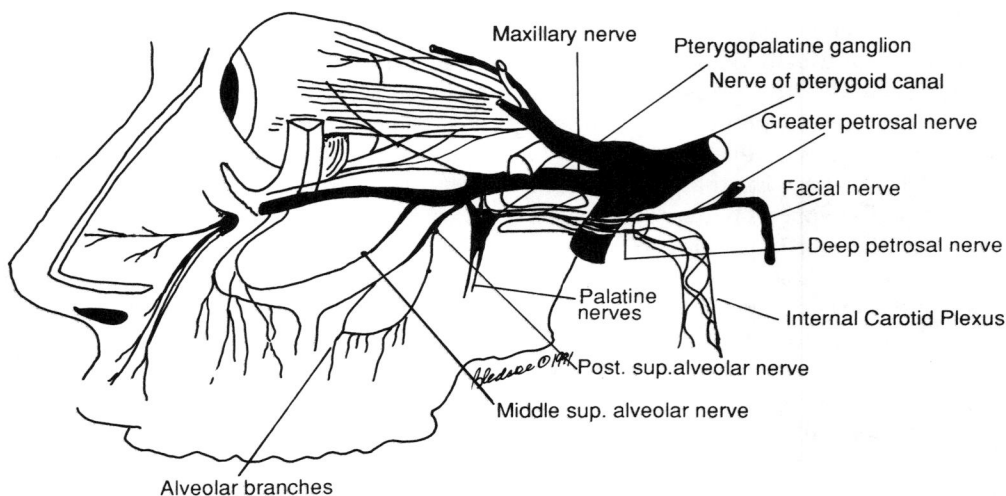

Figure 42.3. The location of the sphenopalatine ganglion and related structures.

glionic parasympathetic fibers from the sphenopalatine ganglion pass through the sphenopalatine branches of the maxillary nerve and are distributed along the peripheral branches of the maxillary nerve. The greater and lesser palatine nerves and the pharyngeal branch of pterygopalatine ganglion are the major peripheral nerves from the sphenopalatine ganglion. In summary, fibers from the ganglion supply sympathetic and parasympathetic innervation (as well as some somatic afferent fibers) to most of the mucous membranes of the pharynx, face, and lacrimal gland.

Clinical Symptoms

Sphenopalatine neuralgia was first described in 1908 by Sluder (64) and again in 1932 by Vail (65), who termed it "vidian nerve neuralgia." The pain of sphenopalatine neuralgia is usually described as burning and aching. It is usually most intense in the periorbital and retroorbital regions but may radiate to the temple, maxilla, and upper gum. Rhinorrhea, lacrimation, and injection of the conjunctiva on the affected side are commonly present during the headache (66). As with cluster headache, ethanol intake and marked ambient temperature changes are considered to be precipitating factors. The symptoms usually begin in the 3rd to 5th decades of life and are more common in females than in males (67).

Sphenopalatine neuralgia certainly accounts for some undiagnosed cases of atypical facial neuralgia and may also be misdiagnosed as a cluster or tension headache. Clinically, the symptoms produced by sphenopalatine neuralgia and cluster headache can be quite similar, and indeed, some authors have claimed that the conditions are interrelated (66). Sphenopalatine neuralgia can usually be differentiated from cluster headache, because of several distinguishing characteristics (67). Headaches associated with sphenopalatine neuralgia tend to be longer, lasting hours to days, and are almost always associated with symptoms of

parasympathetic activity, such as lacrimation and rhinorrhea on the affected side. The pain associated with sphenopalatine neuralgia is usually described as "burning and aching," while that of cluster headache tends to be expressed as "stabbing, tearing, or shooting." Sphenopalatine neuralgia is more common in females; cluster headache is more common in males.

Procedures

Definitive diagnosis of sphenopalatine neuralgia can be made by performing a local anesthetic block of the ganglion. Because of the ganglion's submucosal location, this can easily be accomplished using local anesthetic applied in the nasopharynx over the surface of the ganglion (68). Actual injections of local anesthetic into the sphenopalatine fossa are not necessary for this purpose. A topical anesthetic (4% lidocaine or benzocaine is effective) is first sprayed into the nostril to anesthetize the nasal mucosa over the turbinates. Cotton-tipped applicators saturated with local anesthetic solutions (2% lidocaine is commonly used) are then advanced along the superior border of the middle turbinate, until they reach the area just posterior to the turbinate. They are left in place against the mucosa for 15 to 20 minutes. Alternatively, two applicators may be used, one placed above and one below the posterior end of the middle turbinate. Because of the benign nature of the treatment, it is appropriate for diagnostic purposes, even in cases of probable migraine or cluster headaches, in which it is only occasionally effective. If the treatment is effective, it may be repeated as needed to abort headaches. The side effects of this procedure are limited to epistaxis and occasional cases of temporary orthostatic hypotension.

Neurodestructive procedures of the sphenopalatine ganglion require actual injection into the pterygopalatine fossa. At least 3 techniques for the injection of the sphenopalatine ganglion have been described. The intranasal route of injection was originally described by Sluder (64).

After topical anesthesia of the nasal mucosa, a long (8 to 10 cm) 22-gauge needle is passed through the middle turbinate and directed posteriorly, cephalad, and slightly laterally until bony contact is made (69). The bony wall of the sphenomaxillary fossa is then pierced, and 1 to 2 ml of solution injected. Because this technique is usually quite painful and also may result in profuse bleeding, it is rarely used today.

The ganglion may also be reached via the posterior palate. This approach to the sphenopalatine ganglion requires the use of an angled needle introduced through the posterior palatine foramen into the pterygopalatine canal (68). This foramen is located two-thirds of the distance between the midline of the mouth and the last molar tooth. The needle is advanced cephalad until paresthesias are obtained. Two to 3 ml of local anesthetic are then deposited at this location. This technique may damage the greater palatine nerve, and it requires a great deal of experience to perform successfully.

Most commonly, the extraoral route of injection is used. The procedure is quite similar to that used for maxillary nerve injections (Fig. 42.2). A 22- or 20-gauge spinal needle is usually introduced percutaneously beneath the most prominent portion of the zygoma, perpendicular to the skin, and advanced until the lateral pterygoid plate is reached. Under fluoroscopic imaging the needle is then "walked" cephalad until the pterygopalatine fossa is reached. Paresthesias in the distribution of the maxillary nerve are usually obtained.

The injection of 1 to 2 ml of absolute alcohol or 6% phenol into the pterygopalatine fossa has been reported to destroy the spehnopalatine ganglion and to effectively relieve severe refractory cases of sphenopalatine neuralgia (66). Hypesthesia in the distribution of the maxillary nerve and decreased lacrimation on the affected side are to be expected for variable lengths of time following destruction of the sphenopalatine ganglion. The technique has been reported to be safe (67), but because the maxillary nerve and artery lie in close approximation to the sphenopalatine ganglion, severe complications could occur.

Recently, radiofrequency thermocoagulation of the sphenopalatine ganglion has been reported to be as effective as chemical neurolysis (70). Because of the potential complications associated with the injection of neurolytic chemicals, radiofrequency thermocoagulation of the ganglion should offer superior margins of safety (70). Thermocoagulation at 60 to 65°C for 60 seconds is effective (70). Placement of radiofrequency electrodes for thermocoagulation is performed in the same manner as neurolytic block. Cryoneurolysis (percutaneous freezing) has also been used to successfully destroy the sphenopalatine ganglion (23). Because of the larger size of the cryoprobe (usually 16-gauge), this procedure must be performed via a transnasal approach. This approach is associated with a higher rate of complications (23), and the procedure does not seem otherwise superior to thermocoagulation.

More than half of those patients whose pain is initially relieved by any of the above techniques (71) or following surgical removal of the ganglion (72, 73) will have recurrence of symptoms within 1 year following sphenopalatine neurolysis. However, some authors feel that when pain does return it is less severe than that experienced prior to the procedure (73).

It must be remembered that other neural structures besides the sphenopalatine ganglion are affected by all of these procedures. The sympathetic fibers accompanying the maxillary artery and afferent fibers from the maxillary division of the trigeminal nerve are equally affected because of their close proximity to the sphenopalatine ganglion. It is possible that in some cases neurolytic and local anesthetic injections actually exert a beneficial effect by destroying these structures rather than the sphenopalatine ganglion.

Because of the signs of parasympathetic overstimulation, which also accompany classic cluster headache, many authors have attempted to implicate the sphenopalatine ganglion in the pathogenesis of cluster headache. While results of removing or destroying the sphenopalatine ganglion as a treatment for cluster headache have been generally disappointing, there are at least a few reports of successful termination of cluster headache symptoms following this type of therapy (74). It is possible that these successes actually were cases of sphenopalatine neuralgia misdiagnosed as cluster headache. In cases of true cluster headache, alcohol and glycerol neurolysis (75) as well as radiofrequency thermocoagulation (76) of the sphenopalatin ganglion have all been demonstrated to have low success rates.

MYOFASCIAL TRIGGER POINT HEADACHES

A myofascial trigger point is a painful, palpable mass of spasmed muscle tissue located in a tight band in the muscle body. Palpation of a trigger point will usually reproduce the patient's pain and may actually cause spontaneous twitching in the affected muscle. Headaches associated with myofascial trigger points are extremely common. They may be associated with tension headaches, with generalized myofascial syndromes involving other body parts, or they may be idiopathic. The trapezius, sternocleidomastoid, temporalis, splenius capitus, medial and lateral pterygoid, and semispinalis muscles are all commonly affected. The symptoms and pain referral patterns of the specific myofascial trigger points are covered in depth elsewhere (77). However, careful physical examination of the muscles of the head and neck will usually demonstrate any trigger points during palpation. If the patient's headache pain is exacerbated or reproduced by palpation of such a point, treatment should at least be attempted.

While massage, cooling, and stretching may all benefit trigger point pain, definitive therapy usually consists of trigger point injections. Although "dry needling" may successfully disrupt the trigger point cycle in other parts of the body (78), it is not appropriate in the head and neck area because the large-gauge needles used for this technique are likely to cause significant bleeding. Injection of 1 to 3 ml of dilute lidocaine or bupivacaine through a small (27-gauge) needle will usually provide superior relief with minimal risk of hematoma formation (79). It is not uncommon for the localized pain relief that follows the injection of one trigger point to reveal additional areas that require treatment. Usually, several such secondary trigger points will coexist, and best results will be obtained if all (or as many as possible) are treated simultaneously. One or 2 sets of injections is often sufficient to relieve the patient's pain for weeks or months. Since both emotional and physical stress exacerbate myofascial pain complaints, trigger point injections are most effectively used to provide temporary pain relief while other forms of therapy (psychological or pharmacological) become effective.

HEADACHES WITH SYMPATHETIC NERVOUS SYSTEM INVOLVEMENT

Anatomy

Preganglionic sympathetic neurons innervating the head originate in the T1 to T4 spinal segments, exit the spinal cord with the first 4 thoracic nerve roots, and terminate in the cervical ganglia of the sympathetic trunk. Postsynaptic fibers ascend along the carotid and vertebrobasilar arterial systems. The external carotid plexus provides sympathetic innervation to most of the face, while the internal carotid plexus gives branches to the sphenopalatine ganglion and the ciliary ganglion. The vertebral plexus provides sympathetic innervation to the intracranial arteries and meninges.

Pathophysiology

There have been occasional reports of cranial and facial pain caused by reflex sympathetic dystrophy that has responded to stellate ganglion block (68). Other anecdotal reports have stated that some types of vascular headache may occasionally respond to interruption of the sympathetic pathways to the head (80, 81), but the actual pathophysiology involved is unclear.

Procedure

Stellate ganglion block may be performed by either the paratracheal or lateral approach (82). In the paratracheal approach, the fingers of the practitioner's hand are used to separate the soft tissues of the neck laterally, away from the trachea. A 25-gauge 1-inch needle is then inserted just caudal and lateral to the cricoid cartilage and advanced until bony contact is made with the vertebral body of C7. After careful aspiration, 10 ml of local anesthetic is deposited. In the lateral approach, the sternocleidomastoid muscle and soft tissues are retracted toward the midline. Palpation in this area will reveal the prominence of the C6

transverse process (Chassaignac's tubercle) at approximately the level of the cricoid cartilage. A 25- or 27-gauge needle is introduced at this level and advanced until bony contact is made just caudal to the C6 transverse process. After careful aspiration, 10 ml of agent is deposited at this location. With either approach the needle must be withdrawn slightly after making bony contact, since the longus colli and middle scalene muscles lie between the vertebra and the stellate ganglion.

Stellate ganglion block has many complications and should not be performed by inexperienced personnel. Central neuraxis block (spinal or epidural) is possible if the needle is advanced too far. Numerous blood vessels are present in the area, and intravenous or intraarterial injections may occur. Pneumothorax is more common if the lateral approach is used, especially on the right side where the cupola of the lung is approximately 2 cm higher than on the left (82). The esophagus may be punctured when performing the block using the paratracheal approach. This is more common on the left side, since the esophagus is more lateral in this location (82). For these reasons the authors routinely use the paratracheal approach on the right side and the lateral approach on the left side.

REFERENCES

1. Cox CL, Cocks GR. Occipital neuralgia. J Med Assoc Ala January:1979;23–32.
2. Knox DL, Mustonen E. Greater occipital neuralgia: an ocular pain syndrome with multiple etiologies. Trans Am Acad Opthalmol Otolaryngol 1974;79:513–519.
3. Schultz DR. Occipital neuralgia. J Am Osteopathic Assoc 1977;76:335–342.
4. Hammond SR, Danta G. Occipital neuralgia. Clin Exp Neurol 1978;15:258–270.
5. Vital JM, Grenier F, Dautheribes M, Baspeyre H, Lavignolle B, Senegas J. An anatomic and dynamic study of the greater occipital ner (n. of Arnold). Surg Radiol Anat 1989;11:205–210.
6. Bogduk N. The anatomy of occipital neuralgia. Clin Exp Neurol 1980;17:167–184.
7. Bogduk N. The clinical anatomy of the cervical dorsal rami. Spine 1982;7:319–330.
8. Hunter CR, Mayfield FH. Role of the upper cervical roots in the production of pain in the head. Am J Surg 1949;78:743–749.
9. Adriani J. Regional anesthesia: techniques and applications. 4th ed. St Louis: Warren H. Green, 1985:635.
10. Ehni G, Benner B. Occipital neuralgia and the C1-2 arthrosis syndrome. J Neurosurg 1984;61:961–965.
11. Ehni G. Occipital neuralgia and C1-C2 arthrosis. N Engl J Med 1984;310:127.
12. Poletti CE. Proposed operation for occipital neuralgia: C2 and C3 root decompression. Neurosurgery 1983;12:221–224.
13. Wackenheim A. Functional atlanto-occipital block. Neuroradiology 1971;3:80–81.
14. Fredriksen TA, Hovdal H, Sjaastad O. Cervicogenic headache: clinical manifestation. Cephalgia 1987;7:147–160.
15. Graff-Radford SB, Jaeger B, Reeves JL. Myofascial pain may present clinically as occipital neuralgia. Neurosurgery 1986;19:610–613.
16. Sjaastad O, Fredriksen TA, Stolt-Nielsen A. Cervicogenic headache, C2 rhizopathy, and occiptial neuralgia: a connection? Cephalgia 1986;6:189–195.
17. Cicala RS, Thoni K, Angel JJ. Long-term results of cervical epidural steroid injections. Clin J Pain 1989;5:143–145.

18. Cronen MC, Waldman SD. Cervical steroid epidural nerve blocks in the palliation of pain secondary to intractable tension-type headache. J Pain Symp Manage 1990;5:379–381.

19. Cicala RS, Williams CH. Cervical epidural injections for the treatment of neck pain: a review. Pain Manage 1989;2:141–148.

20. Waldman SD. Complications of cervical epidural nerve blocks with steroids: a prospective study of 790 consecutive blocks. Reg Anaesth 1989;14:149–151.

21. Cicala RS, Westbrook LL, Angel JJ. Side effects and complications of cervical epidural steroid injections. J Pain Symp Manage 1989;4:64–66.

22. White JC, Sweet WH. Pain and the neurosurgeon. Springfield IL: Charles C Thomas, 1969.

23. Cook N. Cryosurgery of headache. Res Clin Stud Headache 1978;5:86–101.

24. Janetta PJ. Arterial compression of the trigeminal nerve at the pons in patients with trigeminal neuralgia. J Neurosurg 1967;26:159–162.

25. Janetta PJ, Gildenberg PL, Loesser JD, Sweet WH, Ojemann GA. Operations on the brain and brain stem for chronic pain. In: Bonica JJ, ed. The management of pain. Philadelphia: Lea & Febiger, 1990.

26. Sweet WH. Trigeminal neuralgias. In: Alling LL, Manan PE, eds. Facial pain. Philadelphia: Lea & Febiger, 1977.

27. Vassilakis D, Phylaktakis M, Selviaridis P, Karavelis A, Sirmos C, Vlaikidis N. Symptomatic trigeminal neuralgia. J Neurosurg Sci 1988;32:117–120.

28. Brisman R. Trigeminal neuralgia and multiple sclerosis. Arch Neurol 1987;44:379–381.

29. Gokalp HZ, Kanpolat Y, Tumer B. Carotid-cavernous fistula following percutaneous trigeminal ganglion approach. Clin Neurol Neurosurg. 1980;82:269–272.

30. Ecker A, Perl T. Alcoholic gasserrian ganglion injection for the relief of tic douloureux. Preliminary report of a modification of Penman's method. Neurology 1958;8:461–466.

31. Harris W. An anlysis of 1,433 cases of paroxysmal trigeminal neuralgia (trigeminal tic) and the end results of gasserian alcohol injection. Brain 1940;63:209–224.

32. Putnam TJ, Hamptom AO. A technique of injection into the gasserian ganglion under roentgenographic control. Arch Neurol Psychiatry 1936;35:92–98.

33. Hakanson S. Trigeminal neuralgia treated by the injection of glycerol into the trigeminal cistern. Neurosurgery 1981;9:638–646.

34. Sweet WH, Poletti CE, Macon JB. Treatment of trigeminal neuralgia and other facial pain by retrogasserian injection of glycerol. Neurosurgery 1981;9:647–653.

35. Van de Velde C, Smeets P, Caemaert J, Van de Velde E. Transoval trigeminal cisternography and glycerol injection in trigeminal neuralgia. JBR-BTR 1989;72:83–87.

36. Spaziante R, Cappabianca P, Peca C, de Divitiis E. Percutaneous retrogasserian glycerol rhizolysis. Observations and results in 50 cases. J Neurosurg Sci 1987;31:121–122.

37. Sweet WH, Poletti CE. Problems with retrogasserian glycerol in the treatment of trigeminal neuralgia. Appl Neurophysiol 1985;48:252–257.

38. Saini SS. Retrogasserian anhydrous glycerol injection therapy in trigeminal neuralgia: observations in 552 patients. J Neurol Neurosurg Psychiatry 1987;50:1536–1538.

39. Fujimaki T, Fukushima T, Miyazaki S. Percutaneous retrogasserian glycerol injection in the management of trigeminal neuralgia: long term follow up results. J Neurosurg 1990;73:212–216.

40. Swerdlow B, Shuer L, Zelcer J. Coronary vasospasm during percutaneous trigeminal rhizotomy. Anaesthesia 1988;43:861–863.

41. Fraioli B, Esposito V, Guidette B, Cruccu G, Manfredi M. Treatment of trigeminal neuralgia by thermocoagulation, glycerolization, and percutaneous compression of the gasserian ganglion and/or retrogasserian rootlets: long-term results and therapeutic protocol. Neurosurgery 1989;24:239–245.

42. North RB, Kidd DH, Piantadosi S, Carson BS. Percutaneous

retrogasserian glycerol rhizotomy. Predictors of success and failure in treatment of trigeminal neuralgia. J Neurosurg 1990;72:851–856.

43. Sweet WH, Wespic JG. Controlled thremo-coagulation of trigeminal ganglion and rootlets for differential destruction of pain fibers. I, Trigeminal neuralgia. J Neurosurg 1974;40:143–156.

44. Wespic JG. Technique for radiofrequency gasserian ganglionectomy. Appl Neurophysiol 1976;39:122–132.

45. Salar G, Job I, Mingrino S. Cortical evoked responses before and after percutaneous thermocoagulation of the gasserian ganglion. Preliminary report. Appl Neurophysiol 1981:44:355–362.

46. Tarlov E. Percutaneous and open microsurgical techniques for relief of refractory tic douloureux. Surg Clin North Am 1980;60:593–606.

47. Piquer J, Joanes V, Roldan P, Barcia-Salorio JL, Masbout G. Long-term results of percutaneous gasserian ganglion lesions. Acta Neurochirurgica 1987;39:139–141.

48. Salar G, Mingrino S, Iob I. Alterations of facial sensitivity induced by percutaneous thermocoagulation of the gasserian ganglion. Surg Neurol 1983;19:126–130.

49. Broggi G, Franzini A, Lasio G, Giorgi C, Servello D. Long-term results of percutaneous retrogasserian thermorhitomy for "essential" trigeminal neuralgia: considerations in 1000 consecutive patients. Neurosurgery 1990;26:783–787.

50. Siegfried J. 500 percutaneous thermocoagulations of the gasserian ganglion for trigeminal pain. Surg Neurol 1977;8:126–131.

51. Lahuerta J, Lipton S, Miles J. Percutaneous radio frequency gangliolysis in the treatment of trigeminal neuralgia. Eur Neurol 1985;24:272–275.

52. Abdou-madi M, Trop D, Morin L, Olivier A. Anaesthetic considerations in percutaneous radiofrequency coagulation of the gasserian ganglion. Can Anaesth Soc J 1984;31:255–262.

53. Lichtor T, Mullan JF. A 10 year follow-up of percutaneous microcompression of the trigeminal ganglion. J Neurosurg 1990;72:49–54.

54. Mullan S, Lichtor T. Percutaneous microcompression of the trigeminal ganglion for trigeminal neuralgia. J Neurosurg 1983;59:1007–1012.

55. Lobato RD, Rivas JJ, Sarabia R, Lamas E. Percutaneous microcompression of the gasserian ganglion for trigeminal neuralgia. J Neurosurg 1990;72:546–553.

56. Frank F, Fabrizi AP. Percutaneous surgical treatment of trigeminal neuralgia. Acta Neurochir 1989;97:128–130.

57. Meglio M, Cioni B, d'Annunzio V. Percutaneous microcompression of the gasserian ganglion: personal experience. Acta Neurochir 1987;39:142–143.

58. Brown JA, Preul MC. Trigeminal depressor response during percutaneous microcompression of the trigeminal ganglion for trigeminal neuralgia. Neurosurgery 1988;23:745–748.

59. Esposito S, Delitala A, Bruni P, Hernandez R, Callovini GM. Therapeutic protocol in the treatment of trigeminal neuralgia. Appl Neurophysiol 1985;48:271–273.

60. Sheldon CM, Pudenz RH, Doyle J. Electrical control of facial pain. Am J Surg 1978;114:209–212.

61. Broggi G, Servello D, Franzini A, Giorgi C. Electrical stimulation of the gasserian ganglion for facial pain: preliminary results. Acta Neurochir 1987;39:144–146.

62. Ruskin AP. Sphenopalatine (nasal) ganglion: remote effects including psychosomatic symptoms, rage reaction, pain and spasm. Arch Phys Med Rehabil 1979;60:353–359.

63. Clemente CG. Gray's anatomy of the human body. 30th Am ed. Philadelphia: Lea & Febiger, 1985:1163,1168,1172–1174.

64. Sluder G. The role of sphenopalatine (or Meckel's) ganglion in nasal headaches. NY Med J 1908;87:989.

65. Vail HH. Vidian neuralgia. Ann Otol 1932;41:837–856.

66. Devoghel JC. Cluster headache and sphenopalatine block. Acta Anaesthesiol Belg 1981;1:101–107.

67. Ryan RE, Facer GW. Spenopalatine ganglion neuralgia and cluster headache: comparisons, contrasts, and treatment. Headache 1977;17:7–8.

68. Waldman S, Waldman K. Reflex sympathetic dystrophy of the face and neck. Reg Anesth 1987;12:8–12.

69. Adriani J. Regional anesthesia: techniques and applications. 4th ed. St Louis: Warren H. Green 1985:145–157.

70. Salar G, Ori C, Iob I, Fiore D. Percutaneous thermocoagulation for sphenopalatine ganglion neuralgia. Acta Neurochir 1987;84:24–28.

71. Brown LA. Mythical sphenopalatine ganglion neuralgia. S Med J 1962;55:670–672.

72. Meyer JS, Binns PM, Ericsson AD, et al. Sphenopalatine ganglionectomy for cluster headache. Arch Otolaryngol 1970;92:475–484.

73. Cepero R, Miller RH, Bressler KL. Long-term results of sphenopalatine ganglionectomy for facial pain. Am J Otolaryngol 1987;3:171–174.

74. Kitrelle J, Grouse D, Seybold M. Cluster headache: local anesthetic abortive agents. Arch Neurol 1985;42:496–498.

75. Ekbom K, Lindgren L, Nilsson BY, Hardebo JE, Waldenlind E. Retro-gasserian glycerol injection in the treatment of chronic cluster headache. Cephalgia 1987;7:21–27.

76. Mathew NT, Hurt W. Percutaneous radiofrequency trigeminal gangliorhizolysis in intractable cluster headache. Headache 1988;28:328–331.

77. Travell J, Simons DG. Myofascial pain and dysfunction: the trigger point manual. Baltimore: Williams & Wilkins, 1983.

78. Gunn CC. Dry needling of muscle motor points for chronic low back pain. A randomized clinical trial with long-term follow up. Spine 1980;5:279–282.

79. Bonica JJ. The management of pain. Phildelphia: Lea & Febiger, 1990:742–744.

80. Kaneko T, Yamamuro M. A case of hemiplegic migraine treated with stellate ganglion block. Jpn J Anesth 1978;27:62–65.

81. Miyazaki T, Kamiyama Y, Kitajima T, Onda M. Clinical study of DHE-45. Jpn J Anesth 1976;25:65–70.

82. Adriani J. Regional anesthesia: techniques and applications. 4th ed. St. Louis: Warren H. Green, 1985:475–479.

43

Neurosurgical Considerations

JOSEPH H. ARGUELLES and KIM J. BURCHIEL

Pain referred to the head is a very common complaint that in most cases signals a benign condition that is best managed medically. However, headache can be a symptom of a life-threatening condition, such as an intracranial mass lesion, or it can be the unrelenting sequela of a structural neurological disease unresponsive to medical therapy. Only in those contexts is treatment of headache within the domain of the surgeon. Indeed, although surgical treatments are quite useful in the treatment of facial neuralgias, there are, to our knowledge, no useful surgical treatments for any of the so-called primary headache disorders.

In the current chapter, we discuss a selected few of the conditions in which headache is a prominent feature and for which the adequate treatment is surgical. These conditions sort into two categories: (a) craniofacial pain disorders in which the pain experience is the major morbidity of the condition (the facial pain syndromes are covered elsewhere in this book and the reader is directed to those sections for further information) and (b) conditions in which significant intracranial pathology results in headache as a chief or sole complaint. No attempt is made to cover these conditions exhaustively. Instead we emphasize the characteristics of surgically significant headaches and discuss the management of a few selected conditions.

HEADACHE ASSOCIATED WITH SIGNIFICANT INTRACRANIAL PATHOLOGY

All physicians should be cognizant of the warning signs that a headache may be associated with significant intracranial pathology, which are

New Onset of Persistent or Recurrent Headache in a Patient without a History of Headaches. In most instances this will herald the onset of a benign headache condition. However, unless there is compelling evidence to the contrary, the presence of a mass lesion must be considered and searched for via computed tomography (CT) or magnetic resonance imaging (MRI).

Sudden or Explosive Onset of Headache. This is frequently seen in conjunction with intracranial bleeding from an aneurysm, vascular malformation, or tumor.

Focal Neurological Deficits. Such deficits in conjunc-

tion with headache demand a thorough workup to define or rule out serious intracranial pathology.

Fever in Association with Headaches. This association is seen in cases of viral or bacterial infection of the central nervous system, but it may also be present when intracranial bleeding has occurred.

Headache in Association with Intracranial Hypertension. Intracranial mass lesions, hemorrhage, hydrocephalus, or infection can all produce intracranial hypertension. Early recognition of this situation is essential because of the potential for death or irreversible neurological damage if appropriate treatment is delayed.

ELEVATED INTRACRANIAL PRESSURE

Some common clinical signs of elevated intracranial pressure are slow or absent pupillary responses, disconjugate or absent eye movements; motor deficits including decerebrate or decorticate posturing, focal weakness, and upper motor neuron signs such as clonus or hyperreflexia; altered level of consciousness or coma; respiratory changes including slow shallow breathing, Cheyne-Stokes respiration, neurogenic hyperventillation, ataxic breathing, and respiratory arrest; and Cushing's triad (bradycardia, hypertension, and widened pulse pressure), which is a late and ominous finding.

Radiologic findings consistent with elevated intracranial pressure include absent or compressed basal cisterns; effacement of the cortical sulci; shift of midline structures; dilation of the ventricular system, and the presence of a significant intracranial mass.

HEADACHE AND TUMOR

Individuals with intracranial tumors will frequently experience headache. It will be the presenting complaint for about one-third of all patients with a supratentorial tumor and for most patients with a posterior fossa mass, other than a cerebellopontine angle tumor, which presents most frequently with hearing loss (1, 2). In most situations, the headache is of little or no value in determining the location of the tumor. It can be expected to approximately overlie the tumor in only about one-third of cases (2).

There are three major mechanisms for the generation of pain by intracranial tumors: the tumor may produce tension in major veins, dural sinuses, or arteries that are richly supplied by pain-mediating afferent fibers; it may directly invade or compress pain-mediating cranial nerves or sympathetic afferents; or it may produce an inflammatory process involving the scalp. In most cases, the headache produced by an intracranial tumor will respond very well to corticosteroid administration. An initial dose of 6 to 24 mg of dexamethasone given IV, followed by a maintenance dose of 2 to 6 mg given two to four times each day will usually provide relief while definitive treatment is planned.

Many attempts have been made to summarize those characteristics of headache that are indicative of the presence and location of an intracranial tumor as well as those that may be of localizing value. However, the qualities that patients ascribe to headaches associated with tumors are greatly varied, and in the absence of other clinical and radiologic data, these headaches cannot be reliably distinguished from benign headaches. For example, nocturnal awakening due to headache is common when an intracranial tumor is present, but it is not diagnostic. Likewise, headache brought on by or exacerbated by cough is often cited as suggestive of tumor (1), but as with exertional headache, it is most often a benign idiopathic condition (3). Therefore, all patients who present with the new onset of persistent or recurring headache or who show a significant change in the quality of their previously diagnosed pattern of headaches should receive a thorough neurological workup, including appropriate imaging studies.

Vomiting, papilledema, impaired mentation, seizures, or focal neurological deficit in conjunction with headache is highly suggestive of an intracranial tumor. A contrast-enhanced CT or MRI scan is mandatory in such cases.

The surgical management of intracranial tumors is complex and beyond the scope of this chapter. Further information may be obtained from any of the standard neurosurgical texts.

HEADACHE AND SUBARACHNOID HEMORRHAGE

Approximately 26,000 people in North America suffer an acute subarachnoid hemorrhage annually. Of these, at least half will die or be significantly disabled (4). In about 75% of these cases, the subarachnoid hemorrhage is due to a ruptured cerebral aneurysm. Six percent are due to ruptured arteriovenous malformations, 6% are due to bleeding disorders, and the remaining 13% are of unknown etiology (5).

This condition can produce the most severe headache known. Patients typically complain of a headache that was explosive in onset and frequently state that it is the "worst headache of my life." The headache is often accompanied by mild fever, stiff neck, photophobia, vomiting, syncope or brief coma, and altered mental status. Brudzinski's and Kernig's signs may develop within a few hours of the onset of the headache. Examination may also reveal visual field anomalies, diplopia, oculomotor paralysis, and hemiparesis. In severe cases, the patient may lapse into coma shortly after the onset of the headache. Confirmation of a suspected subarachnoid hemorrhage should be obtained via CT scan or lumbar puncture. A non-contrast-enhanced CT scan is the study of first choice and is of considerable value. This study will reveal the presence of subarachnoid blood in 90% of cases of subarachnoid hemorrhage, when obtained within 3 days of the event. Beyond the third day this value falls to 30% (6). In addition, CT often provides valuable information regarding the location of the source of hemorrhage. Parasylvian hematomas are suggestive of a ruptured middle cerebral artery aneurysm, whereas a hematoma in the anterior intrahemispheric space is consistent with a ruptured anterior communicating artery aneurysm. When the subarachnoid hemorrhage has resulted from primary intraparenchymal or intraventricular bleeding, the CT scan will demonstrate this in most cases. CT scan can also demonstrate the occurrence of early hydrocephalus, a frequent complication of subarachnoid or intraventricular hemorrhage demanding immediate surgical treatment.

If the CT results are equivocal or if CT is unavailable, the diagnosis of subarachnoid hemorrhage can be made by lumbar puncture. The presence of 100 or more erythrocytes per cubic millimeter of CSF is considered diagnostic of subarachnoid hemorrhage. Lumbar puncture is not without risk in the setting of subarachnoid hemorrhage. Hillman (7) reported significant neurological deterioration in 2.2% of patients undergoing lumbar puncture to diagnose subarachnoid hemorrhage. Lumbar puncture should not be performed if the CT demonstrates subarachnoid blood. However, in cases in which subarachnoid hemorrhage has not occurred, the morbidity associated with lumbar puncture is negligible, and in those cases where subarachnoid hemorrhage has occured, the morbidity associated with misdiagnosis justifies the risk of lumbar puncture. Clinical or radiographic signs of intracranial hypertension as described earlier also represent contraindications to lumbar puncture.

When subarachnoid hemorrhage has been verified by CT or LP, four-vessel angiography should be obtained as soon as possible. An angiogram will fail to demonstrate a lesion in about 4% of cases of subarachnoid hemorrhage verified by CT or lumbar puncture. This can be due to aneurysms that do not fill because of vasospasm or thrombosis; likewise a thrombosed arteriovenous malformation may not be apparent angiographically. Complications occur in about 10% of patients undergoing four-vessel angiography after subarachnoid hemorrhage. These complications are about evenly divided among transient hemiparesis, permanent focal deficits, aneurysmal rupture, and ischemic events (8).

Retrospective studies show that warning headaches may occur in up to 60% of patients with intracranial aneurysms who will eventually suffer a subarachnoid hemorrhage (9, 10). Like the classic headache of subarachnoid hemorrhage, these headaches are usually sudden in onset but are somewhat less severe (11). Approximately one-half of such patients seek medical attention at the time of these headaches. Patients who have a history of benign headache will often describe these warning headaches as different in quality from their usual headaches. Symptoms similar to those of subarachnoid hemorrhage may be seen in conjunction with these warning headaches. The etiology of warning headaches has been the subject of some speculation, however it is most likely that these headaches result from small subarachnoid hemorrhages or "sentinel bleeds." Patients with such headaches should be worked up by CT scan, and lumbar puncture should be performed if the CT scan is negative. It is important to note that the symptoms associated with these sentinel bleeds may be misleading. The headache may be gradual in onset and not severe. Misdiagnosis may occur in 20 to 25% of patients with a subarachnoid hemorrhage. Tension headache, viral syndrome, and migraine headache are common misdiagnoses in this setting (12).

Day and Raskin (13) reported a case of a patient who experienced a headache suggestive of subarachnoid hemorrhage. Both CT and lumbar puncture were negative, yet a subsequent angiogram revealed an aneurysm and associated vasospasm. This raises the question of whether all patients with histories consistent with subarachnoid hemorrhage should undergo angiography regardless of negative CT scans and normal CSF studies. This approach is probably unwarranted. Wijdicks et al. (14) followed a series of 71 patients with sudden severe headache and other signs suggestive of subarachnoid hemorrhage. All patients considered had normal CT scans and no sign of hemorrhage on lumbar puncture. The patients were followed for a mean period of 3.3 years, and none of these patients went on to have a subarachnoid hemorrhage. Serious ischemic complications occur in about 1.3% of cerebral angiograms (15), and the likelihood of missing a subarachnoid hemorrhage on both CT and lumbar puncture is very small. We therefore do not recommend angiography as a routine part of the workup for headache suggestive of subarachnoid hemorrhage in the absence of other confirmatory evidence. Current advances in MRI technology are providing the means for noninvasive angiographic imaging, and these techniques may soon play a valuable role in the diagnosis of subarachnoid hemorrhage (16).

CHRONIC SUBDURAL HEMATOMA

The term *chronic subdural hematoma* refers to a hematoma that comes to medical attention more than 20 days after the inciting trauma (17). Chronic subdural hematoma occurs with an incidence of approximately 1–2/100,000 per year.

Most patients with this disorder are either elderly or in late middle age. Although most of these lesions are the result of trauma, no history of head injury is obtained in a significant number of patients with the disorder. Often there is a history of seemingly insignificant head trauma. In many patients, chronic alcoholism may be a complicating factor. Trauma may not have been a factor in the initial hemorrhage for patients with coagulation disorders.

The onset of symptoms is insidious. The initial hemorrhage into the subdural space may be small or there may be significant coexistent brain atrophy resulting in the absence of mass effect or early clinical signs of intracranial bleeding. The mechanism leading to the symptomatic expansion of these lesions has been a matter of controversy. Within 24 hours, fibroblasts begin to migrate from the dura into the hematoma. Within 3 weeks, the hematoma is encapsulated between membranes. It is likely that the enlargement of these lesions results from the leakage of proteins into the hematoma capsule as well as from recurrent hemorrhage (18–20).

The recognition of the presence of a chronic subdural hematoma is complicated by its variety of clinical presentations. In large series, less than one-half of patients present with impaired consciousness. The only nearly universal feature is persistent headache. It may begin abruptly or in combination with any or all of the following symptoms: vomiting, stiff neck, photophobia, ataxia, apathy, amnesia, focal weakness or sensory anomalies, and seizures. In this way, the presentation of chronic subdural hematoma may mimic tumor, meningitis, dementia, or any variant of cerebrovascular disease. Therefore, the diagnosis of chronic subdural hematoma must be considered whenever a patient beyond the fifth decade presents with a new and persistent headache, even if other signs of neurological disease are absent.

The diagnosis can be confirmed or excluded radiographically. A contrast-enhanced CT scan is the preferred diagnostic study. The non-contrast-enhanced CT appearance of a hematoma will change as time elapses from the initial hemorrhage. When compared with the surrounding brain tissue, the hematoma will appear hyperdense in the first week, isodense for the second and third weeks, and hypodense thereafter. During the period in which the hematoma appears isodense, it can be easily overlooked on a non-contrast-enhanced scan. The presence of midline shift or distortion of the cerebral ventricles can alert the physician to the presence of an isodense subdural hematoma, but bilateral subdural hematomas may obscure even these findings. If the diagnosis is strongly suspected—as it would be in a 60-year-old gentleman with a history of falling 2 weeks prior to the development of headache and other neurological symptoms—a contrast-enhanced CT scan or an MRI scan should be obtained. In the former case, the enhancement of the membranes and cortex surrounding the hematoma may help to define it; in the latter case, the signal from the hematoma is readily distinguished from that of the surrounding brain. Although the MRI scan would be least likely to miss a chronic subdural hematoma, CT scan is the most cost-effective study at most institutions.

Patients with chronic subdural hematomas have been managed successfully without surgery, using diuretics, corticosteroids, and bedrest; however the duration of treatment averages 3 to 5 weeks, and many patients will eventually require operation in spite of maximal therapy (21, 22). Therefore, the prudent course of action is operative drainage of these lesions. A dose of 10 to 12 mg of dexamethasone IV followed by 4 to 6 mg every 6 hours may help to ameliorate the patient's symptoms until definitive measures can be taken.

Craniotomy for drainage with excision of the hematoma membranes has been advocated by some in the past, but drainage via burr holes or twist-drill craniostomy gives an equally good result (23). Of course these simpler procedures are the preferred methods of treatment. When the hematoma is completely liquid, excellent results can be obtained with either method. If there is a solid component to the hematoma, burr-hole drainage must be employed. If necessary, two burr holes can be made, and saline can then be flushed through the subdural space to remove the solid portions of the clot. A drain should be placed in the subdural space and left in place for 24 to 72 hours. The time needed for drainage is determined by the daily output of the drain.

Twist-drill craniostomy is particularly suited to the treatment of the medically frail patient. It can be safely performed at bedside under local anesthesia. A twist-drill hole is made at an oblique angle to the skull, through a scalp incision of 1 cm or less. The dura and outer hematoma membrane is then penetrated using a 14-gauge needle. A small red rubber or other catheter is then passed into the subdural space and connected to a sterile closed drainage system. The drainage bag is placed a few centimeters below the head to allow the hematoma fluid to siphon off slowly. The catheter is typically removed after 24 hours, and the patient mobilized. This procedure should only be used when the hematoma is uniformly hypodense on CT. The hematoma must also be thick enough to allow penetration of the skull and dura without endangering the cortex.

Postoperative CT scanning will frequently reveal residual hematoma. This is of no consequence, since evacuation of a portion of the hematoma is usually all that is needed to relieve symptoms and promote resorption of the remaining fluid. True recurrence of chronic subdural hematoma occurs with a frequency of about 10 to 50% (23). Patients who do not recover promptly or who deteriorate after drainage should be rescanned. The most common cause of recurrence is bleeding from the vascular outer membrane of the hematoma. A small percentage of patients will deteriorate and die after drainage. Infections occur with a

frequency of between 1 and 5% after drainage of chronic subdural hematomas.

The reported mortality after chronic subdural hematoma is variable. In large series, the rate is about 10%. Most patients will return to normal or near-normal function after adequate treatment. The patient's condition at the time of operation is of greater predictive value than the size of the hematoma. However, patients will frequently make a full recovery even if they are in coma at the time of the operation.

BENIGN INTRACRANIAL HYPERTENSION

Pseudotumor cerebri is a syndrome of obscure etiology, involving increased intracranial pressure in the absence of a mass lesion or cerebral edema. The typical patient is an obese young woman who complains of headache, blurred vision, transient visual loss, nausea, and vomiting. Frequently, patients will report that their visual symptoms are exacerbated by a Valsalva maneuver. Focal neurological deficits such as abducens nerve palsy and facial nerve palsy are sometimes present, and papilledema is a common though not universal finding (25). The cerebrospinal fluid pressure as measured by lumbar puncture is typically 20 to 40 cm of water. Values above 60 cm have been reported (26). A significant number of patients will experience a spontaneous resolution of all symptoms within weeks to months of their onset. As a result, pseudotumor cerebri has come to be known as "benign intracranial hypertension" (27, 28). Very little is known about the natural history of this condition, and fulminant cases of pseudotumor cerebri with rapid progression to total blindness have been reported (26). Indeed, although headache is a prominent feature of the condition, the major goal of therapy is to prevent visual loss.

The pathophysiology of pseudotumor cerebri is not well understood. The syndrome has been associated with many conditions, including obstruction of intracranial venous drainage, endocrine dysfunction, hematologic disorders, disorders of vitamin metabolism, and drug reactions (29). Fifteen to 20% of patients with pseudotumor cerebri have no other apparent disorders. It is probable that pseudotumor cerebri is a family of disorders involving abnormalities of the regulation of intracranial pressure. Several studies present evidence for abnormal CSF absorption in patients with pseudotumor cerebri (25, 30, 31).

The diagnosis of pseudotumor is one of exclusion. The CT scan reveals no evidence of a mass lesion, ventricular dilatation, or cerebral edema. Occasionally a contrast-enhanced scan will reveal thrombosis of the sagittal sinus. Lumbar puncture reveals normal protein levels and cell counts in the CSF. The opening pressure may be remarkably elevated, as stated previously. However, several authors report cases of pseudotumor cerebri in which resting CSF pressures were normal (25, 30, 32). Continuous monitoring of such patients reveals the frequent occurrence of transient elevations in CSF pressure that are not related to activity or straining. Fundoscopic evaluation of these patients will frequently reveal florid papilledema or the absence of venous pulsations.

The treatment of pseudotumor is largely empirical. For those patients with associated conditions, medical therapy is directed at those conditions. The use of steroids is controversial, and some authors report that they are of little benefit in the absence of adrenocortical insufficiency (29). Johnston et al. (33) reviewed 134 cases of pseudotumor treated over a 35-year period and reported good results with corticosteroids as the first line of treatment. Several other authors report similar results. We would suggest a trial of corticosteroids in all patients diagnosed with this condition.

All patients with this condition should undergo a full ophthalmologic evaluation. Optic nerve decompression procedures are indicated to facilitate the resolution of visual symptoms and prevent progressive visual impairment due to chronic papilledema.

Serial lumbar puncture may be performed to control the elevated intracranial pressure. Enough fluid is removed to lower the CSF pressure into the normal range. Many patients will need no further therapy. If frequent serial lumbar punctures prove to be of only transient benefit, a theco-peritoneal shunt should be placed. The percutaneously placed lumbar-peritoneal shunt is most frequently used, although cisternal and ventricular shunting procedures have been used to treat pseudotumor.

Shunting procedures are not without risk. Shunt occlusions necessitating revision occur in as many as 50% of patients treated with lumbar peritoneal shunts. Serious but rare complications of lumbar peritoneal shunts include meningitis, disc space infection (34), and cerebellar tonsilar herniation syndromes (35).

CONCLUSIONS

We have discussed four disparate conditions that present clinically with headache. They were chosen to illustrate conditions that may be confused with benign medically treatable headaches. The proper detection of these as well as each of the myriad surgically significant conditions presenting with headache is frequently complicated by the spectrum of symptoms seen in each of these conditions. For instance, the presentation of a small subarachnoid hemorrhage is sometimes less dramatic than the onset of a common migraine headache. Yet even in those cases, there will often be clues to the true etiology of the headache. Recognition of these clues is essential to avoiding the inevitable catastrophe of a second hemorrhage.

In many cases in which headache results from significant surgically approachable intracranial pathology, lost time will correlate with increased morbidity. Therefore, all clinicians dealing with headache patients must have a reasonably high suspicion of serious intracranial pathology whenever they encounter these patients. For the individual physician seeing headache patients, catastrophic misdiag-

nosis is an uncommon event. Neurosurgeons see such cases with some frequency, and unfortunately the morbidity associated with delayed diagnosis is often high.

We believe that the widespread availability and safety of CT and MRI scans dictates their frequent use in the workup of headache patients. Such scans are mandatory in the setting of new onset of persistent or recurrent headaches, headache of explosive onset, headache associated with fever and meningismus, or headache associated with intracranial pathology.

REFERENCES

1. King RB, Young RF. Cephalic pain. In: Youmans JR, ed. Neurological surgery 3rd ed. Philadelphia: WB Saunders, 1990:3856–3879.
2. Wolf HG. Headache and other head pain. 3rd ed., rev. by D'Alessio DJ. New York: Oxford University Press, 1972.
3. Adams RD, Victor M. Headache and other craniofacial pains. In: Principles of neurology. 2nd ed. New York: McGraw-Hill, 1981: 128.
4. Sacco RL, Wolf PA, Bharucha NE, Meeks SL, Kannel WB, et al. Subarachnoid and intracerebral hemorrhage. Natural history, prognosis, and precursive factors in the Framingham study. Neurology 1984;34:847–854.
5. Sahs AL. Subarachnoid hemorrhage. In: Harrison MJG, Dyken ML, eds. Cerebral vascular disease. London: Butterworths, 1983:354.
6. Espinosa F, Weir B, Noseworthy T. Nonoperative treatment of subarachnoid hemorrhage. In: Youmans JR, ed. Neurological surgery. 3rd ed. Philadelphia: WB Saunders, 1990:1661–1688.
7. Hillman J. Should computed tomography scanning replace lumbar puncture in the diagnostic process in suspected subarachnoid hemorrhage? Surg Neurol 1986;26:547–550.
8. Smith RR, Miller JD. Pathophysiology and clinical evaluation of subarachnoid hemorrhage. In: Youmans JR, ed. Neurological surgery. 3rd ed. Philadelphia: WB Saunders, 1990:1644–1660.
9. King RB, Saba MI. Forewarnings of subarachnoid hemorrhage. NY State J Med 1974;74:638–639.
10. Okaware S. Warning signs prior to rupture of an intracranial aneurysm. J Neurosurg 1973;38:575–580.
11. Verweij RD, Wijdicks EFM, van Gijn J. Warning headache in aneurysmal subarachnoid hemorrhage. A case control study. Arch Neurol 1988;45:1019–1020.
12. Adams HP, Kassell NS, Boarini DJ, Kongable G. The clinical spectrum of aneurysmal subarachnoid hemorrhage. J Stroke Cerebrovasc Dis 1991;1(1):3–8.
13. Day JW, Raskin NH. Thunderclap headache: symptom of unruptured cerebral aneurysm. Lancet 1986;2:1247–1248.
14. Widjicks EFM, Kerkhoff H, van Gijn J. Long-term follow-up of 71 patients with thunderclap headache mimicking subarachnoid hemorrhage. Lancet 1988;2:68–70.
15. Dion JE, Gates PC, Fox AJ, Barnett HJM, Blom RJ. Clinical events following neuroangiography: a prospective study. Stroke 1987;18: 997–1004.
16. Masaryk T, Modic MT, Ross JS, Ruggieri PM, Laub GA, et al. Intracranial circulation: preliminary results with three-dimentional MR angiography. Radiology 1989;171:793–799.
17. Rosenorn J, Gjerris F. Long-term follow-up review of patients with acute and chronic subdural hematomas. J Neurosurg 1978;48:345–349.
18. Sato S, Suzuki J. Ultrastructural observations of the capsule of chronic subdural hematoma in various clinical stages. J Neurosurg 1975;43:569–578.
19. Yamashima T, Yamamoto S. How do vessels proliferate in the capsule of a chronic subdural hematoma? Neurosurgery 1984;15: 672–678.

20. Yamashima T, Yamamoto S, Friede RL. The role of endothelial gap junctions in the enlargement of chronic subdural hematoma. J Neurosurg 1983;59:298–303.

21. Suzuki J, Takaku A. Nonsurgical treatment of chronic subdural hematoma. J Neurosurg 1970;33:548–553.

22. Gjerris F, Schmidt K. Chronic subdural hematoma. Surgery or manitol treatment. J Neurosurg 1974;40:639–642.

23. Cooper PR. Post-traumatic intracranial mass lesions. In: Cooper PR, ed. Head injury. Baltimore: Williams & Wilkins, 1987:238–284.

24. Tindall GT, Payne NS II, O'Brien MS. Complications of surgery for subdural hematoma. Clin Neurosurg 1976;23:465–482.

25. Spence DJ, Amacher AL, Willis NR. Benign intracranial hypertension without papilledema: role of 24-hour cerebrospinal fluid pressure monitoring in diagnosis and management. Neurosurgery 1980;7:326–336.

26. Kidron D, Pomeranz S. Malignant pseudotumor cerebri. Report of two cases. J Neurosurg 1989;71:443–445.

27. Amacher AL, Spence D. Spectrum of benign intracranial hypertension in children and adolescents. Childs Nerv Syst 1985;1:81.

28. Gjerriss F, Sorensen PS, Vorstrup S, et al. Intracranial pressure, conductance to cerebrospinal fluid outflow, and cerebral blood flow in patients with benign intracranial hypertension (pseudotumor cerebri). Ann Neurol 1985;17:158–162.

29. Greer M. Pseudotumor cerebri. In: Youmans JR, ed. Neurological surgery. 3rd ed. Philadelphia: WB Saunders, 1990:3514–3530.

30. Sklar FH, Beyer CW Jr, Ramanathan M, Cooper PR, Clark WK. Cerebrospinal fluid dynamics in patients with pseudotumor cerebri. Neurosurgery, 1979;5:208–216.

31. Johnston I, Paterson A. Benign intracranial hypertension: II. CSF pressure and circulation. Brain 1974;97:301–312.

32. Johnston I, Paterson A. Intracranial pressure monitoring in patients with benign intracranial hypertension. In: Lundberg N, Ponten U, Brock M, eds. Intracranial pressure II. New York: Springer-Verlag, 1975:500–502.

33. Johnston I, Paterson A, Besser M. The treatment of benign intracranial hypertension: a review of 134 cases. Surg Neurol 1981;16:218–224.

34. Cabezudo JM, Olabe J, Bacci F. Infection of the intervertebral disk space after placement of a percutaneous lumboperitoneal shunt for benign intracranial hypertension. Neurosurgery 1990;26:1005–1009.

35. Sullivan LP, Stears JC, Ringel SP. Resolution of syringomyelia and chiari malformation by ventriculoatrial shunting in a patient with pseudotumor cerebri and a lumboperitoneal shunt. Neurosurgery 1988;22:744–747.

44

Headache Management in the Patient with Complicating Medical Disorders

GLEN D. SOLOMON

Headache may be the most common pain syndrome seen in medical practice. Due to the prevalence of headache in the population, patients who suffer with headache are also likely to suffer with other illnesses. The management of the headache sufferer with concomitant medical disease demands knowledge of the illnesses that are associated with headache and an understanding of the pharmacology of the medications used in headache therapy.

In clinical practice, most headaches are not caused by underlying pathology. However, it is important to recognize that headache may be the presenting symptom of several medical conditions. Fever, of any etiology, is probably the most common medical problem that causes headache. Less common causes include pheochromocytoma, chronic renal failure, hyperthyroidism, and malignant hypertension. Pheochromocytoma may present with a pounding headache associated with hypertension, diaphoresis, tachycardia, and palpitations (1).

Rheumatologic diseases may have headache as an early manifestation. Headache is common in systemic lupus erythematosus, polyarteritis nodosa, and giant cell arteritis (2). Almost 60% of patients with fibrositis report headache, usually of the tension type. Sjögren's syndrome often is manifest by neuropsychiatric disturbances including depression; one patient had headache as the initial symptom. Most types of vasculitis may also cause headache.

Headache upon awakening may be the initial symptom of sleep apnea syndrome. The headache often will improve as the day progresses. Sleep apnea is most commonly observed in obese, middle-aged males. Associated symptoms include snoring, daytime somnolence, hypertension, and arrythmias.

While patients with headaches caused by an underlying illness constitute less than 1% of the total headache population, it is common for patients with benign headache disorders to have concomitant medical problems.

To evaluate the prevalence of concomitant medical diseases in chronic headache sufferers, Featherstone (3) reviewed 1414 life insurance applications to obtain 200 head-

ache cases and matched controls without chronic headaches. The average age for his groups was 45 years. The groups were equally divided by gender. Headaches were not classified by diagnosis (i.e., migraine, cluster, etc.). Six conditions were found to occur more often in the headache group: hypertension, dizziness (or vertigo), gastroesophageal reflux, depression or anxiety, peptic ulcer disease, and irritable bowel syndrome. Three conditions were significantly more common in the nonheadache population: nephrolithiasis, alcohol abuse in men, and abdominal pain in women. Several conditions had the same prevalence in both headache and nonheadache groups: ischemic heart disease, mitral valve prolapse, cardiovascular disease, central nervous system ischemia, cigarette smoking, emphysema, and previous surgery.

While Featherstone's paper (3) reviewed "idiopathic" headache, other investigators have looked for associations between specific headache diagnoses and medical diseases. Migraine has been associated with an increased prevalence of coronary vasospasm (4, 5), Raynaud's phenomenon (6), aspirin-sensitive asthma (7), mitral valve prolapse (8), and hypertension (9). Cluster headache is associated with a threefold increase in the prevalence of peptic ulcer disease (10). Chronic tension-type headache sufferers have an increased prevalence of depressive symptoms.

PHARMACOLOGY OF HEADACHE MEDICATIONS

Medications That Exacerbate Headache

Many medications can trigger de novo headache or exacerbate headache in patients with an underlying headache disorder. Askmark and colleagues (11) evaluated data from the World Health Organization Collaborating Centre for International Drug Monitoring. Drug-related headache was most frequently reported with the following medications: indomethacin, nifedipine, cimetidine, atenolol, trimethoprim-sulfamethoxazole, zimeldine, nitroglycerin, isosorbide dinitrate, ranitidine, isotretinoin, captopril, piroxicam, metoprolol, and diclofenac. When the frequency of headache was compiled with respect to the amount of drug sold, the drugs most like to cause headache were zimeldine, nalidixic acid, trimethoprim, griseofulvin, ranitidine, and nifedipine.

Certain medications were found to initiate migraine headaches. These included cimetidine, oral contraceptives, atenolol, indomethacin, danazol, nifedipine, diclofenac, and ranitidine. Medications that may aggravate existing migraine include hormonal therapy, such as oral contraceptives, clomiphene, and postmenopausal estrogens, and vitamin A and its retinoic acid derivatives.

Both migraines and cluster headaches may be exacerbated by nitrates and by vasodilators such as hydralazine, minoxidil, nifedipine, and prazocin.

Reserpine depletes catecholamine and serotonin stores within the brain and can cause depression, migraine, and tension-type headaches. Indomethacin, while useful in treating cluster variant headaches, can cause a generalized headache.

Medications Used to Treat Headaches

A wide variety of medications have been used in the prophylaxis of migraine, including methysergide, β-blockers, calcium channel blockers, nonsteroidal antiinflammatory drugs (NSAIDs), tricyclic antidepressants, and cyproheptadine. Medications used in the prophylaxis of cluster headache include ergotamine, corticosteroids, methysergide, verapamil, and lithium carbonate. Treatment of tension-type headache may include antidepressants, both tricyclic and monamine oxidase inhibitors (MAOIs), and NSAIDs. Of the antidepressants, the tricyclic agents are usually the first choice due to the lower incidence of side effects and serious drug interactions compared with the MAOIs.

When selecting a medication for the headache patient with concomitant medical problems, knowledge of the physiological effects of the medication is critical. Effects on the cardiovascular system frequently limit the use of headache drugs in patients with coronary artery disease, congestive heart failure, or arrythmias.

Tricyclic antidepressants have several potential cardiac effects (12). These drugs may cause orthostatic hypotension, although they do not have negative inotropic effects. The orthostatic hypotension is mediated though α-adrenergic receptor blockade, and is most commonly reported with tertiary amines such as amitriptyline and imipramine. Cardiac conduction problems can occur with all tricyclic antidepressants but not with trazadone, fluoxetine, sertraline and bupropion. Tricyclics slow the process of depolarization and prolong repolarization, a quinidine-like effect. On electrocardiogram, there may be prolongation of P-R, QRS, and Q-T intervals. This effect is only of clinical significance in patients with second-degree heart block, right or left bundle-branch block, or intraventricular conduction delays (QRS width >0.11 sec-

onds). In patients with first-degree heart block, treatment with tricyclics does not cause the development of higher degrees of heart block. Patients with advanced heart block or intraventricular conduction delays who require therapy with antidepressant agents should be treated with fluoxetine, sertraline, bupropion, trazedone, or monamine oxidase inhibitors.

β-Blockers are often valued as first-line drugs for the prophylaxis of migraine. While generally well tolerated, they are contraindicated in patients with congestive heart failure, bronchospastic disease (i.e., asthma, emphysema, chronic bronchitis), diabetes mellitus, and Wolff-Parkinson-White syndrome. β-Blockers may also exacerbate Raynaud's phenomenon, a condition found more commonly in migraine sufferers than in normal persons. Side effects of β-blockers include depression, fatigue, and sleep disorders. Depression is more commonly reported with propranolol than with other β-blockers. These side effects may worsen the tension-type headache component of the mixed headache syndrome.

Patients should not abruptly discontinue β-blocker therapy, since abrupt discontinuation may lead to myocardial infarction, even in patients with no prior history of heart disease (13).

In addition to the prophylaxis of migraine, β-blockers have multiple therapeutic uses. They are used in the treatment of angina pectoris, hypertension, and anxiety, and in the secondary prevention of myocardial infarction.

Calcium channel blockers are useful in the prophylaxis of migraine and cluster headache (14). The calcium channel blockers constitute a diverse group of drugs with varying effects on the heart and peripheral vasculature. Verapamil and diltiazem have negative inotropic effects and slow conduction through the A-V node. Therefore, these agents should be avoided in patients with congestive heart failure, advanced heart block, or sick sinus syndrome. The dihydropyradine calcium channel blockers—nifedipine, nicardipine, and nimodipine—have no effect on cardiac conduction but can cause marked vasodilation.

Calcium channel blockers have large number of therapeutic uses. They are indicated for the treatment of hypertension and angina pectoris, including vasospastic angina. Verapamil is also approved for use as an antiarrhythmic for paroxysmal supraventricular tachycardia and for atrial fibrillation and flutter (used with digoxin). Other potential uses of calcium channel blockers (not FDA-approved) include prophylaxis of migraine and cluster headaches, relief of esophageal spasm, prevention of nocturnal leg cramps, treatment of bipolar affective disorder (manic-depressive illness), adjunctive therapy of irritable bowel syndrome, cancer chemotherapy, and secondary prevention of myocardial infarction.

Nonsteroidal antiinflammatory drugs (NSAIDs) are widely prescribed as analgesics and for the treatment of arthritis. They are valuable in both the acute treatment and prophylaxis of migraine headache, and as adjunctive therapy for tension-type headache. Unlike the β-blockers and calcium channel blockers used in migraine prophylaxis, NSAIDs do not lower blood pressure or affect cardiac conduction. Unlike ergotamine or isomethepane preparations used in the acute treatment of migraine, NSAIDs do not cause vasoconstriction.

Adverse effects from NSAIDs are relatively common and may include gastrointenstinal symptoms such as dyspepsia, heartburn, nausea, vomiting, diarrhea, constipation, and generalized abdominal pain. Most NSAIDs can cause bleeding of the upper gastrointestinal tract. Renal effects of NSAIDs may include decreased glomerular filtration rate (GFR) with sodium, chloride, and water retention. These renal problems are most likely to occur in patients who are elderly, who are hypertensive, who have renovascular or advanced atherosclerotic disease, or who take diuretics. Analgesic nephropathy, the most common cause of drug-induced renal failure, has been associated with excessive use of NSAIDs along with phenacetin or acetaminophen.

MANAGEMENT OF CONCOMITANT DISEASES

Hypertension

Several studies have documented an association between hypertension and migraine (3, 9). Additionally, several conditions can present with both elevated blood pressure and headache (1). These include malignant hypertension (hypertensive crisis), pheochromocytoma, hyperthyroidism, vasculitis, chronic renal disease, increased intracranial pressure, and sleep apnea. Medications that can elevate blood pressure and exacerbate migraine include amphetamines, cocaine, estrogens, and oral contraceptives.

Certain medications prescribed for the treatment of hypertension can also exacerbate migraine. These include hydralazine, minoxidil, nifedipine, prazosin, and reserpine. Conversely, several medications used in the treatment of hypertension are effective in the prophylaxis of migraine. These agents include the β-blockers, calcium channel blockers, angiotensin-converting-enzyme inhibitors (ACEIs), clonidine, and guanfacine.

Several β-blockers have been evaluated in controlled studies, and it appears that only those drugs which lack partial agonist activity (intrinsic sympathomimetic activity) are effective in migraine prophylaxis. In his review of β-blockers in migraine, Dalessio (15) concluded that nonselective β-blockers (propranolol, nadolol, and timolol) were somewhat more effective than cardioselective β-blockers (metoprolol and atenolol). The only β-blockers currently approved by the FDA for migraine prophylaxis are propranolol and timolol.

Multiple calcium channel blockers have been approved for the treatment of hypertension, including verapamil, diltiazem, nifedipine, and nicardipine. Several studies have shown verapamil to be effective for the prophylaxis of both migraine and cluster headaches (14). Limited data suggest that diltiazem may be useful in migraine prophylaxis. Nifedipine has significantly greater vasodilating properties than the other calcium channel blockers and may initially exacerbate migraine. With continued use, it does have efficacy in preventing migraine. Nicardipine, a dihydropyridine calcium channel blocker related to nifedipine, has recently been found effective in migraine prophylaxis. The author has also used this agent in cluster headache with good results. None of the calcium channel blockers have been approved by the FDA for the treatment of migraine or cluster headache.

Two calcium channel blockers that are not antihypertensive agents—nimodipine and flunarizine—are effective in the prophylaxis of migraine and cluster headache. Nimodipine is approved for the prevention of cerebral vasospasm following subarachnoid hemorrhage. Its use in headache prevention is limited only by its high price. Flunarizine is widely prescribed in Europe but has yet to be approved by the FDA for use in the United States.

Clonidine, an α-agonist, has been widely used for migraine prophylaxis in Scandinavia. Studies done in the United States have not shown this agent to be particularly effective in migraine. Clonidine is unique in its ability to block the symptoms and signs of opiate withdrawal. This drug is very valuable in the early management of patients with narcotic dependency (16). It is ineffective for barbiturate, ergotamine, or benzodiazepine withdrawal states.

The angiotensin-converting-enzyme inhibitor (ACEI) captopril has been reported to inhibit the enzyme enkephalinase (17). It may thereby slow the breakdown of the naturally occurring opioid enkephalin. Captopril has been reported to be effective in migraine prophylaxis (17) as well as in therapy of tension-type headache (18). The other clinically available ACEIs (lisinopril and enalapril) have not been studied in headache, although the author has found them to be effective in small numbers of patients.

Cardiac Disease

The prevalence of coronary artery disease (ischemic heart disease) was not different in headache sufferers than controls in Featherstone's study (19) of life insurance applications. Featherstone (19) reviewed ECGs from this group and reported that electrocardiographic changes suggestive if ischemic heart disease were less common in headache sufferers than in control patients. In this group of patients, yielding 161 pairs of ECGs, there were no differences in the frequency of smoking, diabetes mellitus, or hyperlipidemia. Ischemic ECG changes were found in 50 control patients and 30 headache patients, a significant difference. Pathological Q waves were found in 21 controls and 14 headache sufferers, while ST-segment depressions were found in 12 controls and 6 headache patients. There were no differences in the frequency of left ventricular hypertrophy, premature ventricular contractions, or conduction defects.

While Featherstone (19) did not report an increase in the prevalence of ischemic heart disease in patients with idiopathic headache, other researchers have found an association between migraine and coronary artery vasospasm (4–6, 20). Fournier and associates (4) reported on one family with both migraine and coronary artery spasm. Kuritzky (5) found transient ST-segment elevations associated with chest pain, suggesting vasospastic angina, during migraine attacks in some patients. Both studies suggest that vasospastic angina is associated with migraine and may be part of a generalized vasospastic disorder. It is suggested that migraine sufferers with chest pain during migraine attacks should undergo further evaluation for vasospastic angina (20). This group would include young females who would not otherwise be considered to be at risk for coronary artery disease. The treatment of choice for a patient with both migraine and vasospastic angina is a calcium channel blocker (20).

Nitrates and nitroglycerin used in the management of coronary artery disease may induce migraine attacks and cluster headaches in susceptible individuals. Because there are no alternative medications for the acute management of angina pectoris (21), these drugs will continue to be used in patients with both coronary artery disease and headaches. For the long-term management of angina pectoris, β-blockers and calcium channel blockers are effective and are useful in the prophylaxis of migraine. Several calcium channel blockers are effective for the prophylaxis of cluster headache, in addition to their value in angina.

The difficulty of managing cluster headache in the patient with coronary artery disease was shown in a paper by Solomon et al. (22). We found that 4 of 14 elderly cluster sufferers had a diagnosis of coronary artery disease, yet 3 of the 4 patients were treated with the vasoconstrictor methysergide. Methysergide is contraindicated in patients with coronary artery disease. Some of these patients may have benefited from treatment with a calcium channel blocker for both their cluster headaches and angina.

Several medications used in the treatment of headache can cause problems for patients with cardiac disease. Ergotamine tartrate and sumatriptan, used in the treatment of both migraine and cluster headache, may exacerbate coronary artery disease. Ergotamine and sumatriptan have been shown to induce coronary vasospasm even in the absence of atherosclerosis (23). Methysergide is a vasoconstrictor that can cause pericardial, pulmonary, and retroperitoneal fibrosis with long-term, uninterrupted use. Tricyclic antidepressants can increase the risk of arrythmias in certain patients (12).

Certain conditions exacerbate the vasoconstrictor properties of ergotamine (and possibly sumatriptan) and may therefore increase the risk of coronary vasoconstriction. These conditions include sepsis, thyrotoxicosis, anemia, and vascular disease (24). Isometheptene mucate, a sympathetic amine found in the drug Midrin, is a weaker vasoconstrictor than ergotamine but should generally be avoided in patients with coronary artery disease. Nonsteroidal antiinflammatory drugs are the migraine abortive agents of choice in patients with ischemic heart disease, since vasoconstrictors like ergotamine and isometheptene are contraindicated. The NSAIDs that are effective in aborting migraine attacks include naproxen sodium (25), flurbiprofen (26), and meclofenamate (27).

Paroxysmal supraventricular tachyarrythmias (PSVT) have also been associated with migraine headache (28). Attacks of PSVT may occur during a migraine attack or may occur as a migraine equivalent (acephalgic migraine). One case report noted improvement in both PSVT and migraine after treatment with digoxin (29).

Leviton and Camenga (30) reported an association between migraine and hyperbetalipoproteinemia. They found that treatment with clofibrate improved both the hyperlipidemia and the frequency of migraine attacks. Because certain fatty acids cause the release of serotonin, it is possible that other abnormalities in lipids may eventually be discovered in migraine sufferers.

Like migraine, mitral valve prolapse (Barlow's syndrome) is a common disorder of young women. Mitral valve prolapse has a population prevalence of about 6% in women without migraine, but Gamberini (8) found a prevalence of mitral valve prolapse of 23% in women migraine patients. In patients with mitral valve prolapse, 51% suffered with migraine, almost twice the expected prevalence rate.

The treatment of choice for symptomatic mitral valve prolapse in patients with migraine is β-blocker therapy. β-Blockers should reduce the chest pain, anxiety, and palpitations of mitral valve prolapse, in addition to reducing migraine frequency.

Asthma

Although there is no increased frequency of asthma in headache sufferers, one study from Poland (7) reported an association between aspirin-sensitive asthma and migraine. The prevalence of migraine in asthma (without aspirin sensitivity) was 13%, while in patients with aspirin-sensitive asthma, the prevalence of migraine was 45.7%. Aspirin-sensitive asthma constitutes 4 to 20% of all asthma cases and constitutes an illness consisting of asthma, anaphylactic reactions to aspirin or NSAIDs, and nasal polyps. Patients with aspirin-sensitive asthma may also be sensitive to tartrazine dye (yellow #5), which is used to color certain medications.

The treatment of migraine in patients with aspirin-sensitive asthma is complicated because NSAIDs may cause anaphylaxis and β-blockers may induce bronchospasm. The migraine prophylactic medication of choice would be a calcium channel blocker. Other agents such as methysergide, ACE inhibitors, or clonidine may be alternatives.

The treatment of asthma in the headache sufferer is not different from the routine management of asthma. Inhaled steroids and β₂-agonist drugs are the agents of first choice. Theophylline and nonspecific β-agonists may trigger headache and should be considered as second-line treatment. Cromolyn sodium is of particular value in patients with atopic asthma. Cromolyn sodium may also have benefit in reducing the frequency of migraine in patients whose headaches are related to diet (31).

Rheumatologic Disorders

Migraine occurs with increased frequency in patients with systemic lupus erythematosus (SLE), Sjögren's syndrome, and Raynaud's phenomenon without underlying connective tissue disease (2). Brandt and Lessell (32) reported that migraine with aura was commonly found in patients with SLE and that the onset of migrainous symptoms often preceded the diagnosis of SLE. They stated that migrainous symptoms were commonly associated with exacerbations of SLE and abated when SLE activity abated. Corticosteroids were more effective than antimigraine therapy (limited to ergotamine, aspirin, narcotics, and propranolol) in controlling the headaches and the aura in their series. Newer agents such as calcium channel blockers and NSAIDs may be more effective than the agents used in this study, but data are lacking.

Lupus anticoagulant, an antiphospholipid antibody, is associated with thrombotic disorders in patients with and without lupus. Several cases of migrainous stroke have occurred in patients with circulating lupus anticoagulant (33). The treatment of patients with lupus anticoagulant is controversial. Asymptomatic patients generally are not treated with anticoagulants, while patients who suffer thrombotic events usually receive long-term anticoagulation.

Sjögren's syndrome, a disorder marked by keratoconjunctivitis sicca, xerostomia, and episodic enlargement of the parotid glands, may present with dementia or depression. The dementia may be caused by either vasculitis or anti-CNS antibodies. Migraine is reported to occur in 46% of patients with primary Sjögren's syndrome (Sjögren's without rheumatoid arthritis) (2). This compares with migraine occurring in 11% of controls, 12% in patients with rheumatoid arthritis/Sjögren's syndrome, and 32% in patients with scleroderma. Treatment of migraine in patients with Sjögren's syndrome should exclude tricyclic antidepressants, since the anticholinergic side effects will worsen the dry mouth and dry eyes. Severe and recurrent headaches may indicate Sjögren's cerebritis, which requires

coticosteroid therapy. Measurement of the sedimentation rate may help differentiate migraine from Sjögren's cerebritis.

Patients with rheumatoid arthritis may suffer headaches from several pathogenic mechanisms (2). Subluxation of the upper cervical vertebrae may lead to tension-type (muscle-contraction) headache. The headache may be localized to the neck or occipital area, or radiate to the temples or retroorbital area. Rheumatoid arthritis often involves the temporomandibular joints, causing pain in the temporal region. Management of the rheumatoid arthritis with NSAIDs, remittive drugs (i.e., gold, methotrexate, d-penicillamine), or, in the case of upper cervical spine subluxation, surgery, will generally relieve the headache.

Patients with Raynaud's phenomenon, in the absence of other rheumatologic disease, have an increased prevalence of migraine (6). Prophylactic treatment of migraine in these patients should include a calcium channel blocker, which can help both conditions, and the avoidance of β-blockers, which can exacerbate Raynaud's phenomenon.

Peptic Ulcer Disease

Featherstone (3) reported that peptic ulcer disease is more common in headache sufferers than in nonheadache control patients. In patients with cluster headache, the prevalence of peptic ulcer disease may be three times greater than control populations.

Aspirin and NSAIDs generally should be avoided in patients with peptic ulcer disease. If NSAIDs are critical to headache therapy, nonacetylated salicylates (i.e., salsalate, choline salicylate, magnesium salicylate, etc.) may be less toxic to the gastric mucosa. Of the traditional NSAIDs, naproxen, ibuprofen, sulindac, and tolmetin have the least propensity to cause peptic ulcerations. An alternative approach is to use a NSAID in conjunction with misoprostel, a prostaglandin that protects the gastric mucosa from NSAID injury. Because prostaglandins may induce abortion, misoprostel must be used with great care in women of child-bearing potential and is contraindicated in pregnant women. The most common side effect of misoprostel is diarrhea.

Medications used to treat peptic ulcer disease may occasionally trigger migraine headache. The H₂-antagonist ranitidine caused a 3% incidence of headache and may exacerbate migraine in susceptible individuals (34). Famotidine causes a 4.7% incidence of headache. Headache from cimetidine is rare. Therefore, the H₂-antagonist of choice for headache sufferers appears to be cimetidine. Sucralfate and antacids are also useful agents in the management of peptic ulcer disease and do not exacerbate headache. Some tricyclic antidepressants, particularly doxepin, have histamine-antagonist properties and may be valuable in the management of peptic ulcer disease.

Recurrent abdominal pain is a disorder of children that

some experts believe to be a migraine equivalent, sometimes called the "recurrent syndrome" (35). Recurrent syndrome is defined as recurrent abdominal pain with or without nausea and vomiting, associated fever, and autonomic symptoms such as pallor and sweating. Amery and Forget (35) reported an increased gut permeability in children with recurrent syndrome. They postulate that increased gut permeability to certain noxious substances can explain the dietary triggers of migraine in select patients.

Obesity

Obesity is a common medical problem, with an estimated prevalence in the United States of 25 to 45% of the population over the age of 30 (36). Diseases associated with obesity include degenerative joint disease, respiratory compromise, cardiomegaly, hypertension, diabetes mellitus, menstrual irregularities, gout, and fatty liver. Obesity is commonly seen in headache sufferers. It is likely that societal attitudes toward obesity may increase the psychological stresses of obese headache patients and further exacerbate their condition. The author has observed numerous patients who discontinued effective headache therapy because the medication used induced weight gain or increased appetite.

Many drugs used in the treatment of headache may increase appetite. Among these are tricyclic antidepressants, monamine oxidase inhibitors, valproic acid, and cyproheptadine. β-Blockers occasionally impair exercise tolerance, with the potential for weight gain.

In obese patients or patients who gain an excessive amount of weight from antidepressive drugs, the antidepressants of choice are fluoxetine, sertraline, trazedone, or bupropion. These agents do not usually cause weight gain and may induce a small weight loss. Patients must also be encouraged to exercise regularly to increase caloric expenditure and reduce caloric intake to achieve weight control.

SUMMARY

As more headache sufferers seek professional help for their problem, it will be incumbent on physicians to consider all of a patient's medical illlnesses in choosing therapy. As new medications are used in the therapy of headache, it will become easier to tailor treatment to specific patient needs. The physician who treats patients with headache and concomitant medical problems must remain cognizant of the pharmacology and adverse effects of therapies, to prevent an exacerbation of either the medical condition or the headaches.

REFERENCES

1. Haber E, Slater EE. High blood pressure. In: Rubenstein E, Federman DD, eds. Scientific American Medicine. New York: Scientific American, 1988;1,VIII:1–30.
2. Pal B, Gibson C, Passmore J, Griffiths ID, Dick WC. A study of headaches and migraine in Sjögren's syndrome and other rheumatic disorders. Ann Rheum Dis 1989;48:312–316.
3. Featherstone HJ. Medical diagnoses and problems in individuals with recurrent idiopathic headaches. Headache 1985;25:136–140.
4. Fournier JA, Fernandez-Cortacero J, Granado C, Gascon D. Familial migraine and coronary artery spasm in two siblings. Clin Cardiol 1986;9:121–127.
5. Kuritzky A, Zehavi I, Appel S, et al. Cardiac arrhythmias in migraine: a 24-hour Holter study. Headache 1985;25:161.
6. Miller D, Waters DD, Warnica W, Szlachcic J, Kreeft J, Theroux P. Is variant angina the coronary manifestation of a generalized vasospastic disorder? N Engl J Med 1981;304:763–766.
7. Grzelewska-Rzymowska I, Bogucki A, Szmidt M, Kowalski ML, Prusinski A, Rozniecki J. Migraine in aspirin-sensitive asthmatics. Allergol FT. Immunopathology 1985;13:13–16.
8. Gamberini G, D'Alessandro R, Labriola E, et al. Further evidence on the association of mitral valve prolapse and migraine. Headache 1984;24:39–40.
9. Gardner JW, Mountain GE, Hines EA. The relationship of migraine to hypertension headaches. Am J Med Sci 1940;200:50–53.
10. Diamond S, Solomon GD, Freitag FG. Cluster headache. Clin J Pain 1987;3:171–176.
11. Askmark H, Lundberg PO, Olsson S. Drug-related headache. Headache 1989;29:441–444.
12. Roose S, Glassman A, Giardina E, Walsh B, Woodring S, Bigger J. Tricyclic antidepressants in depressed patients with cardiac conduction disease. Arch Gen Psychiatry 1987;44:273–275.
13. Psaty BM, Koepsell TD, Wagner EH, LoGerfo JP, Inui TS. The relative risk of incident coronary heart disease associated with recently stopping the use of β-blockers. JAMA 1990;263:1653–1657.
14. Solomon GD. Comparative efficacy of calcium antagonist drugs in the prophylaxis of migraine. Headache 1985;25:368–371.
15. Dalessio DJ. Beta blockers and migraine. JAMA 1984;252:2614.
16. Gold MS, Pottash AC, Sweeney DR, et al. Opiate withdrawal using clonidine. JAMA 1980;243:343–346.
17. Fanciullacci M, Spillantini MG, Michelacci S, Sicuteri F. Pharmacological "enkephalinase" inhibitions in man. Adv Exp Med Biol 1986;198:153–160.
18. Minervini MG, Pinto K. Captopril relieves pain and improves mood depression in depressed patients with classical migraine. Cephalalgia 1987;7(suppl 6):485.
19. Featherstone HJ. Headaches and heart disease: the lack of a positive association. Headache 1986;26:39–41.
20. Wayne VS. A possible relationship between migraine and coronary artery spasm. Aust NZ J Med 1986;16:708–710.
21. Cohn PF, Braunwald E. Chronic ischemic heart disease. In: Braunwald E, ed. Heart disease—textbook of cardiovascular medicine, vol. 2. Philadelphia: WB Saunders, 1984:1347.
22. Solomon GD, Kunkel RS, Frame J. Demographics of headache in elderly patients. Headache 1990;30:273–276.
23. Benedict CR, Robertson D. Angina pectoris and sudden death in the absence of atherosclerosis following ergotamine therapy for migraine. Am J Med 1979;67:177–178.
24. Ziegler DK. The treatment of migraine. In: Dalessio DJ, ed. Wolff's headache and other head pain. New York: Oxford University Press, 1987:90.
25. Johnson ES, Ratcliffe DM, Wilkinson M. Naproxen sodium in the treatment of migraine. Cephalalgia 1985;5:5–10.
26. Awidi AS. Efficacy of flurbiprofen in the treatment of acute migraine attacks: a double-blind cross-over study. Curr Ther Res 1982;32:492–497.
27. Sheftel FD, Rapoport AM, Marriot J, Saper J, Kunkel R, Steinmetzer R. Comparison of Meclomen, ergotamine tartrate with caffeine and placebo for the treatment of acute headaches: a double-blind parallel group multi-center study. Headache 1988;28:299.
28. Johansson BW. Migraine and the heart. Acta Med Scand 1983;213:241–243.
29. Johansson BW. Migraine: effect of digoxin. J R Soc Med 1982;75:215.
30. Leviton A, Camenga D. Migraine associated with hyper-pre-beta lipoproteinemia. Neurology 1969;19:963–965.

31. Monro J, Carini C, Brostoff J. Migraine is a food-allergic disease. Lancet 1984;2:719–721.

32. Brandt KD, Lessell S. Migrainous phenomena in stystemic lupus erythematosus. Arth Rheum 1978;21:7–16.

33. Levine SR, Deegan MJ, Futrell N, Welch KMA. Cerebrovascular and neurologic disease associated with antiphospholipid antibodies: 48 cases. Neurology 1990;40:1181–1189.

34. Epstein CM, Klopper J. Ranitidine headache. Headache 1985;25:392–393.

35. Amery WK, Forget PP. The role of the gut in migraine: the oral 51-Cr EDTA test in recurrent abdominal pain. Cephalalgia 1989;9:227–229.

36. Fitzgerald FT. The problem of obesity. Annu Rev Med 1981;32:221–231.

45

Analgesic Pharmacology in Management of Headache Pain

LAWRENCE M. HALPERN

Headaches often reoccur. Because of the repetitive character of pain paroxysms, opioids (with the possible exception of "weak opioid analgesics," e.g., codeine, propoxyphene) should not be used until all other diagnostic and therapeutic measures have failed. Even then, considerable care must be used to minimize complications of headache management caused by opioid dependence (1).

Recurrent headaches may reflect either underlying physical pathology or severe emotional disturbances in patients who experience them. Migraine headaches, cluster headaches, and vascular headaches are relatively benign when compared with more devastating headaches caused by subarachnoid hemorrhage, cerebellar hemorrhage, meningitis, intercranial masses, temporal arteritis, or other physical causes.

Headaches with underlying and potentially dangerous pathology should be evaluated by careful history, physical examination, and diagnostic testing. For relatively benign headaches, several treatment modalities may be helpful, including nonsteroidal analgesics and oxygen therapy. Prophylaxis with ergot alkaloids may also be effective. Migraine headaches are usually relatively benign, carry little morbidity except for pain and vomiting, and are unusual in pediatric populations. It is important to differentiate migraine and other relatively benign headaches from the potentially more devastating headaches described above.

INITIAL PHARMACOTHERAPY OF MIGRAINE

Dihydroergotamine is the drug of choice for initial therapy of migraine in the emergency room or office. It is usually given with prochlorperazine or dexamethazone. Oxygen may be effective therapy. Analgesics or sedatives can be used for refractory headaches for which a positive diagnosis has been established or a severe pathological diagnosis has been ruled out. Management should be individualized using approaches acceptable in this population after a diagnosis has been established (see Table 45.1.)

INITIAL PHARMACOTHERAPY FOR CLUSTER HEADACHES

Mild to moderate acute episodes of cluster headache may respond to nonsteroidal antiinflammatory agents, such as

aspirin and acetaminophen, and so-called weak narcotic analgesics, e.g., propoxyphene or codeine. Use of "strong" narcotic analgesics (e.g., meperidine) should be avoided because of rebound headache, the likelihood that headaches will be recurrent phenomena, and, because of their potential for physical dependence and addiction. (See Table 45.2.)

USE OF LOCAL ANESTHETICS TO ABORT HEADACHES

Lidocaine 4%, 1 ml topically applied via nostril ipsilateral to the pain (2), so as to enter the sphenopalatine fossa, may rapidly (within 3 minutes) abort acute cluster headache, both spontaneous and nitrate-induced. This finding suggests pain transmission via the sphenopalatine fossa (3).

Cocaine, 5 to 10%, 2 drops 4 times a day in the sphenopalatine region, can abort acute cluster headache. The effect appears to be attributable to the local anesthetic and not the sympathomimetic actions (3). Cocaine is as effective as lidocaine (4) but possesses a risk because of its high abuse potential (2).

PROPHYLAXIS OF CLUSTER HEADACHE

Ergotamine tartrate, a potent vasoconstrictor, can provide prophylaxis or even abort cluster headache if administered 2 mg p.o., 2 hours before an expected attack (5). It may be effective in up to 80% of episodic headaches but is not recommended for chronic cluster headaches (2). General recommendations are shown in Table 45.3.

Major adverse reactions include paresthesias and peripheral vascular insufficiency. Gangrene of extremities occurs rarely. Occasionally patients may complain of angina. At high doses, ergotism may occur. For these reasons, the drug is contraindicated in peripheral vascular disease, severe hypertension, and angina. It should be avoided in peptic ulcer patients, in pregnancy, infection, and in patients with renal or hepatic disease. Dependence to ergotamine may occur.

Dihydroergotamine (0.5 to 1 mg s.c. or IM) will considerably shorten the duration of a cluster headache. It is a hydrogenated derivative of ergotamine used for parenteral (IV or IM) administration. It produces less nausea and

Table 45.1.
Initial Treatment of Migraine in the Emergency Room

	1. Dihydroergotamine 0.5–1 mg IV over 3–4 min, may repeat in 1 hr to maximum dose of 2 mg
either	2. Prochlorperazine 5–10 mg IV
or	3. Dexamethazone 12–20 mg IV or IM; may repeat in 8–12 hr, not to exceed 24 hr from first injection
alternatively	4. Chlorpromazine 6.25–12.5 mg IV bolus q. 15 min; 25–50 mg IM, or 50–100 mg p.r. q6h
	5. Oxygen 4–6 liter/min worthwhile in small percentage of cases
	6. 1–2 liter normal saline IV in adult patients if dehydrated from excessive vomiting

Table 45.2.
Initial Treatment of Cluster Headaches

1. Analgesics: nonsteroidals or "weak opioids"
2. Oxygen 100% 7–10 liter/min for 5–15 min to abort an acute attack of cluster headache
3. Prophylactic: ergotamine tartrate if pattern of episodes is known; 2 mg p.o. 2 hr prior to expected attack; 1–2 mg p.o. each hour at onset of attack (maximum dose 8–10 mg/day)

Table 45.3.
Ergotamine Tartrate Prophylaxis of Episodic Cluster Headache

	1.	2 mg p.o. 2 hr prior to an attack
	2.	1–2 mg (to 8–10 mg/day) p.o. each hour at onset of attack
OR	3.	0.25–0.5 mg IM (to 1–1.5 mg/day) each hour at onset of attack
OR	4.	2 inhalations (0.72 mg) at pain onset
OR	5.	1–2 mg p.r.[a]

[a]Campbell JK. Facial pain due to migraine and cluster headache. Semin Neurol 1988;8:324–331.

vomiting but more pronounced α-adrenergic blockade than ergotamine. The vasoconstrictive action of dihydroergotamine is less prominent than that of ergotamine, and twice the dose is recommended (6).

Adverse reactions are similar to those of ergotamine. Pale or cold hands or feet, blisters on the hands or feet, numbness and tingling of extremities, and swelling of the feet or lower legs may occur. The drug should be used with caution in coronary artery disease, severe hypertension, infection, or impairment of hepatic or renal function.

Methysergide, 4 to 10 mg/day p.o. in two to four divided doses is effective in patients under 30 years old unless tolerance develops (7–9). It is 60 to 65% effective in episodic headaches and is not recommended for chronic cluster headaches (2). Adverse reactions to methysergide include vascular insufficiency, anginal pain, and psychiatric disturbances (hallucinations and increased anxiety). Drug-free periods are recommended because of the capacity to induce dependence, and the drug should be used with caution in patients with angina or severe arteriosclerotic heart disease.

Lisuride, a dopamine and peripheral serotonin-antagonist is an experimental drug (10) that is being investigated as a treatment with fewer side effects. The drug is not yet available in the United States.

Prednisone, 20 to 40 mg every other day for 5 days, can be used in patients who have become refractory to ergots. Success rates of 75 to 90% are claimed (2) for episodic headache and 40 to 90% in those with chronic headaches. Caution should be used for patients with or at risk of peptic ulcer disease, and health care providers should be alert for development of peptic ulcer disease as a consequence of provision of steroids to any patient.

Major adverse reactions to steroids include gastric ulceration and anemia; edema may precipitate heart failure in some patients. Continued high-dose administration without interruption may lead to osteoporosis and aseptic necrosis. The drug is contraindicated in cases of systemic fungal infection. Adrenal suppression may occur at high doses, and diuretic-induced hypokalemia may be exaggerated.

PSYCHOTROPICS IN HEADACHE MANAGEMENT

Chlorpromazine, 75 to 100 mg/day during attack, may be useful for relief of pain (11). The drug has been shown to block α- and β-adrenergic and dopamine receptors and has antihistamine and antiserotonin properties. Dosage reductions are required in hepatic insufficiency, renal failure, and in elderly patients. Caution should be used in patients with epilepsy, glaucoma, liver disease, and pregnancy. Absorption is decreased with concomitant antacids. Chlorpromazine may enhance the effects of phenytoin, antidepressants, and propanolol and may reduce the effects of guanethidine and levodopa. Orthostatic hypotension may occur, requiring blood pressure monitoring prior to and following administration.

Lithium carbonate, 600 to 1500 mg/day p.o. in two to four divided doses (2, 5), may be used for the prophylaxis of chronic cluster headache in patients over 45 years of age. It may eliminate headache, but autonomic symptoms may remain.

Major adverse reactions to lithium include diarrhea, nausea, leukocytosis, SA node abnormalities, hypercalcemia, hypothyroidism, dermatitis, diabetes insipidus, convulsions, renal toxicity, and mental confusion. It is contraindicated in pregnancy or lactation and in patients with renal impairment; it should be used with caution in the elderly or in patients with cardiac disease or organic brain damage or patients on concomitant neuromuscular blocking agents. Lithium levels should be monitored carefully in patients taking diuretics who are on restricted salt intake or with increased insensible water loss from warm environments.

Amitryptyline, 10 to 150 mg/day, is of use in prophylaxis of vascular headache. It may be especially effective in some headache patients, especially if depression coexists (12, 13). Major adverse reactions include orthostatic hypotension, tachycardia, granulocytopenia, confusional reactions, tachycardia, granulocytopenia, convulsions, and hepatotoxicity. Use with caution in the elderly, hyperactive patients, epilepsy, and ischemic heart disease. This drug must be used with caution with concomitant monoamine oxidase inhibitors. It may reduce the effect of guanethidine, clonidine, and reserpine and may enhance the effects of warfarin, phenothiazines, thyroid preparations, or sympathomimetic amines.

Propanolol, 40 to 80 mg/day four times a day, has been shown to be effective prophylaxis against vascular headaches (14). Dosage must be reduced in cases of chronic renal or hepatic insufficiency. Major adverse reactions include congestive heart failure (CHF), bronchospasm, severe bradycardia, peripheral arterial insufficiency, and cardiac arrest. It is contraindicated in bronchial asthma, bradycardia, CHF, cardiogenic shock, and pulmonary hypertension as a consequence of right ventricular failure. Abrupt withdrawal may precipitate angina or acute myocardial infarction (MI).

Cyproheptadine, 4 mg three times a day, has been claimed to be an alternate therapy, while not a drug of choice for headache management.

Calcium channel blockers, nifedipine 60 to 120 mg/day p.o., may be useful in headache prophylaxis (15). Verapamil, 240 mg/day p.o., nifedipine, and nimodipine, reduced headache frequency, and verapamil significantly reduced headache fequency (16).

Histamine desensitization may be a useful alternative for patients with intractable chronic cluster headache (17).

ANALGESICS OVERVIEW: PERIPHERALLY ACTING NONNARCOTIC AGENTS AS ANALGESICS

Peripherally acting analgesics such as the nonnarcotic analgesics, (e.g., salicylates) are useful agents for treating headaches of mild to moderate intensity. Because of risks of rebound headache, addiction, and physical dependence, opioid analgesics, "narcotics," should be used with caution in patients with vascular or cluster headaches (11). Some physicians recommend that narcotics never be used for relief of headache pain. Others feel that their use is justified in certain clinical settings (18). Recommended "weak opioid" analgesics include codeine and propoxyphene.

One useful finding over the last few years of analgesic research is that antiinflammatory agents are all useful as analgesics. The most common ones used in headache management are described below, then placed in context by setting them against the background of all of the nonsteroidals presently available. A discussion of the methods of selection and use of nonsteroidals follows.

PERIPHERALLY ACTING ANALGESICS

Nonsteroidal antiinflammatory agents, including acetaminophen, provide analgesia via inhibition of cyclooxygenase enzymes, a peripheral mechanism, with consequent reduction in further synthesis of inflammatory mediators known as sensitizers or activators of peripheral nociceptors (19). Other as yet undescribed mechanisms may explain disproportionate analgesic and antiinflammatory effects observed with some agents of this class (e.g., acetaminophen, zomepirac, and ketorolac).

Subclasses of peripherally acting analgesics include: p-aminophenols, salicylates, proprionic acids, acetic acids, oxicams, fenamates, and pyazoles (20). Variability in clinical response to different agents in a subclass is marked, and outcome is not easily predicted on the basis of outcome from previous trials with other agents.

Peripherally acting agents produce analgesic responses that are characterized by a ceiling dose above which side effects increase but additional analgesia does not occur. A ceiling dose limits use of peripherally acting agents to those cases where pain is mild to moderate. Equivalent doses are usually derived from studies of clinical populations where patients have a single inflammatory (e.g., arthritis) disease and no other significant complicating medical problems.

With certain clinical exceptions, these agents may be used repeatedly because tolerance and physical dependence are not associated with repetitive or continuous use.

CHOOSING THE APPROPRIATE NONSTEROIDAL DRUG

Peripherally acting analgesics are used independently for mild-to-moderate pain. When combined with opioids, they may provide additional analgesia and can be used for the treatment of more severe pain (21, 22). Drug selection must be individualized for each patient and decisions based upon profiles of adverse effects associated with peripherally acting agents as a class, each of the subclasses, and each individual drug (Table 45.4). Peripherally acting analgesics as a class must be used cautiously if at all in patients with renal insufficiency. If the patients must be treated with a peripherally acting analgesic, data suggest that sulindac has less potential for renal toxicity than other drugs in this class (23). If analgesia is required for mild-to-moderate pain and antiinflammatory action is not essential, acetaminophen may be useful; however, recent studies have shown a potential for renal toxicity from this drug as well (24). The pyrazoles have long been associated with a greater risk of side effects than other agents in this class, and other agents with fewer adverse reactions have replaced them. Nevertheless, these agents continue to be provided in treatment of mild-to-moderate pain despite excessive risk to patients.

Most agents are contraindicated as analgesics in patients with peptic ulcer disease or for whom interruption of blood clotting mechanisms would be a problem. Appropriate drug choices in these cases would include acetaminophen, choline magnesium salicylate, and salsalate. These peripherally acting analgesics have much less ulcer potential than other agents and do not impair platelet aggregation at doses that are used for pain control (25). If there is additional concern about ulcers or gastric irritation, misoprostol may be used in conjunction with these agents.

Misoprostol is a synthetic prostaglandin analogue that has recently become available and can be used to suppress

Table 45.4.
Nonsteroidal Antiinflammatory Drugs

Chemical Class	Generic Name	Approximate Half-Life (hr)	Dosing Schedule	Recommended Starting Dose (mg/day)[a]	Maximum Recommended (mg/day)	Comments
p-Aminophenol derivatives	Acetaminophen[b]	2–4	q4–6h	1400	6000	Overdosage produces hepatic toxicity; not antiinflammatory and therefore not preferred as first-line analgesic or coanalgesic in pts with inflammatory pain; lack of GI or platelet toxicity may be important in some pts; at high doses, platelet counts and liver function tests should be done monthly
Salicylates	Aspirin[b]	3–12[c]	q4–6h	1400	6000	Standard for comparison; may not be tolerated as well as some of the newer NSAIDs[d]
	Diflunisal[b]	8–12	q12h	1000 × 1 then 500 q12h	1500	Less GI toxicity than aspirin[d]
	Choline magnesium trisalicylate[b]	8–12	q12h	1500 × 1 then 1000 q12h	4000	Unlike other NSAIDs, choline Mg trisalicylate and salsalate have minimal GI toxicity and no effect on platelet aggregation, despite potent antiinflammatory effects;
	Salsalate	8–12	q12h	1500 × 1 then 1000 q12h	4000	may therefore be particularly useful in some pts[d]
Propionic acids	Ibuprofen[b]	3–4	q4–8h	1200	4200	Available over-the-counter[d]
	Naproxen[b]	13	q12h	500	1000	Available as a suspension[d]
	Naproxen sodium[b]	13	q12h	550	1100	[d]
	Fenoprofen	2–3	q6h	800	3200	[d]
	Ketoprofen	2–3	q6–8h	150	300	[d]
	Flurbiprofen[b]	5–6	q8–12h	100	300	Experience too limited to evaluate higher doses, though it's likely that some pts would benefit[d]
Acetic acids	Indomethacin	4–5	q8–12h	75	200	Available in sustained-released rectal formulations; higher incidence of side effects, particularly GI and CNS, than proprionic acids[d]
	Tolmetin	1	q6–8h	600	2000	[d]
	Sulindac	14	q12h	300	400	Less renal toxicity than other NSAIDs[d]
	Suprofen[b]	2–4	q6h	600	800	Experience too limited to evaluate higher doses, though it is likely that some pts would benefit[d]
	Diclofenac	2	q6h	75	200	[d]
	Ketorolac	4–7	q4–6h	120	240	Parenteral formulation available; experience too limited to evaluate higher doses[d]
Oxicams	Prioxicam	45	q24h	20	40	Administration of 40 mg over weeks is associated with a high incidence of peptic ulcer, particularly in the elderly[d]
Fenamates	Mefenamic acid[b]	2	q6h	500 × 1 then 250 q6h	1000	Not recommended for use longer than 1 week and therefore not indicated in recurrent pain therapy[d]
	Meclofenamic acid	2–4	q6–8h	150	400	[d]
Pyrazolones	Phenylbutazone	50–100	q6–8h	300	400	Not a first-line drug due to risk of serious bone marrow toxicity

[a]Starting dose should be one-half to two-thirds recommended dose in the elderly, those on multiple drugs, and those with renal insufficiency. Doses must be individualized. Low initial doses should be titrated upward if tolerated and clinical effect is inadequate. Doses can be incremented weekly.
[b]Pain is approved indication.
[c]Half-life of aspirin increases with dose.
[d]At high doses, stool guaiac test should be done bimonthly and liver function tests, BUN, creatinine level, and urinalysis should be checked every 1–2 months.

gastric ulceration from any nonsteroidal agent whose major action is inhibition of cyclooxygenases and which would ordinarily deplete prostaglandins. The drug is especially useful for the prevention of ulcers that often occur during long-term treatment with aspirin-like drugs (26, 27). The drug may produce some diarrhea, which usually doesn't require discontinuation of treatment. Because of its uterotonic action, the drug should not be administered to pregnant women.

All peripherally acting analgesics (with the exception of acetaminophen) may exacerbate encephalopathy in patients with preexisting organic brain syndrome. Acetaminophen is itself hepatotoxic in high doses and should be used with care if at all in patients with hepatic insufficiency.

Other factors may be considered when choosing a non-steroidal drug. A favorable previous response of an individual to a nonsteroidal is reason to choose that agent again, as there is remarkable individual variability in responding to different agents. If compliance becomes an issue, once-a-day (piroxicam) or twice-daily (e.g., naproxen, choline magnesium trisalicylate, diflunisal) drugs may be used. If cost becomes an issue, prices of different drugs at different pharmacies vary widely, and pharmacy prices may be surveyed before drugs are selected.

USING THE DOSE-RESPONSE CURVE TO ENHANCE THERAPEUTIC EFFECTIVENESS OF NONSTEROIDALS

Once a nonsteroidal has been selected for an individual patient, a therapeutic trial is necessary to determine optimal dosage (i.e., maximally effective analgesia with minimal side effects). Some exploration of the dose-response curve should be undertaken. Start at recommended daily doses and increase doses gradually, attempting to identify a ceiling dose that provides maximum benefit at minimum side effects for each headache episode. If there is no increase in analgesia following an increase of dose, then the ceiling dose has been reached for that patient. The dosage should be returned to the previous level and continued, or discontinued. If analgesia improves following an increased dose, the ceiling has probably not been reached, and there may be an improved therapeutic response at a slightly higher dosage. Dose-related toxicity limits the upper end of the dose-response curve and indicates that dose exploration has gone too far and the dosage exceeds that which can be given safely. Maximal increments between 1.5 and 2 times the standard dose provide the best analgesia. The aim of dose exploration is to use the lowest dose that provides the greatest degree of analgesia attainable. Several weeks are required to judge efficacy of nonsteroidal doses in treatment of chronic inflammatory diseases (e.g., arthritis), but a briefer period, perhaps a week, can provide information for the infrequent user. Once a drug is selected and optimal dosage found for an individual patient, the agent can be used for future headache episodes.

Close monitoring is required if higher doses are used or patients continue doses for uninterrupted long intervals. Monitoring should include tests for fecal blood, urinalysis, and evaluation of bound urea nitrogen, and creatinine clearance every 30 to 60 days of continuous use. Episodic use characteristic of some headache patients may relax this requirement somewhat.

Because of variability in patient responses to different nonsteroidals, it is important to understand that failure of a specific NSAID to provide pain relief may be followed by successful analgesia with another drug. Thus, failure with an NSAID should be followed by a trial with another drug from a different subclass of nonsteroidals (e.g., salicylate trial followed by propionic acid trial).

SPECIFIC AGENTS USEFUL IN HEADACHE MANAGEMENT

Ibuprofen, 300 to 400 mg p.o. 3 times a day, may be used to treat headache of mild-to-moderate intensity. In severe headache pain, ibuprofen may not be of value. Limiting adverse reactions may include vertigo, tinnitus, and GI bleeding. The drug is contraindicated in aspirin-intolerant patients and should be used with caution in patients with peptic ulcer or systemic lupus erythematosus.

Aspirin, 650 to 975 mg every 4 to 6 hours, may be useful in treating headache pain of mild-to-moderate intensity. When headache pain is severe, the role of aspirin may be limited (11). As with most nonsteroidals, aspirin may exacerbate uremic symptoms and should be avoided in hepatic insufficiency. Adverse reactions include increased bleeding time and potential bleeding episodes, hypersensitivity reactions such as urticaria and anaphylaxis, hepatotoxicity after high doses, and tinnitus at high doses. Aspirin is contraindicated in bleeding disorders, in the last month of pregnancy, and where hypersensitivity to aspirin exists. Caution should be used in cases of asthma, nasal polyps, and ulcers and in patients receiving anticoagulants. There are many drug-drug interactions for aspirin. Toxic concentrations of aspirin are those above 345 µg/ml.

Acetaminophen, 2 to 3 tablets every 4 to 6 hours, may be useful in treating mild headaches. If pain is excruciating, acetaminophen may be of limited value. Dose reduction is not required in renal failure or geriatric patients. Major adverse reactions include hepatotoxicity (overdose) and thrombocytopenia. This drug must be used with caution in cases of G-6-PD deficiency.

Indomethacin, 50 mg p.o. three times a day, may be useful in treating headache of mild-to-moderate intensity. When intensity escalates, indomethacin is of limited value. Dosage reductions are not necessary in renal insufficiency but are necessary in severe liver disease. Major adverse reactions include blood dyscrasias such as agranulocytosis, aplastic anemia, and leukopenia; hepatitis; severe skin reactions; headache, and dizziness. Indomethacin is contraindicated in pregnancy, breast-feeding period, and in patients with active GI lesions and should be avoided in patients with aspirin intolerance. Indomethacin has been shown to aggravate psychiatric conditions, epilepsy, and parkinsonism. Drug-drug interactions include attenuation of the effect of some β-blockers and increased effects of lithium, furosemide, and thiazide diuretics.

OPIOID ANALGESICS

Although opioids are not recommended for headache management unless alternative diagnostic and therapeutic measures have proven ineffective, some discussion of opioid selection and use should be included here for the sake of completeness. As with the NSAIDS, there is a great deal of individual variability in patients response to individual opioid drugs. Pharmacological and pharmacokinetic factors have a great deal to do with initial selection of an opioid drug. These factors also strongly influence secondary or tertiary choices should changes become necessary (Table 45.5).

Opioids are either agonists (e.g., morphine, meperidine) or agonist-antagonists having mixed actions at various opioid receptors. Agonist-antagonist opioids can be further subdivided into mixed agonist-antagonist (e.g., nallorphine-like agents pentazocine, nalbuphine, and butorphanol) or partial agonists (the long-acting morphine-like agent buprenorphine

Table 45.5.
Opioid Analgesics

	Equianalgesic Doses[a]	Half-Life (hr)	Peak Effect (hr)	Duration (hr)	Toxicity	Comments
Morphine-like agonists						
Morphine	10 IM	2–3	0.5–1	3–6	Constipation, nausea, sedation most common; respiratory depression rare in cancer pts	Standard comparison for opioids; multiple routes available (see Table 45.4)
	20–60 p.o.[b]		0.5–2	4–7		
Controlled-release Morphine	20–60 p.o.[b]	—	3–4	8–12		
Hydromorphone	1.5 IM	2–3	0.5–1	3–4	Same as morphine	Used for multiple routes (see Table 45.4)
	7.5 p.o.	—	1–2	3–4		
Oxycodone	30 p.o.	2–3	1	3–6	Same as morphine	Combined with aspirin or acetaminophen for moderate pain; available orally without coanalgesic
Oxymorphone	1 IM	—	0.5–1	3–6	Same as morphine	No oral formulation
	10 p.r.		1.5–3	4–6		
Meperidine	75 IM	2–3	0.5–1	3–4	Same as morphine + CNS excitation; contraindicated in those on MAO inhibitors	Not preferred for recurrent pain due to potential toxicity of normepizioine
	300 p.o.	—	1–2	3–6		
Heroin	5 IM	0.5	0.5–1	4–5	Same as morphine	Analgesic action due to metabolites, predominantly morphine; not available in U.S.
Levorphanol	2 IM	12–15	0.5–1	3–6	Same as morphine	With long half-life, accumulation occurs after beginning or increasing dose
Methadone	10 IM	15–57	0.5–1.5	4–6	Same as morphine	Risk of delayed toxicity due to accumulation; dosing should start on p.r.n. basis, with close monitoring
	20 p.o.					
Codeine	130 IM	2–3	1.5–2	3–6	Same as morphine	Usually combined with NSAID
	200 p.o.					
Propoxyphene HCl	—	12	1.5–2	3–6	Same as morphine plus seizures with overdose	Toxic metabolite accumulates but not significant at doses used clinically; often combined with NSAID
Propoxyphene napsylate	—	12	1.5–2	3–6	Same as hydrochloride	Same as hydrochloride
Hydrocodone	—	2–4	0.5–1	3–4	Same as morphine	Only available combined with acetaminophen
Mixed agonist-antagonists						
Pentazocine	60 IM	2–3	0.5–1	3–6	Same profile of effects as buprenorphine, except for greater risk of psychotomimetic effects	Produces a withdrawal in opioid-dependent pts; oral preparation combined with naloxone in U.S.; ceiling doses and side-effect profile limits role
	180 p.o.	—	1–2	3–6		
Nalbuphine	10 IM	4–6	0.5–1	3–6	Same as buprenorphine, except for greater risk of psychotomimetic effects, which is lower than pentazocine	Produces withdrawal in opioid-dependent pts; no oral formulation; not preferred for recurrent pain therapy
Butorphanol	2 IM	2–3	0.5–1	3–4	Same profile of effects as nalbuphine	Produces withdrawal in opioid-dependent pts; no oral formulation; not preferred for recurrent pain therapy
Partial agonist						
Buprenorphine	0.4 IM	2–5	0.5–1	4–6	Same as morphine, except less risk of respiratory depression	Can produce withdrawal in opioid-dependent pts; has ceiling for analgesia; sublingual tablet, not yet available in U.S.; may be useful in recurrent pain pts, not naloxone-reversible
	0.8 s.l.		2–3	5–6		

[a]Dose that provides analgesia is equivalent to 10 mg intramuscular morphine.
[b]Extensive survey data suggest that the relative potency of IM:p.o. morphine of 1:6 changes to 1:2–3 with chronic dosing.

is currently the only such agent available). Distinctions concerning opioids can also be based on patterns of interactions with mu, kappa, and sigma receptors (1).

Agonist-antagonist drugs should not be used for treatment of headache pain in patients who have chronic headaches treated with opioid-agonist drugs. Agonist-antagonist agents all have the ability to specifically reverse opioid effects and precipitate narcotic abstinence syndrome in patients physically dependent on opioid-agonist drugs. Mixed agonist-antagonist drugs (especially pentazocine) affect sigma receptors and have a high incidence and potential for psychotomimetic effects. Most mixed agonist-antagonist drugs are not available in an oral formulation, the preferred route of administration in this population. Sublingual buprenorphine, available in many countries, has never been released in the United States. Agonist drugs remain a mainstay of ambulatory pain management.

"WEAK" VERSUS "STRONG" OPIOIDS

The distinction between "weak" and "strong" classes is purely an operational one. Codeine is the standard "weak" opioid, a group that includes propoxyphene, oxycodone-nonsteroidal combinations, hydrocodone, meperidine, and pentazocine. No data from controlled studies suggest that these agents (with the possible exception of pentazocine) have ceiling doses for analgesia or flatter dose-response curves. So-called weak drugs can be used to treat severe pain, but as dosage increases, side effect liability also increases. It is common clinical practice to initiate opioid therapy with a "weak" opioid, either independently or in combination with peripherally acting analgesics. If additional analgesia is sought, so-called strong analgesics (e.g., meperidine or hydromorphone) are then used. Meperidine, while an ever-popular "strong" analgesic, is toxic after repetitive use because of accumulation of nor-meperidine and should not be used repeatedly in patients who require closely spaced episodes of analgesia for severe pain.

Propoxyphene, 65 mg p.o. three to four times a day, may be useful in treating vascular headaches of mild-to-moderate intensity. Cluster headache pain may be excruciating, and therefore the role of propoxyphene may be limited (11). Major adverse reactions include convulsions after high doses, psychosis, dependence, hypoglycemia, hepatotoxicity, and respiratory depression. Dizziness, drowsiness, tremors, mental confusion, and anxiety can occur when it is administered with orphenadrine. Propoxyphene should be used with caution in pregnancy. Chronic use may produce dependence and may enhance the effects of CNS depressants, warfarin, orphenadrine, carbamazepine, and doxepin.

DRUG TOXICITY

As with nonsteroidals, there is remarkable variability in patient response to opioid drugs. This is observed as a difference in response of a single patient to different drugs or a variety of patients to the same drug. Thus, it is desirable to individualize the application of opioids for pain in specific patients. The repeated use of meperidine is complicated by accumulation of a toxic metabolite, nor-mepiridine, with the development of central nervous system actions including hyperactivity, myoclonus, tremulousness, seizures, and mood swings including depression (28). These effects are most likely to occur in patients who receive many doses over long periods of time or who have renal insufficiency. This action essentially contraindicates the repeated use of this drug in individual patients over long periods of time.

PHARMACOKINETIC DIFFERENCES AND CHOICES AMONG OPIOID DRUGS

Terminal elimination half-life is the most important pharmacokinetic factor in individualized drug selection and rational use of opioid agents. Half-lives of 2 to 3 hours have been found for morphine, hydromorphone, oxycodone, meperidine, codeine, pentazocine, and butorphanol. Half-lives of 15 to 57 hours have been determined for methadone and 12 to 15 hours for levorphanol. Four to five half-lives are required for a drug to approach steady-state plasma levels, regardless of drug, dosing interval, or route of administration. Thus, accumulation of drug can occur for many days after dosage adjustment has been accomplished if drugs continue to be administered. Durations of analgesic action are only loosely related to elimination half-life (e.g., doses of meperidine produce peak analgesia at 1.5 hours after administration), and the dosage interval for readministration should be explored for individual patients between 2 and 3 hours. While the half-lives of methadone and levorphanol are relatively long, readministration intervals for methadone are roughly 4 to 6 hours, and for levorphanol, 4 hours. Drugs with long half-lives tend to accumulate and produce respiratory depression, thus, repeated doses of long-acting drugs require careful monitoring of respiratory rate and analgesia (29). Long half-life agents should be used with care if at all in patients predisposed to adverse drug effects, those with major organ failure, those with encephalopathy, those who are not available for frequent follow-up, or those who are not compliant with prescription instructions.

FAVORABLE PRIOR EXPERIENCE IS A REASON TO CHOOSE AN OPIOID FOR READMINISTRATION

With the exception of meperidine, a prior favorable experience with an opioid gives reasonable expectations that repeated use of this opioid will produce a favorable response. With meperidine, the risk of nor-mepiridine toxicity increases dramatically with chronic oral administration, especially at high doses, and prior experience is no guarantee of a salutary repeat experience.

Start with the lowest effective dose. A patient who has little or no prior experience with "strong" opioids should receive a starting dose equivalent to 5 to 10 mg of morphine IM. Understanding the concept of equianalgesic dose or relative potency (30) is important, so health workers can switch between opioid drugs or alter routes of administration.

Titrate the dose up at each administration to the desirable effect or until side effects become dangerous (e.g., respiratory rate depression) or uncomfortable (e.g., persistent nausea and vomiting). Naloxone (Narcan) can be administered if effects of opioids become life-threatening.

Do not discontinue effective nonsteroidals when beginning opioid use. The combined mechanisms of action can be beneficial in reducing the overall dose of opioid finally required to ameliorate headache pain.

BE AWARE THAT TOLERANCE, PHYSICAL AND PSYCHOLOGICAL DEPENDENCE MAY COMPLICATE THE MOST WELL INTENTIONED THERAPY

Repeated doses of opioids will eventually (2 weeks) lead to progressive failure of expected response from a given opioid dose. As tolerance develops, physical dependence develops in parallel. Physical dependence means that following abrupt discontinuation or precipitation by administering an opioid antagonist, uncomfortable and stereotyped withdrawal symptoms called "abstinence syndrome" may occur. The discomfort from perceived withdrawal may cause a patient to develop a headache requiring opioids to ward off impending withdrawal symptoms.

SUMMARY

Rational opioid selection is based on pharmacological principles and clinical experience. Headache patients' drug therapy begins with selection of a nonsteroidal agent, appropriate dose determined for each patient. If headaches persist or are more intense than can be covered by nonsteroidal agents, then nonsteroidals in combination with "weak" opioids should be used. If after completion of diagnostic procedures a decision to use "strong" opioids is made, most of the 2- to 3-hour drugs are candidates for selection. If this regimen is started, physical and psychological dependence must be watched for after repeated administration. Because of the toxicity of its major metabolite, problems with tolerance and physical dependence, and the possibility of "rebound" headache induced by the drug, meperidine (Demerol) should not be used repeatedly or at high dose. It is generally unwise to start headache patients on strong opioids because of difficulties encountered discontinuing these agents.

REFERENCES

1. Gilman AG, Rall TW, Nies AS, Taylor P, eds. Goodman and Gilman's the pharmacological basis of therapeutics. 8th ed. New York: Pergamon 1990.
2. McKenna JP. Cluster headache. Am Fam Physician 1988;37:173–178.
3. Kittrelle JP, Grouse DS, Seybold ME. Cluster headache local anesthetic abortive agents. Arch Neurol 1985;42:496–498.
4. Hardebo JE, Elner A. Nerves and vessels to the pterygopalatine fossa and symptoms of cluster headache. Headache 1987;27:528–532.
5. Kudrow L. Cluster headache: diagnosis and management. Headache 1979;19:142–150.
6. AMA Division of Drugs. AMA drug evaluations. 5th ed. Chicago: American Medical Association, 1983.
7. Graham J. Possible renal complications of Sansert (methysergide) therapy for headache. Headache 1965;5:12–14.
8. Graham J, Parnes L. Possible cardiac and renovascular complications of Sansert therapy. Headache 1965;5:14–18.
9. Kunkel R. Fibrotic syndromes with chronic use of methysergide. Headache 1971;11:1–5.
10. Rafaelli E Jr, Martins OJ. Daqua Filho ADSP Lisuride in cluster headache. Headache 1983;23:117–121.
11. Caviness VS Jr, Obrien P. Current concepts: headache. N Engl J Med 1980;302(8):446–450.
12. Couch J. Amitriptyline in the prophylaxis of migraine: effectiveness and relationship of antimigraine and antidepressant effects. Neurology 1976;22:366–369.
13. Parnell P, Cooperstock R. Tranquilizers and mood elevators in the treatment of migraine: an analysis of the migraine foundation questionnaire. Headache 1979;19:78–89.
14. Weber R, Reinmuth O. The treatment of migraine with propanolol. Neurology 1972;22:366–369.
15. Meyer JS, Hardenberg J. Clinical effectiveness of calcium entry blockers in prophylactic treatment of migraine and cluster headaches. Headache 1983;23:266–277.
16. Meyer JS, Dowell R, Mathew N, et al. Clinical and hemodynamic effects during treatment of vascular headaches with verapamil. Headache 1984;24:313–321.
17. Diamond S, Freitag FG, Prager J, et al. Treatment of intractable cluster. Headache 1986;26:42–46.
18. Olenick JS, Taylor RB. Emergency evaluation and treatment of headache. Prim Care 1986;13:97–107.
19. Vane JR. Inhibition of prostaglandin synthesis as a mechanism of action for aspirin-like drugs. Nature New Biol 1971;234:231–238.
20. Sunshine A, Olsen NZ. Non-narcotic analgesics. In: Wall PD, Melzak R, eds. Textbook of pain. 2nd ed. New York: Churchill Livingstone, 1986:670–685.
21. Ferrerr-Brechner T, Ganz P. Combination therapy with ibuprofen and methadone for chronic cancer pain. Am J Med 1984;77:78–83.
22. Ventafridda V, Fochi C, DeConno F, Sganzeria E. Use of nonsteroidal antiinflammatory drugs in the treatment of cancer. Br J Clin Pharmacol 1980;10:343–346.
23. Swainson CP, Griffiths P. Acute and chronic effects of sulindac on renal function in chronic renal disease. Clin Pharmacol Therap 37:298–300.
24. Sandler DP, Smith JC, Weinberg CR, Buckalew VM, Dennis VW, et al. Analgesic use and chronic renal disease. N Engl J Med 1989;320:1238–1243.
25. Cohen A, Thomas GB, Cohen EE. Serum concentration, safety, and tolerance of oral doses of choline magnesium trisalicylate. Curr Ther Res 1978;23:358–364.
26. Sontag SJ. Prostaglandins in peptic ulcer disease: an overview of current status and future directions. Drugs 1986;32:445–457.
27. Monk JP, Clissold SP. Misoprostol: a preliminary review of its pharmacodynamic and pharmacokinetic properties, and therapeutic efficacy in the treatment of peptic ulcer disease. Drugs 1987;33:1–30.
28. Kaiko RF, Foley KM, Grabinski PY, et al. Central nervous system excitatory effects of meperidine in cancer patients. Ann Neurol 1983;13:1180–1185.
29. Ettinger DS, Vitale PJ, Trump DL. Important clinical pharmacologic considerations in the use of methadone in cancer patients. Cancer Treat Rep 1979;63:457–459.
30. Houde RW. Misinformation: side effects and drug interactions. In: Hill CS, Fields WS, eds. Advances in pain research and therapy, vol 11. New York: Raven Press, 1989:145–161.

46

Acupuncture

GEORGE A. ULETT

HISTORICAL

Acupuncture has long been recognized as a treatment method for headache. Historical documents from China suggest that the procedure arose serendipitously some 4000 years ago. The *Nei Ching* (1), written over 3000 years ago, compiled the observations and metaphysical explanations given by many generations of ancient Chinese healers. As there was no knowledge of physiology and only rudimentary ideas about anatomy, theories to explain the action of acupuncture were based mostly on Taoistic religious beliefs, superstition, and numerology.

Despite the fact that such theories have little relevance in today's scientific world, treatments based upon these traditional theories can produce useful results. Patients are treated with needles, and headaches are relieved. One of the foremost internationally known practitioners of acupuncture, Dr. Felix Mann of London (2), once observed that ancient acupuncturists got good results but for the wrong reasons.

SCIENTIFIC BASIS OF ACUPUNCTURE

In the last two decades, international researchers have made discoveries that have rendered obsolete the ancient meridian hypotheses. The ideas of the ancients have in a sense been validated but now reformulated in scientific terms. Today it is known that acupuncture is essentially a technique for getting a stimulus, preferably a DC current, into the central nervous system. The best points to use are those where nerve fibers are most easily accessed, such as motor points, Golgi tendon organs, or points adjacent to nerve roots or fibers.

Our own early research convinced us that although, as in all of medicine, placebo response is important, the acupuncture effect was not the result of suggestion (3). Poor hypnotic subjects benefit from pain relief by acupuncture as well as good subjects. We also found that while needles alone have some effect on pain, the addition of electric current doubles the effectiveness of the treatments (4).

Shapiro and Stockard (5) recently stated that if we can accumulate good evidence of acupuncture's pathophysio-logical effects we can expect acupuncture to be integrated into Western medical practice. Actually that evidence appears to be at hand. Peng and Greenfield (6) have reviewed recent studies of the physiological effect of needles inserted into muscle tissue. Work of Liu et al. (7) and Gunn (8) have given evidence that the most effective acupuncture points are actually motor points where nerve enters muscle. We have used this concept most successfully clinically and in our teaching (9).

Chang (10) early discovered that the site of analgesic action of morphine was in the brain. Knowledge of nature's own morphine-like substances, the endorphins, opened up a whole new chapter in pain research. In 1973, Solomon Snyder and Candace Pert (11) reported in *Science* that they had located brain receptor sites for opioids, and in 1975, Professor Hans Kosterlitz and Dr. John Hughes (12) discovered enkephalin in the brainstem of rats. The pieces of this scientific jigsaw puzzle began to come together.

Han's group in Beijing had shown that the classical neurotransmitter, serotonin, was most important for mediating acupuncture analgesia (13) and that the central catecholamine norepinephrine had an antagonistic effect upon acupuncture analgesia in the spinal cord. Mayer et al. (14) studied laboratory-induced tooth pain in humans, producing acupuncture analgesia by manual twirling of needles in LI-4, the first dorsal interosseous motor point in the hand. In a double-blind study, he found that naloxone blocks this analgesia while saline does not.

Microinjection studies of naloxone into the periaqueductal gray or intrathecally over the spinal cord showed decreased acupuncture analgesia in rats and rabbits (15). The opioid peptides could be grouped into the enkephalins, endorphins and dynorphins. Working with Terenius, Han (16) used the antibody injection technique to show that enkephalins are mediators for acupuncture analgesia in both the brain and spinal cord, while beta endorphin is effective in the brain but not in the spinal cord. In a carefully conducted experiment, Han also showed that dynorphin antiserum blocks acupuncture analgesia in rabbits (17). Dynorphins are effective in the spinal cord but not in the brain (18).

In summary, it appears that acupuncture releases beta endorphins and enkephalin in the brain and dynorphin and enkephalin in the spinal cord. Important correlates of the endorphin acupuncture analgesia hypothesis are found in the reports of Sjölund et al. (19) that endorphins are increased in cerebrospinal fluid with acupuncture stimulation.

Traditional acupuncturists have observed that needle manipulation at the same point can bring about different results. Needling the anterior tibialis motor point can, for example, treat diarrhea in one case and constipation in another. Presumably the needles are manipulated differently in each case. A possible explanation lies in the fact that low-frequency (2 to 4 Hz) stimulation causes a profound release of metenkephalins, while high-frequency stimulation (80 to 100 Hz) releases endorphins.

The work of Han has clearly shown that it is the frequency rather than the intensity of the stimulation that is of the utmost importance in producing acupuncture analgesia (20), and thus it may be that lack of response to electroacupuncture could well be overcome by finding the proper parameters of stimulation for each individual and each type of headache. Because the acupuncture effect depends upon manipulation of biochemical systems that have widespread effects throughout the central nervous system, it has become apparent that the effectiveness of acupuncture stimulation does not depend upon the specific placement of needles. Rather, this is relative rather than specific.

It is only important perhaps that some locations have a somewhat greater overall effect than others. Thus, a needle placed in the *Hoku* (LI-4), dorsal interosseus motor point of the thumb, or any other motor point distal on the upper extremity may produce widespread analgesic effects through actuating the beta endorphinergic and enkephalinergic systems. Simultaneous stimulation of another point (for example *Tsu-san-li* (ST-36), the tibialis anterior motor point) might produce an additive effect. As the release of dynorphins is most likely to occur at a local level in the central nervous system, it would seem that stimulation of a point in the upper extremity (*Hoku* (LI-4) for example) would be more likely to bring relief of headache than points in the lower part of the body.

Again, however, such stimulation would be greatly affected by the frequency of the stimulus used. Han (20) has clearly shown that different kinds of neuropeptides can be released in the central nervous system simply by changing the frequency of electrical stimulation without moving the needle position. Low-frequency (2 Hz) electroacupuncture activated beta endorphin and metenkephalin activity in the central nervous system. High frequency (100 Hz in the rat and 15 Hz in the rabbit) accelerated the release of dynorphin in the spinal cord. Thus, by selecting the proper parameters of neuroelectric acupuncture, it is possible to create a specific chemical environment in the central nervous system aimed at the treatment of various functional disorders.

In addition to the central opioid analgesia there is also a local physiological effect produced by stimulating in the myotome of the painful area.

In summary, from the above it becomes apparent that to successfully treat headaches and head pain by acupuncture one should place the needles on points in the upper part of the body and/or on the head. Electrical stimulation is of course essential. It has been known since early times that electricity was useful in the treatment of headaches (21). In those prescientific days, migraine was treated by simply placing the two ends of an electric eel across the head. Now we have more sophisticated electronic stimulators from which to choose. Although many acupuncture texts still recommend using only needles placed in the traditional manner, we believe as the result of our own studies, that electrical stimulation should be used in all acupuncture treatments. However, until more is known about the relationship between specific frequencies and different types or locations of headache, it would be well to use a simulator that would alternatively present both high and low frequencies of electrical stimulation.

NEEDLES AND NEEDLING

Acupuncture means literally "sharp-penetration," or the placement of needles through the skin. Originally, needles were of many types made from heavy wire and with wound handles to assist in twirling as they were inserted. Today's acupuncture needles are disposable. They are made of very fine stainless steel in gauges from 26 (0.45 mm) to 32 (0.26 mm). Gauges 28 and 30 are most popular. Needles vary in length from 1 to 10 cm. Needles from 1 to 2 inches are most commonly used. There are different types of disposable needles. One common type has a plastic handle and comes presterilized in a plastic tube that is shorter than the needle handle. For insertion, the tube is simply placed against the skin, and with a sharp tap the needle is painlessly inserted. When the tube is removed, the needle may be pushed to the desired depth.

There is little or no pain associated with proper needle technique. The more rapid the insertion, the better. The fingers and skin area to be penetrated should be cleaned with alcohol prior to needle insertion. The depth of insertion must be governed by the size of the muscle mass to be penetrated to reach the area of stimulation. It is not possible to give a figure for the safe depth of insertion at each point, as there is so much variation from one person to another. A sound knowledge of anatomy is, therefore, necessary for the proper practice of acupuncture. Whenever possible, the tip of the needle should approximate a motor point. When the point is reached, the patient may experience a feeling of pressure, heavy soreness, or distention. Such sensations are termed *De Qi* or *Teh Che*. This results from stimulation of the receptors in the muscle, including those nerves involved in proprioception and mechanoreception. This sensation is not painful and occurs within a few seconds of insertion, and it may remain localized or spread along the distribution of the nerve trunk.

Most needles may be inserted vertically at 90° perpendicular to the skin. To bypass certain bones and organs, etc., a 45° angle of insertion may sometimes be necessary. For points about the face with little muscle mass, needles are often inserted under and even more parallel to the skin surface.

COMPLICATIONS

Acupuncture is a very safe method for the treatment of headaches and facial pain. Complications and side effects are far less than those seen with the administration of most analgesics. If general precautions are taken, no complications occur. As acupuncture is often done by persons with no medical training, the literature describes a number of instances of untoward happenings.

Dizziness and fainting can occur. This vasovagal effect is seen (rarely) in persons who are anxious about receiving acupuncture for the first time. Such patients should lie flat during the treatment. Even more rare is needle-grasp, when muscle tension or gamma reflex makes it difficult to withdraw the needle. This can be overcome by applying a second needle angled toward the tip of the grasped needle.

Should a needle bend, simply change the patient's position and withdraw the needle in the direction of the curve. I have never experienced a broken needle requiring surgical removal. Again, with new disposable needles, this should never occur.

Upon removing the needle, the point of penetration should be inspected for subcutaneous bleeding. This can sometimes occur, even after the delay of a minute or two. Simple surface pressure is sufficient for control. Small ecchymoses may occur some hours later at the point where the needle was inserted. These are of no importance, and the patient should be informed of such possible occurrence. We have treated hemophiliac patients without this complication.

In the hands of unskilled practitioners with poor knowledge of anatomy, penetration of organs has been reported. Atelectasis has occurred following treatment of shoulder areas when the acupuncturist has failed to realize that, particularly in thin females, the apex of the left lung may be within 2 inches of the skin surface. Selection of needles and depth of penetration should always be appropriate to the region being treated.

Some pain or discomfort may occur with clumsy, inept techniques. If the patient moves after needle insertion, small muscle tears and pain may result. It is important, therefore, that the patient be in a position of comfort for the duration of the treatment. The face and ear can be sensitive areas.

STIMULATION OF THE NEEDLES

Traditionally, and especially in Asia and Europe, stimulation of the acupuncture needles is accomplished by manual manipulation of the needles. Also traditionally, to increase the intensity of stimulation, heat was added to the needles by burning a punk-like substance, moxa, on the needle handle. Patients with burn scars on their bodies testify to the ongoing use of such moxibustion treatments.

Modern acupuncture is accomplished by the use of electrical stimulation. Our own studies have shown electrical stimulation to be 100% more effective than simple needling techniques. Because neuroelectric acupuncture produces a stronger stimulation, it is often reserved for the second and subsequent treatments, especially in patients who are initially apprehensive. With electrical stimulation, beneficial treatment can be accomplished due to current spread even if the needles are not precisely located.

Stimulation is brought to the needles by small wire leads from the stimulator. The paired wires are affixed by small clips to the needles that usually are nearby each other, although no definite rule has been established for such placement. The number of needles stimulated depends upon the number of lead jacks in the stimulator. There are usually three or four, and hence, six or eight needles can be connected at one time.

A great deal of investigation remains to be done to ascertain the ideal parameters of stimulation. Currently it is felt that useful stimulation can occur with currents varying from 0.5 to 50 milliamps. Voltages are from 0.3 to 9 volts, usually produced by a 9-volt dry cell source. The wave forms vary but customarily are square waves, exponentially rising or falling, from 0.1 to 0.3 milliseconds duration, occurring in trains. These, thus, are pulsating DC potentials.

Most of the electroacupuncture equipment on the market produces a square wave output. In this case, the "needle sensation" elicited from the negative electrode is much stronger than that induced from the positive lead. Polarization may be induced by long-term stimulation. To overcome such problems, asymmetric biphasic modified square wave currents have been used, but with only partial solution of the problem. A more successful apparatus utilizes identical wave forms with alternating polarity, thus ensuring equally intense stimulation at both electrodes.

Pulses from 1 to 100 Hz have been used. Some workers feel that slow pulsations (1 to 20 Hz) are best for acute pain, while fast (80 to 120 Hz) are for chronic pain. This belief is not universally held. Stimulating equipment usually gives a choice of impulse patterns, with waves being continuous or coming initially in bursts with the impulse frequency being adjustable. In dense disperse (D-D) stimulation, a slow disperse, such as 2 per second, alternates with a burst of dense (80 to 100 Hz) waves. This type of stimulus can act upon both beta and kappa opiate receptors and hence yield pain relief through both beta endorphin and dynorphin mechanisms.

Sessions of stimulation typically last 20 to 30 minutes. Although the few data in the scientific literature do not support any specific amount of stimulation, most reports indicate that improvement will occur within six to eight treatments. Some patients will improve after only one or two treatments, while others require many more. Occasionally, patients get no therapeutic response until after 10 to 12 sessions. Initially, some patients are treated two to three times a week, later one treatment a week is sufficient. In patients with severe pain, treatment may be given two times a day, 5 days a week. In other patients with chronic pain, it has been useful, after an initial course, to continue with maintenance treatments once a month. We have found that such a schedule may prevent relapses. Other patients obtain complete relief after six or eight treatments and do not require more. Pain relief is usually cumulative with successive treatments; although, here too, the course of recovery may be irregular. If there is no relief in 8 to 10 treatments, acupuncture is probably an inappropriate modality for that patient.

The duration of relief from a single treatment varies greatly. Initially the relief may be transient, building up to longer periods of comfort with successive treatments. With chronic pain, at times, the greatest relief may appear 1 or 2 days days after the treatment. On occasion, the pain seems to increase for a few hours following the treatment, before a long period of abatement.

The level of stimulation required varies from patient to patient and for the same patient from day to day. The patient should be able to feel the stimulus, but it should not be uncomfortable. Often there is muscle fibrillation. The current is adequate when either of the above occurs. As treatment progresses, the patient may state that the stimulus is no longer felt. This is simply the result of body accommodation with the level of stimulation remaining the same. Such accommodation is less likely to occur with the dense-disperse type of stimulation, which alternates frequencies. In some patients, reddening of the skin around the needle may be seen, but with careful adjustment of current, burns are not seen.

PATIENT SELECTION AND PREPARATION

We have treated patients of all ages with acupuncture. Although it is usually given in the physician's office, hospitals are increasingly tolerant of acupuncture procedures. Some insurance companies will reimburse, at least in part, for acupuncture, particularly if it is explained in terms of electrical nerve stimulation.

There is no way to predict which patients will respond to neuroelectric acupuncture stimulation. While it has been reported that hypnotizable subjects do better than nonhypnotizable persons, this would seem to be part of the generalization that positive suggestion added to any treatment will improve the result. In our research and that of others, poorly hypnotizable subjects have had good results from acupuncture. A positive attitude is said to be predictive, but we have successfully treated patients who were openly skeptical and who came to the office reluctantly, at the urging of a spouse. Less-positive results are found in patients who have had previous surgery. Success on the first treatment has some positive predictive value.

Patients should be psychologically prepared by some discussion of the nature of acupuncture, the near absence of side effects, no pain, etc. Patients should be placed in a comfortable position and cautioned against any gross body movements. The bladder should be emptied prior to treatment. The patient should have no alcohol or drugs active on the nervous system prior to treatment.

RESULTS—CLINICAL STUDIES

Clinically, the effectiveness of neuroelectric acupuncture has much support. Its value in the treatment of headache and many types of pain has been demonstrated in our own practice and by the experience of others (22). Controlled studies of acupuncture are difficult, as the insertion of needles, even into nonacupuncture points, can reduce pain. The placebo effect alone can account for 30 to 35% relief. Experience worldwide seems to indicate an effectiveness of acupuncture treatments of 75% or more, at least twice the placebo response rate.

Some 30% of patients fail to respond to acupuncture treatments. This is approximately the same number who fail to respond to the administration of morphine. These persons possibly have some inherited defect in their opiate receptor system. The administration of DL-phenylalanine can convert some patients from nonresponders to responders, but more work remains to be done to determine how best to help this group of patients.

The physician who wishes to learn a useful, scientifically based, acupuncture technique faces a dilemma. The many courses that are currently taught by nonphysicians simply continue to support the metaphysical beliefs promulgated in the 3000-year-old *Nei Ching*. Even the very few courses taught by physicians for physicians have hesitated to entirely break away from the metaphysical approach, while giving only passing notice to the new discoveries. A major recent textbook (23), for example, has an excellent introductory chapter on the scientific basis of acupuncture and then proceeds to devote the major portion of the book to a detailed description of traditional Chinese acupuncture. If physicians wish to use acupuncture for the treatment of headache must they spend 3 years learning all the nuances of ancient Chinese medicine including meridian theory and pulse diagnosis? Or should they simply use a cook-book approach? If so, what formulae of points should be selected and from which authority? Or is there perhaps a more scientific approach to the treatment of such patients?

Western physicians, trained in the scientific method, are accustomed to basing their diagnosis and treatment upon a system of factual observations and double-blind studies using modern technology. Few are willing to ignore their scientific training and adopt the metaphysics of traditional Chinese medicine. Some have accomplished the difficult psychological task of maintaining these two completely different systems of medicine in two apparently logic-tight compartments. They thus, unquestioningly accept the concepts of traditional Chinese medicine and practice it within the setting and atmosphere of modern medicine. They state with naiveté that "someday we will find an explanation of how acupuncture works," blind to the fact that we already have!

A Western-trained physician might well experience some confusion upon reading a description of the various types of headache given in the tradition of ancient Chinese medicine. For example, a respected German physician stated in a recent article (24),

> According to traditional ideas, chronic headache and migraine are attributed to a blockage of *Qi* in the *Yang* channels of the head. The blockages causing pain are mostly dependent on an internal disturbance of organs and channels and seldom on external influences caused by weather factors. According to the character of pain, *Shi* excess, or *Xu* deficiency-type disturbances may be present.

He further states that in accord with these ancient concepts there are four types of headache: (*a*) gallbladder channel type (pain above the eyes), *Shao-Yang* headache; (*b*) pain in the temple, *Yang-Ming* headache; (*c*) pain along the urinary bladder channel (pain between the eyebrows), *Tai Yang* headache; and (*d*) pain related to the liver channel (in the vertex), *Du 20 Baihui* headache. Such a description is of little help to a Western-trained physician.

A workable compromise, acceptable to many physicians, has been the "formula approach." Here Western-style diagnoses are used, and physicians trustingly accept a certain set of traditional Chinese acupuncture points that have been suggested as useful for the condition they wish to treat. Taking one common condition, headache for example, we have explored the latter approach (25). We examined the recommendations that various authorities gave in six texts and 27 journals as to which points were the best for various types of headache. Such results may be complicated by the fact that there are different traditions and different styles of traditional acupuncture. Clinicians from different schools recommend different choices of points and techniques.

The articles we examined referred to headache either by location: general, vertex, occipital, or frontal, or by the Western descriptions of migraine (vascular), tension, or simply "headache." In the articles, 20 separate acupuncture points were listed in various combinations in the different formulae suggested by authors as effective for the treatment of various types of headache. Thus no univer-

sally accepted treatment formula was found for any of the types of headache studied. GB-20 and LI-4 were the most popular points, with the other 18 points recommended in various combinations by the different authors.

Physiological justification for the two most popular points might be the following:

GB-20 is a point just lateral to the trapezius muscle at its insertion into the occipital bone. Stimulation here is of the greater and lesser occipital nerves. It is also likely that stimulation here would affect the Golgi tendon organs at the insertion of the superior trapezius and the sternocleido-mastoid muscles.

LI-4 stimulates the motor points of the dorsal interosseus and adductor muscles of the thumb. This is the most widely used of all acupuncture points, particularly for afflictions of the upper body. It is the primary activator for opposing the thumb to the other digits and hence the basis of an action that permits man to remain civilized. It has a significantly large representation on the surface of the cerebral cortex.

Needle electrodes can be inserted bilaterally into these points. If the needles are then stimulated with a current that alternates between 2 to 8 Hz and 80 to 100 Hz, beta endorphin, metenkephalin, and dynorphin receptors can be stimulated with the activation of those neurohormones essential for the modulation of pain.

In conclusion, from this sampling and from our own experience in the treatment of headaches, we customarily use GB-20 and LI-4. Occasionally, we will place a needle in the area of complaint, as for example using GV-20 at the top of the scalp for headache located at the vertex, or ST-8 for a temporal headache. We suspect, however, that location at the area of the patient's complaint of pain has more of a placebo value by way of treating the patient "where it hurts." With a more physiological motivation, we often use needles placed generally in the concha of each ear. As described in my text (9), needles so placed and electrically stimulated have a demonstrable vagal effect, producing a lowering of blood pressure, slowing of pulse, and a general calming effect relieving the anxiety and stress that are so commonly etiological factors in headache.

For the treatment of pain in the facial region such as trigeminal neuralgia, atypical facial pain, TMJ syndrome, and others, the same principles are followed. We routinely use LI-4 bilaterally because, as previously described, this is the most powerful point for pain in the region of the head. We also, bilaterally, use needles in the conchae of the ears. Other needles may be placed about the face in accord with the area of pain or pathology. Points used are shown in the accompanying diagrams (Fig. 46.1) and described in Table 46.1. They include ST-7, SI-19, LI-20, and ST-6.

These points are often used bilaterally, on the side of the pain, or if this is too sensitive for treatment, good results have been achieved by using the opposite side of the face or head. The stimulating wires may be attached in any convenient manner.

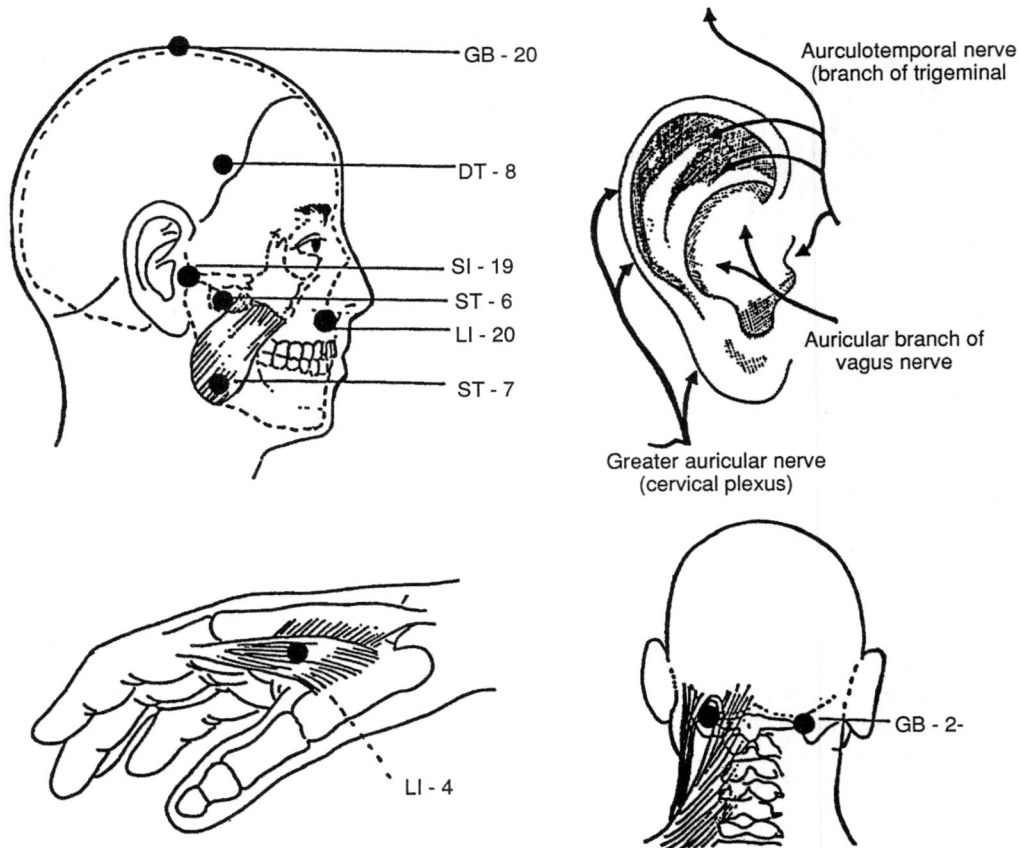

Figure 46.1. Various acupuncture points. (From Ulett GA. Principles and practice of physiologic acupuncture. St. Louis: Warren Green, 1982. With permission.)

Table 46.1.
Description of Acupuncture Points Seen in Figure 46.1

Name	Anatomical Location
LI-4	Motor points of first dorsal interosseus and adductor pollicus muscles
GB-20	At the common tendon point of insertion into the occipital bone of the muscles trapezius and sterno-cleidomastoid; activating the Golgi tendon organs; stimulates the greater and lessor occipital nerves
ST-7	Under the zygomatic arch in front of the condyle of the mandible; in the hollow that fills upon opening the jaw; stimulates branches of the temporal and internal pterygoid nerves
ST-8	In the depression between the tragus and the mandibular joint with the mouth slightly open; stimulates branches of the facial and temporal nerves
GV-20	Bisection of sagittal line with line joining tragi; stimulates the greater occipital nerve
SI-19	In front of the tragus at the depression made when the mouth is slightly open; stimulates the auriculotemporal branch of V and the facial nerve
ST-6	Junction of upper ⅔ and lower ⅓ of the masseter muscle at its motor point; stimulates the greater auricular, facial, and masseteric nerves
LI-20	Nasolabial fold within the fold of cheek at level of inferior edge of ala nasi; stimulates infraorbital branch of V and buccal branch of VII

REFERENCES

1. Veith I. The yellow emperor's classic of internal medicine. Berkley: University of California Press, 1949:260.
2. Mann F. Personal communication.
3. Ulett GA. Acupuncture is not hypnosis. Recent physiological studies. Am J Acupunct 1983:11(1):5–13.
4. Parwatikar S, Brown M, Stern J, Licett G, Sletten I. Acupuncture, hypnosis and experimental pain, I Study with volunteers, II Study with patients. Acupunct Electro-ther Res 1978;3:161–201.
5. Shapiro R, Stockard H. Electroencephalographic evidence demonstrated altered brainwave patterns by acupoint stimulation. Am J Acupunct 1989;17:25–29.
6. Peng A, Greenfield W. A precise scientific explanation of acupuncture mechanisms: are we on the threshold? Editoral review. Acupunct Sci Int J 1990;1:28–29.
7. Liu YK, Varela M, Oswald R. The correspondence between some motor points and acupuncture loci. Am J Chin Med 1975;3:347–358.
8. Gunn CC. Motor points and motor lines. Am J Acupunct 1978;6:55–58.
9. Ulett GA. Beyond yin and yang: how acupuncture really works. St. Louis: Warren Green, 1992.
10. Chang HT. Integrative action of thalamus in the process of acupuncture for analgesia. Sci Sin 1973;16:25–60.
11. Pert CB, Snyder SH. Opiate receptors demonstration in nervous tissue. Science 1973;179:1011–1014.
12. Kosterlitz HN, Hughes J. Some thoughts on the significance of enkephalin, the endogenous ligand. Life Sci 1975;17:91–96.

13. Han JS. The neurochemical basis of pain relief by acupuncture, A collection of papers 1973–1987. Beijing Medical University, 1987.

14. Mayer DJ, Price DD, Raffii A. Antagonism of acupuncture analgesia in man by the narcotic antagonist naloxone. Brain Res 1977;121:368–372.

15. Zou ZF, Du MY, Han JS, et al. Effect of intracerebral microinjection of naloxone on acupuncture and morphine analgesia in the rabbit. Sci Sin 1981;24:1166–1178.

16. Han JS, Xie GX, Zhou ZF, et al. Enkephalin and β-endorphin as mediators of electro-acupuncture analgesia in rabbits. An antiserum microinjection study. Adv Biochem Psychopharmacol 1982;33:369–377.

17. Han JS, Xie GX. Dynorphin: important mediator for electroacupuncture analgesia in the spinal cord of the rabbit. Pain 1984;18:367–377.

18. Han JX, Xie GX, Goldstein A. Analgesia induced by intrathecal injection of dynorphin B in the rat. Life Sci 1984;34:1573–1579.

19. Sjölund B, Terenius L, Eriksson M. Increased cerebrospinal fluid levels of endorphins after electroacupuncture. Acta Physiol Scand 1977;100:382–384.

20. Han JS, Sun LS. Differential release of enkephalin and dynorphin by low and high frequency electroacupuncture in the central nervous system. Acupunct Sci Int J 1990;1:19–27.

21. Scribonius Largus. (Compositiones medicamentorum). Argentorati. 1786.

22. Ulett G. Scientific acupuncture: peripheral electrical stimulation for the relief of pain, Part I Basics, Part II, Clinical aspects. Pain Manage 1989;2:128–134,185–189.

23. Stux G, Pomeranz B. Acupuncture textbook and atlas. Berlin: Springer-Verlag, 1987.

24. Stux G. Migraine treatment with acupuncture and moxibustion—pilot study on 50 patients. Acupunct Sci Int J 1990;1:16–18.

25. Ulett G, Johnson M. Two kinds of acupuncture. The digest of chiropractic economics. (In press).

47

Inpatient Headache Treatment Units

SEYMOUR DIAMOND

Most patients consulting a physician for treatment of headaches will be effectively managed on an outpatient basis. However, some patients are refractory to conventional forms of therapy or have concomitant medical or psychological problems that preclude outpatient therapy. An alternative must be available to attain resolution or at least some relief of their problem. Inpatient therapy, facilitated by a multidisciplinary team, may be indicated for these patients.

A set of criteria has been established for admission to a specialized inpatient unit for headache treatment (Table 47.1). The physician treating the chronic headache patient should be cognizant of these categories, to seek the appropriate management program for the headache sufferer.

PATIENT SELECTION

Prolonged Headache with Severe Associated Symptoms

The first category described in the admission criteria is the patient with prolonged, unrelenting headache. This patient is also suffering accompanying symptoms such as nausea and vomiting. Continuation of these symptoms could jeopardize the patient's general health. The risk of dehydration due to these symptoms or excessive consumption of analgesics indicates a need for immediate hospitalization. The patient with prolonged headache and vomiting may require fluid and electrolyte replacement therapy. Aggressive analgesic therapies, including narcotics, may cause extreme sedation and possible respiratory depression. The patient receiving these agents must be closely monitored, a process most appropriately achieved in an inpatient setting.

Status Migraine

The patient with status migraine is also a suitable candidate for admission to an inpatient headache unit. Status migraine, or status migrainosus, has been defined by the Headache Classification Committee of the International Headache Society (1) as an "attack of migraine with headache phase lasting more than 72 hours despite treatment. Headache free intervals of less than 4 hours (sleep not included) may occur." Because of the prolonged nature of this attack, standard therapies may have failed or the patient may have become tolerant of the analgesics. The ergotamine derivatives are the drugs of choice in migraine abortive therapy. The use of these agents is not advisable on the second, third, or fourth day of an attack, to prevent rebound phenomena. Also, the headache may be accompanied by copious vomiting that poses further risk of dehydration. Corticosteroid therapy is the treatment of choice for these patients. The use of intravenous dihydroergotamine (DHE-45) has been recommended by Raskin and Raskin (2). The intravenous administration of this drug and monitoring of these patients is best accomplished in an inpatient setting.

Analgesic Dependence

For the patient with chronic, unrelenting headaches, habituation to analgesics is a primary hazard. These habituating agents range from simple over-the-counter (OTC) analgesics to narcotics, barbiturates, and tranquilizers. Patients may also be consuming excessive amounts of caffeine in OTC products and beverages and may develop caffeine-withdrawal headaches. Discontinuation of these agents may cause troublesome, and sometimes serious, side effects. Detoxification is most successfully achieved in a specialized inpatient headache unit.

Ergot Habituation

Migraine patients may be taking excessive amounts of ergotamines or using the agents on a daily basis, risking potential rebound phenomena. Withdrawal from ergotamine derivatives may be difficult to accomplish because of the severe and debilitating headaches resulting from discontinuation of these agents.

Complications of Therapy

As with any type of therapy, the potentiality of adverse reactions is a constant threat. The patient using aspirin or aspirin products daily may induce gastrointestinal symptoms, including minor gastric bleeding. Chronic use of acetaminophen is implicated in chronic liver disease. Pa-

Table 47.1.
Admission Criteria: Inpatient Headache Unit

1. Prolonged, unrelenting headache, with associated symptoms such as nausea and vomiting, which, if allowed to continue, would pose a further threat to the patient's welfare
2. Status migraine
3. Dependence on analgesics, caffeine, narcotics, barbiturates, or tranquilizers; withdrawal from these agents must be undertaken in an inpatient setting
4. Habituation to ergots; ergots taken daily, when stopped, will cause a rebound headache
5. Pain accompanied by serious adverse reactions or complications from therapy; continued use of such therapy aggravates pain
6. Pain in the presence of significant medical disease; appropriate treatment of headache symptoms aggravates or induces further illness
7. Chronic cluster headaches unresponsive to treatment
8. Treatment that requires copharmacy with drugs that may cause a drug interaction and necessitates careful observation within a hospital milieu. For example, concomitant therapy using monoamine oxidase inhibitors (MAOIs) and β-blockers
9. Patients with probable organic cause of their headaches, requiring the appropriate consultations and perhaps neurosurgical intervention
10. Headache in the presence of ergot or analgesic toxicity
11. Severe headache in the presence of severe psychiatric disease
12. Severe headache necessitating frequent parenteral medication

tients on some pharmacological agents used in headache therapies, such as lithium or the anticonvulsants, may incur toxicity that requires immediate intervention. Therapies used for concomitant medical conditions may aggravate headaches. For example, antihypertensives, such as reserpine or apresoline, are known to exacerbate headaches. Discontinuation of these therapies and inauguration of appropriate treatment may require hospitalization.

Concomitant Medical Illness

Some coexisting medical conditions may be complicated by the recommended headache therapy. The use of β-blockers is contraindicated in diabetic patients who are insulin-dependent or are using oral hypoglycemics. The patient with headaches may also require referral to other medical specialists, such as a cardiologist. Hospitalization may afford the patient the convenience of consulting these various specialists. The proximity of other practitioners may also ease the burden of the headache specialist in selecting appropriate therapy for the patient with concomitant medical disorders.

Chronic Cluster Headache

The patient with chronic cluster headache has usually been refractory to conventional prophylactic therapies for cluster headache. Some of these patients may require histamine desensitization, involving the intravenous infusion of histamine phosphate over several days. This treatment is most effectively completed in an inpatient setting. Histamine desensitization also involves potentially serious adverse effects, including severe gastrointestinal disturbance, which can be carefully monitored in a hospital unit.

Hospitalization may be indicated for the patient with cluster headache who has become suicidal due to the severity and regularity of the headaches.

Initiation of Concomitant Therapies

Some refractory headache patients will require multiple therapeutic agents, which necessitates cautious monitoring. The patient with the mixed headache syndrome (i.e., daily tension-type (muscle-contraction) headaches with a recurrent migraine headache) may require pharmacological agents for each headache disorder. For example, concomitant therapy with β-blockers and monoamine oxidase inhibitors (MAOIs) may cause a serious drug interaction and should only by inaugurated in a setting in which the patient can be carefully observed.

Headaches due to Organic Causes

When an organic disorder is suspected in a headache patient, the patient may require complex and invasive testing. Although these tests can be accomplished on an outpatient basis, the probability of immediate neurosurgical intervention indicates the need for hospitalization. Also, the proximity of other specialties within the hospital setting may greatly benefit the patient, and facilitate treatment.

Headache in the Presence of Ergot or Analgesic Toxicity

Patients consuming excessive amounts of ergotamine may precipitate ergotism. In an inpatient setting, the patient can be closely observed for signs of ergotism, including vasoconstriction, paresthesias of the lower limbs, coldness of the extremities, or exertional pain in the calves or heels. Ergotism requires immediate medical intervention.

The chronic use of excessive amounts of analgesics, such as aspirin or acetaminophen, may cause renal or hepatic toxicity. Withdrawal from these agents is essential to prevent further complications of treatment. In addition to careful observation of the signs and symptoms of toxicity, these patients will require monitoring during withdrawal.

Severe Headache in the Presence of Severe Psychiatric Disease

Some patients with major and minor depressive illness may present with intractable migraine. Depressive illness may also manifest as daily headaches, which, if left untreated, could lead to addiction or habituation problems. Patients with chronic anxiety and panic states are more prone to development of habituation problems with tranquilizers, sedatives, and prescription and OTC analgesics.

These disorders are impossible to manage on an outpatient basis. The headache treatment may be unsuccessful until the psychiatric disorder is confronted. The convenience of a staff psychologist and consulting psychiatrist on a specialized inpatient headache unit will enhance the care of these difficult patients.

Headache Necessitating Frequent Parenteral Medications

In some cases, patients experience acute headaches that are refractory to standard analgesics. Parenteral analgesics at frequent intervals may be indicated, and hospitalization provides the appropriate milieu for the management of these prolonged, acute attacks. Careful observation of these patients will prevent complications of therapy. Hospitalization also aids in preventing habituation to these parenteral agents.

DEVELOPMENT OF THE INPATIENT HEADACHE UNIT

The concept of specialized inpatient units for chronic pain disorders evolved naturally from the developing interest in the management of pain. Bonica and his colleagues began their multidisciplinary team in a specific unit of the University of Washington Medical Center during the 1960s (3). Fordyce cited these pioneering facilities in his work on operant conditioning for pain disorders (4). These early units focused on all types of chronic pain. Bonica did note that these units must be dedicated solely to treatment of chronic pain and could not be combined with other areas of the hospital (3). He also noted the formation of major comprehensive pain centers that would treat all types of pain disorders and the development of syndrome-oriented pain centers, which focus on the treatment of specific disorders, including low back pain, facial pain, and headaches.

Establishing a separate unit for headache disorders derived naturally from the reported success of these early multidisciplinary pain management centers (5). The Diamond Headache Clinic Inpatient Unit was originally established in 1979, and was moved to its present site, Louis A. Weiss Memorial Hospital, an affiliate of the University of Chicago Hospitals, in 1983. This 35-bed unit adapted the multidisciplinary approach advocated by the center at the University of Washington to fulfill the treatment needs of the chronic headache patient.

MULTIDISCIPLINARY TEAM APPROACH

The patient with chronic headaches who has been refractory to all previous forms of therapy can greatly benefit from a multidisciplinary approach. The members of the inpatient health care team (Table 47.2) focus on the general needs of all patients on the unit as well as cooperatively develop a management approach for the individual patient.

As stated previously, the hospital facility affords the patient the proximity of the attending and consulting staff. Adequate nursing staff is also essential for the success of an inpatient headache unit. These nurses should be thoroughly instructed on the diagnostic and therapeutic approach to the headache patient. The nursing staff should

Table 47.2.
Inpatient Headache Unit: Health Care Team

Staff physicians
Consulting physicians
Nursing staff
Psychologists
Consulting psychiatrists
Social workers
Biofeedback technicians
Leisure activity therapists
Dietitians
Pharmacists
Physical therapists

also be cognizant of the nonpharmacological treatment modalities used in headache therapy.

An important feature of a dedicated inpatient headache unit is the presence of staff psychologists and psychiatrists. The period of hospitalization provides an excellent opportunity for psychological testing and counseling, if required. The psychologist can also present group sessions that confront psychological issues facing the headache patient, such as stress management. A consulting psychiatrist, interested in headache therapy, may enhance the inpatient care of the headache patient, if this type of intervention is indicated.

Biofeedback is a significant aspect of the inpatient care of the headache patient. The period of hospitalization affords the patient adequate time for biofeedback and relaxation training. Biofeedback technicians working on the inpatient unit are also exposed to the overall treatment of the headache patient and can function as a cooperative member of the health team.

The role of diet in headache has been regularly debated in the literature. Clinically, I have observed patients relating food items as headache triggers. All patients on the Diamond Headache Inpatient Unit receive a tyramine-free diet and attend a class presented by a hospital dietitian. The tyramine-free diet is reviewed, and the patients are provided with appropriate menus and recipes. Other nutritional issues are presented, including low-cholesterol and low-calorie diets. These classes provide the patients with a forum in which they can address questions regarding the "headache" diet as well as other nutritional concerns.

A class led by a hospital pharmacist is also a fundamental segment of the multidisciplinary approach. The complexities of the pharmacological management of headache is often confusing to the patient. The pharmacist's class enables them to address their questions about therapy and may also enhance patient compliance. Education often prevents management dilemmas, such as the patient abruptly discontinuing a β-blocker, an action that can trigger morbid consequences.

Discharge planning should be addressed during the hospitalization, and an essential issue is leisure planning. Patients must be aware of alternative activities when they are feeling better. Throughout the hospitalization, well-behavior is promoted. The recreational therapist reinforces this behavior by allowing the patients to express themselves in a nonpain endeavor. Art therapy is one particular activity in which patients can express their pain in a creative manner. The proximity of the physical therapy department provides for easy referral, if needed. During their hospitalization, patients may also use the exercise equipment located in this department.

Each member of the health care team is expected to attend a weekly staff meeting. At this meeting, treatment issues concerning each patient are addressed. This meeting gives each staff member an opportunity to discuss the individual patients and provide insight into the treatment approach. The progress of previous patients may also be discussed, and diagnostic problems may be addressed. Unusual cases may be reviewed, especially patients with organic causes of headache. Other issues confronting the health care team can also be addressed, such as problems with the physical facility or with other hospital departments.

These meetings also provide an opportunity for continuing education in headache diagnostic and treatment issues. Specific headache disorders may be addressed. By providing this forum for discussion, the staff is continually challenged to maintain the quality and to make efforts to improve the unit.

INPATIENT TREATMENT PROGRAM

Because of the complex nature of the headache disorders being treated at the inpatient units, the approach to therapy will involve several modalities (Table 47.3). Some of these treatment programs, such as biofeedback, pharmacological management, and diet have been previously described.

Detoxification

Many of the patients admitted to the inpatient unit must undergo detoxification from habituating drugs. The patient must be withdrawn from these agents to obtain maximum efficiency from the proposed therapy. Detoxification usually begins immediately at admission, with the discontinuation of the suspect drugs, such as narcotics, barbiturates, benzodiazepines, ergots, caffeine-containing agents, and simple OTC analgesics.

During detoxification, careful observation of the patients is essential. Some of these agents, particularly the narcotics, will produce withdrawal symptoms that may have serious consequences. If an opiate is discontinued, withdrawal symptoms may manifest as sweating, yawning, twitching, aching, muscle pain, irritability, mydriasis, and increased respiratory rate. These symptoms usually occur within 24 hours after discontinuation of the offending drug. Within the next 48 hours, the patient may experience nausea, vomiting, tachycardia, hypertension, insomnia, and abdominal

Table 47.3.
Inpatient Headache Unit: Treatment Program

Medical intervention
Diagnostic testing
Detoxification
Nursing care
Biofeedback
Group dynamics
Dietary instruction
Pharmacy education
Group psychotherapy
Leisure activity therapy
Art therapy
Relaxation therapy
Stress management
Exercise class
"Doctor's Bag"
Individual psychotherapy
Physical therapy
Medical/surgical consults
Discharge planning

cramps. The withdrawal process will gradually subside over the next 5 to 10 days. Symptomatic treatment will be required, and careful observation of the patient and continual support are essential. These symptoms may also appear after the discontinuation of codeine and pentazocine, two drugs that are considered relatively safe in regard to habituation problems. Clonidine, an α-agonist, has been used successfully in migraine prophylaxis and has also been reported to be effective in suppressing the symptoms of opiate withdrawal (6). Bakris et al. observed that the use of clonidine effectively alleviated withdrawal symptoms, including tachycardia, hypertension, perspiration, agitation, and opiate-seeking behavior.

Many prescription analgesics used in the abortive therapy of headache contain barbiturates. Typically, the patient discontinuing barbiturates demonstrates anxiety, insomnia, hyperreflexia, diaphoresis, nausea, vomiting, tachycardia, tachypnea, and fever. If the patient was consuming high doses of barbiturates, severe symptoms, such as delirium and convulsive states including grand mal seizures may ensue. The symptoms associated with withdrawal of the benzodiazepines are similar to those of the barbiturates. Patients on high doses of these drugs will experience tremors and sometimes seizures when the drugs are discontinued.

The daily use of the ergotamine derivatives by migraine patients will produce a rebound phenomenon. When a dose of the ergotamine is missed or omitted, the patient experiences a severe rebound headache. Withdrawal from the ergots is especially difficult due to the severe headaches that ensue. These patients may require potent analgesics and possibly phenothiazines for the accompanying GI symptoms. If the vomiting is not controlled, these patients may require fluid replacement therapy. A study by Mathew (7) noted that noproxen may be beneficial for ergotamine-withdrawal symptoms.

Consumption of excessive amounts of caffeine in either

drugs or beverages can also produce rebound headaches. The caffeine-withdrawal headache is often observed on weekends and holidays when patients decrease the amount of coffee normally ingested during the work week. Large amounts of caffeine are present in both OTC and prescription analgesics. The amount required to produce dependence on caffeine depends on the individual's tolerance (8). Withdrawal from caffeine also requires aggressive analgesia for the headache patient. For patients discontinuing these agents, withdrawal symptoms may include grogginess, malaise, rhinorrhea, nausea, depression, and rebound headaches. In addition to standard pharmacological therapies, relaxation methods may be especially beneficial for the patient discontinuing caffeine-containing analgesics. Dietary instruction is essential for these patients in discharge planning, as they must be cognizant of the food products and beverages containing caffeine.

The availability of OTC products containing aspirin or acetaminophen increases their potential for abuse. To determine a patient's possible habituation to one of these products, I will inquire how long a bottle of 100 tablets would last. If it is less than 1 month, the patient should be admitted to the inpatient headache unit for detoxification. Excessive or repeated use of these agents can cause liver or renal toxicity. The risk of ulcer and other GI disturbance is well established with aspirin use. These patients especially must be instructed on alternative methods of dealing with pain and stress. Biofeedback and relaxation exercises may be beneficial.

Psychological Intervention

The patient admitted to the inpatient unit will present with chronic headache as well as a variety of emotional and psychological problems. An important aspect of the inpatient treatment program is the promotion of well-behavior to disrupt the chronic pain behavior.

During hospitalization, the patient is encouraged to participate in the activities on the unit, such as the group sessions with the psychologist and psychiatrist, stress-management class, art therapy, leisure planning (arts and crafts) activities, relaxation training, and the diet and pharmacy classes. A weekly calendar is provided to each patient, listing the various activities on the unit (Table 47.4). The patients are advised to wear street clothes while hospitalized and to eat their meals as a group. Interaction between patients is especially helpful, as many chronic headache patients have felt alone with their pain problem. It is often enlightening to find that other people have suffered similar pain and have also felt misunderstood by family and friends. At the Diamond Headache Inpatient Unit, a weekly session, "Doctor's Bag," is presented by one of the staff physicians. At this session, patients are encouraged to ask general questions about diagnosis, therapy, and other issues concerning their headache problems. It also provides another opportunity to educate the patients about alternatives in therapy, such as relaxation or identifying headache triggers.

During the stress-management classes and group psychotherapy sessions, the patients are instructed on specific stressors and coping mechanisms. These patients must be advised that pharmacological therapies are not the only solution to their headache problem. Specific issues may be addressed during these sessions, such as assertiveness training. Again, the psychologist and staff focus on positive reinforcement of well behavior.

The period of hospitalization provides ample opportunity for psychological testing, if required. Tests such as the MMPI can render excellent insight into the various personality conflicts affecting these headache patients. Neuropsychological testing, if indicated, is an important aspect of psychological testing and complements a neurological examination. If an organic cause is suspected, the

Table 47.4.
Inpatient Headache Unit: Activity Schedule

Time	Sunday	Monday	Tuesday	Wednesday	Thursday	Friday	Saturday
8 am	Breakfast	Breakfast	Breakfast	Breakfast	Breakfast	Breakfast	Breakfast
9 am			Doctor's Bag		Psychologist group I		
10 am		Biofeedback group	Psychiatrist group	Psychologist group II		Warm-up group	
11 am	Visiting hours	Shopping excursion	Walk	Orientation group	Walk	Shopping excursion	Visiting hours
12 noon	Lunch	Lunch	Lunch	Lunch	Lunch	Lunch	Lunch
1 pm			Stress management	Arts & crafts	Relaxation training	Arts & crafts	
2 pm		Dietitian class	Relaxation training	Group therapy (social worker)	Therapeutic art		
3 pm				Pharmacy class			
4 pm		Physical Rx	Exercise class	Physical therapy	Exercise class	Physical Rx	
5 pm	Dinner	Dinner	Dinner	Dinner	Dinner	Dinner	Dinner
7 pm	PBS headache video				PBS headache video	Movies	Movies

8:30 AM–11:50 AM & 1:00 PM–5:00 PM: Biofeedback sessions per physician's orders neuropsychologist may be consulted to determine whether a specific brain function is impaired. These tests may offer a clue to the diagnosis, although traditional diagnostic testing such as CT scan, MRI, skull x-ray, or EEG have been negative. Functional deficits may be identified during administration of the test, enabling the neuropsychologist to localize specific neurological deficits, and the degree of impairment may be assessed. These tests may also be used to establish differential diagnosis, document the course of a condition, provide behavioral foundations for rehabilitation and training, and facilitate patient care plans. The Halstead-Reitan battery and Luria Nebraska battery are the most widely used neuropsychological tests.

If indicated, the patient receives individual psychotherapy to address issues contributing to the headache problem. The psychologist may also observe a need for continuing psychotherapy following discharge. Hospitalization also offers the opportunity for the patient to meet with the consulting psychiatrist, if required. The need for family therapy may also be demonstrated during the hospitalization. The patient's family is often involved in the positive reinforcement of well-behavior. Too often, family members have offered the patient a secondary gain for the chronic pain, such as lavishing attention on a spouse or child when a headache occurs and ignoring the person during a headache-free period.

Pharmacological Therapy

As stated previously in this chapter, many forms of therapy should be initiated under strict supervision. The inpatient headache unit furnishes an environment in which this close monitoring can occur. Because many of these refractory patients are suffering from the mixed headache syndrome, the use of "copharmacy" is indicated. The intricacies of these concomitant therapies require careful observation. These patients also need the support of a highly trained staff when starting complex therapies.

Some pharmacological therapies should only be administered in a hospital setting. For example, the patient receiving histamine desensitization will be receiving IV infusion for several days. The ramifications of these types of therapy are best observed in a controlled environment. Patients receiving IV medications for status migraine and other continuous, unrelenting headaches should also be supervised in an inpatient setting.

LONG-TERM RESULTS

To determine the benefits of inpatient treatment of headache, a retrospective study was undertaken at the Diamond Headache Clinic. A survey was sent to 372 consecutive patients admitted to the inpatient headache unit (9). A 41% response rate was achieved.

Patients were asked to rate the effects of hospitalization on headache frequency, severity, and treatment, immediately following discharge and in the month in which they received the survey. A greater than 50% reduction was noted by 54% of the respondents. It was noted that 10% of the responders stated that they had remained completely headache-free.

The patients were also asked which treatment modality was most beneficial to them following the hospitalization. Medical intervention and nondrug therapies, such as dietary instruction, were viewed as most helpful. Seventy-two percent found psychological therapies to be beneficial, and 54% rated biofeedback as useful. Although the patients did not directly identify the multidisciplinary approach as beneficial, they considered the multiple modalities extremely valuable in their progress.

SUMMARY

The establishment of inpatient headache units has offered excellent opportunities for the treatment of refractory headache patients. A controlled environment is essential in initiating complex therapy as well as achieving detoxification. Through these units, the patient is exposed to a multidisciplinary approach by the health care team, who have insight into the intricacies of headache therapy. Admission into these units also offers the patient an opportunity to receive support and care from the consulting staff. Psychological intervention is easily undertaken on the inpatient headache unit, and patients are offered coping methods to personally manage their headache problems. Continuity of care, through the entire health care team, certainly enhances the progress of patients previously refractory to all forms of conventional therapy. This success also decreases the number of physician visits, medication consumption, and days missed from school or work. The economic ramifications of this progress are startling.

REFERENCES

1. Olesen JS. Classification and diagnostic criteria for headache disorders, cranial neuralgias and facial pain. Cephalalgia 1988;8(suppl 7):1–96.
2. Raskin NH, Raskin KE. Repetitive intravenous dihydroergotamine for the treatment of intractable migraine. Neurology 1984;34(suppl 1):245.
3. Bonica JJ. Multidisciplinary/interdisciplinary pain programs. In: Bonica JJ, ed. The Management of Pain, vol. 1. Philadelphia: Lea & Febiger, 1990.
4. Fordyce WE. An operant conditioning method for managing chronic pain. Postgrad Med 1973;53:123–128.
5. Diamond S. Inpatient treatment of headache. Clin J Pain 1989;5:101–103.
6. Bakris GL, Cross PD, Hammarsten JE. The use of clonidine for management of opiate abstinence in a chronic pain patient. Mayo Clin Proc 1982;57:657.
7. Mathew NT. Amelioration of ergotamine withdrawal symptoms with naproxen. Headache 1987;27:102–106.
8. Elkind AH. Drug abuse and headache. Med Clin North Am 1991;75:717–732.
9. Diamond S, Freitag FG, Maliszewski M. Inpatient treatment of headache: long-term results. Headache 1986;26:189–197.

Index

Page numbers in italics denote figures; those followed by "t" denote tables.

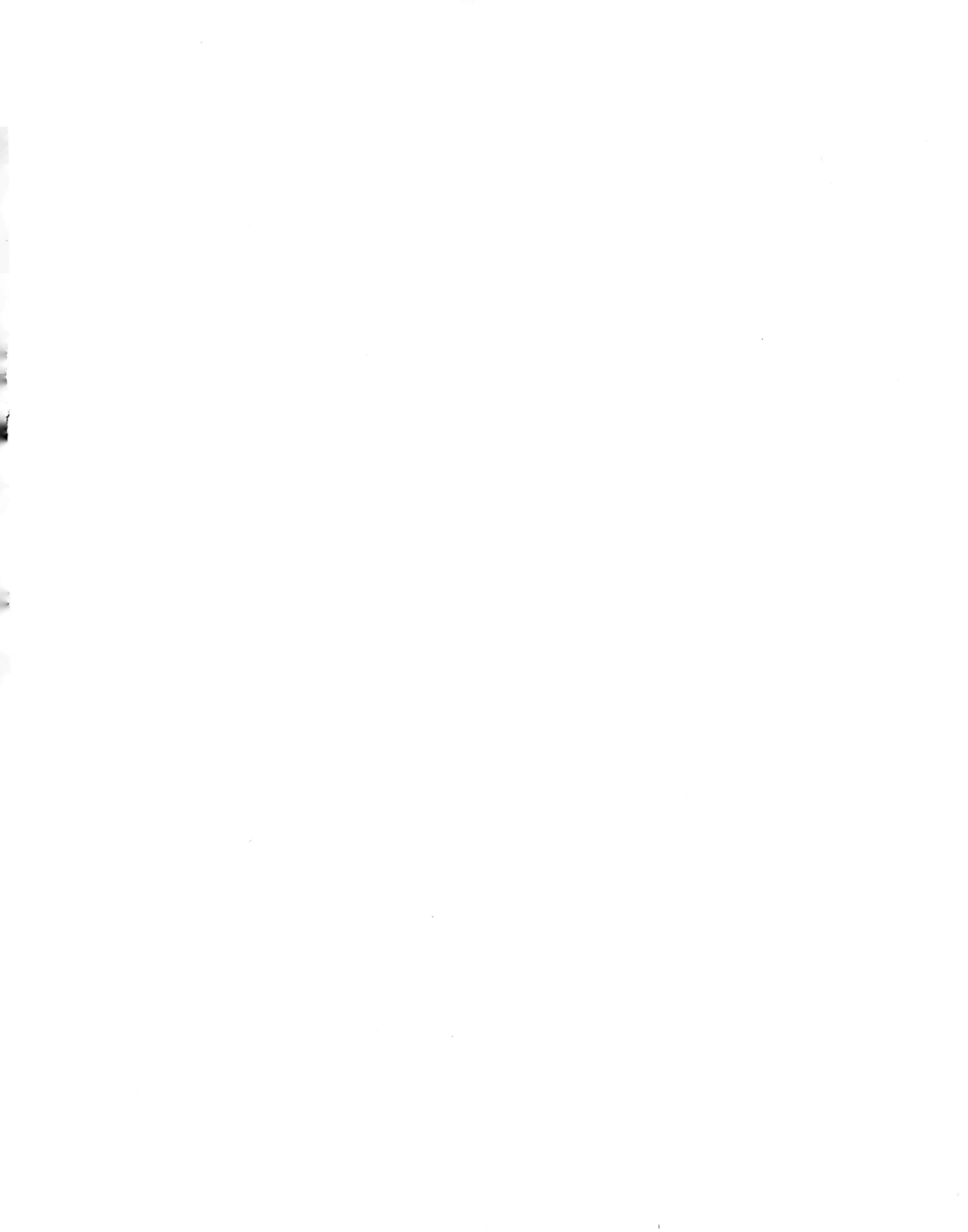

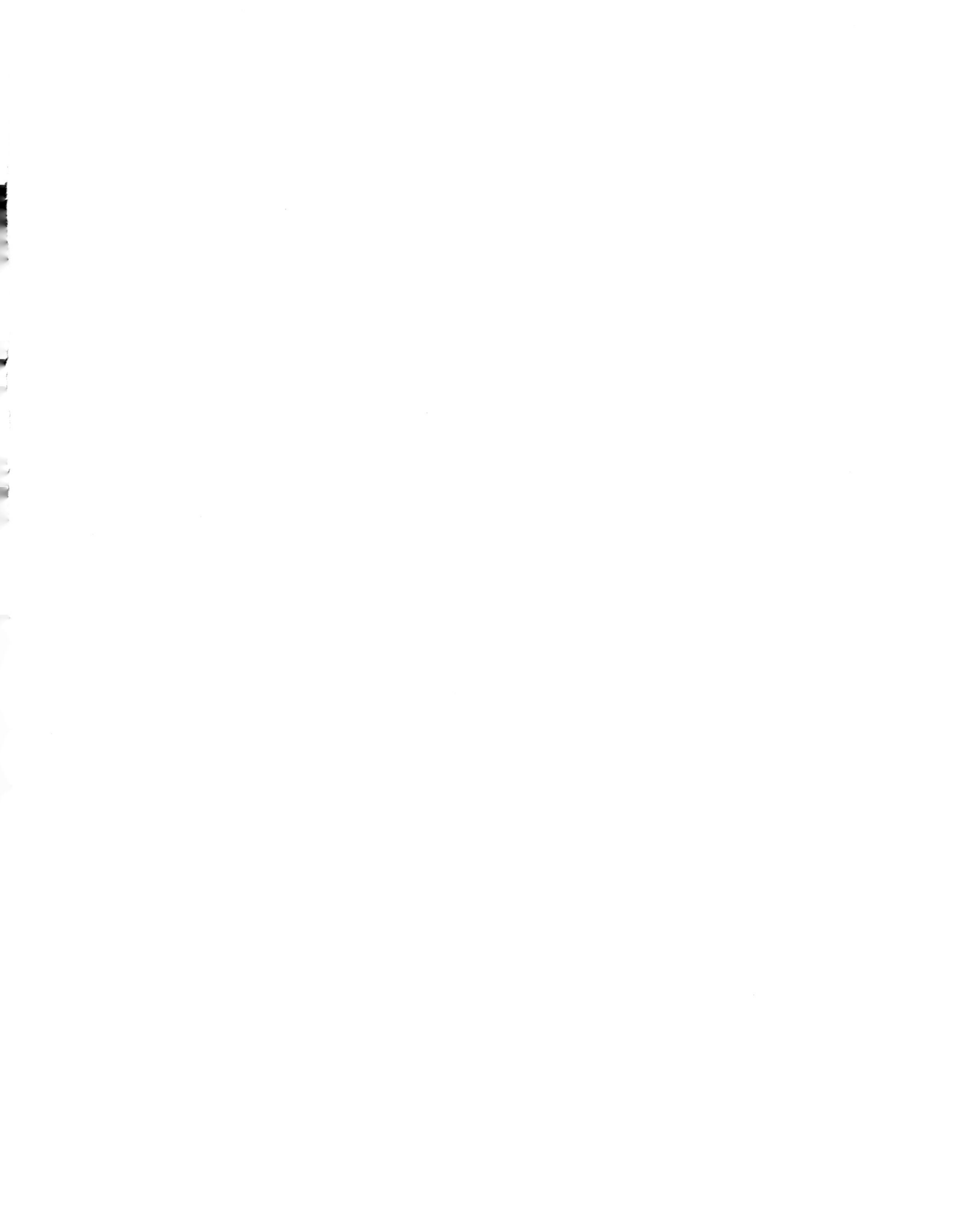